Introduction to Communication Disorders

A LIFESPAN EVIDENCE-BASED PERSPECTIVE

ROBERT E. OWENS, JR.
College of St. Rose

KIMBERLY A. FARINELLA
Northern Arizona University

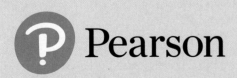 Pearson

330 Hudson Street, NY NY 10013

8064

KH

Director and Publisher: Kevin M. Davis
Executive Portfolio Manager: Julie Peters
Managing Content Producer: Megan Moffo
Content Producer: Faraz Sharique Ali
Portfolio Management Assistant: Maria Feliberty and Casey Coriell
Development Editor: Carolyn Schweitzer
Executive Product Marketing Manager: Christopher Barry
Executive Field Marketing Manager: Krista Clark
Manufacturing Buyer: Deidra Smith
Cover Design: Carie Keller, Cenveo
Cover Art: Portra Images/DigitalVision/Getty Images; KidStock/Blend Images/Getty Images
Media Producer: Autumn Benson
Editorial Production and Composition Services: SPi Global, Inc.
Full-Service Project Manager: Sree Meenakshi.R, SPi Global
Editorial Project Manager: Shiela Quisel, SPi Global
Text Font: ITC Mendoza Roman Std

Credits and acknowledgments borrowed from other sources and reproduced, with permission, in this textbook appear on this page or on appropriate page within text.

To obtain permission(s) to use material from this work, please visit https://www.pearson.com/us/contact-us/permissions.html

Cataloging-in-Publication Data is available on file at the Library of Congress.

1   18

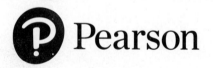

ISBN-13: 978-0-13-480147-6
ISBN-10:   0-13-480147-4

2\22\19

To Our Many Friends with Communication Disorders

ntroducing a new edition is always exciting and exhausting. We have taken great pains to reach a balance that we hope will please our various readers, from professors to students. We hope that those of you who are familiar with the previous editions will agree with us that this edition is a worthy introduction to the field of speech pathology and audiology and one that contributes meaningfully to the education of speech-language pathologists and audiologists.

Within each chapter, we have attempted to describe a specific type of disorder and related assessment and intervention methods. In addition, we have included lifespan issues and evidence-based practice to provide the reader with added insights. Each type of disorder is illustrated by personal stories of individuals with that disorder. Further knowledge can be gained through the suggested readings provided at the conclusion of each chapter.

NEW TO THIS EDITION

This sixth edition of *Introduction to Communication Disorders* has many new features that strengthen the existing material in the previous edition. These include the following:

- Chapters have been reorganized and rewritten to help conceptualize the information differently so as to conform more to current clinical and educational categories. Several chapters have been reworked entirely, specifically Chapters 5, 8, 9, and 11.

- As always, the material in each chapter has been updated to reflect the current state of clinical research. Special attention has been paid to the growing body of evidence-based research and literature. A quick perusal of the references will verify the addition of hundreds of new professional articles.

- As in the past, we have worked to improve readability throughout the book and to provide the right mix of information for those getting their first taste of this field. Several professors and students have commented favorably on our attempt in previous editions to speak directly to the reader, and we have continued and expanded this practice.

- We have continued to provide evidence-based practices in concise, easy-to-read boxes within each chapter. This demonstrates our commitment to this practice begun in the previous edition. As with all the rest of the text, these boxes have been updated to reflect our best knowledge to date.

- Users of previous editions may be pleased to find that we have attempted in the Augmentative and Alternative Communication (AAC) chapter to shift the focus. In the past, this chapter has been primarily one that explains AAC rather than approaching the topic from the disorder orientation found in the other chapters. Some explanation is inherent in the topic, but it has been softened in the current edition.

- Each chapter has been reorganized so that chapter Learning Objectives are reflected in the organization of the chapter.
- In our ever-changing field, terminology is constantly in flux. We have updated each chapter to use the most up-to-date terms.
- Anatomy figures are now in color, and new medical photographs were added to Chapter 9.
- Along with new video examples that outline careers in the field of communication disorders, show how different disorders affect speech, and explain speech development, in this edition new Video Exercises provide opportunities for students to watch a video, answer questions about it, and read feedback to gain a greater understanding of the content.
- Thought Questions have been updated and appear in both the print and eText versions to generate critical thinking on a variety of concepts and techniques.
- Chapters structured around Learning Outcomes include assessment items for each major section so that students can check their understanding of the content they've just read about.
- Case studies were rewritten, and clinical application questions pertaining to each case study can be accessed in the "Check Your Understanding" assessment, with comprehensive feedback to each question provided.

The eText Advantage

The eText is an affordable, interactive version of the print text. Publication of *Introduction to Communication Disorders* in an eText format allows for a variety of advantages over a traditional print format, including a search function allowing the reader to efficiently locate coverage of concepts. **Boldface** key terms are clickable and take the reader directly to the glossary definition. Index entries are also hyperlinked and take the reader directly to the relevant page of the text. Navigation to particular sections of the book is also possible by clicking on desired sections within the expanded table of contents. Finally, sections of text may be highlighted, and reader notes can be typed onto the page for enhanced review at a later date.

To further enhance assimilation of new information, *Video Examples* are interspersed throughout chapters to demonstrate text concepts in action. *Video Exercises* pose clinical application questions and provide comprehensive feedback to deepen understanding of key ideas. At the end of major sections, readers can access multiple-choice or true/false *Check Your Understanding* questions to assess comprehension of text concepts. Immediate feedback is provided on the appropriateness of responses. *Thought Questions* are placed in the margins, fostering reflection and building connections between text concepts.

To learn more about the enhanced Pearson eText, go to www.pearsonhighered.com/etextbooks.

We hope that you'll agree with us that this is a more user-friendly and informative text than the previous editions. Please feel free to contact us with suggestions for further strengthening our work.

ACKNOWLEDGMENTS

Robert Owens

I am most deeply indebted to my co-author Kim Farinella, Ph.D., who is a dedicated professional and a tireless worker. Despite being a new mom and a fulltime faculty member, she has put in a herculean effort on this new edition. I am truly blessed to have had such an indefatigable co-author through this sometimes very trying task of producing a new edition. I can never acknowledge her contribution enough, but—from the bottom of my heart—thanks, Kim.

I would like to thank the faculty of the Department of Communication Sciences and Disorders and the entire faculty and administration at the College of St. Rose in Albany, New York. What a wonderful place to work and to call home. The college places a premium on scholarship, student education, professionalism, and a friendly and supportive workplace environment, and recognizes the importance of our field. I am indebted to all for making my new academic home welcoming and comfortable. I am especially thankful to President Carolyn Stefanco, School of Education Dean Margaret McLane, my chair Jim Feeney, and my colleagues in my department, fellow faculty members Dave DeBonis, Dierdre Muldoon, Jack Pickering, Anne Rowley, and Julia Unger, and fellow clinical faculty members Director of Clinical Education Jackie Klein, Robin Anderson, Elizabeth Baird, Nina Benway, Marisa Bryant, Sarah Coons, Jessica Evans, Colleen Fluman, Elaine Galbraith, Julie Hart, Barbara Hoffman, Melissa Spring, and Lynn Stephens. You have all made me feel welcomed and valued.

I would be remiss if I did not acknowledge the continuing love and support I receive from my best buddy Addie Haas. She was with us in the first and second editions and continues to be a source of inspiration.

Finally, my most personal thanks and love goes to my spouse and partner, who supported and encouraged me and truly makes my life fulfilling and happy. I'm looking forward to our life together.

Kimberly Farinella

I want to thank Dr. Bob Owens for continuing to include me as a co-author on this textbook. It is an honor to work alongside one of my favorite former professors and mentors. His course was my first introduction to the field of speech-language pathology over 20 years ago. I continue to be inspired by this great man, and hope to have the same positive influence on my students.

I want to thank my former student, Niki Knight, for recruiting her dad, Steven R. Knight, CRNA APRN to take medical photographs for us for over a year, which he provided for use in the current edition of this textbook. I am forever grateful for the amount of time and effort that Mr. Knight devoted to helping us make this edition more clinically useful.

I would also like to thank my dear friend, Margo Zelenski, and the Mayo Clinic in Scottsdale, Arizona for contributing the swallowing videos to us for use in this edition. I'm also grateful to the clients and their families who were willing to share their audio and video samples with us so that students can learn from them.

I want to thank the Pearson editorial management team, specifically, Julie Peters, Carolyn Schweitzer, Shiela Quisel, and Faraz Sharique Ali, who worked closely with us to make this edition stellar. Thank you also to Jon Theiss for editing the audio and video samples.

Finally, I want to thank my husband, Tom, for his love and support of me and our family, and his willingness to be a full-time daddy so that I could work and complete this project. It has been quite an experience and I'm enjoying every minute.

The following reviewers offered many fine suggestions for improving the manuscript: Tausha Beardsley, Wayne State University; Wendy Bower, State University of New York at New Paltz; Louise Eitelberg, William Paterson University; Adrienne B. Hancock, The George Washington University; Susan McDonald, Cerritos College. Their efforts are sincerely acknowledged.

BRIEF CONTENTS

CONTENTS

CHAPTER 8   Fluency Disorders   **225**

Introduction to Communication Disorders

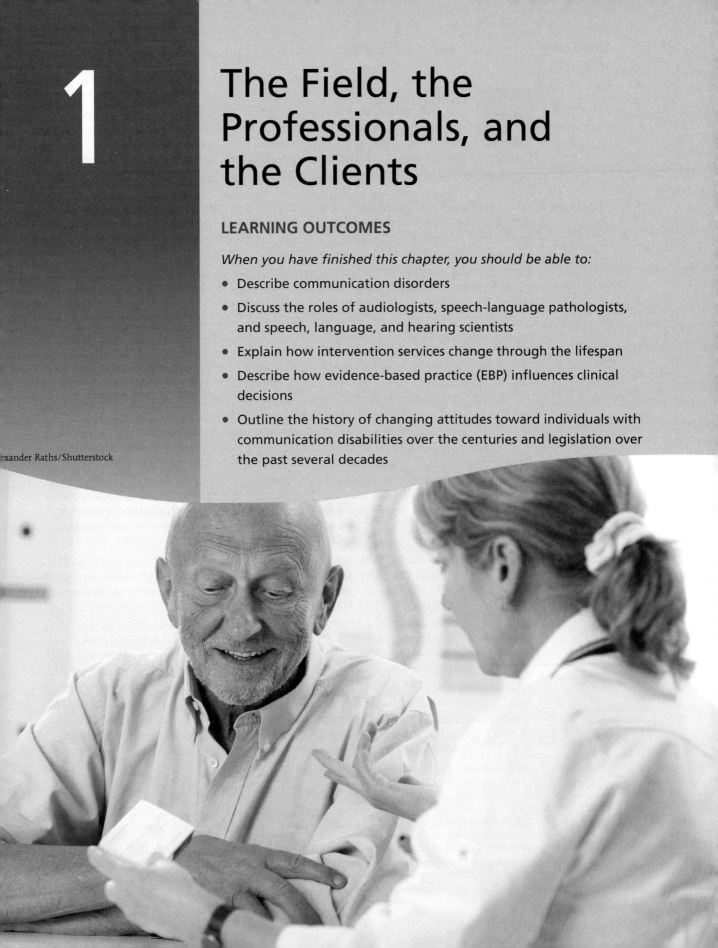

1

The Field, the Professionals, and the Clients

LEARNING OUTCOMES

When you have finished this chapter, you should be able to:

- Describe communication disorders
- Discuss the roles of audiologists, speech-language pathologists, and speech, language, and hearing scientists
- Explain how intervention services change through the lifespan
- Describe how evidence-based practice (EBP) influences clinical decisions
- Outline the history of changing attitudes toward individuals with communication disabilities over the centuries and legislation over the past several decades

Alexander Raths/Shutterstock

C an you imagine life without communication? No talking, no listening, no interacting with others? Communication is part of what makes us human. Even minor or temporary problems with communication, such as temporary laryngitis, are often frustrating. Imagine problems with eating and swallowing. We've all experienced the temporary inconvenience of trying to eat with a sore throat. What would life be like if these problems were more lasting?

Valery has loved baseball for as long as she can remember. She got it from her dad, a devoted Yankees fan. She loves to watch it and talk about it, but most of all she loves playing it. Unfortunately, she now believes because of her head injury in an auto accident that she'll never be able to even express how much she misses it. Even so, today may be momentous. Her speech-language pathologist (SLP), Pam, plans to introduce Valery to an assistive technology device that has a speech generator. Who knows what we'll hear from Valery next?

Valery is just one of millions of people who face daily communication challenges. We hope through this text to explore these challenges to communication, as well as to feeding and swallowing.

In this first chapter, we'll introduce this topic and the professionals who work with individuals who have communication and feeding and swallowing challenges. These highly trained professionals are called audiologists, speech-language pathologists, or speech/language scientists. We'll explore their roles and explain the need for evidence-based practice (EBP) and why it's important to intervention. EBP is one of the bases of this text. In addition, this first chapter provides a historical perspective and outlines the laws that mandate appropriate care for those in need. Finally, along the way, we'll explore why people choose these careers.

In the remainder of the text, we'll begin with some background material so we have a similar understanding of what comes next. We take a **holistic** approach to diagnosis and treatment of people with communicative impairments and examine the sometimes perplexing contrast between "typical" and "impaired." There are separate chapters that discuss speech characteristics such as voice, fluency, and phonology. We also provide chapters that are organized on the basis of etiology, such as neurogenic and craniofacial disorders. Within each chapter, we examine the interconnectedness of age, time of onset, social and cultural factors, and cause of the presenting disorder, and we describe evidence-based assessment and treatment practices. We recognize that it's common for an individual who demonstrates difficulties with one aspect of communication to be affected in other areas as well.

Why does someone decide to become a speech-language pathologist (SLP) or audiologist? It is mostly because of the satisfaction this person receives from helping others to live a fuller life. Many—maybe even you—first became interested through a personal or family encounter with a communication disorder or through work or volunteer experience with individuals having communication disorders. SLPs and audiologists may also have chosen their careers because they want to be useful to society, to contribute to the general good.

COMMUNICATION DISORDERS

We've mentioned communication disorders, but we haven't been very specific. It's always good to agree on our topic in any type of communication, so let's begin here.

A **communication disorder** impairs the ability to both receive and send, and also process and comprehend concepts or verbal, nonverbal, and graphic information. A communication disorder may affect hearing, language, and/or speech processes; may range from mild to profound severity; and may be developmental or acquired. One or a combination of communication disorders may be presented by an individual, and may result in a primary disability or may be secondary to other disabilities.

That's a lot. In short, a communication disorder may affect any and all aspects of communication, even gesturing. A communication disorder may affect hearing, language (the code we use to communicate), and/or speech (our primary mode or manner of communication). This is reflected in the American Speech-Language-Hearing Association's (ASHA) name. (The Appendix describes ASHA's professional role in more detail.) Although they work primarily with people having communication disorders, SLPs are not limited to just speech and language. As mentioned, SLPs are involved in feeding and swallowing disorders and non-speech (called *nonverbal*) forms of communication

A **speech disorder** may be evident in the atypical production of speech sounds, interruption in the flow of speaking, or abnormal production and/or absences of voice quality, including pitch, loudness, resonance, and/or duration. For example, when you had laryngitis your voice was temporarily affected. A **language disorder**, in contrast, is an impairment in comprehension and/or use of spoken, written, and/or other symbol systems, such as English. Finally, a **hearing disorder** is a result of impaired sensitivity of the auditory or hearing system. No doubt you've heard individuals referred to as deaf or hard of hearing. In addition, auditory impairment may include **central auditory processing disorders**, or deficits in the processing of information from audible signals.

It's appropriate to note here that communication disorders do not include communication differences, such as dialectal differences or speaking another language. If you've been to a country where you don't speak the language well, you know that this definitely can impede communication. While these differences may lead to communication difficulties, they are differences, not disorders, and cannot be treated by SLPs as if they are.

Another communication variation is **augmentative/alternative communication** systems. Far from being communication impairments, these systems, whether signing or the use of digital methods, are attempts often taught by SLPs to compensate and facilitate, on a temporary or permanent basis, for impaired or disabled communication disorders.

Finally, we would be remiss if we didn't at least note that an SLP's responsibility also extends to feeding and swallowing disorders. These vary from the preterm infant with a weak sucking response to the adult patient recovering from a stroke and slowly regaining the motor control needed to chew and swallow easily.

As you can see, communication and feeding and swallowing disorders cover a wide range of problems with varying severities and are related to several other disorders. Our purpose in preparing this text is to help you understand and appreciate the many varied disorders that are the charge of the SLP and audiologist.

Maybe a few pages ago you had some vague recollection of an SLP in your elementary school who mostly worked with children correcting their production of difficult speech sounds. That's part of disordered communication, but it's only a small part, as you are about to find out.

Check Your Understanding 1.1

Click here to check your understanding of the concepts in this section.

THE PROFESSIONALS AND THEIR ROLES

Opportunities for SLPs and audiologists include serving individuals of all ages from infancy through the aged with varied disorders, from mild to profound, in a wide assortment of settings.

Today, professionals who serve individuals with communication disorders come from several disciplines. They often refer clients to one another or work together in teams to provide optimal care. Specialists in communication disorders are employed in early intervention programs, preschools, schools, colleges and universities, hospitals, independent clinics, nursing care facilities, research laboratories, and home-based programs. Many are in private practice. Although it is still in its infancy, **telepractice**—provision of language assessment and intervention via the Internet—is slowly expanding, especially in underserved geographical areas (Waite et al., 2010).

 Video Example 1.1

Before you begin, you might want to check out this video on becoming an audiologist or speech-language pathologist. https://www.youtube.com/watch?v=_OIcPbndZMo

Audiologists

Audiologists are specialists who measure hearing ability and identify, assess, manage, and prevent disorders of hearing and balance. They use a variety of technologies to measure and appraise hearing in people from infancy through old age. Although they work in educational settings to improve communication and programming for people with hearing disabilities, audiologists also contribute to the prevention of hearing loss by recommending and fitting protective devices and by consulting with government and industry on the detrimental effects and management of environmental noise. In addition, audiologists evaluate and assist individuals with **auditory processing disorders (APD)**, sometimes called central auditory processing disorders. They also select, fit, and dispense hearing aids and other amplification devices and provide guidance in their care and use (DeBonis & Moncrieff, 2008). Licensed audiologists are independent professionals who practice without a prescription from any other health care provider (ASHA, 2001b). Box 1.1 contains an audiologist's comments on some of the challenges and rewards of the profession. As you will note, being a good detective, or problem solver, is one of the skills that is needed. Websites of interest are found at the end of the chapter.

Credentials for Audiologists

At the present time, the educational requirement for an audiologist is 3 to 5 years of professional education beyond the bachelor's degree. An audiologist's studies will culminate in a doctoral degree that may be an audiology doctorate (AuD) or a doctor of philosophy degree (PhD) or doctor of education degree (EdD) in audiology.

After a person has earned a doctorate, obtained the required preprofessional as well as paid clinical experience, and passed a national examination, she or he is eligible for the Certificate of Clinical Competence in Audiology (CCC-A) awarded by ASHA. The ASHA CCC-A (sometimes referred to as ASHA "Cs") is the

BOX 1.1 | An Audiologist Reflects

I chose to become an audiologist because I enjoyed the challenge. Most clients come in and are frightened or apprehensive. I try to set them at ease while I explain each test I will perform. At each step, I try to bring the client along and make sure that he or she understands what I will be doing and why. Children are often the biggest challenge and sometimes refuse to cooperate. This is when I have to be at my best. If I confirm the presence of a hearing loss, then my task becomes one of counseling and referral. It takes time to walk a client through the results and the possibilities. Older clients are often not willing initially to accept a diagnosis of hearing loss. Counseling is very important, especially for family members. It is all too easy for family members to adopt an "I told you so" attitude, but we must be sensitive to the needs of the client with the loss who will need time to adjust to his or her now-diagnosed disorder. It is this detective work and the counseling that give me satisfaction and motivate me to come to work every day.

generally accepted standard for most employment opportunities for audiologists in the United States. In addition, states require audiologists to obtain a state license. The requirements for state licensure tend to be the same as or similar to the ASHA standards (ASHA, 2001b, 2001c).

You can further explore a career in audiology at three websites. The Acoustical Society of America (http://asa.aip.org) has materials of special interest to hearing scientists and audiologists. The American Academy of Audiology (www.audiology.org) provides consumer and professional information regarding hearing and balance disorders as well as audiological services. Finally, ASHA (www.asha.org) provides information for professionals, students, and others who are interested in careers in audiology or hearing science. Simply click on "Careers" in the upper-left corner of the website.

 Video Example 1.2

Although audiologists work with both children and adults, you might find this video to be especially interesting and informative. https://www.youtube.com/watch?v=Ah_53tDcV64

Speech-Language Pathologists

Speech-language pathologists (SLPs) are professionals who provide an assortment of services related to communicative disorders. The distinguishing role of an SLP is to identify, assess, treat, and prevent communication disorders in all modalities (including spoken, written, pictorial, and manual), both receptively and expressively. This includes attention to physiological, cognitive, and social aspects of communication. SLPs also provide services for disorders of swallowing and may work with individuals who choose to modify a regional or foreign dialect. Like audiologists, licensed SLPs are independent professionals who practice without a prescription from any other health care provider (ASHA, 2000a, 2000b, 2000c). Box 1.2 contains reflections by two SLPs; the first one has been in private practice as a clinician for over 25 years. Although sometimes frustrated by the lack of support in his work setting, he believes in setting his imagination free and not giving up in the challenge to help others.

BOX 1.2 | **A Speech-Language Pathologist Reflects**

For me, the exciting part of my job is the problem solving and the satisfaction of helping others. Similar to a fictional detective who collects all the clues, synthesizes the information, and deduces the guilty party, I evaluate each client and determine the best course of intervention. The more severe the impairment, the greater the challenge, and I love a challenge. How can I help a young man who attempted suicide, and is now brain injured, to access the language within him? How can a young child with autism begin the road through communication to language? How can I help parents communicate with their infant who has deafness, blindness, and cerebral palsy? When is the best time to introduce signing with a nonspeaking client? These are all challenges for me and the children and adults I serve. We work together as I try to solve each communication puzzle and propose and implement possible intervention strategies. Sometimes I'm very successful and sometimes I have to reevaluate my methods, but as I said, I love a challenge.

Credentials for Speech-Language Pathologists

With technology, the task of an SLP is changing. Technologies for digital speech recording and analysis are now readily available, as are new and exciting assistive technologies for those with great difficulty communicating via speech (Ingram et al., 2004). SLPs have a master's or doctoral degree and have studied typical communication and swallowing development; anatomy and physiology of the speech, swallowing, and hearing mechanisms; phonetics; speech and hearing science; and disorders of speech, language, and swallowing.

Three types of credentials are available for SLPs:

1. Public school certification normally stipulates basic and advanced course-work, clinical practice within a school setting, and a satisfactory score on a state or national examination. At the least, prospective school SLPs need a bachelor's degree, although in most states, a master's degree either is the entry-level requirement or is mandated after a certain number of years of employment. The exact requirements to become a school SLP vary from state to state. ASHA encourages the same standards for SLPs in all employ-ment settings, as described in the following paragraph.

2. ASHA issues a Certificate of Clinical Competence in Speech-Language Pathology (CCC-SLP) to an individual who has obtained a master's degree or doctorate in the field, completed a monitored clinical fellowship year, and successfully passed a national qualifying examination. Ongoing pro-fessional development must be demonstrated through a variety of continu-ing education options. Since 2004, the United States, the United Kingdom, Australia, and Canada have allowed mutual recognition of certification in speech-language pathology (Boswell, 2004).

3. Individual states have licensure laws for SLPs that are usually independent of the state's department of education school certification requirements. A license may be needed if you plan to engage in private practice or work in a hospital, clinic, public school, or other setting. Most states accept a person with a ASHA CCC-SLP as having met licensure requirements, although you will need to check with your state licensing board on the specifics.

Table 1.1 shows the credentials that are needed in the professions of audiology and speech-language pathology. These are also found on the ASHA website.

If you want to further explore a career in speech-language pathology, check out the ASHA website (www.asha.org). You'll find a wealth of information, as well as discussion of various disorders that affect children and adults who may benefit from the help of a SLP. Type in the disorder you wish to explore in the search box in the upper right of the website. If you wish to read about a career as a SLP, click on "Careers" at the top left of the website.

 Thought Question 1.1

Were you surprised by the scope of possible intervention for SLPs and audiologists? Did you begin reading thinking only of speech and hearing? What surprised you the most, and why?

 Video Example 1.3

Watch this video that explores the SLP's scope of practice. https://www.youtube.com/watch?v=CX7zPnBEbWE

Speech, Language, and Hearing Scientists

Individuals who are employed as speech, language, or hearing scientists typically have earned a doctorate degree, either a PhD or an EdD. They are employed by universities, government agencies, industry, and research centers to extend our knowledge of human communication processes and disorders. Some may also serve as clinical SLPs or audiologists.

What Speech, Language, and Hearing Scientists Do

Speech scientists may be involved in basic research exploring the anatomy, physiology, and physics of speech-sound production. Using various technologies, these researchers strive to learn more about typical and pathological communication. Their findings help clinicians improve service to clients with speech disorders. Recent advances in knowledge of human genetics provide fertile soil for continuing investigation into the causes, prevention, and treatment of various speech impairments. Some speech scientists are involved in the development of computer-generated speech that may be used in telephone answering systems, substitute voices for individuals who are unable to speak, and fulfill many new purposes. Box 1.3 contains some observations by a speech-language scientist who enjoys the interdisciplinary nature of his work.

The professions of speech-language pathology and audiology require lifelong learning. Clinicians need to be able to intelligently use relevant research findings in their practice.

TABLE 1.1

Credentials for speech-language pathologists and audiologists

Credentialing Organization	Speech-Language Pathologist	Audiologist
American Speech-Language-Hearing Association (ASHA)	Certificate of Clinical Competence in Speech-Language Pathology (CCC-SLP)	Certificate of Clinical Competence in Audiology (CCC-A)
State department of education	Certification as teacher of students with speech and language disabilities*	—
State professional licensing board	License as speech-language pathologist	License as audiologist

*The title for the school-based speech-language pathologist varies from state to state.

BOX 1.3 | **A Speech-Language Scientist Reflects**

I work as a speech scientist and college professor specializing in voice science. In this profession I'm able to combine my love of communication with my interest in biology. As a student I hadn't realized the possibilities that would be open to me in this profession. I instruct students in the structure and functioning of the speech mechanism and in voice disorders. In the clinic, I use instrumentation to measure different parameters of voice. This enables me to objectify my diagnosis and provide accurate measurement of speech changes that may result from any number of disorders as varied as laryngeal cancer and neuromuscular dysfunction. I also work with transgender clients, helping them adopt a new voice. I love my work because it combines science and technology with speech-language pathology.

Language scientists may investigate the ways in which children learn their native tongue. They may study the differences and similarities of different languages. Over the past half a century or so, the United States has become increasingly linguistically and culturally diverse; this provides an excellent opportunity for cross-cultural study of language and communication. Some language scientists explore the variations of modern-day English (dialects) and how the language is changing. Others are concerned with language disabilities and study the nature of language disorders in children and adults. An in-depth knowledge of typical language is critical to understanding language problems.

Hearing scientists investigate the nature of sound, noise, and hearing. They may work with other scientists in the development of equipment to be used in the assessment of hearing. They are also involved in the development of techniques for testing the hard-to-test, such as infants and those with severe physical or psychological impairments. Hearing scientists develop and improve assistive listening devices such as hearing aids and telephone amplifiers to help people who have limited hearing. In addition, hearing scientists are concerned with conservation of hearing and are engaged in research to measure and limit the impact of environmental noise.

It's never too early to think about graduate school. Whether you eventually choose to become an audiologist, an SLP, or a speech, language, or hearing scientist, you will need advanced training. Consider cost, location, faculty, and practicum opportunities. Two websites can be helpful. The ASHA site (www.asha.org) lists graduate programs. Click on "Careers" to explore further. The Peterson's Guide site (www.petersons.com) can assist you with helpful advice about graduate school and a student planner. Type "speech-language pathology," "audiology," or "speech, language, or hearing science" in the *Find the School of Scholarship That's Right for You* box in the middle of the opening section of the website.

Related Professions: A Team Approach

Specialists in communication disorders do not operate in a vacuum. They work closely with family members, regular and special educators, psychologists, social workers, doctors and other medical personnel, and occupational, physical, and music therapists. They may collaborate with physicists and engineers. Box 1.4 contains a SLP's schedule, showing a tremendous amount of teamwork.

BOX 1.4 | **A Team Approach**

Alicia is the senior speech-language pathologist in a community-based rehabilitation center in New York State. During the mornings, Alicia works with infants, preschoolers, and school-age children at the center. In the afternoons, she directs the Augmentative/Alternative Communication Program and assists severely impaired individuals of all ages to improve their communication abilities. The schedule outlined below has a bit more collaboration than is normally found in any one day, but it suggests the kinds of activities that are typical within a workweek.

8:30 A.M.	Education staff meeting for preschool children: classroom teacher, psychologist, social worker, occupational therapist, physical therapist.
9:00	Preschool class activity: eight children ages 3–4, one classroom teacher, two aides.
10:00	Individual half-hour therapy sessions with children in the preschool and school programs.
11:30	Combined physical and speech therapy for Jeramy, age 4, diagnosed with spastic cerebral palsy; work with physical therapist.
noon	Lunch
12:30 P.M.	Prepare for the afternoon.
1:00	Consult with engineer on wheelchair switch for Lucretia, age 7, who is multiply disabled.
1:30	Outpatient, David, aged 24, had been in a motorcycle accident and experiences some speech and language difficulties.
3:00	Conference with Sally Brown, Bettina's foster mother, and Barbara Sloane, the social worker for the family.
3:30	Communication Disorders Department meeting. Malcolm, an audiologist, reports on a 3-hour course he took on Saturday on cochlear implants.
4:30	The workday is officially over, but Alicia stays until 5:00 to read the professional journal *Language, Speech, and Hearing Services in the Schools,* which arrived today. Alicia is especially interested in the article about using children's books in working with preschoolers, and photocopies it to share with other staff members.

Check Your Understanding 1.2
Click here to check your understanding of the concepts in this section.

SERVICE THROUGH THE LIFESPAN

This text mentions two things—lifespan and evidence-based practice—in the subtitle. Before we move on, let's discuss each one briefly and why it's important.

Individuals with communication and swallowing disorders may be of any age, and professionals address their needs from birth through old age. According to U.S. Census Bureau reports, 1 in 5 people has a disability. This translates into over 65 million people in the U.S. In general, the likelihood of having a disability increases as we age. Although the exact number of individuals in the United States who have speech, voice, and swallowing and/or language disorders is difficult to determine (ASHA, 2008), they are in the tens of millions.

The U.S. Census Bureau reports that about 2% of all children born in the United States have some existing disabling condition, and that hearing loss occurs more often than any other physical problem (Brault, 2005). All infants in the United States must be screened for hearing loss. Babies and toddlers may exhibit developmental delay and have physical problems, including those involving movement, hearing, and vision, that may impact their communication and feeding abilities.

An interdisciplinary approach is necessary in the assessment and treatment of young children, and an Individualized Family Service Plan (IFSP), developed for each child treated, must address the needs of the entire family, with sensitivity to that family's language and culture. Early identification and intervention has been demonstrated to be highly valuable in facilitating optimum results and potentially preventing later difficulties. Some children will be diagnosed as having developmental difficulties not evident at birth.

Preschoolers with communication difficulties must also be identified and helped. For some, services begun earlier may now be handled by different agencies. The youngster may be placed in a special preschool, and professionals may continue to assist the family in addressing the child's needs.

Almost half of all SLPs are employed by school systems. They work with youngsters in all grades, addressing a full range of communication and swallowing problems. These are described in the chapters that follow. School-age children with communication difficulties often experience academic and social difficulties, which add additional urgency to the work of communication experts. Some young adults, such as those who were identified earlier as being developmentally delayed or with physical disabilities, may continue to receive certain services until they are 21 years old.

Other individuals may find themselves in need of communication services for the first time later in life. For example, between 1.5 and 2 million Americans sustain traumatic brain injury each year in the United States (see Chapters 4 and 7) stemming from bicycle, motorcycle, or car accidents; falls; or firearms. As a result, they may have cognitive and/or motor problems that interfere with their ability to communicate and/or eat. The SLP plays an important role in rehabilitative efforts.

Among those over age 65, stroke, neurological disorders, and cognitive impairments may interfere with effective communication and swallowing. Hearing loss may affect at least one-quarter of people in this age group, creating a need for assessment and treatment. SLPs and audiologists work directly with such individuals. They often also work with spouses and children, as well as staff members of nursing homes and other adult facilities in providing counseling and guidance directed toward improving quality of life in these later years (Lubinski & Masters, 2001).

 Thought Question 1.2

As you think about intervention across the lifespan and working as a member of a team, think about variations in this arrangement. Are there ages of clients or severities of disorders in which you as an SLP might work alone with a client, times when you might consult with other specialists, and still other times when you might serve as a member of a team?

 Check Your Understanding 1.3
Click here to check your understanding of the concepts in this section.

EVIDENCE-BASED PRACTICE

As in other professions, SLPs and audiologists use evidence-based practice to provide the best services possible.

Throughout this text, we'll try to report the best information we can, based on the research evidence available. As an SLP or audiologist (if that is your career choice), it will be your responsibility to provide the best and most well-grounded research-based intervention that is humanly possible. In other words, you should do what works best and is most effective.

Deciding on the most efficacious intervention is a portion of something called evidence-based practice (EBP). EBP is an essential part of effective and ethical intervention. The primary benefit is the delivery of optimally effective care to each client (Brackenbury et al., 2008). Using EBP, clinical decision making becomes a combination of scientific evidence, clinical experience, and client needs. In other words, research, specifically the small portion of research directly relevant to decisions about practice, is combined with reason when making decisions about treatment approaches (Dollaghan, 2004).

EBP is based on two assumptions (Bernstein Ratner, 2006):

- Clinical skills grow not just from experience but from the currently available data.
- An expert SLP or audiologist continually seeks new therapeutic information to improve efficacy.

Professional journals, called peer-reviewed journals, in which each manuscript is critiqued by other experts in the field and accepted or rejected on the basis of the quality of the research, are the best sources of clinical research-based evidence.

The philosophy and methods of EBP originated in medicine, but have now been adopted in many other health care professions and related services. Ideally, EBP is a work in progress with updates as we learn more. New information may come to light through research that changes previous assumptions about that evidence. None of this relieves SLPs and audiologists of the responsibility to provide the best, most efficacious assessment and intervention possible. See the ASHA online resource at the end of the chapter.

In this discussion, we've used two terms: *efficacy* and *effectiveness*. These are sometimes difficult to discern, given the heterogeneous nature of the existing research studies, so it's important that you understand the generally accepted meanings of these terms from a clinical and research perspective. Technically, **efficacy** as it relates to clinical outcomes is the probability of benefit from an intervention method under ideal conditions (Office of Technology Assessment, 1978). There are three key elements to this definition:

- It refers to an identified population, such as adults with global aphasia, not to individuals.
- The treatment protocol should be focused, and the population should be clearly identified.
- The research should be conducted under optimal intervention conditions (Robey & Schultz, 1998). Of course, results in real-life clinical situations may differ somewhat.

Of interest is the therapeutic effect or the positive benefits resulting from treatment. The ideal treatment, then, would seem to be the one that results in the largest changes to meaningful client outcomes, with only limited variability across clients (Johnson, 2006).

Unfortunately, in the fields of speech-language pathology and audiology, only a small percentage of the research articles address intervention directly. Making clinical decisions, therefore, is not particularly easy, especially given potentially competing claims, varying clinical expertise, and client values. Still, SLPs are tasked with determining which treatment approach is best for each client. It is also important for SLPs to recognize that efficacy is never an all-or-nothing proposition (Law et al., 2004; Rescorla, 2005).

Effectiveness is the probability of benefit from an intervention method under average conditions (Office of Technology Assessment, 1978). The effectiveness of treatment is the outcome of the real-world application of the treatment for individual clients or subgroups. In short, effectiveness is a measure of "what works." Valid clinical studies must be realistically evaluated for the feasibility of applying them to intervention with specific populations and individuals (Guyatt & Rennie, 2002).

One way of determining potential effectiveness, but not the only one, may be a clinical approach's reported **efficiency** (Kamhi, 2006a). Efficiency results from application of the quickest method involving the least effort and the greatest positive benefit, including unintended effects. For example, an unintended benefit of working to correct difficult speech sounds is that it improves the production of untreated easier sounds, although the reverse is not true (Miccio & Ingrisano, 2000). Targeting more difficult sounds would seem to be more efficient.

Other factors in decision making include the clinician's expertise and experience, client values, and service delivery variables. In addition to clinical experience and expertise, individual SLP factors such as attitude and motivation are important. Clients vary widely and respond differently to intervention based on each client's unique characteristics, such as family history and support, age, hearing ability, speech and language reception and production, cognitive abilities, and psychosocial traits, such as motivation. Finally, service delivery factors include the targets and methods selected, the treatment setting, participants, and the schedule of intervention.

An SLP or audiologist must carefully discuss possible intervention options with a client and/or family, including an explanation of the research evidence. The goal is to provide sufficient information to enable the client and/or family to make an informed choice or to collaboratively plan and refine the options to suit the client and/or family preferences.

Making good clinical decisions is not always easy. High-quality evidence-based research must be evaluated critically by each SLP and applied to specific clients with specific communication disorders. EBP requires the judicious integration of scientific evidence into clinical decision making (Johnson, 2006). Although EBP can improve and validate clinical services, we must acknowledge that it can be difficult to incorporate into everyday clinical settings because of the time required for SLPs to comb through relevant research. In addition, evidence may be limited, contradictory, or nonexistent (Brackenbury et al., 2008). In the last analysis, however, the necessity of providing the best intervention services possible must be the foremost professional concern.

You can explore EBP further at two websites. The ASHA site (www.asha.org) describes EBP and offers guidance for clinical practice. Click on "Practice Management" to find the "Practice Portal" which will take you to a choice of disorders you may wish to explore. The National Institute on Deafness and Other Communication Disorders (NIDCD) site (www.nidcd.nih.gov) contains relevant health and research information. Just type the disorder in the search box in the upper right of the website.

 Check Your Understanding 1.4
Click here to check your understanding of the concepts in this section.

COMMUNICATION DISORDERS IN HISTORICAL PERSPECTIVE

It is believed that many early human groups shunned less able individuals. They sometimes abandoned children who were malformed or who had obvious physical disabilities. Groups also often abandoned, deprived of food, or even killed aged people who could no longer contribute. There is also archaeological data to suggest that in some early cultures those with physical disabilities were sometimes considered to have special powers.

Over the centuries, attitudes have changed somewhat. By the late 1700s to early 1800s in some parts of the world, societal efforts were being made to help those who were unable to care for themselves. Individuals began to be classified and grouped according to their disorder. Special residences for individuals with deafness, blindness, mental illness, and intellectual limitations were established, although most were little more than warehouses providing no services other than what was necessary to keep the residents alive (Karagiannis et al., 1996).

The first U.S. "speech correctionists" were educators and others in the helping or medical professions who took an interest in speech problems (Duchan, 2002). These were accompanied by a few "quacks" who promised curing therapies or drugs. The more legitimate therapists came from already established professions. Among them were Alexander Melville Bell and his father, Alexander Graham Bell, of telephone fame. Other Americans trained with famous "speech doctors" in Germany and Austria or became interested in speech correction because of their own difficulties, often with stuttering. The first professional journal, *The Voice*, which appeared in 1879, focused primarily on stuttering research and intervention.

Early interest groups were formed primarily among teachers within the National Education Association and among physicians and academics belonging to the National Association of Teachers of Speech. The latter group formed the American Academy of Speech Correction in 1925, a precursor to ASHA, and attempted to promote scientific inquiry and to set standards for training and practice. ASHA has had varying names over the years; it finally settled on American Speech-Language-Hearing Association in 1978.

The profession of audiology originated in the 1920s, when *audiometers* were first designed for measuring hearing. Interest surged in the 1940s when returning World War II veterans exhibited noise-induced hearing loss due to gunfire or prolonged and unprotected exposure to noise. Others had psychogenic hearing loss as a result of trauma. The Veterans Administration provided hearing testing and rehabilitation.

Gradually, ASHA was able to establish professional and educational standards and to advocate for the rights of individuals with disabilities. During the 1960s in the United States and elsewhere, intense energy was directed toward the advancement of civil rights for all people. Just as the rights of women, ethnic minorities, gays, and lesbians have been and are being recast, the status of individuals with disabilities has been reevaluated, and bold reforms have been initiated. The American Coalition of Citizens with Disabilities was created in 1974; legislative action on behalf of all Americans with disabling conditions began in earnest around the same time. In many cases, people with disabilities occupied leadership roles in the push for change. As a result of this work, providing opportunities for individuals with disabilities to develop to their full potential was no longer simply an ethical position. It became federally mandated through a series of laws.

A series of laws passed by the U.S. Congress over the past 50 years mandates appropriate treatment for individuals with disabilities.

Congress enacted the Education for All Handicapped Children Act (EAHCA) as Public Law 94–142 in 1975. It mandated that a free and appropriate public education must be provided for all children with disabilities between the ages of 5 and 21. Several years later, Public Law 99–457 extended the age of those served to cover youngsters between the ages of birth and 5 years. In 1990, Congress reauthorized the original law and renamed it the Individuals with Disabilities Education Act (IDEA). IDEA addressed the multicultural nature of U.S. society. The needs of English language learners (ELLs) and those from racial and ethnic minorities were targeted for special consideration. Reauthorized in 2004, IDEA established birth-to-6 programs as well as new early intervention services. ASHA has been a vital advocacy agency throughout this long legislative process.

 Check Your Understanding 1.5

Click here to check your understanding of the concepts in this section.

SUMMARY

Speech-language pathologists, audiologists, and other specialists work together to assist those with communicative impairments. They work in a variety of settings and with people of all ages. They are rewarded by contributing to the well-being of others. Professionals who are engaged in clinical service for those with communication disorders must have a master's or doctoral degree and supervised clinical experience. They must have earned the American Speech-Language-Hearing Association Certificate of Clinical Competence (ASHA-CCC) in their area of specialization.

Services are provided to individuals from birth through advanced age. The American Speech-Language-Hearing Association (ASHA) is the largest organization of professionals working with communication disorders. ASHA's missions include the scientific study of human communication, provision of clinical service in speech-language pathology and audiology, maintenance of ethical standards, and advocacy for individuals with communication disabilities. As a result, federal legislation currently mandates services for people with disabilities.

SUGGESTED READINGS/SOURCES

American Speech-Language-Hearing Association. (2017a). *Careers That Grow With You: The Future of Audiology and Speech-Language Pathology.* Accessed on April 25, 2017 at http://www.asha.org/Careers/Careers-That-Grow-With-You/.

American Speech-Language-Hearing Association. (2017b). *Learn About the CSD Professions: Make A Difference, Make A Change.* Accessed on April 25, 2017 at http://www.asha.org/Students/Learn-About-the-CSD-Professions/.

Nicolosi, L., Harryman, E., & Kresheck, J. (2003). *Terminology of communication disorders: Speech, language, hearing* (5th ed.). Baltimore: Williams & Wilkins.

2

Typical and Disordered Communication

LEARNING OUTCOMES

When you have finished this chapter, you should be able to:

- Explain the role of culture and environment in human communication

- Describe the different aspects of human communication

- Demonstrate how communication disorders may be classified, including the names and frequency of occurrence of different types of communication disorders

- Describe in general the assessment and intervention process

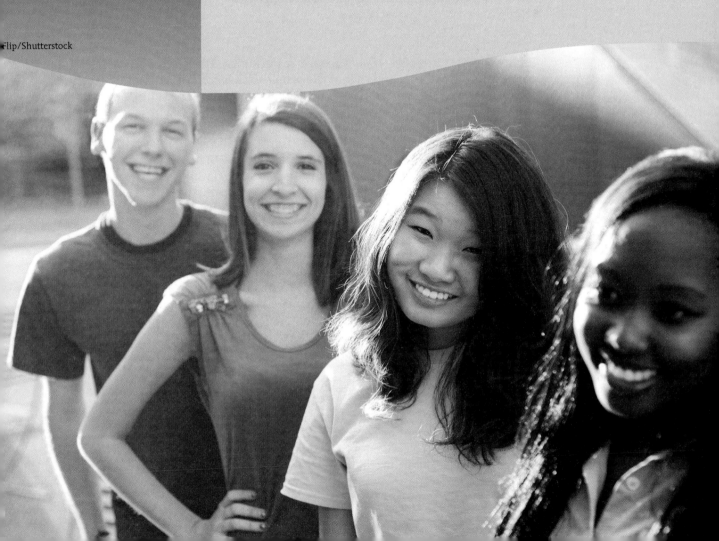

What is **communication**? It's important for us to answer that question before we can explore communication disorders. In general, we can say that communication is an exchange of ideas between sender(s) and receiver(s). It involves message transmission and response or feedback.

ROLE OF CULTURE AND THE ENVIRONMENT

Humans are social beings. Possibly the worst punishment for a prisoner is to be sentenced to isolation. Milder discipline for a teenager might include limitations on texting or email use. These restrictions are punitive because we humans are social beings. We have powerful drives to be with and to communicate with others.

It is axiomatic to say "We cannot *not* communicate" (Watzlawick et al., 1967, p. 48). Even a lack of response to someone sends a message to "leave me alone."

We communicate to make contact or to reach out to others, and to satisfy our needs, to reveal feelings, to share information, and to accomplish a host of purposes. Communication is interactive; it is a give-and-take. The importance of effective communication is highlighted when it fails or is hindered in some way. Think about how frustrated you get by a temporary lapse in Internet or cellphone service. Now imagine if that was a permanent, semi-permanent, or recurring condition.

Several variables affect communication and its success or failure. These include cultural identity, setting, and participants, to name a few. The study of these influences on communication is called **sociolinguistics**.

Cultural Identity

Each of us is a member of a language community. The more you understand about your own culture and that of the people with whom you communicate, the more effective your interaction will be. Perhaps you have traveled to a country in which a language that you did not know was spoken. You might have been able to communicate by gesture and pantomime; however, you would have to agree that while you could exchange some meaning, it fell far short of optimal communication. If this text were written in perfectly good Mandarin Chinese and you could not read that language, it would communicate nothing meaningful to you. Speakers and listeners must share competence in a common language if they are to communicate fully.

Even when two people come from the same language background, "perfect" communication is rare. This is because successful communication depends not just on language and speech but on related factors, such as age, socioeconomic status, geographical background, ethnicity, gender, and ability.

 Thought Question 2.1

As the U.S. population diversifies, it's good to think about the impact of culture on communication and on disorders. Can you think of any communication differences that might be culturally based but might seem to the unaware person to be a disorder? Most of these, but not all, will affect pragmatics or language use.

The location and the participants also influence the nature of communication. Where you interact affects how and what you'll say. You communicate differently at home, in school, in a noisy restaurant, and at a ballgame. Similarly, you might speak quite differently to your best friend, your mother, your father, your boss, your grandmother, and large audiences.

The Environment

Not only does communication reflect the cultures of the speakers but it also occurs within an environment or context. In fact, the act of communication often only makes sense within a context. "Can you take out the garbage on the way?" would seem odd if uttered during a haircut. Likewise, "You're hilarious!" would seem out of place at a funeral. There are places to ask questions and places where it would seem inappropriate.

The communication environment includes not only the location in which communication occurs, but also the people involved and the event in which they are involved. Often, the communication itself is the context. "Sure, honey" would only work as a response to the request about garbage but wouldn't make sense as a reply to being called hilarious at a funeral, especially if you had just met the individuals involved. Even when we write, we must consider the reader and must build the context on paper from the language available to us.

 Check Your Understanding 2.1
Click here to check your understanding of the concepts in this section.

ASPECTS OF COMMUNICATION

As noted in Chapter 1, communication takes many forms and can involve one or a combination of our senses, including sight, hearing, smell, and touch. It can include both verbal, such as the spoken or written word, and nonverbal means, such as naturalistic gestures, facial expressions, or signs. The primary vehicle of human communication is language, and speech is the primary means of language expression for most individuals.

Language

Language is a socially shared code that is used to represent concepts. This code uses arbitrary symbols that are combined in rule-governed ways (Owens, 2016). Taken together, the characteristics of language are that it is:

- A socially-shared tool
- A rule-governed system
- An arbitrary code
- A generative process
- A dynamic scheme

Let's discuss each aspect of language separately.

Language is a social tool for relating to others and for accomplishing a variety of objectives. As pointed out earlier, others must share the language code if communication is to occur. When an infant utters "ga da da ka," we cannot call this "language" because this "code" is not shared.

Many people are so accustomed to their own language that they fail to recognize its arbitrary nature. Is there anything in the sound combination or the written letters of the word *water* that resembles the wet stuff? No, words are arbitrary. Is the French word *l'eau* or the Italian *l'acqua* any more or less moist? The equivalent of the English word *butterfly* is *farfalla* in Italian, *mariposa* in Spanish, and *Schmetterling* in German—four very different renditions for that graceful creature. Some words have no equivalent in other languages. For example, the Spanish word *salsa* has no one-word English equivalent, so in the U.S. we use the Spanish word.

Parents often assume that their infant's earliest "ma ma" or "da da" are uttered in reference to themselves. These sound combinations are not considered true words unless there is evidence that they are used meaningfully.

Each language, in addition to being composed of arbitrary but agreed upon words, consists of rules that dictate how these words are arranged in sentences. In English, an adjective precedes a noun; for example, we say, "brown cow." In French, as in many other languages, this sequence is reversed, and French speakers say, "le vache brun" ("the cow brown"). The rules of a language make up its **grammar**. Interestingly, you do not have to be able to explain the rules to recognize when they have been broken. Take, for example, the sentence "The leaves of the maple green tree in the breeze swayed." You know intuitively that the sentence doesn't sound correct.

Language is **generative**; this means that you can create new utterances. As a speaker, you don't just quote or repeat what you heard before. Instead, you present your own ideas in an individual way. Imagine trying to have a conversation if all you could do was imitate your conversation partner.

Languages are also **dynamic**; they change over time. The Academie Française has tried to keep French "pure" and true to its origins by attempting to keep "foreign" words from infiltrating. For example, it has tried to ban the English words "jet" and "drugstore." But "le jet" is apparently easier to use than the French "l'avion à réaction," and so it stays. No academy, no school, no law, and no army can keep languages from being modified. American English adds five or six new words each day, many from other languages. Pronunciation, grammar, and ways of communicating also change.

 Video Example 2.1

Environmental changes influence the evolution of language. Watch this video about how the Internet is changing the English language. https://www.youtube.com/watch?v=P2XVdDSJHqY

All human languages consist of similar basic ingredients. The primary inter-related components have been labeled form, content, and use. See Figure 2.1.

Form

Form consists of phonology, morphology, and syntax. **Phonology**, or the sound system of English, consists of about 43 phonemes, or unique speech sounds. Although different languages use many of the same phonemes, variations exist. Spanish and German, to name only two, do not use the English "th."

Figure 2.1 Components of language.

FORM
Syntax
Morphology
Phonology

CONTENT
Semantics

USE
Pragmatics

Sources: Data from Owens (2012) and Shadden & Toner (1997).

Speech sounds are not combined arbitrarily. **Phonotactic** rules specify how sounds may be arranged in words. Like rules of grammar, phonotactic rules are not universal. For example, "k" and "n" cannot be blended in spoken English. For this reason, the "k" in "knife" and "Knoxville" is silent for native English speakers.

Morphology, the second aspect of form, involves the structure of words. A **morpheme** is the smallest grammatical unit within a language. Words contain both **free morphemes** and **bound morphemes**. A free morpheme may stand alone as a word. For example, *cat*, *go*, *spite*, *like*, and *magnificent* are all free morphemes. If you attempt to break them into smaller units, you lose the meaning of the word. In contrast, *cats*, *going*, *spiteful*, *dislike*, and *magnificently* each contain one free morpheme and one bound morpheme. The bound morphemes *-s*, *-ing*, *-ful*, *dis-*, and *-ly* change the meanings of the original words by adding their own meanings. Bound morphemes cannot be used alone, and must be attached to free morphemes.

Syntax pertains to how words are arranged in a sentence and to the ways in which one word may affect another. In an English declarative sentence, the subject comes before the verb: "John is going to the opera." When we reverse the order of the subject and the auxiliary or helping verb *is*, we change the meaning of the sentence and end up with a question: "Is John going to the opera?" One word can also change another. We say "I walk" but "She walks." The *s* on the verb occurs because of the pronoun *she*. This also occurs with *he*, *it*, and singular nouns, such as *puppy*. "I walk" but "The puppy walks."

Content

Because language is used to communicate, it must be about something, and this is its content, meaning, or **semantics**. **Semantic features** are the pieces of meaning that come together to define a particular word. For example, *girl* and *woman* share the semantic features of *feminine* and *human*, but *child* is generally considered a feature in *girl* and not in *woman*. You'll notice that we said "generally" because, although most of us think of a girl as being young, it is common among some groups of people to refer to any woman as a "girl." Each word has multiple meanings, as you can quickly verify by looking in the dictionary. It is the other aspects of language, such as use and form, that determine which of these definitions is appropriate in context.

Use

If you are beginning to think that this is complicated, you're right. As we said earlier, social and cultural factors influence the way language is used. Use, or **pragmatics**, is the driving force behind all aspects of language. We speak for a reason. It is the purpose of our utterance that primarily determines its form and content. For example, if you are with a friend and are hungry, you might say, "Let's get something to eat." If the purpose were a simple biological drive, then simply "Eat" might suffice. Remember Cookie Monster? "Cookie!" But who and where you are, whom you are with, and the time of day also influence what you say. If you are at your home, and you have invited a friend to dinner, you might say, "Dinner is ready." If you are working with someone as noon approaches, you might suggest, "Let's break for lunch."

While all aspects of language are important, it is the use or the purpose of communication that dictates form and content.

Video Example 2.2

Pragmatics may be difficult to understand. Watch this video about pragmatics that includes a brief overview. https://www.youtube.com/watch?v=0xc0KUD1umw

Pragmatic rules vary with culture. For example, in the United States business meetings tend to be very task-oriented. Very little time is spent on social exchanges; the work to be done has center stage. In Saudi Arabia, however, when two people meet for the first time for business purposes, they might spend the entire session talking about family and friends and not get to the meat of the business until the second meeting. The rules for business conversations in each of these societies are different. A few general rules for speakers of American English are presented in Figure 2.2.

Speech

Speech is the process of producing the acoustic representations or sounds of language. Features such as articulation, fluency, and voice interact to influence speech production. The final product reflects the rapid coordination of movements associated with each of these features.

Articulation

Articulation refers to the way in which speech sounds are formed. How do we move our tongue, teeth, and lips to produce the specific phonemes of a language? How do we combine these individual sounds to form words? Chapter 8 explains the nature of speech sound production and describes the problems that may occur.

The component of speech that includes rate and rhythm is referred to as prosody. Prosodic features are known as suprasegmentals. *Supra-* means "above" or "beyond," so suprasegmental features go beyond individual speech sounds (or segmental units) and are applied to words, phrases, or sentences. Stress and intonation are also suprasegmental features of speech production that are discussed later in this chapter.

Figure 2.2 A sampling of pragmatic rules for speakers of american english.

1. Only one person speaks at a time. Each person should contribute to the conversation.
2. Speakers should not be interrupted.
3. Each utterance should be relevant.
4. Each speech act should provide new information.
5. Politeness forms reflect the relationship of the speakers.
6. Topics of conversation must be established, maintained, and terminated.
7. The speaker should be sensitive to successfully communicating the message, avoiding vagueness and ambiguity.
8. The listener should provide feedback that reflects comprehension of the message.

Although most of the time we attempt to use a clear, sufficiently loud voice, sometimes our meaning may be more effectively communicated by a whisper, a whine, or a throaty rasp. When you are upset, your voice might sound angry to the point where someone says, "Don't use that tone of voice with me." Clearly, tone communicates information.

Fluency

Fluency is the smooth, forward flow of communication. It is influenced by the rhythm and rate of speech. Every language has its own rhythmic pattern, or timing. Do we pause after each word that we speak? Do we pause after each sentence? If we do, how long do the pauses last? What is our phrasing? You'll note that timing is not an isolated feature of speech. A word or syllable that is held tends to be emphasized and said more loudly.

The speed at which we talk is our **rate**. Overall rate can reveal things about us. It may provide clues about where we come from. For example, people from New York usually speak more rapidly than those from Georgia. However, if you habitually speak very quickly, it may suggest that you are in a hurry, are impatient, or have a great deal to say. By contrast, slow speech may connote a relaxed or casual demeanor.

Voice

Voice can reveal things about the speaker as well as about the message. A person with a hoarse voice might (correctly or not) communicate to others that she or he smokes. A person with a soft, high-pitched voice might be communicating youth or immaturity. A deep, throaty voice might connote masculinity or authority.

Both the overall level of loudness and the loudness pattern within sentences and words are important. A generally loud voice may communicate strength; a soft one may suggest timidity. By stressing different words within a sentence, you are also conveying different meanings. Say the following sentence in each of the ways listed here, with the emphasis or increased loudness on the underlined word. Notice how the meaning changes:

I got an "A" on my Physics final.

I got an "A" on my Physics final.

I got an "A" on my Physics final.

I got an "A" on my Physics final.

Placing the stress on different syllables within certain words also changes the meaning. Stressed syllables often have long vowels, as in the first word in each of the following pairs:

record   record

recess   recess

present   present

You might have noticed that as you vary the stress, the pitch, duration, and pronunciation of different speech sounds may also change. The pitch tends to go up as the loudness is increased. Similarly, you are likely to prolong the syllable that receives stress.

The symbols /ɛ/, /ə/, and /l/ represent phonemes, or speech sounds to be described in more detail in Chapter 9.

Pitch is a listener's perception of how high or low a sound is; it can be physically measured as frequency or cycles per second, called hertz. **Habitual pitch** is the basic tone that an individual uses most of the time. Women usually have higher-pitched voices than men, and children have higher voices than adults of both sexes. So our habitual pitch tells something about who we are.

Pitch movement within an utterance is called **intonation**. Say the following sentence by bringing your pitch down for the last word and then say it by raising your pitch at the end:

She wants to do the dishes.

A rising intonation can turn a statement into a question.

You'll notice that intonation influences meaning. You should also observe that as you alter intonation, your rhythm and loudness patterns also change.

Punctuation and font type and size may contribute to the meaning of an email. A century ago, perfumed letter paper modified the written word.

Nonverbal Communication

Although most humans rely heavily on spoken communication, some researchers report that about two thirds of human exchanges of meaning take place nonverbally. The term *nonverbal* encompasses both the suprasegmental aspects of speech that we described in the previous section and the **nonvocal** (without voice) and nonlinguistic (nonlanguage) aspects of communication.

Artifacts

The way you look and the way you have decorated yourself and your personal environment communicate something about you. People make assumptions about our personalities and trustworthiness on the basis of our possessions, clothing, and general appearance.

Kinesics

Kinesics refers to the way we move our bodies, called *body language*. This includes overall body movement and position as well as gestures and facial expression. Gestures such as a "brush-off" and facial expressions such as a frown have explicit meanings, and they support and contribute to the larger speech system. By contrast, signing may be a primary means of communication for someone who has deafness. ASL is described in greater detail in Chapter 12 and Chapter 13.

Space and Time

The study of the physical distance between people as it affects communication is called **proxemics**. Proxemics not only reflects the relationship between people but is also influenced by age and culture. Infants, children, people from Middle Eastern and Latin cultures, and those with strong emotional attachments, such as lovers, tend to interact in intimate or close proximity, very near one another.

Tactiles are touching behaviors. Who touches whom and how and where on the body the touch occurs can reveal a great deal. Although children in our society learn that touching others is usually not appropriate and are told early on to "keep your hands to yourself," infants' earliest interactions normally include considerable parental and caretaker touch.

Speech-language pathologists recognize the heterogeneous nature of the U.S. population and strive to be sensitive to both verbal and nonverbal variations.

Chronemics is the effect of time on communication. Again, cultural and age factors influence this aspect of communication. People from German and Scandinavian backgrounds tend to be exactingly prompt, while those from Latin and African cultures may permit greater time flexibility. Status and context also affect chronemics. You might be kept waiting at the doctor's office, but your doctor does not expect to have to wait for you. Promptness is part of the U.S. work ethic. If you are routinely late to class or to a job, you've violated a chronemic norm and might have to pay a price in terms of a lowered grade or lost employment.

Age, sex, education, and cultural background influence every aspect of communication. These natural variations in communication are not impairments. Differences reflect regional, social, cultural, or ethnic identity and are not a disorder of speech or language.

As we mature, our communication changes. The crying of an infant may become the call "Mommy" within a year. Table 2.1 offers a sampling of typical communication features at different life stages. We describe communication impairments in the next section.

Communication Through the Lifespan

The most complex and challenging task newborns face is learning the abstract code called "language" that those around them use to communicate. To do this, infants must first learn the rudiments of communication and begin to master the primary means of language transmission, called "speech." The early establishment of communication between children and their caregivers fosters the development of both speech and language, which in turn influences the quality of communication. This intricate pattern is fostered by physical, cognitive, and social development as a child matures. In a seeming reversal, language proficiency is critical to development of higher cognitive and social skills (Oller et al., 2001).

The key to an infant becoming a communicator is being treated as one. The process of learning speech and language is a social one that occurs through interactions of children and the people in their environment. Although both speech and language depend on physical and cognitive maturation, neither is sufficient to account for the rapid developments in children's communication.

Speech and language are learned within routines and familiar activities that shape children's days and within conversations about food, toys, and pets and later about school, social life, and the like. A young child uses a variety of speech cues and patterns to break continuous speech into more readily interpretable chunks (Sanders & Neville, 2000). For example, no words in American English begin with the "ks" (written /ks/) sound, but that same combination can signal the end of a word.

In different cultures, the type of child–caregiver interaction, the model of language presented to the child, and the expectations for the child differ, but each is sufficient for the learning of the language of the culture. Learning to become an effective communicator is a dynamic and active process in which children in our culture become involved in the give-and-take of conversations. Even the more formal educational processes of learning to read and write are initially social and occur within early book-reading activities in the home involving children and caregivers.

Every person's speech and language continue to change until the end of life. Communication reflects the changes occurring in us and around us. Even the

TABLE 2.1

A lifespan view of typical communication

Age Range	Receptive Communication	Expressive Communication							Nonverbal Communication	
		Language			Speech			Artifacts	Kinesics	Space/Time
		Form	Content	Use	Articulation	Fluency	Voice			
Infancy	Quiets/turns to human voice; Distinguishes speech sounds	Prelinguistic sound-making	No "true" speech; vocalizations; body movement focus on here and now	Obtain assistance; imitate, respond to others	Gurgles, coos, babbles	Rhythm and rate begin to resemble that of surrounding language toward end of year	Varies volume, rate, pitch	Toys, materials given to child; may "give" objects to others	Gestures precede meaningful spoken language	Close proximity/immediacy
Toddler	Responds to some verbal commands	Vocabulary growth from 4 to 300 words; moves from single word to short utterances	Familiar names, actions	Imitate, greet, protest, question	Simplified phonology		High (childish) pitch, more variability than adults	Toys; begins to construct things; start of imaginary play	Gestures slowly take second place to spoken language	Proximity decreases; begins to comprehend "now" and "later"
Preschool	Comprehension far exceeds expression; enjoys stories, books; follows increasingly complex commands; comprehends simple humor	Vocabulary grows from 1,000 to more than 2,000 words; uses complete sentences	Immediate to imaginary; includes past, present, and future	Greet, request, protest, inform, pretend, entertain	Almost all speech sounds correctly produced by the end of this period	Part-word, whole word, and phrase repetition not uncommon	Adjusts to listener; often used effectively to enhance verbal communication	Tremendous variability; reflects social/cultural background	Gestures used to enhance verbal communication	Begins to understand personal space

TABLE 2.1
(Continued)

Receptive Communication		Expressive Communication							Nonverbal Communication	
		Language			Speech					
Age Range		Form	Content	Use	Articulation	Fluency	Voice	Artifacts	Kinesics	Space/Time
School-age	Reading skills improve; receptive language grows to 50,000 words by sixth grade, 80,000 words end of high school; comprehension becomes adult-like	Vocabulary grows to 25,000 to 30,000 words; slang important; written language more complex than spoken language	Very broad; includes distant as well as near and abstract concepts	May enjoy talking, sharing thoughts, raising and answering personal as well as abstract questions; narrative skills expand	Speech sounds correctly produced	Rate may be rapid; fluency is good	Pitch drops to adult levels with puberty; voice used to supplement verbal message	Clear indication of what is wanted; reflect peer group, gender	Gestures used in wide array of means to supplement speech	Becomes territorial; mature understanding of space and time
Early and middle adulthood	Comprehension increases	Education and occupation may be reflected in vocabulary	Full range of topics; written language continues in importance and sophistication	Instructing; directing others may be added if not there earlier	Mature articulation	Use of rhythm and rate to enhance message	Mature pitch; full-bodied vocal quality	Tremendous variety dependent on sociocultural and individual variables	Body movement and gestures continue to supplement verbal communication	Space may reflect relative "importance" in environment as well as cultural factors
Advanced age	Comprehension may decrease with hearing loss	Vocabulary may reflect "older" generation	May focus more on past than future	May have limited communication partners; speech may be major way to achieve companionship	Normally not impaired	Rate may be slow	Pitch may increase; vocal quality may become "thinner"	Old/familiar items may become increasingly treasured	Body movement may be less forceful	May crave touch, as significant others become less available

Sources: Data from Owens (2012) and Shadden & Toner (1997).

Note: This is a sampling of communication behaviors. Variability within each age group is the norm.

Communication is established very early between child and caregiver.

means of communication can change. Your grandparents began life without a computer and had to learn this new means of communication. We, the authors, had to learn to use computers to communicate when we were young adults. You, in contrast, grew up with the Internet and cellphones. Many preschoolers now have tablets and Kindles.

Languages change, too. New words and phrases have entered American English within your lifetime, such as *Internet*, *Bluetooth*, *iPod*, *smartphone*, *texting*, *hip-hop*, and *hybrid vehicle*. Other cultures and languages have contributed *mullah*, *sushi*, *bodega*, and *tsunami*. A competent communicator continues to adapt to changes in the language and in the communication process.

Children become communicators because we treat them as if they already are.

 Check Your Understanding 2.2

Click here to check your understanding of the concepts in this section.

COMMUNICATION AND SWALLOWING IMPAIRMENTS

Now that you have an idea of the complexity and varied nature of communication, it should be easy to see that much can go wrong. Let's expand on what we discussed in Chapter 1. We can further define communication disorders as consisting of disorders of speech (articulation, voice, resonance, fluency), oral neuromotor patterns of control and movement, feeding and swallowing disorders, language and/or literacy impairment, cognitive and social communication deficits, and hearing and processing difficulties. This definition does not confine itself to speech communication and includes other communication systems. That's a lot! Although communication disorders may be categorized on the basis of whether reception, processing, and/or expression is affected, the three dimensions are often intertwined, reflecting the integration of the processes. Figure 2.3 presents various systems for categorizing speech and language disorders. In similar fashion, swallowing disorders could be classified based on the type and severity of the impairment.

The American Speech-Language-Hearing Association (ASHA) website (www.asha.org) discusses various disorders that affect children and adults who may benefit from the help of an SLP or audiologist. Type in the disorder you wish to explore in the search box in the upper right of the website.

Etiology, the cause or origin of a problem, may be used to classify a communication problem. Disorders may be due to faulty learning, neurological impairments, anatomical or physiological abnormalities, cognitive deficits, hearing impairment, damage to any part of the speech system, or a combination.

Sometimes a dichotomy is made between **congenital** and **acquired** problems. Congenital disorders are present at birth; acquired ones result from illness, accident, or environmental circumstances anytime later in life. An individual may have a disorder that is either congenital or acquired, or both. Finally, an individual's disorder may range from borderline or mild to profoundly severe.

Speech-language pathologists are concerned with both verbal and nonverbal disorders of communication.

As mentioned in Chapter 1, typical variations in communication and swallowing are not disorders. For example, **dialects** are differences that reflect a particular regional, social, cultural, or ethnic identity, and are not disorders of speech or language. Likewise, differences found in the speech and language of English language learners (ELLs) are not disorders.

Figure 2.3 Possible speech, language, and hearing disorders.

Speech communication disorders can have various causes which are congenital and/or acquired and severities ranging from mild to severe. Nonverbal and literacy impairments can further complicate communication impairments.

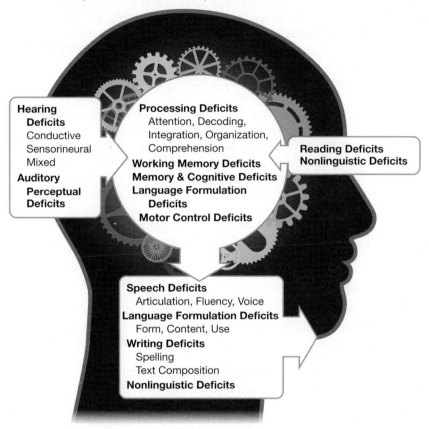

 Video Example 2.3

Before we begin to discuss disorders, watch this video. As you watch, note the behaviors that often accompany stuttering as you listen to what the children have to say. What characteristics of this type of communication disorder did you observe and hear the children describe? Might some characteristics be shared with other communication disorders? https://www.youtube.com/watch?v=da6xnm5feV4&index=4&list=PLEBC36C3D7AA1E348

Language Disorders

In this section, we give you an overview of different types of disorders. This will give you the basics for later, more in-depth discussions. Although we focus on form, content, and use, language impairments tend to cross these boundaries. A deficit in one area tends to affect the others.

Disorders of Form

As explained earlier, language form includes phonology, morphology, and syntax. An error in sound use, such as not producing the ends of words ("hi shi i too sma" for "his shirt is too small"), constitutes a disorder of phonology. This in turn, might affect morphology if a child omits the plural -s or the past tense -ed. Syntactical errors include incorrect word order and run-on sentences (for example, "I want to go mall and go skate and buy peanuts and you come with me 'cause I want you to but not Jimmy 'cause he's not big enough to go skate"). These errors in school-age children may affect both academic achievement and social well-being.

Disorders of form may be due to many factors, including sensory limitations such as hearing problems or perceptual difficulties such as learning disabilities. Limited exposure to correct models may also hinder a child's language development. For many children who are delayed in their production of mature language forms, the cause is not apparent. Neurological disorders caused by stroke or traumatic brain injury may result in a loss of access to language even though language remains intact.

Patterns that seem like errors at first are sometimes a reflection of a particular speech dialect or the influence of another language. An SLP must distinguish between dialectal or second language variations and disorders.

Disorders of Content

Children and adults with limited vocabularies, those who misuse words, and those with word-finding difficulties may have disorders of content or semantics. Similarly, limited ability to understand and use abstract language, as in metaphors, proverbs, sarcasm, and some humor, suggests semantic difficulties. A persistent pattern of avoiding naming objects and referring instead to "the thing" is another indication of a disorder of content. Although limited experience or a concrete learning style may contribute to this problem in youngsters, among older people cerebrovascular accidents (strokes), head trauma due to accidents, and certain illnesses, such as cognitive impairment (previously called dementia), may result in word-retrieval problems and other content-related difficulties.

Disorders of Use

It is not uncommon for an individual to have an impairment in more than one aspect of communication.

Pragmatic language problems may be related to limited or unacceptable conversational, social, and narrative skills; deficits in spoken vocabulary; and/or immature or disordered phonology, morphology, and syntax. Examples of impaired pragmatic language skills might include difficulty staying on topic, providing inappropriate or incongruent responses to questions, and constantly interrupting the conversational partner. Culture, group affiliations, setting, and participants described earlier in this chapter play a major role in judgments regarding pragmatic competence.

Speech Disorders

As mentioned earlier, disorders of speech may involve articulation (the production of speech sounds), fluency (rhythm and rate), or **voice** (pitch, loudness, and quality). They may affect people of all ages, be congenital or acquired, be due to numerous causes, and reflect any degree of severity.

Disorders of Articulation

Production of speech requires perception and conceptualization of the speech sounds in a language as well as motor movements to form these sounds in isolation and in connected speech. You must have both a mental/auditory image of the sound you are going to say and the neuromuscular skills to produce the sound. The cognitive and theoretical concepts of the nature, production, and rules for producing and combining speech sounds in language is known as *phonology*, which we know from the previous section is an aspect of language. The actual production of these sounds is called **articulation**.

It is not always easy to determine whether an individual's speech-sound errors indicate an impairment of phonology or articulation. To sort this out, SLPs identify the phonemes that are incorrectly produced and look for error patterns that may point to phonological disturbances. The sound system of a language is usually fully in place by age 7 or 8. Children with multiple speech-sound errors past age 4 may have *phonological* difficulties. The causes of phonological disorders are often not known but may result from faulty learning due to illness, such as ear infections, hearing or perceptual impairments, or other problems in the early years.

An SLP is interested in a client's ability to move the structures needed in speech, such as the jaw, lips, and tongue. The causes of articulation disorders include neuromotor problems such as cerebral palsy, physical anomalies such as cleft palate, and faulty learning. When paralysis, weakness, or poor coordination of the muscles for speech result in poor speech articulation, the disorder is called **dysarthria**. In contrast, apraxia of speech, although also poor articulation due to neuromotor difficulties, appears to be due to programming the speech mechanism, not muscle strength. Dysarthria and apraxia can affect both children and adults. Assessment and treatment of phonological and articulatory disorders are described in Chapter 10.

Disorders of Fluency

As we described earlier, fluency is the smooth, uninterrupted flow of communication. Certain types of fluency disruptions are fairly common at different ages. For example, many 2-year-olds repeat words: "I want-want-want a cookie." Around age 3, youngsters often make false starts and revise their utterances: "Ben took . . . he broked my crayon." Because this speech pattern is so common, it is sometimes referred to as **developmental disfluency**. Even typically fluent adults occasionally use **fillers** ("er," "um," "ya know," and so on), **hesitations** (unexpected pauses), **repetitions** ("g-go-go"), and **prolongations** ("wwwwell"). When these speech behaviors exceed or are qualitatively different from the norm or are accompanied by excessive tension, struggle, and fear, they may be identified as **stuttering**. Appropriate diagnosis and intervention when warranted are the task of an SLP (Yairi et al., 2001).

Fluency disorders are generally first noticed before 6 years of age. If remediation efforts are not made or are unsuccessful, this condition might continue and even worsen by adulthood. Adult onset of disfluency also occurs. Advancing age, accidents, and disease can all disrupt the normal ease, speed, and rhythm of speech. The causes of nonfluent speech are typically unclear; this is explored further in Chapter 8.

Speech-language pathologists use several indices to differentiate developmental disfluency from early stuttering.

Disorders of Voice

As in other areas of speech, voice matures as a child gets older. From uncontrolled cries to carefully modulated whispers, shouts, and variations in pitch, the development of voice follows a predictable pattern. Although occasionally children are born with physiological problems that interfere with normal voice, more common is the pattern of **vocal abuse**. It is characterized by excessive yelling, screaming, or even occasional loud singing that results in **hoarseness** or another voice disorder.

Habits such as physical tension and excessive yelling, coughing, throat clearing, smoking, and alcohol consumption can disrupt normal voice production. These behaviors may result in polyps, nodules, or ulcers on the vocal folds where voice production begins. Disease, trauma, allergies, and neuromuscular and endocrine disorders can also affect voice quality. For example, individuals with Parkinson's disease, a progressive neurological disorder affecting the range of muscle movement, may have a soft voice with limited pitch and loudness variation.

Hearing Disorders

A hearing disorder results from impaired sensitivity in the auditory or hearing system. It may affect the ability to detect sound, to recognize voices or other auditory stimuli, to discriminate between different sounds, such as mistaking the phoneme /s/ for /f/, and to understand speech.

Deafness

When a person's ability to perceive sound is limited to such an extent that the auditory channel is not the primary sensory input for communication, the individual is considered to have deafness. Deafness may be congenital or acquired.

Universal neonatal hearing screening is mandated by law in many states. In this way, congenital deafness can be identified and addressed very early.

Total communication, including sign, speech, and speechreading, is often considered the most effective intervention for deafness. **Assistive listening devices (ALD)**, **cochlear implants**, and **auditory training** may be helpful. These are explained in Chapter 12.

Hard of Hearing

A person who is hard of hearing, in contrast to one who is deaf, depends primarily on audition for communication. Hearing loss may be temporary due to an illness, such as an ear infection, or permanent, caused by disease, injury, or advancing age. Hearing loss is usually categorized in terms of severity, laterality, and type. The severity of a hearing loss may range from mild to severe. It may be bilateral, involving both ears, or **unilateral,** affecting primarily one ear. Finally, the loss may be **conductive**, **sensorineural**, or **mixed**. A conductive loss is caused by damage to the outer or middle ear. People with this type of loss usually report that sounds are generally too soft. A sensorineural loss involves problems with the inner ear and/or auditory nerve. This type of damage is likely to affect a person's ability to discriminate and consequently understand speech sounds, although they may "hear" them. It's typical for some older people to report that they hear just fine but wish others would not mumble. Mixed hearing loss, as the name implies, is a combination of both conductive and sensorineural loss (see Chapter 12 for further discussion).

Auditory Processing Disorders

An individual with an auditory processing disorder (APD) may have normal hearing but still have difficulty understanding speech. Individuals with APDs struggle to keep up with conversation, to understand speech in less-than-optimal listening conditions (i.e., degraded speech signal, presence of background noise), to discriminate and identify speech sounds, and integrate what they hear with nonverbal aspects of communication (DeBonis & Moncrieff, 2008). These difficulties are sometimes traced to tumors, disease, or brain injury, but often the cause is unknown. APDs can occur in both children and adults. A special battery of auditory diagnostic tests is used to determine or rule out APDs; however, there is currently no "gold standard" to ensure correct identification of the disorder (McFarland & Cacase, 2006). APDs may coexist with other disorders, including attention-deficit/hyperactivity disorder (ADHD) and speech-language and learning disabilities (ASHA, 2005c).

Swallowing Disorders

Difficulty swallowing is called **dysphagia**, and stated simply it means difficulty moving food or liquid from your mouth to your stomach. In some cases dysphagia may be associated with pain, or swallowing may be impossible. Persistent dysphagia may indicate a serious medical condition. Although swallowing difficulties may occur at any age, dysphagia is more common in older adults. The causes of swallowing problems vary, and treatment depends on the cause. These causes are usually associated with other neuromuscular disorders.

How Common Are Communication Disorders?

Before we attempt to estimate the numbers of people who have disorders of communication and swallowing, we should examine the concept of normalcy.

What Is "Normal"?

A recent cartoon showed an empty room and a sign reading "Meeting of Members of Functional Families." The implication was that there are no functional, or "normal," families. Likewise, we could ask, "Is anybody normal?" If anything, variability is the norm. We humans are remarkable in our diversity. Just as no two snowflakes are identical, no two individuals, even twins, are exactly alike. Our faces, fingerprints, and manner of communication are unique.

Most measures of humans, such as the number of individuals at varying heights, will result in what is called a "bell-shaped curve." We see this phenomenon with test scores as well. Most people will cluster near the average or the *mean* and will be considered "normal," typical, or average. Higher or lower scores are above or below average. An individual performing in the lowest 5% to 10% would have a score considered to be significantly below average. If we are testing language ability, such a low score may indicate a language disorder.

Because the word *normal* suggests "without problems," we, the authors, prefer to use the term *typical* when we mean "like most others of the same age and group." Classifying people on the basis of statistical percentage is little more than a numbers game. A more valid approach requires clear definitions of speech and language disorders and a thorough analysis of performance.

Communication and Swallowing Disorders as Secondary to Other Disabilities

Most communication disorders are secondary to other disabilities. For example, children with a cleft palate have physical health problems as well as voice and articulation disorders. People with cerebral palsy typically have motor deficits beyond speech and swallowing. Children with learning disabilities are especially likely to

Thought Question 2.2

At this point, you've had a very brief introduction to communication and swallowing disorders. Which areas interest you most? Why?

Thought Question 2.3:

Although we prefer the term *typical* rather than *normal*, what does "normal" mean to you? Does it matter to you? If so, how would you define "normal"?

Figure 2.4 The normal curve, percentile equivalents, and standard scores.

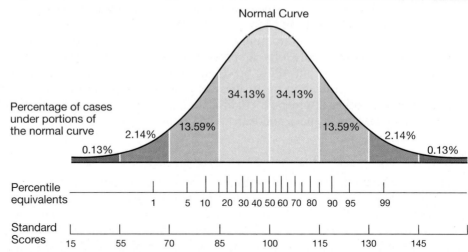

Source: Based on information from *Assessing and Screening Preschoolers*, by E. V. Nuttall,
I. Romero, and J. Kalesnik, 1992, Boston: Allyn & Bacon; and *Measurement and Assessment*,
by E. H. Wiig and W. A. Secord, 1992, Chicago: Riverside Publishing Co.

have language difficulties, but may also have articulation, voice, fluency, and/or hearing deficits. In addition, they experience academic and social difficulties.

Estimates of Prevalence

Prevalence refers to the number or percentage of people within a specified population who have a particular disorder or condition at a given point in time. If you determined the prevalence of stuttering in the entire U.S. population, among first-grade children, among college seniors, among U.S. males, or among U.S. females, you would get different prevalence figures in each case. For this reason, prevalence statistics must specify the population on which they are based.

The terms *incidence* and *prevalence* are often confused. Incidence refers to the number of *new* cases of a disease of disorder in a particular time period. Prevalence is the number of *new and old* cases in a particular time period.

Current estimates suggest that about 17% of the total U.S. population have some communicative disorder. About 11% have a hearing loss, and approximately 6% have a speech, voice, or language disorder. Many of those with hearing losses also have speech, voice, or language disorders.

The percentage of people with hearing loss increases with age. Between 1% and 2% of people under 18 years of age have a chronic hearing loss, compared with approximately 32% of those over age 75. Exposure to noise has contributed to the hearing loss in about a third of those affected.

Communication disorders vary with gender. For example, certain disorders, such as autism spectrum disorder, are four times as prevalent in males as in females.

Impairments of speech-sound production and fluency are more common in children than adults and more common among males than females. Speech disorders due to neurological disorders or brain and spinal cord injury occur more often among adults. It has been estimated that anywhere between 3% and 10% of Americans have voice disorders; the percentage is greater among school-age children and among people over age 65.

Language disorders occur in 8% to 12% of the preschool population; the prevalence decreases through the school years. Language deficits in older adults may be associated with stroke or cognitive impairment. It is likely that 5% to 10% of people over age 65 experience language disabilities related to these disorders.

It is estimated that 6 to 10 million Americans (about 3% of the population) have dysphagia. Although these figures may seem relatively low, it is likely that more, generally mild, cases are not reported (Tierney et al., 2000). The prevalence of dysphagia varies based on age, the definition that researchers use, and the population studied. For example, the prevalence of pediatric dysphagia among otherwise typically developing children has been reported to be 25%–45%, and to be higher for children with developmental disabilities (Arvedson, 2008; Bernard-Bonnin, 2006; Brackett, Arvedson, & Manno, 2006; Lefton-Greif, 2008; Linscheid, 2006; Manikam & Perman, 2000; Rudolph & Link, 2002).

Among adult populations prevalence is higher in seniors (Barczi, Sullivan, & Robbins, 2000; Bhattacharyya, 2014; Cabré et al., 2014; Roden & Altman, 2013; Sura, Madhavan, Carnaby, & Crary, 2012). In part, accurate data collection is complicated by the many disorders that can lead to dysphagia (Bhattacharyya, 2014). Estimates range from 13% of older adults living independently to 68% of long-term care facility residents (Kawashima, Motohashi, & Fujishima, 2004; Serra-Prat et al., 2011).

Table 2.2 highlights some communication and swallowing disorders that may appear through the lifespan.

TABLE 2.2

Communication disorders that may manifest themselves through the lifespan

Age Range	Disorders	Receptive Communication	Expressive Communication	Swallowing
Infancy	Hearing impairment Fetal alcohol or drug-exposure syndrome Parental neglect/abuse Cerebral palsy	Limited response to sound/speech Limited response to others Atypical physical postures and movement Deaf infants vocalize normally for first 6 mos. Others may have little vocalization Passivity	Atypical birth and other early cries	May have difficulties with breast or bottle; later problems with solid foods
Toddler	Autism/pervasive developmental disorder may be identified (hypersensitive to stimuli) Mental retardation not suspected earlier may now become apparent Brain injury due to falls	Comprehension of spoken language limited	Delay in first spoken word Utterances limited May use objects ritualistically	Rigid food preferences/dislikes Caution needs to be taken to prevent putting small objects in mouth that may be swallowed/choked on

(continued)

TABLE 2.2
(Continued)

Age Range	Disorders	Receptive Communication	Expressive Communication	Swallowing
Preschool	Delays that were suspected earlier may become more pronounced Fluency difficulties may emerge Specific language disabilities Middle ear problems common	Interactions with peers and others may be difficult	Inappropriate use of toys/objects Vocabulary may be limited, utterances short Alternative/augmentative communication may be recommended Excessive disfluency; delayed phonology and grammatical development	Food preferences may be more entrenched
School-age	Language learning problems Attention-deficit/hyperactivity disorder Brain injury due to falls and other accidents	Difficulties in attending, following directions, speech and reading comprehension	Narrative and other pragmatic skills may be affected	Inappropriate eating habits may become established
Young adulthood	Brain injury due to bike, motorcycle, car, and other accidents most prevalent in these years	Comprehension affected, generalized confusion, abstract thinking impaired	Pragmatic skills affected Life plans altered Dysarthria and apraxia may affect speech intelligibility	Neuromotor injury may impact swallowing
Middle adulthood	Hearing often starts to decline Life-threatening illnesses such as cancer may be diagnosed Neurogenic problems may appear; multiple sclerosis, ALS, Parkinson's, and Alzheimer's diseases; stroke (aphasia)	Speech in noise may be difficult to comprehend Aphasia and Alzheimer's may result in comprehension difficulties	Illness-related depression may affect expressive communication Dysarthria and apraxia may impair speech intelligibility Alzheimer's and aphasia cause language difficulties	Eating/swallowing may be impaired initially following stroke; swallowing difficulties often present in degenerative neuromotor diseases (e.g., multiple sclerosis, ALS)
Advanced age	Hearing deficits common Neurogenic problems become progressively worse	Difficulty understanding speech may cause "tuning out"	Voice may be weak Word-finding problems Inappropriate speech Perseveration	Disinterest in food, swallowing impairments may lead to aspiration pneumonia

Sources: Data from from Owens (2014) and Shadden & Toner (1997).

Note: This is a sampling of problems that may be seen. Variability within each age group is the norm.

Check Your Understanding 2.3
Click here to check your understanding of the concepts in this section.

ASSESSMENT AND INTERVENTION

An SLP, perhaps you someday, has many responsibilities for the management of communication and swallowing disorders. At the top of the list would be assessment to ascertain the presence of a disorder and to describe the extent and intervention to ameliorate any disorder identified. Other responsibilities include prevention and advocacy and serving as a clinician counselor.

The Role of the SLP in Prevention

As an SLP, you'll be involved in prevention of communication disorders as well as assessment and intervention. The goal of ASHA is that SLPs can help eliminate the causes and onset of communication disorders and foster optimal communication. This can be accomplished through education and the identification of potentially harmful and unhealthy situations, such as smoking and noise abatement. Secondary to prevention is early identification and intervention to forestall more serious conditions. A key lifespan concept is *wellness* or the optimal level of communication competence at all stages of life. To this end, SLPs take part in classroom education, community forums, wellness fairs, and counseling activities. If you go to the ASHA website (http://www.asha.org/) and type in prevention in the search box, you'll be able to read all the different ways in which SLPs are involved in prevention activities.

Assessment of Communication and Swallowing Disorders

Not everyone is assessed for communication disorders. Formal assessment occurs only after someone recognizes the possibility of a problem. Selection for assessment may come from referral by another professional or concerned adult, such as a pediatrician or parent, or from screening. Adults may also refer themselves if they feel they have a communication disorder or dysphagia.

The purpose of screening is to determine whether a problem exists. Children between the ages of birth and 36 months may be brought to special centers for screening for speech, language, hearing, motor, and other functions. Older children are screened in preschools and schools. In addition, every state in the United States requires that hearing screening tests be given to infants at their birthing facility or as soon after birth as possible.

Specialists in communication disorders may encourage referrals from other professionals and concerned individuals by publicizing the nature of the services that they provide.

Defining the Problem

Assessment of communication disorders is the systematic process of obtaining information from many sources, through various means, and in different settings to verify and specify communication and swallowing strengths and weaknesses, identify possible causes of problems, and make plans to address them.

If a problem is identified, an SLP may make a **diagnosis**, which distinguishes an individual's difficulties from the broad range of possible problems. Although a diagnostic report might include a label such as *dysphonia*, it more importantly contains a complete description of this disorder that reflects the person's ability to communicate, variability of symptoms, severity, and possible causes.

A person who has been identified during screening may have a communication disorder. A screening is not a diagnostic evaluation. Screenings simply suggest which individuals should receive further evaluation.

Assessment Goals

The goals of assessment are listed in Figure 2.5. The primary goal of diagnosis is determining the nature of the disorder. Sometimes **diagnostic therapy** is suggested. In this case, the SLP will work with the client for a time and will obtain a clearer picture of the person's communication abilities and limitations in the process.

As mentioned earlier, communication impairments may involve hearing, speech, language, processing, and/or swallowing, or, more likely, some combination of these. During assessment, specifics of all of these are probed. Both the client's communicative strengths and limitations are noted. An SLP provides data reporting the consistency of behaviors and, where appropriate, indicates how the client compares with more typical individuals.

> Clinicians may differ in their judgments of the severity of a disorder. Use of objective criteria ensures more consistency in this determination.

If a problem exists, an SLP will want to describe its severity. Exactly what determines a particular severity rating is related to several factors. Although published tests often suggest severity ratings depending on a client's performance scores, these must be used with caution. There is a broad range of typical communication behavior, and an SLP should not rely overly on any single test.

> Family members and clients are often eager to know the prognosis. They will ask questions such as "Will my child outgrow this problem?" or "How long will it take to correct this disorder?"

Whenever possible, an SLP should try to ascertain the reason(s) for the communication and/or swallowing deficit, especially if the cause persists. The cause is referred to as the **etiology**. There may be **predisposing causes** that underlie the problem, such as genetic factors, **precipitating causes** that triggered the disorder, such as a stroke, and **maintaining** or **perpetuating causes** that continue or add to the problem. Whether the etiology is known or not, an SLP must thoroughly describe the client's communication behavior.

Figure 2.5 Goals of assessment.

A communication disorders specialist is charged with answering the following questions when assessing an individual:
1. Does a communication problem exist?
2. What is the diagnosis?
3. What are the deficit areas? How consistent are they?
4. What are the individual's strengths?
5. How severe is the problem?
6. What are the probable causes of the problem?
7. What recommendations should be made?
8. What is the prognosis (likely outcome) without and with intervention?

Source: Based on Lund, N., & Duchan, J. (1993). Assessing children's language in naturalistic contexts (3rd ed.). Englewood Cliffs, NJ: Prentice Hall.

Recommendations for addressing the client's communicative and/or swallowing deficiencies are often the most-read portions of assessment reports. In making a plan, the first decision is whether intervention is warranted. If it is, then its nature must be described. Treatment recommendations can be thought of as a "working hypothesis" that may need to be altered as intervention proceeds. Assessment continues throughout treatment, in the forms of data collection and probes of behavior.

An SLP obtains background information about a client from a written case history completed by the client, parent, or significant other; an interview; and reports from other professionals.

In communication disorders, an SLP makes a **prognosis** regarding whether the problem will persist if no intervention occurs and what the likely outcome is if a course of therapy or other treatment plan is followed. A prognosis is an informed prediction of the outcome of a disorder, both with and without intervention, and is based, in part, on the nature and severity of the disorder; the client's responsiveness to trial therapy during assessment; and the client's overall communicative, intellectual, and personal strengths and weaknesses. The client's home and school environments are also important factors that can affect the outcome.

> An SLP makes a determination about a client's current functioning and the nature of the problem from multiple sources and clinical intuition.

Assessment Procedures

Assessment may take many forms. Ideally, a clinician should sample a broad variety of communication skills through multiple procedures in several settings. The focus should be on the collection of **authentic data**—that is, actual real-life information—in sufficient quantity to be able to make meaningful and accurate decisions.

Each client has individual needs. An SLP must attempt to determine which needs are paramount at a particular time and then develop a plan to meet these needs.

The need for the use of a variety of procedures should be readily apparent. How often as a student have you said that a test did not accurately measure what you know or what you can do? The same is true for individuals with communication impairments. By using multiple measures and reports, an SLP or audiologist tries to obtain the most accurate description of a child's communication possible. These methods may include:

- A case history filled out by a parent, family member, professional, or the client
- A questionnaire completed by a parent, family member, professional, or the client
- An interview with a parent, family member, and/or the client
- A systematic observation of the client's communication and/or swallowing skills
- Testing with more than one assessment tool and including a hearing screening and an **examination of the peripheral speech mechanism**
- **Dynamic assessment**
- Communication sampling and analysis

> Formal test results during assessment differ from baseline data. During formal testing, a wide range of communicative skills are evaluated. Baseline data reveal an individual's performance level with regard to a few selected potential targets.

Most tests are **norm-referenced**, meaning they yield scores that are used to compare a client with a sample of similar individuals. Norm-referenced instruments should be chosen carefully to fit the characteristics of each individual child. In contrast, a **criterion-referenced** test evaluates a client's strengths and weaknesses with regard to particular skills and does not make comparisons to other children. This more descriptive method is usually reserved for dynamic assessment and sampling.

Dynamic assessment includes probing to explore a client's ability to modify behavior by producing previously misarticulated sounds, learning a language rule, reducing disfluencies, and the like. The goal is to mesh more flexible nonstandardized approaches with more formal, structured methods found in most tests. Dynamic assessment often takes the form of a *test–teach–test* paradigm to examine the "teachability" of a communication feature. The child's potential for learning is assessed by giving small amounts of assistance and determining the difficulty for the child of performing the newly learned behavior.

Most clinicians also use a **speech** and/or **language sampling** technique when assessing the communication of both children and adults. Guidelines for sample collection and analysis are described in Chapter 4. With adult clients, sampling can be accomplished while reviewing the case history with clients or asking them to explain how they spent their day or to tell about their last vacation (Duffy, 2005).

Although patients who have dysphagia may have a variety of complaints, they usually report coughing or choking, or an abnormal sensation when trying to swallow. The evaluation often involves a team of specialists, including an SLP. A case history can be extremely important in identifying the cause(s). General health information should also be reviewed, including illnesses, current medications, and alcohol and tobacco use. A case history can help identify the location of the difficulty. Other evaluations may include a neurological assessment of neuromuscular control, motor and sensory assessment, a guided eating assessment including a variety of liquids and solids, an oral examination, and laboratory tests as needed to screen for infections and inflammatory conditions.

Evidence-Based Practice

Most ASHA assessment guidelines relate to specific disorders and are described in the following chapters. Still, some general guidelines can be deduced from these evidence-based analyses. These are included in Box 2.1.

Intervention with Communication and Swallowing Disorders

Each child brings his or her sense of self to the therapeutic situation. Most of this self-concept has grown out of interactions with family members and individuals in the immediate community. An SLP's failure to recognize and include these dimensions of an individual's social identity can negatively impact intervention (Demmert, McCardle, and Leos, 2006).

Intervention for individuals with communication and swallowing disorders is influenced by the nature and severity of the disorder, the age and status of the client, and environmental considerations, as well as personal and cultural characteristics of both client and clinician. Despite this, some general principles and procedures can be identified.

Providing culturally responsive intervention is extremely important for children from culturally and linguistically diverse (CLD) backgrounds. SLPs can integrate culturally based materials into intervention.

As mentioned in Chapter 1, ASHA has taken a proactive position stressing the need to integrate research and clinical practice (Kamhi, 2006a; Katz, 2003; Ramig, 2002; Wambaugh & Bain, 2002). ASHA's Code of Ethics requires clinicians to "provide services that are based on careful, professional reasoning" (Apel & Self, 2003, p. 6). Evidence-based practices ensure that "clinicians abide by these

BOX 2.1 | **Evidence-Based Practice in Assessment of Individuals with Communication Impairments**

Developmental Level

- Early identification may be especially important for young children with significant communication disorders.
- The form of communication varies with a child's age and developmental status, and should be reflected in the communication features assessed.

Difference vs. Disorder

- Multilingualism and dialectal variations in the home and other care environments affect the way in which language is learned and used, and should be considered in an assessment.
- Bilingual clients should be assessed in both languages in order to provide an accurate picture of speech and language strengths and weaknesses.

Format

- Significant others who interact with the client on an ongoing daily basis should be included in the assessment process.

- Assessment and analysis should be multifaceted and in depth because the dividing line between typical and disordered speech and language is not always clear.
- Assessment materials and strategies should be appropriate to the culture and language of the client and family.
- The setting of the assessment should be appropriate to the developmental stage and/or overall health of the client and be comfortable for both the client and significant others.
- Assessment materials and strategies should reflect the developmental level or condition of the client.

Source: From Clinical Practice Guideline. Published by New York State Department of Health.

ethical codes while best serving their clients" (Apel & Self, 2003, p. 6). ASHA has established the National Center for Treatment Effectiveness in Communicative Disorders and is currently coordinating a National Institutes of Health–funded effort to promote clinical research that will support EBP.

Intervention can take a variety of forms based on the type of disorder, the aspects of communication affected, the age of the client, and the severity of the disorder, to name just a few of the variables. As you watch this video of one of the highly respected professionals in this field, notice the many different disorders addressed and the varying approaches with each.

Objectives of Intervention

Regardless of the specific nature of a problem, intervention in speech-language pathology has as its overriding goal the improvement of the client's communication and swallowing skills:

1. The client should show improvement not just in a clinical setting; progress should generalize to his or her real-world environments, such as home, school, and work.

2. The client should not have to think about what has been learned; in large part, it should be **automatic.**

3. The client must be able to **self-monitor**. Although modifications should be automatic, they will still require monitoring. The client should be able to listen to and observe himself or herself, and make corrections as needed without the therapist's being present.

4. The client should make optimum progress in the minimum amount of time.

5. Intervention should be sensitive to the personal and cultural characteristics of the client.

Target Selection

Even young and relatively low-functioning individuals are more responsive to therapy when they understand the goals.

The assessment report should provide recommendations for long-term goals and short-term objectives for communication intervention. The clinician, however, will have to decide which specific targets should be addressed and in what sequence. The client's personal needs and the potential for intervention to generalize to everyday use are most relevant in making meaningful choices. Likelihood of success and typical behavior of others of the client's age and gender might provide additional insights.

Baseline Data

Before beginning a program of intervention, an SLP obtains **baseline data**; that is, the SLP tries to elicit the target behavior(s) multiple times and under multiple conditions, and records the accuracy of the client's responses. This gives the SLP information about the client's starting point. Baselines are essential in determining a client's progress and the success of a treatment program.

Behavioral Objectives

Once a clinician has obtained baseline data, he or she develops short-term objectives. These are the targets for each treatment session or for several sessions. A behavioral objective is a statement that specifies the target behavior in an observable and measurable way. To do this requires that the clinician identify what the client is expected to do, under what conditions, and with what degree of success. The letters ABCD might help you to remember the format for writing behavioral objectives:

A. *Actor.* Who is expected to do the behavior?

B. *Behavior.* What is the observable and measurable behavior?

C. *Condition.* What is the context or condition of the behavior?

D. *Degree.* What is the targeted degree of success?

For example, *John* [Actor] *will describe pictures* [Behavior] *using both the correct noun and verb* [Condition] *with 90% accuracy* [Degree]. Goals and objectives enable an SLP to observe and measure progress in intervention (Roth, 2011). Poorly written objectives make it difficult to determine efficacy. Specific goals and objectives are required for individualized family service plans (IFSPs) used with infants and toddlers and their families, individualized education plans (IEPs) used in the schools, and for third-party payers, such as insurance companies and government agencies.

Clinical Elements

Successful intervention is multifaceted and includes a variety of elements. This may include, but is not limited to, direct and incidental teaching, counseling, and inclusion of the family and family environment.

Intervention for communication disorders occurs in many settings. Broadening the base for treatment helps to ensure that what is learned in a clinical setting is transferred to a variety of real-world contexts.

Treatment Plan. As with writing goals and objectives, conscious selection of specific intervention techniques also allows for accountability. SLPs select what they believe and what evidence has shown to be the best intervention approach, types of materials, and logical steps to follow to take the client from where he or she is now to the objective selected. Successful intervention builds on what the client can do at present.

Direct Teaching. Part of the role of an SLP is being a teacher. Traditional clinical methods include explaining or reviewing the target and guided practice. **Behavior modification** training approaches have been shown to be successful for a broad variety of communication disorders. Behavior modification is a systematic method of changing behavior. During training, the SLP attempts to elicit the desired response from the client by providing a **stimulus**. The client is expected to *respond*, and the clinician **reinforces** this response if correct or provides corrective feedback if it is not.

Incidental Teaching. Behavior modification follows a highly structured format that an SLP directs. A low-structured or more client-led approach may also be used. In this method, the SLP follows the client's lead but teaches along the way. This is referred to as **incidental teaching**. The SLP manipulates the environment so that communication occurs more naturally. For example, imaginary play with a young child or a cooking or art project with one who is older may serve as situations in which therapy occurs.

Counseling. In addition to direct work with the client on a communication problem, an SLP can provide a supportive environment for the client and other key people in the client's life. A person with a communication disorder may experience a host of feelings including embarrassment, anger, depression, and inadequacy. Family members may have similar emotions regarding the client's communication and may also feel pity or guilt, perhaps blaming themselves for the problem.

Family and Environmental Involvement. An individual might spend 2 hours a week with an SLP and 110 awake hours alone and with other people, often family. Depending on the family circumstances, family members may be asked to help the client with specific activities at home to foster carryover to everyday situations. A spouse may be critical in assisting therapy for an adult who had a stroke or has a voice problem due to recent accident or illness. An SLP must recognize the significant others in the client's life, from infancy through advanced age, and engage them in productive ways. **Support groups** consisting of individuals who have similar difficulties often provide an avenue to practice what has been learned in therapy, to share feelings related to the disability, and to maintain communication skills once formal treatment has been terminated.

 Thought Question 2.4

You probably envisioned SLPs and audiologists working with individual clients or small groups of clients, helping them change communication and swallowing behaviors. Did you imagine yourself being a counselor or working with parents or spouses? When might you wish to do either or both?

Measuring Effectiveness

An SLP determines readiness for dismissal from therapy largely by assessing its effectiveness. Did the client meet the long-term goals and short-term objectives? SLP-designed **post-therapy tests** similar to those used to determine baselines are normally used to answer this question. In addition, it is essential that the client has gained a degree of *automaticity* in the use of the communication target. Errors will occur, however, and the client should be able to *self-monitor* and self-correct when needed. If therapy has been effective, the client has been successful in *generalizing* learned skills to the out-of-clinic world.

Follow-up and Maintenance

After a client has been dismissed from therapy, an SLP must take steps to ensure that the progress that was achieved is not lost. This is done in two ways: Upon dismissal, the client or family should be encouraged to return when anyone feels a need. More reliable is the establishment of a regular follow-up schedule. The client may be contacted by telephone or email every 6 months for a period of 2 years or so after the termination of therapy. If warranted, retesting may be suggested, and **booster treatment** may be provided if needed.

 Check Your Understanding 2.4

Click here to check your understanding of the concepts in this section.

SUMMARY

Communication is an exchange of ideas; it involves message transmission and response. Human communication is remarkable and may take many forms. It is strongly influenced by culture and environment. Not only do people speak different languages, but within language groups, age, gender, socioeconomic status, geographical background, ethnicity, and other factors influence our communication.

The primary vehicle of human communication is language. It may be spoken, written, or signed and has been described in terms of form, content, and use. Form refers to the sound system, or phonology; word structure, or morphology; and syntax, or how the words are arranged in sentences. Content is semantics or meaning, and use is the purpose or pragmatics of the communication. Communication is also transmitted by nonverbal behaviors and characteristics.

A breakdown can occur in any aspect of communication. When communication is unimpaired, we tend to take it for granted; but when it fails, we may feel frustrated and isolated. About 17% of the U.S. population currently experience some limitation of hearing, speech, and/or language. An additional 3% may have dysphagia. See the ASHA website to learn more about various disorders: www.asha.org.

Assessment of communication and swallowing disorders requires an understanding of both in context. Communication behaviors can be viewed as occurring on a continuum from typical to disordered. With each case, an SLP must decide where the demarcation is.

Referrals and screenings are the primary ways in which individuals are selected for assessment. During assessment, an SLP verifies and defines the client's problem, identifies deficits and strengths, probes causality, makes a treatment plan, and provides a prognosis for improvement. This is achieved through multiple techniques, including sampling of communicative and swallowing behaviors in several settings.

Assessment and treatment function in a cyclical fashion, with one influencing the other. In many ways, an SLP is assessing the client each time the client is seen in therapy. Successful intervention often uses a team approach that involves family members as well as professionals. Provisions for follow-up ensure that the gains made in therapy are maintained. In the chapters that follow, techniques for assessment and treatment of specific communication and swallowing disorders are described.

SUGGESTED READINGS/SOURCES

Hirsh-Pasek, K., & Golinkoff, R. (1999). *The origins of grammar: Evidence from early language.* Cambridge, MA: MIT Press.

Levinson, S. C. (2015). Turn-taking in Human Communication – Origins and Implications for Language Processing. *Trends in Cognitive Science*, 20, 6-14. Access at http://www.cell.com/trends/cognitive-sciences/fulltext/S1364-6613(15)00276-4

Ruben, B., & Stewart, L. (2006). *Communication and human behavior* (5th ed.). Boston: Pearson Education.

Tomasello, M. (2010). *Origins of human communication.* Cambridge, MA: MIT Press.

3

Overview of the Anatomy and Physiology of the Speech Production Mechanism

LEARNING OUTCOMES

When you have finished this chapter, you should be able to:

- Describe the structures, muscles, and physiology of the respiratory system

- Describe the structures, muscles, and functions of the laryngeal system

- Describe the structures and functions of the articulatory/resonating system

- Explain the speech production process

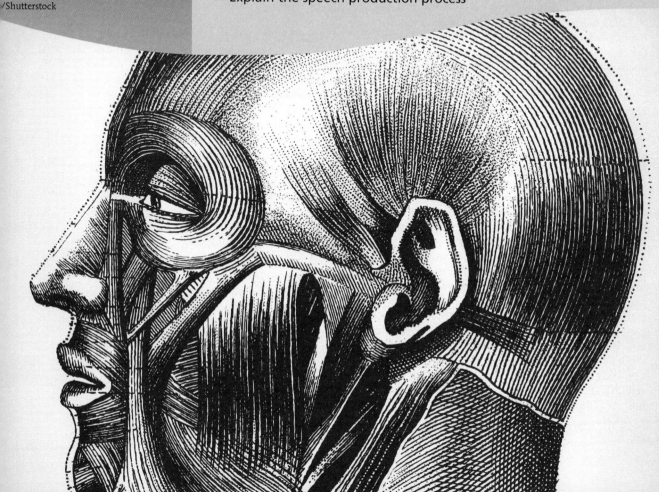

P eople often take for granted speech production as a biological function that takes care of itself; your thoughts and ideas are expressed with little or no apparent effort. But for all its apparent simplicity, the production of speech requires an incredibly complex coordination of biophysical events involving hundreds of muscles and millions of nerves. It is paradoxical that such complex physiological behavior appears to be so effortless. This natural paradox, however, is probably necessary. If we had full conscious comprehension of what we are doing when we speak, we would probably be unable to utter a single word. Monitoring all the nerves and muscles, the tone of the voice, facial expression, and word order would be an impossible intellectual feat.

For many individuals, however, speech production is anything but effortless. Sometimes abnormalities of anatomical structures and physiological systems that support speech interfere with the speech production process. Case Study 3.1 describes an unfortunate incident in which a person's speech and swallowing are

---

CASE STUDY 3.1

Case Study of a Young Man with Severe Damage to the Face and Mouth: Rickey

Rickey is 23 years old, and currently works in construction alongside his dad and uncle building and remodeling homes. He has been helping out with the family business since he was 13 years old. On the side, he volunteers his time for Habitat for Humanity building small, affordable homes for low-income families.

Several long-time construction crew members that Rickey has worked alongside since he was a young teenager are heavy smokers. Rickey started smoking when he was 14, and continues to smoke at least a pack of cigarettes a day, sometimes more. He recently married his high school sweetheart, and they are expecting their first child this summer. Rickey is very aware of the dangers of secondhand smoke, particularly for pregnant women and young children. Rickey has been trying to quit smoking for the past 6 months but to no avail. He heard about electronic cigarettes from a friend and thought that switching to these "e-cigarettes" might help him quit, as well as reduce exposure of secondhand smoke to his pregnant wife.

One morning, after charging the e-cigarette in his car, Rickey arrived at a worksite and "lit up" just before stepping out of his car. As he pushed the "on" button while inhaling, the e-cigarette exploded and caught fire. The construction crew called emergency medical services, and Rickey was taken by ambulance to the hospital. The explosion fractured his maxilla (upper

jaw), lacerated his soft palate, and caused the loss of several teeth. The fire caused first-degree burns to his face, mouth, and neck.

Rickey underwent maxillary surgery followed by immobilization of his jaw; he remained in the hospital for several days for post-surgical monitoring and wound care for his burns. He was evaluated by a speech-language pathologist for speech and swallowing difficulties as a result of his injuries. The speech-language pathologist provided him with a white board and dry-erase markers so he could communicate by writing when speech was too painful or laborious. His diet was modified to accommodate the post-surgical immobilization of his jaw as well as pain associated with the oral-facial burns and lacerated soft palate. After his injuries healed, Rickey underwent dental implant surgery to replace his missing teeth.

As you read this chapter and subsequent chapters in this text, think about:

- How speech is affected when damage occurs to one or more of the physiological subsystems that support speech (respiratory, laryngeal, and articulatory/resonating).
- What specific eating and speaking difficulties Rickey might have had as a result of his injuries.
- How the speech-language pathologist might have evaluated Rickey's speech and swallowing function.

disrupted as a result of damage to structures necessary for these daily life activities. Knowledge of the anatomy and physiology of the speech mechanism is fundamental to understanding many different communication disorders that are evaluated and treated by speech-language pathologists (SLPs). Successful treatment of voice and swallowing disorders, laryngectomy (the surgical removal of the larynx), and cleft palate requires a thorough understanding of the anatomy and physiology of the speech mechanism.

Anatomy is the study of the structures of the body and the relationship of these structures to one another. **Physiology** is a branch of biology that is concerned with the functions of organisms and bodily structures.

Three physiological subsystems are involved in speech production: (1) the **respiratory system** provides the driving force for speech by generating positive air pressure values beneath the vocal folds; (2) the vocal folds, anatomical structures in the **laryngeal system** or *larynx*, vibrate at high rates of speed, setting air molecules in the vocal tract into multiple frequencies of vibration; and, finally, (3) the **articulatory/resonating system** acts as an acoustic filter, allowing certain frequencies to pass into the atmosphere while simultaneously blocking other frequencies.

In this chapter, we discuss the basic structures, muscles, and physiology of the subsystems of speech production and address the changes in each across the lifespan.

THE RESPIRATORY SYSTEM

The primary biological functions of your respiratory system are to supply oxygen to the blood and to remove excess carbon dioxide from the body. This process is automatic, and is controlled by the respiratory centers located within the brainstem of the central nervous system. Although the primary function of respiration is to sustain life, it also serves as the generating source for speech production. Air is inhaled into your lungs to become the potential energy source for sound production. The air is then expelled in a controlled manner, to be modified by your vocal folds and articulators to generate speech sounds.

Structures of the Respiratory System

The primary components of the adult respiratory system include (1) the pulmonary apparatus, which is further subdivided into the lungs, the trachea (windpipe), and the pulmonary airways, and (2) the chest wall (thorax), comprising the rib cage wall, the abdominal wall, the abdominal content, and the diaphragm (Hixon & Hoit, 2005). The structures of the chest wall surround and encase the pulmonary apparatus, and together they form a single functional unit (Hixon et al., 2014).

The **lungs** are a pair of air-filled elastic sacs that change in size and shape and allow us to breathe. The left lung is smaller than the right to allow room for the heart. Air moves to and from the lungs via the **trachea** and the intricate network of branching tubes called bronchi (Figure 3.1).

Muscles of the Respiratory System

The respiratory muscles are divided functionally into muscles of inspiration and muscles of expiration. Inspiratory muscles are generally found above the diaphragm; expiratory muscles are located below the diaphragm. With the exception

Figure 3.1 Anterior view of the trachea and bronchi (a) and anterior view of the bronchi entering the right and left lungs (b).

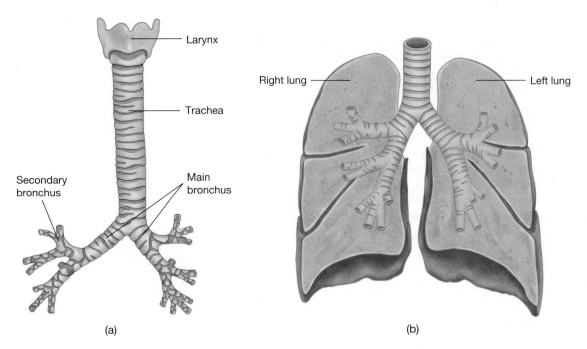

(a)   (b)

of the diaphragm, all respiratory muscles are paired (i.e., located on both the right and left sides of the body).

Muscles of Inspiration

The diaphragm is the principal muscle of inspiration. It is a dome-shaped structure composed of a thin, flat, nonelastic central tendon and a broad rim of muscle fibers that radiate up to the edges of this central tendon. The central tendon is in direct contact with each lung, as shown in Figure 3.2a. The diaphragm separates the thorax (chest) from the abdomen. At rest, it looks like an inverted bowl (Hixon & Hoit, 2005). Figure 3.2b shows the relative position of the diaphragm at rest. When the diaphragm contracts during inspiration, it pulls downward and forward, thus enlarging the thorax.

In addition to the diaphragm, numerous thoracic and neck muscles contribute to inspiration. These muscles are illustrated in Figure 3.3.

Muscles of Expiration

Expiration allows carbon dioxide to be expelled from the body via the lungs and for speech to be produced. The most important muscles of expiration are located in the front and on the sides of the abdomen. During expiration, these muscles, depicted in Figure 3.4, assist the diaphragm's movement back to its relaxed dome-shaped configuration.

Numerous other muscles located on the front and back of the thorax may also contribute to respiration. The use of other muscles during inspiration and expiration may be related to body position, certain pathological states, and environmental conditions.

Figure 3.2 Anterior view of the relationship of the diaphragm to the lungs (a) and anterior view of the diaphragm at rest (b).

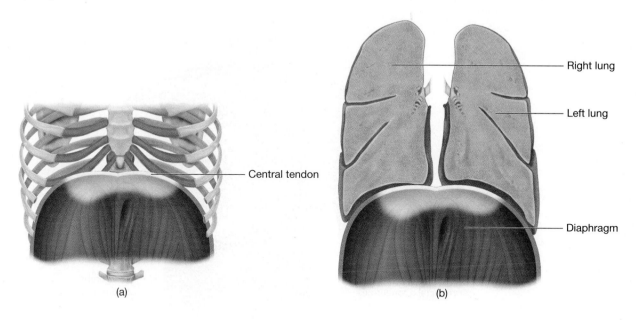

(a)

(b)

Central tendon

Right lung

Left lung

Diaphragm

Figure 3.3 Anterior view of thoracic muscles.

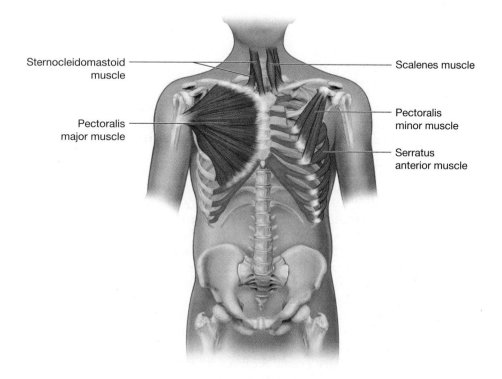

Sternocleidomastoid muscle

Scalenes muscle

Pectoralis major muscle

Pectoralis minor muscle

Serratus anterior muscle

Figure 3.4 Anterior view of abdominal musculature. Muscles are cut to illustrate the different layers of muscle.

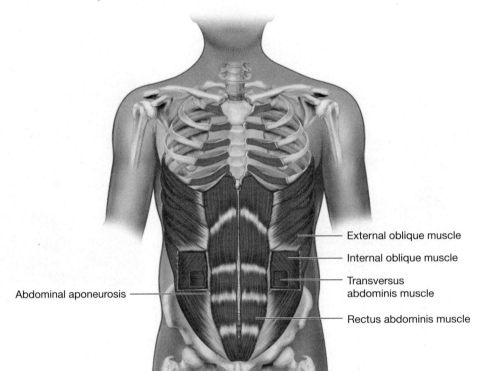

External oblique muscle

Internal oblique muscle

Transversus abdominis muscle

Rectus abdominis muscle

Abdominal aponeurosis

The Physiology of Tidal Breathing and Speech Breathing

Quiet breathing, or **resting tidal breathing**, is breathing to sustain life. As you are reading this chapter, you are using tidal breathing. The rate and depth of breaths taken during tidal breathing are determined by your body's oxygen needs and the amount of carbon dioxide in the blood. Resting tidal breathing involves contraction of the diaphragm, moving it downward and slightly forward, which in turn expands the rib cage wall and moves the abdominal wall outward (Hixon & Hoit, 2005). Expansion of the rib cage wall also causes expansion of the lungs. This results in an increase in lung volume and a decrease in **alveolar pressure** (i.e., pressure within the lungs) below that of atmospheric pressure. Air then rushes into the lungs, equalizing alveolar pressure with atmospheric pressure. Approximately 0.5 L of air is inhaled during quiet breathing.

When the resting tidal inspiratory cycle ends, expiration (or exhalation) begins. Expiration results from the decrease in the size of the rib cage wall, and thus compression of the lungs, which in turn increases the pressure within the lungs (Hixon & Hoit, 2005). Air then rushes out of the lungs until equilibrium with atmospheric pressure is reached. Expiration during quiet breathing is a relatively passive event, achieved by gravity and the natural tendency (i.e., passive recoil) of the pulmonary-chest wall unit to return to its relaxed state. However, in the upright body position, the abdominal wall muscles remain active throughout the resting tidal breathing cycle (Hixon et al., 2014). A respiratory cycle is defined as one inhalation followed by one exhalation. During resting tidal breathing, the duration of inspiration and expiration are relatively equal.

Breathing for purposes of speech production differs from resting tidal breathing in a number of ways. First, contraction of the diaphragm produces rapid, forceful inspirations. Furthermore, the time spent inhaling is short relative to the time spent exhaling, which is much longer. You may inhale as much as 2 L of air during speech breathing, depending on the specific demands of the utterance. Unlike expiration during quiet breathing, active muscle contraction of both inspiratory and expiratory muscles is needed during speech to prevent all the air from rushing out of the lungs too quickly.

Speech breathing differs from quiet breathing in many ways, but the oxygen and carbon dioxide ratio in the blood is the same for both types of breathing.

 Thought Question 3.1

How might breathing patterns differ while singing?

Lifespan Issues of the Respiratory System

At birth, you had a rest breathing rate between 30 and 80 breaths per minute. By age 3, your tidal breathing rate had decreased to values between 20 and 30 breaths per minute. This change in rate is due to the fact that newborns have very few alveoli, the areas where gas exchange occur in the lungs. Alveoli increase in number with age, such that by adulthood there are several hundred thousand (Kent, 1997; Zemlin, 1998). Watch preschool children and make note of their more frequent and deeper inhalations relative to adults. By age 7 the number of alveoli approaches adult values, and by 10 years of age the respiratory system functions in a more adultlike fashion. Tidal breathing rates are between 17 and 22 breaths per minute, and lung and abdominal wall volumes and lung pressures during speech production more closely approximate those used by adults (Hoit & Weismer, 2018).

As children grow, the structures of the respiratory system increase in size, and in turn lung capacity increases. Maximum lung capacities are reached in early adulthood and remain fairly constant until middle age. Respiratory function for speech breathing purposes becomes less efficient beginning in the seventh or eighth decade of life.

Respiratory function is also affected by exercise, health, and smoking. It is estimated that smoking in older people could result in a 500 mL (approximately 1 pint) cumulative loss in pulmonary function every 10 years (Kent, 1997).

 Check Your Understanding 3.1

Click here to check your understanding of the concepts in this section.

THE LARYNGEAL SYSTEM

The primary biological function of the larynx is to prevent foreign objects from entering the trachea and lungs. In addition, the larynx can impound air for forceful expulsion of foreign objects that threaten the lower airways.

Structures of the Laryngeal System

The primary structure of the laryngeal system is the **larynx**, which is an air valve composed of cartilages, muscles, and other tissue. It is the principal sound generator for speech production and is colloquially known as the "voice box." The larynx sits on top of the trachea and opens up into the pharynx (throat). The larynx appears to be suspended from the **hyoid bone**, a horseshoe-shaped structure that serves as the point of attachment for both laryngeal and tongue musculature.

The larynx consists of the thyroid, arytenoid, and cricoid cartilages connected to one another by ligaments and membranes (Figure 3.5). The **thyroid cartilage** is the largest laryngeal cartilage. It forms most of the front and sides of the laryngeal skeleton and protects the inner components of the larynx. The upper part has a V-shaped depression called the thyroid notch. It can be felt by palpating the front of the neck. Just below this notch is a jutting protrusion called the **thyroid prominence**, or Adam's apple (Hixon et al., 2014), which can be very prominent in some adult males.

The larynx houses the vocal folds, which are attached at the front near the midline of the thyroid cartilage and at the back to the arytenoid cartilages via the vocal ligament. When viewed from above, the paired vocal folds appear to be ivory-colored bands of tissue. They abduct (move apart) during respiration and adduct (move together) during voice production, or phonation. The space between the vocal folds is called the **glottis**.

Figure 3.5 Anterior view of the skeletal framework of the larynx.

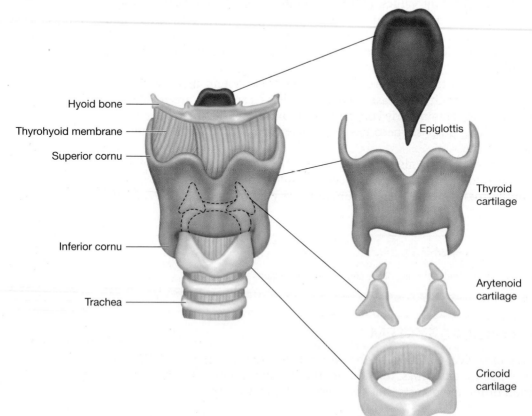

Muscles of the Larynx

The *thyroarytenoid* muscle forms the bulk of each vocal fold. This muscle extends from the angle of the thyroid cartilage to the arytenoid cartilage; contraction of the thyroarytenoid reduces the distance between the thyroid and arytenoid cartilages, causing a shortening and thickening of the vocal folds. The *cricothyroid* muscle directly opposes the action of the thryoarytenoid muscle, stiffening and lengthening the vocal folds; these muscles are therefore called agonist-antagonist muscle pairs (Titze, 1994). The action of the cricothyroid muscle serves to increase vocal pitch, the perceptual correlate of *fundamental frequency* discussed later in this chapter.

Vocal fold **adduction** (moving together) is accomplished by contraction of the *lateral cricoarytenoid* and *arytenoid* (transverse and oblique) muscles. The lateral cricoarytenoid brings the front portion of the vocal folds together, while the arytenoids bring the back portion of the vocal folds together (Hoit & Weismer, 2018). The *posterior cricoarytenoid* muscle is the primary muscle of vocal fold **abduction** (moving apart). Its action directly opposes the action of the lateral cricoarytenoid; therefore, these muscles are also agonist-antagonist pairs (Titze, 1994). Figure 3.6 depicts the laryngeal muscles important for adducting and abducting the vocal folds, and altering vocal fold length, tension, and thickness.

Lifespan Issues of the Laryngeal System

The laryngeal system also goes through significant changes as a function of age. In a newborn, the larynx is small and positioned very high in the neck. The high position of the larynx near the hyoid bone allows the newborn to breathe and nurse simultaneously, while protection of the airway is maintained. The larynx begins to move downward in the neck during the first year of life. It reaches its final position between 10 and 20 years of age (Hixon et al., 2014).

The laryngeal cartilages increase in size and become less pliable with age. The hyoid bone ossifies (turns to bone) by 2 years of age. The vocal folds are approximately 4 to 6 mm long in a newborn. By age 6, they increase to about 8 or 9 mm in length. The increase in length of the vocal folds is equal in boys and girls until puberty. During puberty, the vocal folds increase to approximately 12 to 17 mm in

Figure 3.6 Laryngeal muscles responsible for phonation, and changing vocal fold length, tension, and thickness.

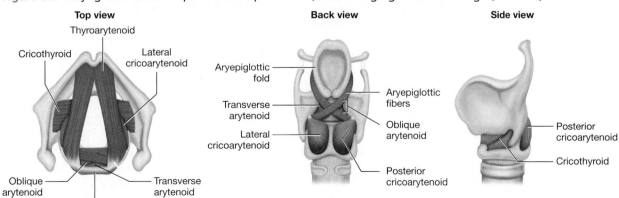

girls and 15 to 25 mm in boys. By adulthood, females' vocal folds are about 21 mm in length; males' are about 29 mm in length (Kent, 1997). The sex difference in adult vocal fold length accounts for the fact that men normally have lower-pitched voices than women.

With advancing age, laryngeal cartilages begin to ossify, although the female larynx, unlike that of males, never completely ossifies. The vocal folds begin to lose muscle tissue (atrophy) while the more superficial layers of vocal fold tissue thicken and lose their elasticity. As a result, the vocal folds become stiffer and less flexible with age. Age effects are realized in men as an increase in pitch, likely due to muscle atrophy and loss of mass of the folds. Women, in contrast, experience a decrease in pitch with age, likely due to hormone-related changes associated with menopause (Stoicheff, 1981).

 Check Your Understanding 3.2
Click here to check your understanding of the concepts in this section.

THE ARTICULATORY/RESONATING SYSTEM

The articulatory/resonating system extends from the opening of the mouth to the vocal folds and comprises the oral cavity, the nasal cavity, and the pharyngeal cavity, as shown in Figure 3.7. Together these three cavities form the vocal tract, which is a resonant acoustic tube that shapes the sound energy produced by the respiratory and laryngeal systems into all of the English speech sounds (Kent, 1997). Structures important for speech production such as the teeth, tongue, and velum (soft palate) are housed within these three cavities.

Structures of the Articulatory/Resonating System

The articulatory/resonating system consists largely of the 22 bones that make up the facial skeleton and cranium (braincase). Some of these bones are shown in Figure 3.8. With the exception of the *mandible* (lower jaw), the bones of the face and cranium are fused tightly together by sutures. The mandible articulates with the temporal bone by means of a complex joint known as the *temporomandibular joint (TMJ)*. This joint allows the mandible to move up and down and side to side, which is necessary for chewing.

Teeth

Adults have a total of 32 teeth that are held within the *alveolar processes* (thick spongy projections) of the mandible and *maxilla* (upper jaw) inside the oral cavity. The obvious biological function of teeth is chewing food, but the teeth are also important for production of some English speech sounds.

Horizontal bones of the maxilla form the bony hard palate, which comprises the front two thirds of the roof of the mouth. Figure 3.9 shows the structures of the bony hard palate and the relationship of the maxillary teeth.

Figure 3.7 Schematic of the human vocal tract.

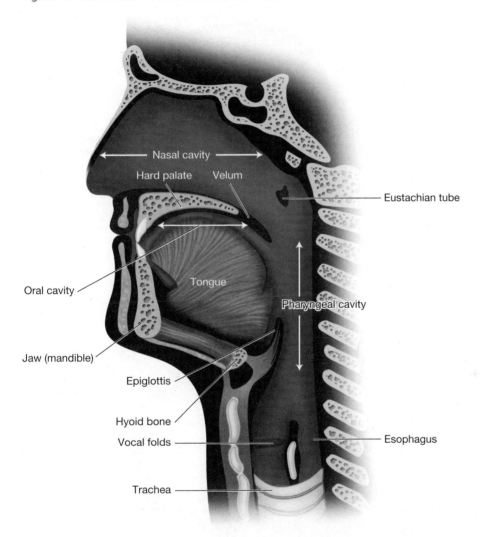

Tongue

The principal structure within the oral cavity important for speech production is the tongue. The tongue is a muscular hydrostat, meaning it has no bone or cartilage, much like an elephant's trunk. It provides its own structural support through contraction of its muscles, but also has a "soft skeleton" of connective tissue that surrounds and separates its different components (Hixon et al., 2014; Kent, 1997).

Velum

The velum, or soft palate, located in the pharynx, is an important structure for both speech and swallowing. You can see a portion of your velum by looking into a well-illuminated bathroom mirror. You will see a structure projecting downward called the **uvula**; the uvula is the termination of your velum.

Figure 3.8 Anterior (a) and lateral (b) views of skull bones.

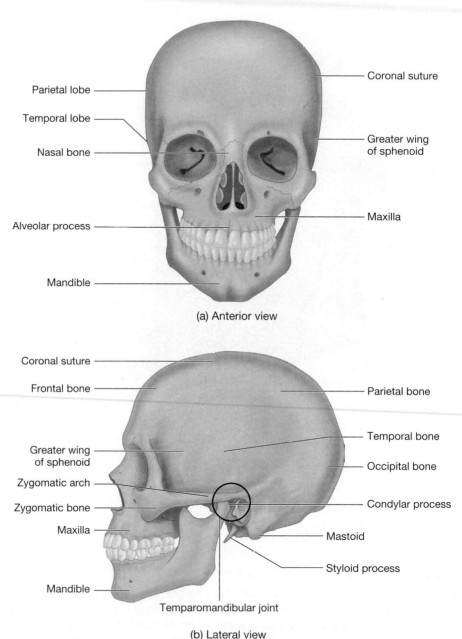

(a) Anterior view

(b) Lateral view

When you breathe through your nose, the velum hangs like a curtain from the posterior aspect of the bony hard palate. During swallowing and speech production, the velum elevates and decouples (separates) the nasal cavity from the pharyngeal cavity, leading to **velopharyngeal closure**, or contact of the velum with the posterior and lateral pharyngeal walls (Kuehn & Henne, 2003). Failure

Figure 3.9 Inferior view of an adult bony hard palate and teeth.

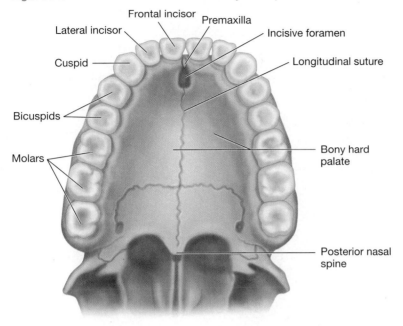

to separate these cavities during swallowing would result in food passing through the nasal cavity.

During speech production, velar elevation is necessary to prevent air from escaping through the nose and to allow sufficient air pressure to build up in the oral cavity for production of pressure sounds (e.g., /p/, /b/). Any air that escapes through the nose during speech can result in a nasal-sounding resonance (quality). Figure 3.10 is a front view of the soft palate and uvula.

Lifespan Issues of the Articulatory/Resonating System

The bones of the skull grow rapidly during the first years of life, and reach adult size by about 8 years of age. At birth, the newborn has 45 separate skull bones that ultimately fuse into 22 bones by adulthood. Once they fuse together, the cranium appears to be one solid bone.

The bones of the lower portion of the face grow at a much slower rate than bones of the skull. These lower facial bones do not reach maximum adult size until about 18 years of age. Because of these different growth patterns of the skull bones and the facial bones, the face is able to grow downward and forward relative to the cranium (Kent, 1997).

Dentition in the infant begins to emerge at about 6 months of age. This first set of teeth is temporary and is usually referred to as primary, or deciduous, dentition. Emergence of the primary dentition is usually complete by 3 years of age. At approximately 5 years of age the primary teeth begin to fall out, and the permanent, or secondary, teeth begin to appear. The emergence of the secondary teeth is usually complete by 18 years of age.

Figure 3.10 Front view of the soft palate and uvula.

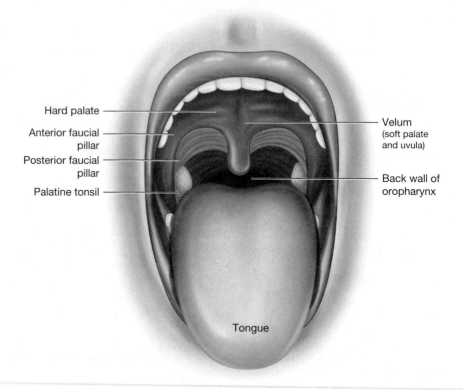

Hard palate

Anterior faucial pillar

Posterior faucial pillar

Palatine tonsil

Velum (soft palate and uvula)

Back wall of oropharynx

Tongue

The tongue of the newborn occupies most of the oral cavity (Kent, 1997). During the first several years of life, the posterior portion of the tongue descends into the pharyngeal cavity. The tongue reaches its mature size at about 16 years of age. In general, the growth of the tongue is similar to the growth of the mandible (lower jaw) and to the lips (Kent, 1997).

At birth, the velum is in close proximity to the epiglottis (i.e., the large, leaf-shaped cartilage attached at its lower end to the thyroid cartilage of the larynx, just below the thyroid notch), causing the infant to have to breathe through his nose. As a result, the velopharynx is open during cry and noncry vocalizations, causing the infant to sound nasalized; that is, sound energy is directed through the nasal cavity rather than through the oral cavity (Hixon et al., 2014; Kent, 1981). By 2 months of age, infants are able to close the velopharynx for syllable productions, but this closure is not consistent. At some point between 6 months and 3 years of age, children consistently achieve airtight velopharyngeal closure for production of oral speech sounds. Adult patterns of velopharyngeal closure are achieved by age 3, and are subsequently maintained throughout the lifespan (Hixon et al., 2014). Aging has been shown to have minimal impact on velopharyngeal function as it relates to speech production (Hoit et al., 1994; Zajac, 1997).

Finally, as one ages the length and volume of the oral cavity increases. This anatomical change influences the overall resonant characteristics of the vocal tract in males and females by lowering the frequencies at which the vocal tract naturally resonates (Xue & Hao, 2003).

> ✅ Check Your Understanding 3.3
>
> Click here to check your understanding of the concepts in this section.

THE SPEECH PRODUCTION PROCESS

The production of speech begins with the sound produced by vocal fold vibration, or **phonation**. Phonation is initiated by approximating or adducting the vocal folds and closing the glottis or opening. Once the vocal folds are closed, air pressure generated by the respiratory system, called *alveolar pressure*, increases beneath the vocal folds.

The air pressure from below displaces the lower edges of each vocal fold laterally (apart). This is followed by lateral displacement of the upper edges of each vocal fold until the vocal folds are fully separated, opening the airway (frames 1, 2, 3, and 4 of Figure 3.11). Following maximum opening of the folds, the vocal folds' natural elastic restoring forces cause the lower edges of the folds to begin to move inward toward the midline, followed by the upper edges, until the vocal folds collide with each other, closing off the airway (frames 5, 6, and 7 of Figure 3.11). The entire process is repeated in a cyclical fashion at the average **fundamental frequency** of vibration, or the number of cycles (i.e., opening and closing of the vocal folds) per second (Story, 2002).

Earlier theories of vocal fold vibration (i.e., Van den Berg's 1958 "Myoelastic aerodynamic theory of voice production") described the importance of the "Bernoulli effect" as the primary mechanism responsible for sustained vocal fold vibration. The "Bernoulli effect," based on Bernoulli's principle, states that high air velocity through a narrow opening (the glottis) creates a negative pressure that sucks the vocal folds together; afterwards, air pressure builds up below the closed vocal folds and then blows the vocal folds apart; the process then repeats itself. We know now that the "Bernoulli effect" plays a very minor role in vocal fold vibration (c.f., Story, 2002; Van den Berg, 1958).

For each vibratory cycle the air in the vocal tract is set into vibration, and sound is produced. The sound that results from vocal fold vibration is complex, consisting of a fundamental frequency, or the lowest-frequency component that corresponds to the rate of vocal fold vibration and approximately 40 additional higher frequencies called **harmonics**. The harmonic frequencies are whole-number multiples of the fundamental frequency. For example, when the fundamental frequency is 100 Hz, the second harmonic is 200 Hz, the third is 300 Hz, and so on. Figure 3.12 is a stylized spectrum of the complex sound produced by vocal fold

Figure 3.11 Anterior view of the vocal folds during one cycle of vibration. Air from the lungs creates pressure beneath the vocal folds (1, 2, and 3). This pressure causes the vocal folds to separate (4). The natural elastic restoring forces of the vocal folds and the time delay with respect to the upper and lower portions of the vocal folds causes the vocal folds to begin to close (5 and 6). The vocal folds close the glottis to end the cycle, and the next cycle begins (7).

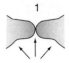
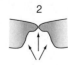
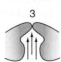

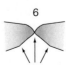
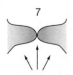

Figure 3.12 A spectrum illustrating a fundamental frequency of 200 Hz and related harmonics (a) and a spectrum of a fundamental frequency of 100 Hz and related harmonics (b).

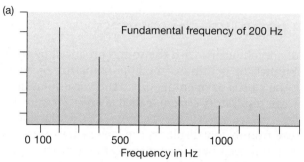

(a)

Fundamental frequency of 200 Hz

0 100   500   1000

Frequency in Hz

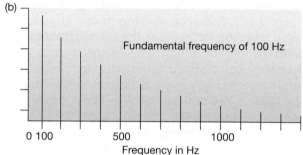

(b)

Fundamental frequency of 100 Hz

0 100   500   1000

Frequency in Hz

Air-filled cavities are acoustic resonators. The frequency or frequencies at which a filled cavity will resonate are determined by the volume of the cavity, the area of the opening of the cavity, and the length of the opening of the cavity.

 Thought Question 3.2

You are drinking water from a bottle. After you have taken a few sips, you blow air across the opening on the top of the bottle, and a sound is produced. After taking a few more sips, you again blow across the opening. Was the sound different the second time you blew across the top of the bottle? The bottle is a resonator. What characteristics of the resonator changed, and how did those changes influence the sound that was produced?

vibration. A spectrum represents the frequencies of a complex sound along the horizontal (x) axis, and their relative intensity is represented on the vertical (y) axis. Note that the relative intensity decreases systematically with increases in harmonic frequency. Download PRAAT for free at www.praat.org to perform your own spectral analysis.

The vocal tract is an acoustic resonator that will modify the quality of the sound produced by the larynx. In any acoustic resonator some frequencies are reduced or attenuated and other frequencies are enhanced, depending on certain physical aspects of the resonator.

Movement of the tongue, lips, and larynx will change the shape of the vocal tract, and in turn modify the sound emanating from the larynx. Produce the vowels /i/ (as in the word "bee") and /u/ (as in the word "boot"). Try to sense how your tongue and lips change position for the production of these two vowels. Changes in the position of your lips and tongue in turn change certain physical characteristics of the vocal tract that directly affect the quality of the sound that emanates from your mouth.

Figure 3.13 represents how changes of vocal tract shape influence which frequencies are enhanced and which are attenuated. A complex sound is produced by vocal fold vibration (a), and the vocal tract acts as a filter attenuating some frequencies and enhancing others (b). The sound that emanates from the mouth during vowel production (c) is related directly to the general shape of the vocal tract determined largely by tongue position. Note that for the /u/ vowel low frequencies are enhanced, whereas high frequencies are somewhat attenuated. For the /i/ vowel low frequencies are somewhat attenuated, whereas high frequencies are enhanced.

Figure 3.13 Spectra of glottal sound source (a) that sets the air in the vocal tract (b) into vibration. The vocal tract filters the glottal sound source differently for the vowels /i/ and /u/, as seen in the radiated spectra (c).

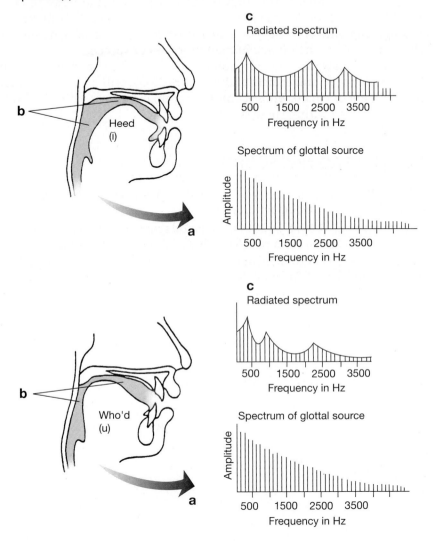

During consonant production, your tongue is sometimes used to momentarily occlude your vocal tract for the production of stop sounds such as /t/, /d/, /k/, and /g/. Production of sounds such as /s/ and /sh/ require your tongue to form a constriction in the vocal tract that will produce frication noise when air is passed through the constriction.

 Check Your Understanding 3.4

Click here to check your understanding of the concepts in this section.

SUMMARY

This chapter provides a general overview of the anatomy and physiology of the speech and voice mechanism. The study of the structures that are used to produce speech and their function is extensive and complex. It is important to remember that although anatomy is static, these structures are capable of dynamic movement that can result in the unique human processes of speech.

The study of anatomy and physiology is essential for a speech-language pathologist. Knowledge and understanding of this topic will assist in the evaluation and treatment of clients whose communication disorder is a direct or indirect result of a breakdown within these systems.

SUGGESTED READINGS/SOURCES

Hixon, T. (2006). *Respiratory function in singing: A primer for singers and singing teachers.* Tucson, AZ: Redington Brown.

Hixon, T., Weismer, G., & Hoit, J. (2014). *Preclinical speech science: Anatomy, physiology, acoustics, and perception* (2nd ed.). San Diego, CA: Plural Publishing.

Hoit, J., & Weismer, G. (2018). *Foundations of speech and hearing: Anatomy and physiology.* San Diego, CA: Plural Publishing.

4

Childhood Language Impairments

LEARNING OUTCOMES

When you have finished this chapter, you should be able to:

- Describe language development through the lifespan
- Characterize language impairment and associated disorders
- Explain the process of assessment in language impairment
- Describe the overall design of language intervention

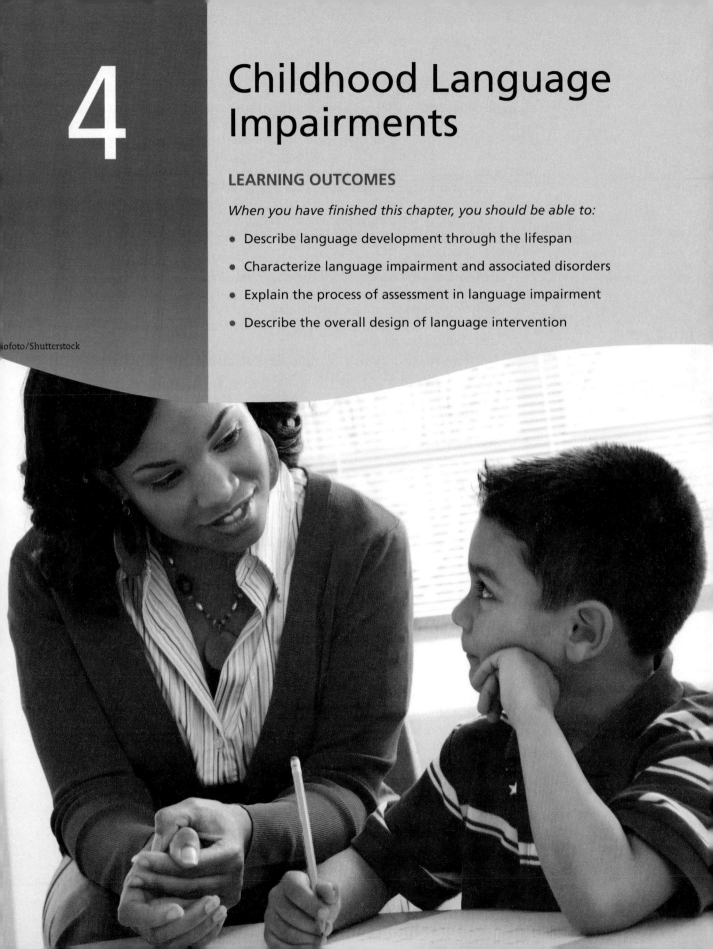

L anguage impairments are a complex group of diverse disorders and delays with a wide range of characteristics, levels of severity, and causes. Some children may exhibit disorders in which language is inappropriate, inefficient, or ineffectual; others use language that is seemingly immature. A word of advice before we begin: It might be helpful to review the parts of language, such as syntax and semantics, mentioned in Chapter 2.

The term **language impairment (LI)** applies to a heterogeneous group of developmental and/or acquired disorders that principally affect the use of spoken or written language for comprehension and/or production and may involve the form, content, and/or function of language. Consider the following about this definition of LI:

- Individuals with LIs are very different from each other. The impairment may occur at any time within the lifespan, and individuals vary in terms of symptoms, manifestations, effects, and severity over time. The communication context, content of the communication, and learning task are also contributing factors to LIs.

- The impairment may be a result of developmental abnormalities and/or may be acquired as a result of accident, injury, or other environmental factors.

- Deficits and/or immaturities may exist in one or more means of communication. For example, preschoolers with LI are often less able to recognize and copy letters. They are also less likely to write and draw, to pretend to read, and to ask questions during parental reading (Marvin & Wright, 1997). In short, young children with language impairments are at risk for literacy difficulties when they later attend school (Nathan et al., 2004).

- One or more aspects of language—form, content, and use—may be affected. For example, as a group, children with LIs use shorter, less elaborate sentences than typical children their age (Greenhalgh & Strong, 2001).

Case Study 4.1 presents the story of one child with LI.

Box 4.1 presents an example of the somewhat scrambled language that we might find exhibited by some children with LI. It is unclear whether most children with LIs exhibit impairments in other areas of development as well, but language deficits persist at least through the primary school years for many children (Tomblin et al., 2003). In the classroom and even on the playground, children with LI, especially boys and those with severe receptive language deficits, may be reticent to speak and may lack social maturity and exhibit behavioral problems (Hart et al., 2004; Huaquing Qi & Kaiser, 2004).

Noticeably absent from our definition of LI are language differences, such as those found in some dialectal speakers and in English language learners (ELLs). Differences do not in themselves constitute a disorder and do not require clinical intervention by a speech-language pathologist (SLP), although elective intervention is possible at the client's request.

You can find easy-to-read guides to LI and other communication disorders at the American Speech-Language-Hearing Association website (www.asha.org). Scroll to the bottom of the page and click on "Public" and then click on "Speech and Language Disorders and Diseases."

To guide you through this complicated topic, this chapter briefly looks at typical language development followed by a discussion of the major disorders

CASE STUDY 4.1

Case Study of a Child with Language Impairment: Kassandra

Kassandra, an active 5-year-old, is an engaging child and an enthusiastic kindergartner. Born 1 month preterm and weighing only slightly over 4 pounds, she was kept in the hospital for postnatal care and observation for several weeks. The team of specialists who worked with Kassandra in the hospital recommended to her parents that she receive early intervention services, first in the home and later at a local clinic. The team was concerned because Kassandra was at risk of having later developmental problems.

By 18 months, Kassandra was not talking, and the team recommended to her parents that she attend a special language-intensive preschool where she would receive both individual and group intervention services. Working together, the speech-language pathologist, developmental specialist, and classroom teacher conducted a thorough evaluation of Kassandra's early communication behaviors, motor skills, and cognitive abilities. Although Kassandra's speech and language were delayed, she appeared to have motor and cognitive abilities that were close to those of typical children.

The speech-language pathologist worked closely with both the classroom teacher and Kassandra's parents to ensure that there was consistency across different communication environments in the way others interacted with the girl and in the communication requirements. Kassandra's program was individualized to include words and phrases for entities in her environment. Once she began to use single words, Kassandra quickly learned to combine them into longer and longer phrases. When she entered kindergarten, she demonstrated language abilities in the low normal range.

As you read the chapter, think about:

- Possible explanations for Kassandra's delay
- Possible evaluative procedures that could be used to measure Kassandra's language
- Possible targets that the intervention team might choose to help Kassandra develop and use language

BOX 4.1 | Example of a Conversation with a Language-Impaired Child

Teacher: Does your family have a pet?

Child: Yeah.

Teacher: Tell me about this pet.

Child: Got a pet.

Teacher: Um-hm, tell me about the pet.

Child: Got a pet.

Teacher: Yes, and I really want to hear about him.

Child: Got with my . . . ah, go with my . . . Dad go with . . .

Teacher: Your dad walks the pet.

Child: No, me.

Teacher: Oh, you and your dad walk the pet.

Child: No, me.

Teacher: Oh, just you walk the dog.

Child: No, me.

Teacher: I'm confused.

Child: Me dog.

Teacher: Oh, it's your dog. Who walks your dog?

Child: With one of them things, you know.

Teacher: What things? Who walks your dog?

Child: With them things like this.

Teacher: Yes, you use a leash.

Theoretically, all speakers of a language should be able to communicate. Some differences may be so great as to impair communication but not qualify as a disorder.

associated with LI. Of necessity, this discussion is an overview, with details left for further study.

LANGUAGE DEVELOPMENT THROUGH THE LIFESPAN

As you already know, language is complex; thus, any attempt to describe its development is also very complicated. In the following sections, we cover only the highlights of child and adolescent development and relate these to some of the disorders to be discussed later in the chapter. An outline of language development is presented in Table 4.1.

Pre-Language

Children become communicators because they are treated as if they are communicators.

Much of your first year of life is spent learning to communicate. Parents talk to a newborn as if he or she understands what the adults are saying. Later on, as children begin to comprehend language in limited ways, parents and caregivers modify their style of talking to maximize comprehension and participation by the child.

Shortly after birth, you became actively involved in a reciprocal process with your family. Sensitive mothers vary their rate of speech based on their infants' rate of responding (Hane et al., 2003). To maintain attention, a parent exaggerates her or his facial expressions and voice and vocalizes more often. In turn, an infant responds with eye contact or sound-making or vocalizing.

As an infant you were a full partner in this interaction, and your behavior was influenced by the communication behavior of your caregivers. Gradually, infant babbling becomes more speechlike and mature, containing syllables rather than individual sounds.

During the first 3 months, caregivers' responses teach children the "signal" value of specific behaviors, and infants learn a stimulus–response sequence. If they

TABLE 4.1

Language development through the lifespan

Age	Accomplishments
3 months	Responds vocally to partner.
8 months	Begins gesturing.
12 months	First word spoken. Words fill intentions previously signaled by gestures.
18 months	Begins combining words on the basis of word-order rules.
2 years	Begins adding bound morphemes. Average length or mean length of utterance (MLU) is 1.6–2.2 morphemes.
3 years	More adultlike sentence structure. MLU is 3.0–3.3 morphemes.
4 years	Begins to change style of talking to fit conversational partner. MLU is 3.6–4.7 morphemes.
5 years	Ninety percent of language form learned.
6 years	Begins to learn visual mode of communication with writing and reading.
Adolescence	Able to participate competently in conversations and telling of narratives. Knows multiple meanings of words and figurative language. Uses a gender style, or genderlect, when talking.

Source: Based on information found in Owens (2016).

signal—by crying, for example—caregivers respond. In addition, they learn that a relatively constant stimulus or signal, such as a bottle, results in a predictable response, such as feeding. The bottle "signals" feeding.

By 3 to 4 months, rituals and game playing have emerged. Rituals, such as feeding and diaper changing, provide children with predictable patterns. As they learn that interactions can unfold in predictable ways, they begin to form expectations of events and to participate more. In addition, games such as "peekaboo" and "I'm gonna get you" have many of the aspects of communication. There is an exchange of turns, rules for each turn, and particular slots for words and actions.

At about 8 to 9 months, you developed **intentionality** in your interactions, primarily through gestures. For the first time, your behavior was meant to influence the other person. The intention to communicate is signaled in gestures accompanied by eye contact with a partner, the use of consistent sound and intonational patterns for specific intentions, and persistent attempts to communicate. These intentional vocalizations or sounds are different from the "private speech" infants use in solitary activities like play (Papaliou & Trevarthen, 2006).

As an infant, you probably used your first meaningful word to express an intention at around 12 months. Real words are used with or without gestures to accomplish the communication purposes, such as requesting, that were previously filled by gestures.

To develop spoken language, children must be able to store sounds, use this information for later comparison and identification, and relate these sounds to meaning. During the first year, an infant learns the sound patterns of the native language. Better speech perception at 6 months of age is related to better word understanding, word production, and phrase understanding later (Tsao et al., 2004). An infant's perceptual ability is usually restricted to his or her native language's speech sounds and syllables by 8 to 10 months of age.

The task of learning language and learning to represent and to symbolize is strongly related to cognitive abilities. **Representation** is the process of having one thing stand for another. For example, in play a hand towel might be used as a blanket for a doll. **Symbolization** is using an arbitrary symbol, such as a word or sign, to stand for something.

> Games and rituals share many characteristics with conversations.

> Early intentions, such as attracting attention, are established in gestures, and first words fill these same functions, often with the accompanying gesture.

Toddler Language

By 18 months you, like many other children, probably could produce approximately 50 single words and were beginning to combine words in predictable ways. Within a few short months, three- and four-word combinations appeared. Accompanying the increases in utterance length and vocabulary is a decrease in the use of babbling, or sound making.

Use

People who are unfamiliar with young children's language often think that children either imitate all first words or use them only to name. In fact, single words are used to make requests, comments, inquiries, and more.

As mentioned, words are acquired first within the intentions that the child is able to express in previously acquired gestures. Several early intentions are presented in Table 4.2. Note all the uses or intentions expressed in the conversation presented in Box 4.2.

TABLE 4.2

Examples of early intentions of children

Intention	Example
Wanting demand	Says the name of the desired item with an insistent voice. Often accompanied by a reaching gesture.
Protesting	Says "No" or the name of the item while pushing it away, turning away, and/or making a frowning face.
Content questioning	Asks "What?" or "That?" or "Wassat?" while pointing and/or looking at an item.
Verbal accompaniment	Speech accompanies some action, such as "whee-e-e" when swung or "Uh-oh" when something spills.
Greeting/farewell	Waves hi or bye with accompanying words.

Note: A fuller list can be found in Owens (2014).

BOX 4.2 | **Example of Toddler Language**

Stacy and her mother are talking while they are coloring. Note that the language concerns the task. Stacy's mom keeps her utterances short and cues Stacy to respond by asking questions. Stacy participates by talking about the task, often incorporating part of the previous utterance into her own:

Mom: What are you making?

Stacy: Doggie.

Mom: Are you making a doggie? Oh, that's nice, Stacy.

Stacy: Where more doggie?

Mom: Is there another doggie underneath?

Stacy: Yeah.

Mom: Where? Can you find the picture? Is that what you're looking for, the picture of the doggie? Where's a doggie?

Stacy: A doggie. Color a doggie.

Mom: Okay, you color the doggie.

Stacy: Mommy color crayon.

Mom: Mommy has crayons. Mommy's coloring. What's mommy making?

Stacy: Doggie.

Mom: A doggie.

Stacy: Okay.

Mom: All right, I'll make a doggie. Is this the doggie's tail?

Stacy: Doggie's tail. More.

Mom: More doggie?

Stacy: Okay.

Mom: Can Stacy color? Hum?

Stacy: More doggie there. More doggie daddy.

Mom: More doggie daddy?

Stacy: Want a more doggie. More doggie. Put more doggie there.

Mom: Okay, you color the doggie on this page. What color's your doggie?

Stacy: Blue. Color this page, mommy.

Content and Form

Vocabulary growth is slow for the first few months, but then increases rapidly. Although the ability to comprehend words develops gradually, it is highly context dependent at first (Striano et al., 2003). Eighteen-month-olds are capable of learning new word-referent associations in as few as three exposures (Houston-Price et al., 2005). By age 2, a toddler has an expressive vocabulary of about 150 to 300 words. Two-year-olds with larger vocabularies also use a greater range of grammatical structures (McGregor et al., 2005).

Each toddler has his or her own **lexicon**, or personal dictionary, containing words that reflect that child's environment. In general, toddlers' definitions are not the same as those of adults because they are based on each child's limited experience.

Early word combinations follow predictable patterns. Some individual words are joined with other individual words, such as "Throw ball." Neither word may be combined with other words. In contrast, some words are combined with several others, as in "Eat cookie," "Eat cracker," "Eat candy," and the like. Finally, other words are used flexibly in several different combinations, as in "Mommy drink," "Drink juice," and "More drink." A child's short utterances represent a complex interaction of syntactic knowledge, cognitive ability, communicative goals, and the structure of the conversation (Valian & Aubry, 2005).

> Adult and toddler definitions are very different. Toddler definitions are based almost exclusively on experience, whereas adult definitions are based more on meanings shared with others.

Preschool Language

For preschoolers, most communication occurs within the framework of conversations with caregivers. With increased memory, children expand their conversational skills to include recounting the past and remembering short personal stories. This memory and recall are aided by the child's increased language skills.

> Language rule learning is a lengthy process that involves identifying patterns, hypothesis testing, and refinement.

A high percentage of preschool children's utterances differ only slightly from utterances produced previously. For example, a child might say, "Doggies are yucky," "Kitties are yucky," "Cows are yucky," and the like, substituting different words in the same frame (Lieven et al., 2003).

From interaction with others, children form hypotheses about the rules of language and use these to produce ever more complex language. This process takes time, and begins one utterance at a time. Caregivers in each child's environment provide feedback and models for further growth (Chouinard & Clark, 2003). For example, in a **reformulation** an adult might respond to "Tommy come 'morrow my birthday" with "Yes, tomorrow your cousin Tommy is coming to your birthday party with all the other kids."

Some children—maybe you—are risk takers who attempt new structures and make mistakes. Other children may make few errors because they attempt to produce new structures infrequently (Rispoli, 2005).

Use

In conversations with caregivers, preschool children introduce topics and maintain them for an average of two to three turns. It is often easier for a preschool child to introduce a new topic than to continue an old one, as in the following example:

Child:	I got a new bike.
Partner:	What color is it?
Child:	Red.
Partner:	Did you ride it on your birthday?
Child:	Mommy saw a spider.

In conversations, preschool children begin to consider that the listener needs to know certain information and the amount of information needed, and that there is a need to change conversational style when speaking to younger children. Style of talking is also reflected in role-playing and narration or storytelling. Four-year-old children can tell simple sequential stories, usually about past events.

Content

Children's expressive vocabularies grow to approximately 300 words by age 2, then mushroom to 900 and 1,500 at ages 3 and 4, respectively (see Box 4.3). They may comprehend two or three times that many words in context.

Words are learned quickly through a process called **fast mapping**, in which the child infers the meaning from context and then uses the word in a similar manner. Fuller definitions evolve over time.

In addition to single words, preschool children acquire words and phrases that are used to join other words and create longer units of language. These include locational terms such as *in, on,* and *under*; temporal terms such as *first* and *last*; quantitative terms such as *more than*; qualitative terms such as *bigger than*; familial terms such as *brother*; and conjunctions such as *and, if, so, but,* and *because*.

Adultlike forms of many sentences evolve during the preschool years.

BOX 4.3 | Example of Preschool Language

G and B are young 4-year-olds. They are playing with firefighter hats, dishes, and dolls. Notice how different this sample is from the toddler language in Box 4.2. Each child supports her portion of the conversation. The syntax seems adultlike, but the content is pure preschool. The rapid change of topics gives this sample a nonsensical quality. With no adult to maintain a cohesive topic structure, this is a free-for-all with only one or two turns on each topic before it shifts:

G: And I gonna wear both of these.

B: At the same time? No, I'm wearing this one.

G: I'm wearing this one.

B: And then I do this.

G: You wear this and I'll wear this.

B: Two colored cups. You drink out of this one. I drink out of the big one. I'm putting the box up there.

G: Okay, I will I have this and you have this.

B: Stay up there.

G: She doesn't look too happy.

B: Uh-oh. Why did I spill it?

G: Mine will only stand.

B: Mine sat.

G: All done with supper. What kind of spoon is this?

B: A plastic one, what else? Now it's time for me to make my own dinner.

G: Time for me too. I have to use this. My baby has to go to bed now. We have to first change their diapers.

B: No we don't.

G: Come here, look.

B: There's a button. I want something to drink.

G: Okay, I'll give you some. Look at this. Watch this. I'm gonna try and make this stand. Do you think this is a girl or a boy?

B: A boy.

G: Oh, cause the boy has the pants on and the girl has the dress on.

B: Happy birthday to you.

G: Grab everythin' up. I'm grabbing most of the doll stuff.

In part, semantic development reflects cognitive development. For example, 4-year-olds demonstrate categorization skills that seem to indicate more advanced procedures for storage of learned information than are seen in younger children.

Form

During the preschool years, changes in language form are very dramatic. Beginning with two- to four-word sentences when you were age 2, you probably acquired 90% of adult syntax by age 5. For English-speaking preschoolers, language becomes more complex as it becomes longer. We can describe children's language development by calculating the average, or **mean length of utterance (MLU)**, in morphemes. The calculation of MLU is discussed later in this chapter. Some MLU values are presented in Table 4.1.

The simple constructions found in the utterances of 18- to 24-month-olds form the basis for a more elaborate grammar, and by age 3 most children's utterances contain both a subject and a verb. This basic structure is elaborated with the addition of articles, adjectives, auxiliary verbs, prepositions, pronouns, and adverbs.

In addition, adultlike negative, interrogative, and imperative sentence forms evolve. For example, a toddler negative consisting of *No cookie* is modified by words such as *no, not, can't, don't,* and *won't* being placed between the subject and verb, as in *Mommy can't catch me.* Other negatives such as *wouldn't, couldn't, is not,* and *isn't* are added later.

Similarly, interrogatives or questions go from single words—such as *Doggie?* and *What?* or *Wassat?*—to more complex questions that ask *what* and *where;* followed developmentally by *who, which,* and *whose;* and, finally, *when, why,* and *how,* and a more mature form in which the verb or auxiliary verb and subject are reversed from the statement "She is happy" to form "Is she happy?" or "Why is she happy?" Repeatedly hearing caregiver questions can have a beneficial effect on a preschooler's development of adultlike questions (Valian & Casey, 2003).

Early sentences consist of only one clause. A clause, like a sentence, has both a subject and a verb. By the end of preschool, children are joining two or more independent clauses together to form compound sentences. Late preschoolers can also attach dependent clauses to independent clauses to form complex sentences such as *I didn't liked the big dog that barked at grandpa last night.* "That barked at grandpa last night" is a clause but not a sentence, so it's called a dependent clause and must be attached to an independent clause, which can stand alone and can be a sentence. These structures appear infrequently in preschool; they develop slowly and are refined throughout the school-age years.

Several bound morphemes are added during the preschool years. These include the progressive verb ending *-ing,* as in *jumping;* plural *-s,* as in *cats;* possessive *'-s* (or *-s'*), as in *mommy's;* and the past tense verb ending *-ed,* as in *talked.* As might be expected, it takes children some time to acquire the use of these morphemes, and it is not uncommon to hear words such as *eated, goed, sheeps,* and *foots.*

 Thought Question 4.1

At what ages would you say children are able to participate in communication, comprehend language, or hold up their end in a simple conversation? On what would you base these decisions?

School-Age and Adolescent Language

When children begin to attend school, they start the long process of establishing their identity independent of their family. Most communication now occurs in conversations outside the home. In part, the status of adolescents within their own social grouping is determined by communication skills.

The means of communication change in school as children learn to read and write. In turn, this skill enables children to use computers, tablets, and cellphones, and it opens a whole new world of information. This development is discussed in Chapter 6.

Reading and writing development is related to **metalinguistic skills**, which enable a child to consider language in the abstract, to make judgments about its correctness, and to create verbal contexts, such as in writing. Younger children are unable to make such judgments, especially without a supporting nonlinguistic context.

Five-year-olds use very adultlike language form, although many of the more subtle syntactic structures are missing. In addition, these children have not acquired some of the pragmatic skills that are needed to be truly effective communicators.

Over the next few years, language development slows and begins to stabilize, but it will be nonetheless significant. Many complex forms and subtle linguistic uses are learned in the adolescent period. The preschool emphasis on development of language form becomes less prominent, and semantic and pragmatic development blossom.

Conversation continues to be the primary locus of communication, and children and adolescents learn to be more effective and efficient communicators. Interactional lessons from the family form a basis for the deepening relationships with peers (Whitmire, 2000).

Use

During the early school-age years, children's language use changes in two ways: Conversational skills continue to develop, and conversational narratives expand and gain all the elements of mature storytelling. Children learn effective ways to introduce new topics and to continue and to end conversations smoothly and appropriately. While in a conversation, they make relevant comments and adapt their roles and moods to fit the situation. In addition, school-age children learn to make even more and increasingly subtle assumptions about the level of knowledge of their listeners and to adjust their conversations accordingly.

> Even with the development of writing, conversation is still the predominant use for language.

Within conversation, teens demonstrate more affect and discuss topics infrequently mentioned at home. The number of turns on a topic increases greatly. Although interrupting increases, it evolves into behaviors, such as asking pertinent questions, that serve to move the topic along.

Narratives, both in conversation and in writing, gain the elements needed in our culture to be considered satisfying. English literate narratives contain an introductory setting statement and a challenge or challenges that the characters—often the speaker—overcome. Events are organized both sequentially and by cause and effect.

Content

Vocabulary continues to grow, but number of words is only the most superficial measure of semantic change. First-graders have an expressive vocabulary of approximately 2,600 words but may understand as many as 8,000 root English words, such as *happy*, and possibly 14,000 when various derivations are included, such as *unhappy* and *happily*. Aided in school, this receptive vocabulary expands to approximately 30,000 words by sixth grade and to 60,000 words by high school. As a bright young adult, you may have close to 100,000 words in your receptive store.

Definitions become more dictionary-like, which means they become less experiential or less based on individual experience and more shared, more categorical (as in *An apple is a kind of fruit*), and more precise. Multiple word meanings are also acquired. The ability to provide definitions is related to the acquisition of metalinguistics, mentioned previously (Benelli et al., 2006). The increasing size of children's vocabularies requires more precision and an organization into categories for easy retrieval.

School-age children also learn to understand and use **figurative language**. Unlike literal meanings, figurative language does not always mean what it seems to mean. For example, *idioms* are expressions that often cannot be understood literally, such as "hit the road" or "off the wall." Figurative language enriches communication, requires higher language functions of interpretation, and correlates with adolescent literacy skills (Dean Qualls et al., 2003). Some forms are not comprehended until adulthood.

Form

Following the rapid development of language form in preschool, there is a gradual slowing, although development continues. Many forms continue to develop into adolescence.

By age 5, children use most verb tenses with common verbs and auxiliary or helping verbs, such as *would*, *should*, *must*, and *might*; possessive pronouns (*his, hers, yours*); and the conjunctions *and, but, if, because, when*, and *so*. They still have some difficulty with multiple auxiliary verbs, as in *should have been*. Five-year-old children also have limited use of the comparative *-er*, as in *bigger*, and superlative *-est*, as in *biggest*; relative pronouns used in complex sentences (I know *who* lives next door); gerunds (We go *fishing*); and infinitives (I want *to eat* now).

Many syntactic structures appear slowly, and children may struggle with acquisition well into the school years (Eisenberg et al., 2008). During the school years, children gradually add passive sentences, such as *The cat is chased by the dog*, in which the entity performing the action is placed at the end rather than the beginning of the sentence; reflexive pronouns, such as *myself, yourself, himself*, and *themselves*; conjunctions, such as *although* and *however*; and variations of compound and complex sentences. It frequently takes a child several years of practice to gain complete control of these linguistic structures. And children may use some, such as conjunctions, correctly in speech before they fully understand the relationships expressed (Cain et al., 2005).

Morphological development focuses on derivational suffixes—word endings that change the word class, such as adding *-er* to a verb to make a noun, as in *paint/painter*—and prefixes. Development of prefixes, such as *un-*, *ir-*, and *dis-*, will continue into adulthood.

 Check Your Understanding 4.1

Click here to check your understanding of the concepts in this section.

LANGUAGE IMPAIRMENTS AND ASSOCIATED DISORDERS

As you can see, language and its use are extremely complex. It stands to reason, then, that language impairment or LI would be even more so. So many things can go wrong at so many junctures that each child with LI represents a unique set of circumstances.

In this section, we discuss several disorders types of LI. Of necessity, we'll discuss groups of children under different categories. Although categories are helpful for discussion of shared characteristics, they are not the same as individuals. Each of us and each child with LI is unique.

The effect that any disorder has on communication and on language development varies with the severity of the disorder and the age of the child. As individuals mature, the communicative requirements change.

We'll make some general statements about LI before we get more specific. Children with expressive vocabulary delays at 24 months of age are at increased risk for later speech/language problems and need for SLP services. The risk of being a late talker at 24 months is strongly associated with being a boy, low socioeconomic status, not being a single child, older maternal age at birth, moderately low birth weight, low quality parenting, receipt of no day care or for less than 10 hr/week, and hearing and attention problems (Harrison & McLeod, 2010; Scheffner Hammer, Morgan, Farkas, Hillemeier, Bitetti, & Maczuga, 2017). Researchers are also identifying important genetic factors that account for variance in children's conversational language skills (DeThorne et al., 2008). Late talkers have an ongoing weakness in language that continues through preschool years and into early adulthood (Rescorla & Turner, 2015).

In addition, research indicates sustained attention deficits in children with LI. Although found in both auditory and visual modalities, attention problems are more pronounced for auditory stimuli, the primary input for language learning (Danahy Ebert & Kohnert, 2011).

Although some disorders that we will discuss are characterized by difficulty with specific aspects of language, most children with LI have difficulty in more than one area. For example, many children with pragmatic difficulties also demonstrate poor receptive vocabulary and poor picture-naming abilities. In addition, many of these children make more semantic errors, nonrelated errors, and omissions and circumlocutions than their typically developing (TD) peers (Ketelaars et al., 2011). Circumlocution is talking to bypass or go around a word, as in "It's that . . . that going round thing".

It's easy to assume from these data that children with LI perform like younger children with similar language skills. That would be incorrect, and would overlook the struggles of children with LI.

The long-term effects of LI for many children are not good, especially without intervention. Children who are identified as late talkers at 24–31 months still have a weakness in language-related skills in late adolescence (Rescorla, 2009). Although most perform in the average range on all language and reading tasks at 17 years of age, they do significantly more poorly in vocabulary/grammar and verbal memory than socioeconomic status (SES)-matched TD peers. Looking at other aspects of life, a nationwide longitudinal study in the United Kingdom found that when compared to TD peers, children with LI had poorer outcomes in literacy and also in mental health, as well as employment, even at 34 years of age (Law et al., 2009).

We will not be discussing all children with LI. The largest group to be excluded are individuals with hearing impairments. Those individuals are discussed in Chapter 12. Children may also exhibit impairments such as aphasia or loss of language as a result of localized brain injury, as discussed in Chapter 7.

One last caution before we move on: The names of some of the disorders we will discuss are in flux. Where this is occurring, we warn you. For example, *intellectual disability* (*ID*) used to be called *mental retardation*. Although many professionals now use *ID,* the term, strictly speaking, includes any cognitive disorder, including traumatic brain injury and Alzheimer's disease. This muddies the picture some. You've been warned; let's go. We'll begin with disorders that primarily affect language and then discuss disorders in which LI is a co-occuring condition.

Specific Language Impairment

As the name implies, children with **specific language impairment (SLI),** increasingly called primary language impairment (PLI), have a disorder primarily characterized by issues with language. These children are at risk for academic failure when they begin school because they will not have the basic language skills for reading and writing in first grade (Choudhury & Benasich, 2003).

Approximately 10% to 15% of middle-class U.S. children may be "late bloomers" whose early language development is delayed. About half outgrow it. Other children may continue to have problems, primarily SLI (Dale et al., 2003).

Children with SLI exhibit significant limitations in language functioning that cannot be attributed to deficits in hearing, oral structure and function, general intelligence, or perception. In other words, no obvious cause seems to exist. Children with SLI exhibit language performance scores that are significantly lower than their intellectual performance on nonverbal tasks. Among those with SLI, nonverbal intelligence, birth and delivery, hearing, and self-help and motor skills all seem to be within normal limits. SLI affects males more than females, and the oral and written language deficits of SLI appear to be cross-generational (Flax et al., 2003). There is an increased prevalence of SLI in families with a history *of speech and language problems.*

> There is no single, obvious cause for SLI.

Brain imaging of children with SLI indicates brain symmetry in the left and right hemispheres, unlike the usual asymmetry of left-side predominance in language processing regions (Ors et al., 2005). Further investigation using magnetic resonance imaging (MRI) suggests that children with SLI exhibit different patterns of brain activation and coordination, reflecting less efficient patterns of functioning, including reduced activation in the brain areas critical for communication processing (Ellis Weismer et al., 2005; Hugdahl et al., 2004). In general, children with SLI have increased integration of the parietal lobe and decreased integration of the frontal lobe on encoding and decreased integration of the parietal lobe on decoding.

Many but not all children with SLI show marked deficits in working memory abilities (Archibald & Joanisse, 2009) and executive function. **Working memory (WM)** is an active process that allows limited information to be held in a temporary accessible state while cognitive processing occurs (Cowan et al., 2005). Tasks that are particularly demanding from either a storage and/or a processing perspective result in fewer resources being available for other aspects of the task. Children with WM deficits, such as those with SLI, exhibit learning difficulties (Swanson & Beebe-Frankenberger, 2004). Relative to age-matched TD peers, many children with SLI show several significant limitations in WM mechanisms and in processing speed. Deficits in WM and processing speed in children with SLI can, in turn, have a negative impact on language learning and functioning.

Executive function, located in the frontal lobe of the brain, is the organizing and directing function of the brain. These functions will vary depending on the cognitive task. Preschool children with SLI demonstrate executive function deficits in both visual and linguistic tasks and in less ability to shift tasks and inhibit behaviors (Yang & Gray, 2017). Other examples of deficits in executive function include problems with both inhibition control and cognitive flexibility (Pauls & Archibald, 2016). Children with SLI also have difficulty controlling auditory attention in both quiet and noisy situations (Victorino & Schwartz, 2015).

This can all be very confusing. The Merrill Advanced Study Center at the University of Kansas has an easy-to-read guide titled "Top 10 things you should know . . . about children with specific language impairment." Simply go to the Merrill website (http://merrill.ku.edu). You'll find "Top 10 Things" under "In the Know" in the middle of the page.

Lifespan Issues

SLI affects between 4% and 7% of preschool children (Law, Boyle, Harris, Harkness, & Nye, 2000). As preschool children, those with SLI are perceived negatively by their peers (Segebart DeThorne & Watkins, 2001). In addition, children with SLI exhibit poor social skills (Conti-Ramsden & Botting, 2004).

SLI is usually diagnosed at preschool age because of severely delayed or impaired language with no known cause (Bishop, 2014; Leonard, 2014). Many children initially thought to have SLI are later identified as having a learning disability, a disorder we'll discuss later. Lingering effects of SLI may result in reading difficulties that reflect difficulty with earlier language skills, such as rhyming, letter naming, and concepts related to print. In general, children with SLI exhibit slower and poorer processing of both linguistic and nonlinguistic material in elementary school (Miller et al., 2001; Weismer et al., 2000). Children with SLI are less successful than TD peers at initiating play interactions; thus, they engage in more individual play and onlooking behaviors (Liiva & Cleave, 2005). Teachers rate these children as exhibiting more reticence and solitary-passive withdrawal (Hart et al., 2004).

Long-term data on children with SLI are sparse. Studies have indicated later academic difficulties, especially with language-based activities. For example, at age 14 children with SLI still exhibit slower response times in language tasks than TD children (Miller et al., 2006). Reticence and extreme aloneness may lead to rejection and bullying by others in middle and high school (Conti-Ramsden & Botting, 2004; Rubin et al., 2002). Many adolescents with SLI perceive themselves negatively and are less independent than their TD peers (Conti-Ramsden & Durkin, 2008; Jerome et al., 2002). For example, adolescents with SLI exchange text messages less often than their TD peers (Conti-Ramsden et al., 2010). This suggests that social difficulties may be restricting use, which in turn curtails opportunities to develop social networks and to make arrangements for peer social interaction.

Deficits in the vocabulary system of young adults with SLI persist even among those who attend college. These deficits are noticeable in semantic flexibility and productivity, especially in those with more severe LI (Hall, McGregor, & Oleson, 2017). These types of problems are characteristic of deficits in executive function.

Language Characteristics

In general, children with SLI have difficulty (1) extracting regularities or patterns from the language around them, (2) constructing word-referent associations for vocabulary growth, and (3) registering different contexts for language. As a result, these youngsters experience difficulties with expressive and/or receptive language, morphological and phonological rule formation, vocabulary development, and language use (Leonard, 2014; Redmond, 2003). Pragmatic problems seem to result from an inability to use language forms appropriately. In addition, children with SLI have deficits in their ability to recognize the impact of and to express emotions (Brinton et al., 2007).

Difficulty with grammatical morphemes, such as plural –*s*, suggests language-processing deficits in phonological working memory where words are held while processed, resulting in less capacity to store phonological information (Corriveau et al., 2007; Montgomery & Leonard, 2006). Imagine having limited ability to hold and process information while communication continues at a rapid rate, thus overwhelming and slowing the entire process. You begin to lose information as more comes in. Expressively, children with SLI may speak more slowly and have frequent speech disruptions (Guo et al., 2008). Even as adolescents, children with SLI continue to struggle with morphological markers and exhibit an ongoing maturational lag compared to TD age-matched and language-matched peers (Rice et al., 2009).

Multiple words must be held and integrated in working memory to reveal the meaning of a sentence as it unfolds in time. Therefore, the processing of semantic information in sentences is much slower in preschool children with SLI compared to their TD peers (Montgomery, 2006; Montgomery & Evans, 2009; Pijnacker, Davids, van Weerdenburg, Verhoeven, Knoors, & van Alphen, 2017). The processing of verbs becomes more difficult as the surrounding context becomes more complex (Andreu, Sanz-Torrent, & Guardia-Olmos, 2012; Thordardottir & Ellis Weismer, 2002).

Both semantic and phonological deficits contribute to word-learning difficulties in children with SLI (Gray, 2004). They are less efficient in using syntax to aid in vocabulary acquisition (Rice et al., 2000). Although word learning is difficult for children with SLI, comprehension seems to be easier than production.

Children with SLI have smaller receptive vocabularies throughout childhood and into early adulthood compared to TD individuals. Differences are less for females, those with higher nonverbal IQs, and those having mothers with higher education (Rice & Hoffman, 2015).

Auditory processing problems may also result in difficulties with shorter words such as prepositions and articles (e.g., *a, the*), auxiliary verbs, and pronouns. Children with SLI exhibit persistent problems with morpheme use (Bedore & Leonard, 2001; Redmond & Rice, 2001).

Word retrieval problems of children with SLI reflect the limited semantic knowledge of these children and difficulty inhibiting activation of non-target competing words (Mainela-Arnold et al., 2008, 2010; McGregor et al., 2002). For example, when a child tries to find a given word, rhyming words, similar words, and those with the same initial sound may all crowd for attention. In addition, a significant subgroup of children with SLI demonstrate deficits in semantic organization (Sheng & McGregor, 2010). If words are poorly organized into categories, they're harder to retrieve.

Although language is the most notable problem, there are often problems in selective attention (Spaulding, Plante, & Vance, 2008), working memory (Vugs, Hendriks, Cuperus, & Verhoeven, 2014), and motor skills (Hill, 2001). These differences may account for the lower performance of children with SLI even on non-language based tasks (Gallinat & Spaulding, 2014).

Social Communication Disorder

You might be asking, "Isn't all communication social?" The answer, of course, is "Yes." We can define social communication as "social interaction, social cognition, pragmatics (verbal and nonverbal), and receptive and expressive language processing" (Adams, 2005, p. 182). That's a mouthful. In general, it's the ability to communicate with a variety of partners in various situations not only through language but through nonlinguistic means, such as facial expression and eye contact (Curenton & Justice, 2004; Inglebret, Jones, & Pavel, 2008). These behaviors vary by culture, and also with situations and partners. For example, lack of eye contact may signal disinterest in general American culture but be considered polite in others.

Social communication disorder (SCD) is persistent difficulty in the social use of verbal and nonverbal communication and may include problems in all those areas. As such, social communication disorder can occur alone or with other disorders such as autism spectrum disorder (ASD) or SLI. In ASD, social communication problems are one of the defining features of the disorder. This is not to suggest that the two disorders are the same. In SCD we do not find the repetitive movements, such as rocking or spinning, or the fixated interests found in ASD.

SCD is relatively new, recognized as a separate disorder only in 2013 in DSM-V, the *Diagnostic and Statistical Manual of Mental Disorders* (5th edition) of the American Psychiatric Association. The presence of SCD can limit effective communication and social participation, negatively affect relationships, and lead to academic and vocational problems.

The causes of SCD may be many and varied, and reflect related disorders of which SCD is a part. Causes may be biological or may reflect neurological conditions, mental disorders and/or overall developmental delays.

Although there is no firm data on the prevalence of SCD, Bishop and McDonald (2009) estimated that 4% of all children exhibit characteristics of SCD. Others have given higher estimates (Murphy et al., 2014). We do know the prevalence of other disorders in which SCD is a characteristic. For example, the Centers for Disease Control and Prevention estimates the prevalence of ASD at 1 in 68 children (CDC, 2014). Mok and colleagues (2014) estimated that 23% of children with SLI also had SCD. Given these figures and the presence of SCD as a separate disorder and its presence within other disorders, we're safe in saying that a significant percentage of children exhibit SCD.

Lifespan Issues

A young child with SCD may not respond differentially to the faces of others or to games or sound-making activities. As infants, these children may prefer aloneness and not respond to or imitate others. They may not initiate interactions or gesture to express their intentions. In general, children with SCD may not form strong attachment bonds with their parents and family. Emotional behaviors may be difficult for others to interpret or may be expressed through tantrums and other challenging behavior.

Given the social nature of language development, a child with SCD may be slow to develop language. At age 4, when TD children are becoming aware of their own and others' ability to think and reason, children with SCD may fall behind in emotional understanding and expression. Because delayed development may mirror a number of disorders or simply reflect typical individuality, it is difficult to diagnose SCD in young children. Diagnosis of SCD is rare before age 4. Children with mild SCD may not be diagnosed until adolescence.

As preschool and school-age children, those with SCD may become socially isolated. The lack of both language and social skills makes them less desirable play and study partners. Their poor language skills, especially the pragmatics of conversation and storytelling, result in difficulties with literacy. They may be inflexible in conversation, and talk *at* rather than *with* their peers. As teenagers, children with SCD may be bullied by other students because of their lack of social skills.

Language Characteristics

In general, the characteristics of SCD include problems with communication for social purposes. These include deficits in interactional skills, social cognition, pragmatic, and language. Interactional skills include adjusting your communication style to your partner. For example, as speakers, we talk differently with young children than we do to older adults. Children with SCD may have difficulty adjusting to different partners, especially in politeness and role recognition. Cooperative tasks such as play and conflict resolution may be difficult.

Social cognition includes understanding and regulating our emotions as they affect others, and involves something called Theory of Mind or ToM. ToM is an evolving notion in children that others have a mind and emotions that differ from their own and that these must be considered in communication. Children with SCD may have difficulty understanding their own emotions and those of others. They may have difficulty directing their behavior to accomplish goals and to share attention with others. A deficit in ToM means that a child may have difficulty figuring out what information a communication partner needs in order to participate in a conversation. For example, a child with SCD might say "She did it" with little other reference to help his or her conversational partner know to whom and what *she* and *it* refer.

In addition, not all communication is explicit. As a participant, you sometimes must infer meaning. When a partner says, "Do you think it's warm enough in here?" she or he may be subtly asking you to turn up the heat. Children with SCD may be very literal in their interpretations of such indirect comments.

Pragmatic, as you've learned is the use of language. This includes using language to accomplish our intentions and clearly signaling our intention to our conversational partner. This is accomplished through language but also through nonlinguistic means such as body language. Pragmatic difficulties also include a lack of understanding or adherence to the rules for conversation and conversational storytelling. Children with SCD may experience difficulty interpreting the intentions of others and encoding their own intentions. Conversations may be incoherent, with frequent abrupt topic shifts. Events may be related in a confused manner, and there may be less flexibility in changing conversational style. As mentioned, nonlinguistic behaviors may be inappropriate or odd, sending confusing messages that may not match the words spoken. Children with SCD may also have difficulty interpreting the gestures, facial expressions, and other body language of others.

Finally, language may reflect the child's general social deficits as mentioned. Words and meanings may be misunderstood unless explicitly stated. Syntax may not reflect a child's intended meaning, and there may be frequent communication breakdowns.

Intellectual Disability

The American Association on Intellectual and Developmental Disabilities (AAIDD) defines **intellectual disability (ID)**, as consisting of the following:

- Substantial limitations in intellectual functioning;
- Significant limitations in adaptive behavior consisting of conceptual, social, and practical skills
- Originating before age 18 (AAIDD, 2009)

Taken together, and with an attempt to be more holistic, we could say that the characterization of ID is based on overall developmental level of an individual. The key is "development." Other forms of cognitive impairment, such as Alzheimer's disease, occur after the developmental period.

Accounting for approximately 2.5% of the population, people with ID vary based on causality and other factors, such as the amount of home support, the living environment, education, mode of communication, and age.

Several websites provide more information on ID. The National Institute of Child Health and Human Development website (www.nichd.nih.gov) is a good place to begin your research of intellectual and developmental disabilities. Type "IDDs overview" in the search box.

Severity classifications are usually based on the level of IQ and range from mild (IQ 52–68) to profound (IQ below 20). IQs in individuals may result in very different skill levels. The use of IQ as a measure of severity is slowly changing. Newer severity measures are based on the amount of assistance an individual needs to get through his or her daily life. This measure is more holistic and considers a client's entire life.

Causes of ID are almost as varied as individuals. Two large categories of possible causal factors are biological and socioenvironmental. These factors may be complicated by cognitive limitations that can affect the processing of incoming and outgoing information such as speech and language. Biological factors include the following:

- Genetic and chromosomal abnormalities
- Maternal infections during pregnancy
- Toxins and chemical agents
- Nutritional and metabolic causes
- Gestational disorders affecting development of the fetus
- Complications from pregnancy
- Complications from delivery
- Brain diseases

Socioenvironmental factors include a stimulation-impoverished environment, poor housing, inadequate diet, poor hygiene, and lack of medical care. The effect of each of these factors varies with each child.

IQ is not the entire picture. For some individuals with ID there may be other cognitive processing differences. Incoming sensory information, such as sounds, are processed by first attending to a stimulus, then perceiving differences and likenesses, organizing and storing the information, and finally retrieval from memory. When compared to TD peers, some individuals with ID do not rely on organizational strategies that link words and concepts to one another. Nor do they spontaneously

---

Intellectual disability means more than just low IQ. Values such as IQ usually measure past learning only.

rehearse information for easy retrieval. Information stored poorly can lead to memory or retrieval problems. To some extent, memory is affected by the type of input. In general, individuals with ID have more difficulty with auditory input, especially linguistic, than with visual input.

Incoming linguistic information undergoes several types of decoding. Simultaneous synthesis occurs all at once and extracts overall meaning. Successive synthesis is more linear, occurring one at a time. Although individuals with ID exhibit some difficulty with both types, those with Down syndrome have much greater difficulty with successive processing, possibly reflecting poor auditory working memory.

> Individuals with intellectual disability may process incoming sensory information differently from those without disability.

Lifespan Issues

Some newborns and infants with ID are identified early because of obvious physical factors, such as syndromes or anatomical anomalies, at-risk indicators such as low birthweight or poor physical responses, or delayed development. Intervention may begin at home or in special early intervention (EI) programs in which a child is seen by a team of medical and educational specialists. It is best for the child if intervention begins as soon as possible. EI focuses on sensorimotor skills such as eye-hand coordination, physical development, and social and communicative abilities. An Individualized Family Service Plan (IFSP) specifying services is written in collaboration with caregivers.

Some children with ID are not identified until age 2 or 3. These youngsters, along with those previously identified, will likely attend a special preschool. They may receive intervention services, such as physical therapy, special education, or speech-language therapy, in either the home or school.

Depending on the severity of a school-age child's ID, she or he may either attend a regular education class and receive special services or receive education in a self-contained, special classroom. Education and training will focus on academic skills, daily living and self-help activities, and vocational needs, depending on the abilities of the child.

Only children with the most profound ID accompanied by other disabilities reside in developmental centers. Generally, children who cannot reside at home live in community residences with 8 to 10 other children their age and with houseparents.

Mike, a man with profound ID and cerebral palsy, lived at home with his older parents as an infant and preschooler. As he matured and his parents aged, Mike was placed in a community residence with other young adults with ID. He received daily care at this center and was able to continue his education at the same school. Most of his training involved daily living skills and use of a communication board to communicate.

> Very few individuals with intellectual disability live in large institutions. Since the 1970s, a philosophy called deinstitutionalization has been responsible for the movement of individuals with ID into small community residences.

In adulthood, living and working arrangements vary widely. People with milder ID often live in the community and work competitively in minimally skilled jobs. More severely involved individuals may live with family members or in community residences containing a small group of similar adults. They may work in a special workshop or be enrolled in a day treatment program in which education and training continue to be the focus.

Language Characteristics

Children with ID vary greatly in their communication abilities. For example, children with Down syndrome (DS) and fragile X syndrome (FXS) have moderate to severe delays in communication development in all areas of language (Roberts et al., 2001). In phonology, boys with FXS make errors similar to those of younger typically developing youth, whereas those with DS have more significant phonological differences than might be expected by delayed development alone (Roberts et al., 2005). In contrast, boys with FXS produce longer, more complex utterances than do boys with DS (Price et al., 2008).

For many individuals with ID, language is the single most important limitation. For approximately half of the population with ID, language comprehension and/or production is below the level of cognition. This might be indicative of cognitive processing problems that accompany ID. For example, those with DS exhibit auditory working memory deficits (Seung & Chapman, 2000).

In initial language development, individuals with ID follow a similar but slower developmental path than that of typically developing children. Even so, these children often produce shorter, more immature language forms (Boudreau & Chapman, 2000). In later development, the paths begin to differ more from typical development. All areas of language exhibit some delay and disorder in children with ID.

Learning Disabilities

According to the National Joint Committee on Learning Disabilities (1991), the term *learning disability* (*LD*) refers to a heterogeneous group of disorders that are manifested by significant difficulties in the development and use of listening, speaking, reading, writing, reasoning, or mathematical abilities. The disorders reflect difficulties in the central nervous system that are not caused by other conditions or environmental influences. Although similar, the definition of LD found in the fifth edition of the *Diagnostic and Statistical Manual* (DSM-5) of the American Psychiatric Association (APA, 2013) calls LD *learning disorder*. If the disorder is focused in one area, such as reading and writing, it is termed a "specific learning disorder" in that affected area.

Children with learning disabilities have difficulty learning and using symbols for speaking, listening, reading, and writing.

Approximately 15% of children with LD have their major difficulty with motor learning and coordination, while more than 75% primarily have difficulty learning and using symbols (Miniutti, 1991). In either case, symbol learning and use are affected.

Approximately 3% of all individuals have LD, but the severity varies widely. Learning disabilities affect males four times as frequently as they do females.

A good place to begin your online exploration of LD is the Learning Disabilities Association website (www.ldaamerica.us). If you click on "For Teachers" or "For Professionals," you will find a wealth of information on intervention. The site also offers links to several other sites. Simply click on "Resources."

 Video Example 4.1

You can find an introduction to and overview of LD and how these disabilities affect language in this video. https://www.youtube.com/watch?v=GoM5HcfQBwE

The characteristics of LD fall into six categories: motor, attention, perception, symbol, memory, and emotion. Few children exhibit all the characteristics described. Motor difficulties may include either hyperactivity or hypoactivity. Hyperactivity, or overactivity, is more prevalent, especially among boys. This results in difficulty attending and concentrating for more than very short periods. Children with hypoactivity may be deficient in their sense of body movement, definition of handedness, eye–hand coordination, and space and time conceptualization.

Attentional difficulties include a short attention span, inattentiveness, and distractibility. Irrelevant stimuli may capture the child's attention, and overstimulation easily occurs. Some children become fixed on a single task or behavior and repeat it compulsively, a process called *perseveration.*

Perceptual difficulties of children with LD involve interpretation of incoming stimuli, although this is not a sensory disorder like deafness and blindness. Children with perceptual disabilities often confuse similar sounds, similar-sounding words, and similar-looking printed letters and words. In addition, children with LD may have difficulty both in determining where to focus their attention and in integrating sensory information from different sources, such as vision and hearing. Those children have particular difficulty in comprehending printed symbols and producing written symbols. It's estimated that as many as 80% of children with LD have some form of reading problem, and that the incidence of these problems in the overall population may range from 5% to 17% (Sawyer, 2006).

Memory difficulties affect short-term retrieval, as in remembering directions, and long-term retrieval, as in recalling names, event sequences, and words. Some children exhibit word-finding problems that result in blocks and the use of fillers ("Ah, ah, you know . . . ") or circumlocutions.

Emotional problems are usually a factor that accompanies LD, and not a causal factor. They are a reaction to the frustration that these children feel. Although most children with LD have normal intelligence, they perform poorly on language-based tasks, and their parents or teachers may tell them that they are not trying or that they're lazy or stupid. Emotional outbursts may result in children being described as aggressive, impulsive, unpredictable, withdrawn, and/or impatient. These youngsters may exhibit poor judgment, unusual fears, and/or poor adjustment to change.

> LDs are not caused by emotional disorders; rather, emotional problems result from misperception and from frustration.

Those who have hyperactivity and attentional difficulties but do not manifest other characteristics of LD, especially perceptual difficulties, may be labeled as having **attention-deficit/hyperactivity disorder (ADHD)**. Children with ADHD have an underlying neurological impairment in executive function that regulates behavior; as a result, they are impulsive. Although ADHD is not a learning disability, children with ADHD often experience problems in social relations that are explained in part by their accompanying pragmatic problems with language use (Leonard et al., 2011). Children with ADHD may not be identified on language testing that ignores pragmatics.

Possibly because of difficulties attending, children with ADHD are less accurate in their interpretations of speech (Nilsen, Mangal, & MacDonald, 2013). These difficulties could lead to more miscommunication.

The fact that LD occurs more frequently in families with a history of the disorder and in children who had a premature or difficult birth suggests possible biological causal factors. A central nervous system dysfunction may involve a breakdown along the neural pathways that connect the midbrain with the frontal cortex, an area that is responsible for attention, regulation, and planning of cognitive activity.

Although not a causal factor, socioenvironmental factors may account for at least some of the behaviors seen in children with LD. For example, misperceptions by a child affect interactions, which influence the child's development, especially language development. Language difficulties, in turn, affect the child's interactions.

Information-processing difficulties are characterized by an inability to use certain strategies or to access certain stored information. In general, children with LD exhibit poor ability to attend selectively or have difficulty deciding on the relevant information to which to attend. As we have seen, discrimination is also extremely difficult. Information that is poorly attended to and poorly perceived will be poorly organized. The cognitive organization of children with LD reflects this confusion. In short, the organization is too inefficient for easy retrieval, so memory is less accurate and retrieval is slower.

Several websites discuss LD. The Learning Disabilities Association of America website (www.ldanatl.org) has a brief checklist of symptoms for parents. Simply go to the site, click on "Parents" at the top. Under "New to LD," click on "Learn more about LD," and then find and click on "Seeing the signs" at the top. This will take you to common behaviors with LD.

Lifespan Issues

As preschoolers, children with LD may exhibit little interest in language or even in books. When a child reaches school, the linguistic demands of the classroom are often well above her or his oral language abilities. The result is often academic underachievement.

Most learning disabilities are not discovered until children go to school, although some children may be enrolled in special preschool programs or may receive therapy services because of poor motor coordination, hyperactivity, or failure to develop language typically. When they reach school, with its accompanying demand for language skills, many children with LD require the services of special educators, speech-language pathologists, and reading specialists. Some children might not be identified in early grades. Very bright children may "learn" to read by memorizing word shapes rather than using phonics-based word-attack skills, as discussed in Chapter 6.

> Attentional, discriminatory, and memory deficits, along with both receptive and expressive symbol use problems, can result in many communication breakdowns.

Children with LD often receive special services while being included in regular classrooms. They can be successful if the teacher makes some adaptation, such as repeating instructions or allowing for a quiet work space, to accommodate their needs. Case Study 4.2 tells the story of one child with a learning disability.

Some children with LD seem to outgrow aspects of their disability. For example, hyperactivity seems to lessen in some adolescents. Other adolescents succeed well

---

CASE STUDY 4.2

Personal Story of a Child with Learning Disabilities

Darren's learning disability went undetected until second grade. As a preschooler, Darren had some difficulty with speech sounds and displayed little interest in books, letters, or drawing. His mother considered his lack of interest and his overactivity to be a "boy thing." Darren received no preschool education. In first grade, he was slow to learn to read and write, as were several of his classmates.

When Darren still seemed to be struggling in second grade, his teacher suggested an evaluation to determine whether he had a learning disability. The school psychologist, a reading specialist, a special education teacher, and a speech-language pathologist evaluated him. They found that Darren's mother had received little, if any, prenatal care and that Darren was born preterm, weighing only 4 pounds, 10 ounces.

After a stay in the hospital of several days, Darren went home with his mother. The rest of his preschool years were uneventful, and he remained at home with his older sister and younger brother, experiencing occasional middle ear infections and childhood illnesses. Although his sister exhibits no signs of LD, Darren's younger brother does exhibit hyperactivity.

At age 11, Darren is a very active child who enjoys sports, especially soccer, which he plays with his best friend, Carlos. Darren has great difficulty reading and writing, and letter and word reversal and transposition are common in both. He has great difficulty sounding out new words. His speech is characterized by word retrieval problems and a limited vocabulary, peppered with "Ya know," "thing," and "one," as in "An' I got that one, ya know, that thing that goes like this."

Darren has had some difficulty behaving in school. His attention easily wanders, and he fidgets in his seat often. If he is not kept busy, he bothers the other students and keeps them from working. He finds himself frequently in fights in school, usually because he has misunderstood some comment of another student. His temper flares easily, possibly because school can be very frustrating.

Although his schoolwork has improved somewhat, he is still well behind his classmates in his ability to read, write, and work independently. This deficit, in turn, has inhibited his ability to solve problems and to think critically in class. He continues to receive tutoring in reading and writing and to see a speech-language pathologist weekly to work on vocabulary, word retrieval, and language use skills.

enough to continue their education and graduate from college. We know adults with LDs who are chemists, engineers, teachers, and speech-language pathologists, although some have lingering vestiges of LD that require lifelong adaptations.

Other adults continue to have difficulty. Matt received special services throughout his school years and finished high school. His language difficulties were complicated by a volatile temper and frequent misinterpretations of the communicative intentions of others. After being fired from a series of jobs, he hit on the idea of informing his new boss that he was "partially deaf" and needed all instructions and feedback repeated face to face. He no longer flies off the handle when given a simple directive by his supervisor, and is gainfully employed. Harry, on the other hand, is in his fifties but has never held a job that required either reading or writing.

Language Characteristics

All aspects of language, spoken and written, usually are affected in children with LD. These children experience difficulty with the give-and-take of conversation and with the form and content of language. Deducing language rules is particularly difficult, resulting in delays in morphological rule acquisition and in the development of syntactic complexity. As a result, overall oral language development may be slow, and frequent communicative breakdown is possible. Word-finding problems may exist, resulting in the child needing more time to respond verbally.

Autism Spectrum Disorder (ASD)

For a child or an older individual to be diagnosed as having **autism spectrum disorder (ASD)**, he or she must have all of the following:

- Persistent problems in social communication and interaction across different contexts. Deficits do not result from general developmental delays, such as those in ID. Problems are seen in all of the following:
- Social-emotional reciprocity

 Thought Question 4.2

If you understand the underlying cause for a type of language disorder, you can often predict the aspects of language that will be difficult. Let's take two different disorders with similar outcomes. Children with SLI and those with LD both tend to omit morphological endings but for different reasons. With limited capacity, children with SLI tend to not remember endings. Those with LD often misperceive morphological endings or do not notice them at all.

- Nonverbal communicative and social interaction behaviors
- Developing and maintaining relationships appropriate for maturity level
- Restricted, repetitive patterns of behavior, interests, or activities characterized by two or more of the following:
  - Stereotyped or repetitive motor movements, use of objects, or speech
  - Excessive reliance on routines, ritualized patterns of behavior, or resistance to change
  - Highly fixated and restricted, abnormally intense interests or focus
  - Hyper- or hypo-sensitivity and reactivity to environmental input, or unusual interest in sensory information

Taken together, these characteristics limit and impair daily functioning. What it means is that many children with ASD, but not all, have abnormal social interactions and failure in the give-and-take of conversation; poorly integrated verbal and nonverbal communication, including eye contact and body language; difficulty adjusting to different social situations and stereotypical motor patterns; and echolalia, or repetition of others' speech, repetitive use of objects, and repetition of certain expressions. For example, when the teacher says, "It's time to clean up," the child may "echo" or repeat the phrase over and over again. In general, the more severe the symptoms, the poorer the individual's language and overall development (Pry et al., 2005).

Motor patterns of behavior may include rocking and a fascination with lights or spinning objects. In addition, a child may insist on certain routines or be preoccupied with specific objects, foods, or clothing. Paired with these preferences, a child with ASD may have an adverse reaction to other sounds or textures. One child known by the authors had approximately a half-dozen outfits consisting of exactly the same articles of clothing. Another would eat only foods of certain colors and textures.

ASD is much more common than previously believed. In 2012, after a national survey, the U.S. Centers for Disease Control and Prevention (CDC) announced the following:

- The incidence of ASD among children was 1 in 88.
- Boys are five times more likely than girls to display ASD characteristics.
- Most children with ASD have IQs above 70 (above the cutoff for ID).

Approximately 25% of children with ASD also exhibit intellectual disability (Chakrabarti & Fombonne, 2001; Fombonne, 2003).

At present, many researchers are trying to identify the early signs of ASD. Early identification can lead to early intervention. The Autism Spectrum Disorder Foundation website (www.myasdf.org/site/) provides some possible early warning signs. Click on "About Autism" and then "Identifying the Disorder."

The primary causal factors in autism are biological. Approximately 65% of all individuals with ASD have neurological differences, and 20% to 30% experience seizures. In addition, some researchers have found unusually high levels of serotonin, a neurotransmitter and natural opiate. They have also discovered abnormal development of the cerebellum, which regulates incoming sensations, and of sections of the temporal lobe responsible for memory and emotions.

At least 15% of children with ASD have a genetic mutation not inherited from their parents (Sebat et al., 2007; Zhao et al., 2007). This is even higher for those with more severe forms of the disorder. Interestingly, the mutations are not similar for all children with ASD. In addition, between 2% and 6% of children with ASD also have fragile X syndrome, a genetic mutation of the X chromosome associated with ID (Belmonte & Bourgerone, 2006).

The incidence of ASD is highest among males and those with a family history of autism. The family pattern suggests a genetic basis for the disorder.

Neural studies suggest that the eye and face detection processing of children with autism may be delayed, explaining in part the early failure to bond with caregivers (Grice et al., 2005). In addition, infants with autism show no difference in brain response to familiar and unfamiliar faces, supporting the notion of facial processing impairment (Dawson et al., 2002).

Differences in processing incoming information also suggest a neurological basis for ASD. Individuals with ASD experience difficulty in analyzing and integrating information. Their responding is often very overselective, resulting in a tendency to fixate on one aspect of a complex stimulus—often some irrelevant, minor detail. As a result, discrimination is difficult.

Overall cognitive processing by children with ASD has been characterized as a *gestalt* in which unanalyzed wholes are stored and later reproduced in identical fashion. The storage of unanalyzed information may account for the way in which individuals with ASD become quickly overloaded with sensory information. Storage of unanalyzed wholes also might hinder memory. It's difficult to organize information on the basis of relationships between stimuli if those stimuli remain unanalyzed. Lack of analysis would also hinder transferring or generalizing learned information from one context to another.

 Video Exercise 4.1

Recognizing Autism Spectrum Disorder

Click on the link to a watch a video of a child with mild ASD, and complete an exercise.

Lifespan Issues

At present, children with ASD are identified by the time they are 2 or 3 years of age. Although early intervention (EI) is critical to maximizing outcomes for children with ASD, EI is often difficult to obtain because of the late age of most diagnoses. Although no babbling or gesturing by 12 months is an early sign, it's not possible at this time to make a definitive diagnosis prior to 24 months of age (Woods & Wetherby, 2003). Although symptoms are present in early childhood, they may not manifest fully until social demands exceed a child's limited capacities

School-age children and adolescents with ASD may be included in regular education classes or be in special classes, depending on the severity of the disorder. In some children, the severity of ASD lessens with age. For example, as Jeffery became a teenager his behavior seemed to be less disruptive, and there were fewer outbursts. Although he could engage in conversation easily, he continued to become annoyed and to begin flapping his hands if more than one person spoke at a time.

People with milder forms of the disorder may be able to live on their own and hold competitive employment. For example, Dr. Temple Grandin, a woman with ASD, is employed as a college professor. Unfortunately, the vast majority of people with ASD are not so successful and require supervision and care. Many with severe ASD have adult life patterns similar to those of adults with ID. Case Study 4.3 presents the story of a child with ASD.

CASE STUDY 4.3

Personal Story of a Child with Autism Spectrum Disorder (ASD)

Just like other new parents, Jayden's mom and dad awaited their first child with heightened anticipation. He was born full term, with no complications, and seemed healthy. Although he had some difficulties nursing and seemed uninterested in eating, these problems were attributed to his being a generally fussy baby who seemed unable to be comforted.

As Jayden developed, he met physical developmental milestones but seemed to lag slightly in social and cognitive development. The pediatrician assured his parents that there is wide variability across infants and that boys often develop more slowly than girls. His mother described him as irritable and quick to cry. He often had temper tantrums, especially when it was time to eat, bathe, or go to bed. Because of these increasing behavior outbursts, Jayden's parents took him from the home less often than they had previously.

When Jayden had not spoken by 18 months, his parents took him to a speech-language pathologist (SLP) for a speech and language evaluation. They were surprised by the many questions the SLP asked concerning Jayden's early social development. She explained speech and language development to them, especially the early acquisition of intent to communicate, which is expressed initially in gestures.

Although the SLP did not diagnose Jayden as having ASD, she recommended that he be enrolled in a social play group for late talkers and strongly suggested that they should have him evaluated at a local hospital by an ASD team, if only to rule out ASD as a cause of his delay and his increasing acting out behavior.

Today Jayden, who was diagnosed with ASD, is enrolled in a special preschool for children with ASD. He receives speech and language services in the classroom daily, and his parents continue intervention at home under the direction of an SLP. Intervention is primarily in the form of play. Jayden signs approximately 50 single words and says about 10 for a variety of purposes.

His parents use signs to inform him about routine changes such as dinner time. His own use of signs seems to have decreased his frustration and acting-out behaviors. Jayden prefers to be alone, and even in his preschool class he rarely interacts with other children, seeming to prefer the company of adults.

Language Characteristics

As a group, children with ASD demonstrate significant delays in language and communication, especially in pragmatics (Tager-Flusberg et al., 2005). A communication problem is often one of the first indicators of possible ASD. Between 25% and 60% of individuals with severe ASD remain nonspeaking throughout their life. Some autistic children who use speech and language demonstrate some immediate or delayed echolalia, which is a whole or partial repetition of previous utterances, often with the same intonation. For example, Mickey would say little during the day but store things said to him during the day and repeat them in sequence before he went to sleep at night. In contrast, Adam would echo immediately. For some children, echolalia might either be a language-processing strategy or signal agreement with the previous utterance. Even when echolalia decreases, other problems, especially those related to pragmatics, persist in the child's language. Most children with ASD who learn to talk go through a period of using echolalia (Prizant et al., 1997).

ASD affects pragmatics and semantics more than language form. Syntactic errors seem to represent a lack of underlying semantic relationships. Prosodic features or suprasegmentals, such as stress, intonation, loudness, pitch, and rate, are often affected, giving the speech of children with ASD the sometimes mechanical quality mentioned. Individuals with ASD often have peculiarities and irregularities in the pragmatics of conversation. The range of intentions is often very limited and may consist solely of demands and, in severe cases, unintelligible vocalizations. Some individuals incorporate entire verbal routines, called *formuli*, into their communication. For example, a child might repeat part or all of a television commercial to indicate a desire for the item that had been in the advertisement. A formula represents the person's attempt to overcome the difficulty of matching the content and form of language to the communicative context. Adults with mild ASD who have good language skills might still misinterpret some of the subtleties of conversation.

> Individuals with autism, even those with seemingly typical language, have continuing problems with pragmatics.

As with any other disability, ASD offers a challenge to parents. The National Institute of Mental Health website (www.nimh.nih.gov/index.shtml) has a helpful parents' guide to ASD. Click on "Health & Education" at the top, scroll down to "Publications," locate "Find Publications by Topic" in the center, and then click on "Autism." There are several other disorders you can also explore on this site.

Video Example 4.2

As you watch this video of a child with severe ASD in an extreme situation, try to look at the child's behavior in light of what you know so far about autism. We have caught him at a bad moment. https://www.youtube.com/watch?v=zSp9k2jISNc

Video Example 4.3

Contrast the first video with this one. What similar behaviors, beyond the tantrums, did you notice in the second video? https://www.youtube.com/watch?v=UvPly9yIkLA

Brain Injury

Impaired brain functioning can result from **traumatic brain injury (TBI)**, cerebrovascular accident or stroke, congenital malformation, convulsive disorders, or encephalopathy, such as infection or tumors. Among children, the most common form of injury is TBI. Cerebrovascular accidents and a fuller discussion of TBI are presented in Chapter 7.

Approximately a million children and adolescents in the United States have experienced TBI, which may be either localized or diffuse brain damage as the result of external force, such as a blow to the head in an auto accident, a fall, or a gunshot wound. Individuals with TBI differ greatly from one another as a result of the site and extent of the injury, the age at onset, and the age of the injury. In general, the smaller the damaged area, the better the chance of recovery. Some individuals recover fully; others remain in a vegetative state. People with TBI exhibit a range of cognitive, physical, behavioral, academic, and linguistic deficits, any of which may be long term.

Cognitive deficits include difficulties in perception, memory, reasoning, and problem solving. Deficits vary and may be permanent or temporary, and may partially or totally affect functioning ability. Children with TBI tend to be inattentive and easily distractible. All aspects of cognitive organization—categorizing, sequencing, abstracting, and generalization—may be affected. Children with TBI have difficulty perceiving relationships, making inferences, and solving problems. They struggle to formulate goals, plan, and achieve their ends. Memory is also affected, although long-term memory before the trauma is often intact.

Psychological maladjustment or "acting out" behaviors, called *social disinhibition,* may occur, in which a person is incapable of inhibiting or controlling impulsive behavior. Other characteristics of TBI may include a lack of initiative, distractibility, inability to adapt quickly, perseveration, low frustration levels, passive-aggressiveness, anxiety, depression, fear of failure, and misperception.

Lifespan Issues

After a cranial accident, some children with TBI may be unconscious for a few minutes or much longer. Upon regaining consciousness, a child usually experiences some disorientation and memory loss. Memory loss may involve only the time of the immediate accident or may be more extensive, including long-term memory loss. TBI may be accompanied by physical disability and personality changes.

Neural recovery over time is often unpredictable and irregular, and the variables that affect recovery of children with TBI are extremely independent. In general, a better recovery is signaled by a shorter, less severe period of unconsciousness following the injury, a shorter period of amnesia, and better posttraumatic abilities.

The age of the injury can be an inaccurate prognosticator. In general, the older the injury, the less chance of change, although this can be complicated by the delayed onset of some deficits. For example, some neurological problems might not be manifested until later in recovery, making neural recovery unpredictable and irregular over time.

When stabilized, a child with TBI begins a long recovery process that can take years. Within the first few months, she or he might experience spontaneous recovery when large gains in ability are made.

Young children often recover quickly, but experience difficulties learning new information and may exhibit severe, long-lasting problems. Older children and adolescents have more to recover from their memory but less new information to learn.

Although the brains of younger children are more malleable or more adaptable than those of older people, this does not mean that younger children will always recover more fully. In addition to recovering the language lost, younger children may still have much language to learn, a task that is possibly made more difficult by the brain injury.

> Even individuals who have made a seemingly full recovery may lack subtle cognitive and social skills. For example, although Jane had been injured in an auto accident but made a seemingly full recovery, she began to exhibit learning problems later when she attended elementary school. Unfortunately, her lack of success in school translated into disciplinary problems later on.

Language Characteristics

Language problems may be evident even after mild cognitive injuries. Some deficits, especially in pragmatics, remain long after the injury, even when general improvement is good. Individuals with severe TBI and resultant deficits in executive function or ability to focus the brain demonstrate problems with pragmatics (Douglas, 2010). More specifically, these individuals have difficulty regulating the amount and manner of conversational participation as well as the relevance of their contributions. A child with TBI may lose the central focus or topic in conversation. Utterances are often lengthy, inappropriate, and off topic, and fluency is disturbed, especially if there are accompanying motor problems.

Language comprehension and higher functions such as figurative language and dual meanings are also often impaired, although language form is relatively unaffected. Semantics, especially concrete vocabulary, is also relatively undisturbed, although word retrieval, naming, and object description difficulties may be present. Narration, especially maintaining story structure and providing enough information, may also pose a problem.

Other Language Impairments

Although we've touched on some of the most prevalent LIs, we have by no means exhausted the discussion. Other forms of LI include but are not limited to

- Nonspecific language impairment (NLI);
- Children who are late talkers;
- Those with childhood schizophrenia, selective mutism (SM), or middle ear infections (otitis media);
- Children who have received cochlear implants; Those who have been exposed to alcohol and drugs in utero, and
- Those who have experienced abuse and neglect.

Children with NLI have a general delay in language development, a nonverbal IQ of 86 or lower, and, as with SLI, no obvious sensory or perceptual deficits but few common characteristics (Rice et al., 2004). Although child health is an important factor among late talkers, most early language delay is due to environmental factors such as poverty and/or homelessness.

Childhood schizophrenia, a serious psychiatric illness that causes strange thinking, odd feelings, and unusual behavior, is uncommon, occurring in approximately 1 of every 14,000 children younger than 13 years of age. Approximately 55% of children and adolescents with schizophrenia have language abnormalities, including language delay especially in pragmatics (Mental Health Research Association, 2007; Nicolson et al., 2000).

Selective mutism (SM) is a relatively rare disorder in which a child does not speak in specific situations, such as school, although she or he may speak normally in others. From 0.2% to 0.7% of all children may have SM at some time, and girls are nearly twice as likely as boys to be affected (Bergman et al., 2002; Kristensen, 2000).

Many young children suffer from chronic otitis media. In general, the cumulative effect of recurrent otitis media can be a significant factor in delayed language development (Feldman et al., 2003).

Those who receive cochlear implants develop language in a manner similar to typically developing children. Although children implanted later have an initial advantage of maturity that enhances language growth, those who receive implants at an earlier age begin to develop spoken language at an ever-increasing rate that soon eclipses that rate for children receiving implants later in childhood (Ertmer et al., 2003).

Fetal alcohol spectrum disorder (FASD) accounts for 1 in every 500 to 600 live births. Alcohol interferes with embryonic development, and infants with FASD often have low birthweight and exhibit central nervous system problems. Later, these children demonstrate hyperactivity, motor problems, attention deficits, and cognitive disabilities. The limitations noted at birth remain with the child for life and can result in poor academic achievement and antisocial behavior. Children with FASD exhibit language problems characterized by delayed development of language, echolalia or inappropriate repetition, and comprehension problems.

Children with FASD and those with fetal drug exposure are behind their peers in reading and other academic tasks.

Prenatal cocaine exposure (PCE) is a continuing problem in children's language development, even into adolescence (Lewis, Minnes, Min, Wu, Lang, Weishampel, & Singer, 2013). As a group, children with PCE have mild but persistent deficits in syntax and phonological processing, which in turn adversely affects reading ability. In addition, caregiver variables, such as low maternal vocabulary, more psychological symptoms, and a poor home environment are also contributing factors.

Finally, each year in the United States approximately 900,000 children are maltreated sufficiently for the neglect and/or abuse to be reported to the authorities (U.S. Department of Health and Human Services [DHHS], 2007). Although neglect and abuse are rarely the direct cause of communication problems, the context in which they occur directly influences a child's development. Poor maternal health, substance abuse, poor or nonexistent pediatric services, and poor nutrition can all affect brain development and maturation.

In general, maltreated children demonstrated consistently poorer language skills with respect to receptive vocabulary, expressive language, and receptive language (Lum, Powell, Timms, & Snow, 2015). Maltreated and abused children are less talkative and have fewer conversational skills than their peers. Their utterances and conversations are shorter, with less complex language, than are those of non-maltreated children (Eigsti & Cicchetti, 2004). Although all aspects of language are affected, it is in pragmatics that children who have been neglected or abused exhibit the greatest difficulties.

So many disorders are associated with LI that they probably all have begun to look similar to you. In actual practice, SLPs treat each child as an individual, not as a member of a category. Of importance is each child's behavior and language features, not group characteristics.

Although this section has focused on disorders, it does not address all the factors that may be related to language impairment. Factors such as poverty, nutrition, child and maternal health, and maternal sensitivity to and stimulation of a child are also important. For example, most children and mothers living in homeless shelters exhibit language deficits for a variety of reasons (La Paro et al., 2004; O'Neil-Pirozzi, 2003). Unfortunately, Black children, poor children, and children who are ELLs are less likely to receive services when compared to White, middle class, English-speaking children (Morgan, Scheffner, Hammer, Farkas, Hillemeier, Maczuga, Cook, & Morano, 2016).

Aspects of Language Affected

In addition to the etiological categories we have just described, language impairments can also be characterized by the language features affected. For example, a child may have difficulty with word recall and conversational initiation, or may possess a limited vocabulary and seem to talk nonstop. Another child may have poor syntax and very short sentences, or withdraw from conversational give-and-take. Figure 4.1 presents the most common language features associated with language impairments. In evaluations, SLPs assess many language features to determine where to begin intervention.

To understand the range of responsibilities of an SLP in various disorders, check the ASHA website (www.asha.org). Type "scope of practice" in the search field and then click on the communication disorder you want to explore.

Thought Question 4.3

Why is pragmatics or language use so frequently the aspect of LI seen in several disorders? Is it related to the nature of pragmatics and how it differs from other aspects of language?

Children with FASD and drug exposure have many learning problems similar to those of children with learning disabilities.

Figure 4.1 Most common language characteristics of children with language impairments.

Pragmatics

Difficulty answering questions or requesting clarification

Difficulty initiating, maintaining a conversation, or securing a conversational turn

Poor flexibility in language when tailoring the message to the listener or repairing communication breakdowns

Short conversational episodes

Limited range of communication functions

Inappropriate topics and off-topic comments; ineffectual, inappropriate comments

Asocial monologues

Difficulty with stylistic variations and speaker-listener roles

Narrative difficulties

Few interactions

Semantics

Limited expressive vocabulary and slow vocabulary growth

Few or decontextualized utterances, more here-and-now; more concrete meanings

Limited variety of semantic functions

Relational term difficulty (comparative, spatial, temporal)

Figurative language and dual definition problems

Conjunction (*and, but, so, because,* etc.) confusion

Naming difficulties may reflect less rich and less elaborate semantic storage or actual retrieval difficulties

Syntax/Morphology

Short, uncomplex utterances

Rule learning difficulties

Run-on, short, or fragmented sentences

Few morphemes, especially verb endings, auxiliary verbs, pronouns, and function words (articles, prepositions)

Overreliance on word order over word relationships

Difficulty with negative and passive constructions, relative clauses, contractions, and adjectival forms

Article (*a, the*) confusion

Phonology

Limited syllable structure

Fewer consonants in repertoire

Inconsistent sound production, especially as complexity increases

Comprehension

Poor discrimination of units of short duration (bound morphemes)

Impaired comprehension, especially in connected discourse such as conversations

Reliance on context to extract meaning

Wh- question confusion

Overreliance on nonlinguistic cues for meaning

 Check Your Understanding 4.2

Click here to check your understanding of the concepts in this section.

ASSESSMENT

An SLP's first task in assessment is to distinguish between children who have a disorder and those who do not. Accurate diagnosis is a prerequisite to ensuring that scarce financial and personnel resources, especially in schools, are allocated in the most beneficial way.

Assessment and intervention overlap and are parts of the same process.

As with other diagnostics, language assessment is a systematic process of discovery and information gathering. Good clinical practice requires that the boundary between assessment and intervention be permeable. A portion of any good assessment is attempting to determine possible avenues for intervention. In turn, each intervention session should contain some assessment of a child's current skill level.

Assessment should be sufficiently broad and deep so that all areas of possible concern are identified and described as accurately as possible. For example, assessment of semantics must include more than receptive understanding and expressive vocabulary size. A thorough examination might also include areas such as word learning abilities and word storage and retrieval (Brackenbury & Pye, 2005).

Bilingual Children, English Language Learners, and Dialectal Speakers

According to the U.S. Census Bureau (2013), 21% of the U.S. school-age population speaks a language other than English at home. Approximately one-third of these children are English language learners (ELLs). In addition, many children speak dialects that differ from the majority American English dialects that teachers use for instruction. For example, African American children make up approximately 17% of the children enrolled in public schools (Fry, 2007). Some professionals have attributed the reported academic underachievement of some of these children, who are often from families with low income, to the African American English (AAE) dialect that many of them speak.

Any assessment of children with culturally and linguistically diverse backgrounds must recognize the possible risk for LI. For example, children from low-SES backgrounds with poorer maternal education have an increased incidence of LI (Schuele, 2001). The task of an SLP is to differentiate LI from language difference.

ELLs and children with dialectal differences are more likely to be identified as needing special education services (de Valenzuela et al., 2006). This is most likely related to performance on standardized tests, many of which may not be appropriate for these children. Clearly, there is a critical need to develop language assessment measures and/or procedures that are appropriate.

Assessment of children who are non-native speakers of English, called English Language Learners (ELLs), pose a challenge for SLPs. As we mentioned, language difference is not a disorder, but deciding whether a child has LI or simply a language difference can be difficult. We do not have tests in most languages and we have few SLPs who speak languages which infrequently occur in the U.S. ELLs with LI have significantly poorer performance than typically developing ELLs on most measures of language except vocabulary (Paradis, Schneider, & Sorenson Duncan, 2013). The greatest difference seems to be on non-word repetition and verb tense morphology.

Diagnostic methods for children from culturally and linguistically diverse backgrounds vary widely, and no single measure or procedure is adequate (Dollaghan & Horner, 2011). Diagnosis should include published tests in both languages if possible, spontaneous and elicited language samples in various settings with differing partners, and dynamic assessment procedures that are more open-ended and include descriptions of a child's use of both English and the child's first language. In dynamic assessment, an SLP modifies procedures to explore the optimal strategies to enhance a child's performance. Dynamic assessment can provide a systematic way to measure learning processes and learning outcomes (Peña, Gillam, & Bedore, 2014).

Referral and Screening

Referral for a communication evaluation may occur at any point in an individual's lifespan. Children, such as those with identifiable syndromes or those who are at risk for developing LI, might be referred at birth or in early infancy; those with LD might go undetected until they begin school; and those with TBI may be referred at the age when injury occurs. Although parents can be effective referral sources for children with more severe language problems, they are less reliable in identifying mild impairment (Conti-Ramsden et al., 2006). Instead, referral may come from a health care professional, such as the family physician.

In a public school, an SLP may decide to test a child on the basis of results of screening testing or teacher referral. Screening tests, used to determine the presence or absence of language problems, are routinely administered to all kindergarten and first-grade students. Screening tests must be chosen and administered very carefully. Even though a test is generally considered nonbiased, some items should be interpreted with caution because they may be problematic for children with differing cultural or linguistic backgrounds (Qi et al., 2003).

Children who are late talkers but appear to have recovered by age 4 are at modest risk for continuing difficulties in elementary school. This risk is no greater than that for other 4-year-olds who have similar language performance at age 4. This indicates that the language of all children in the low normal range at age 4 should be monitored in an ongoing way, including periodic screening (Dale, McMillan, Hayiou-Thomas, & Plomin, 2014).

Surveys and parental questionnaires are also effective diagnostic tools. They compare favorably with other language measures and are part of a thorough well-rounded assessment (Patterson, 2000; Rescorla & Alley, 2001; Thal et al., 2000).

In some settings, an interdisciplinary team of child specialists may handle referral and subsequent evaluation. The nature of many of the disorders mentioned previously may necessitate input from a pediatrician, a neurologist, an occupational therapist, a physical therapist, a developmental psychologist, a special education teacher, an audiologist, and/or an SLP. An interdisciplinary assessment that includes families as active participants and collaborators has been shown to be effective with young children with ASD (Prelock et al., 2003).

> Information from referrals, questionnaires, and interviews provides needed background from which to begin investigating for possible language impairment and determining what that impairment entails.

Case History and Interview

Administering a case history questionnaire and conducting an interview are the first steps in a formal information-gathering process. In addition to asking questions about birth and development, an SLP asks more specific questions relevant to LI. Questions relate to language development, the language environment of the home, and possible causes for LI. Possible questions are presented in Figure 4.2.

Observation

Language is heavily influenced by the context in which it occurs. It is helpful, therefore, to observe a child using language in as many contexts as possible. For example, a school-based SLP might observe in the classroom while a clinic-based SLP might observe on a home visit, in a waiting room, or during a free-play period between the mother and child. Subsequent testing and sampling can provide additional observational periods.

Figure 4.2 Possible questions for questionnaires/interviews when a language impairment is suspected.

Language Use

How does your child . . .

Ask for information?

Describe things in the environment?

Discuss things in the past, future, or outside of the immediate context?

Express emotions or discuss feelings?

Request desired items?

Request attention?

Direct your attention?

Conversational Skills

How does your child . . .

Initiate conversations or interactions with others? What are the child's frequent topics?

Join in when others initiate?

Get your attention before saying something?

Take turns easily while talking? Are there long gaps between your utterances and the child's responses?

Demonstrate an expectation that you will respond when he or she speaks?

Act if you do not respond?

Ask for clarification when confused?

Respond when asked to clarify?

Demonstrate frustration when not understood?

Relay sequential information or stories?

Respond when you say something?

Express emotions?

Are your child's responses meaningful, mismatched, off-topic, or irrelevant?

Form and Content

Does your child . . .

Know the names of common events, objects, and people in the environment?

Seem to rely on gestures, sounds, or immediate environment to be understood?

Speak in single words, phrases, or sentences? How long is a typical utterance? Does the child leave out words?

Use words such as *tomorrow, yesterday,* or *last night?*

Follow simple directions?

How does your child . . .

Talk about past, present, and future events?

Put several sentences together to form complex descriptions and explanations?

Source: Based on Owens, R. E. (2014). Language disorders: A functional approach to assessment and intervention (5th ed.). Boston: Allyn & Bacon.

Behaviors that are observed vary with the age of the child and the reported disorder. In addition to observing a child's communicative behavior, an SLP is also concerned with a child's interests, topics, style, and methods of communicating. With young children, an SLP will also want to note parental sensitivity to a child's communication attempts and parental responding to these attempts. Figure 4.3 presents some behaviors that might be observed during an assessment.

An SLP must remain focused during observation. This requires that she or he define very carefully the behaviors and/or language features that are observed and fully describe the events preceding and following them. Hypotheses about a child's LI are formed during observation. These are either confirmed or negated during the remainder of the assessment and further modified throughout intervention. For example, one adolescent with ID would scream "Don't hit me" repeatedly. It was observed that this occurred when she was asked a question, but the behavior was inconsistent. It was hypothesized that the type of question influenced the response. The hypothesis was confirmed later in the assessment through careful data collection in which the type of question was modified systematically.

Figure 4.3 Possible behaviors to observe during an assessment of language impairment.

With whom the child communicates

Purposes for the child's communication

Effectiveness of the child's communication:

   Obvious patterns of breakdown

Maturity of the child's language:

   Utterance length

   Verb usage

   Complexity

Relative amounts of initiative versus responsive communication

Relative amounts of nonsocial versus social communication

Responsiveness of caregiver

Turn allocation, relative size of child's and caregiver's turns

Testing

SLPs should consult test manuals carefully and select tests that are sensitive and specific to language disorders. Although standardized, norm-referenced tests are appropriate for determining whether a problem exists, they are less useful in identifying specific language deficits. More descriptive measures allow an SLP to explore a child's strengths and weaknesses. In addition, descriptive results can provide useful information for intervention planning.

After building rapport with a child, an SLP can begin testing. It is best to use a series of testing tasks to ensure that many features of language are assessed. One study found that a combination of tasks using children's books, such as shared story retelling in which a familiar story element is altered and comprehension questions, were effective in identifying 96% of children with LI (Skarakis-Doyle et al., 2008). At the very least, receptive and expressive aspects of language form, content, and use should be tested or sampled in some way.

Tasks should be varied, based on their potential effect on different children. Some children can remain on a given task, while others are highly distractible. Others may be reticent to talk or be withdrawn.

Test methodology varies widely. Children may be asked to form syntactically similar sentences, to make judgments of correctness, to reconfigure scrambled sentences, or to imitate exactly what they hear. They may have to supply definitions, form sentences, or point to words named. All these tasks require different language skills. Unfamiliar tasks may unintentionally prejudice the results against the child. Examples of language test tasks are presented in Figure 4.4. Testing is an atypical situation for most children. Typical language use is most likely to be displayed in language sampling.

During testing, an SLP probes a child's performance to try to identify possible effective intervention procedures. Of interest are strategies that either increase production or result in more correct production of a certain language feature

Figure 4.4 Examples of language test tasks.

Test Procedure	Example
Grammatical completion	I'm going to say a sentence with one word missing. Listen carefully, then fill in the missing word. *John has a dish and Fred has a dish.* *They have two _____.*
Receptive vocabulary	Look at the pictures on this page. I'm going to name one, and I want you to point to it. *Touch (Show me) the officer.*
Defining words	I'm going to say some words. I want you to tell me what each word means or use it in a sentence in a way that makes sense. For example, if I said "coin," you might respond "money made from metal" or "I put my coin in the vending machine."
Pragmatic functions	I'm going to tell you a story and ask you to imagine what the person in the story might say. *Mary lost her money and she must call home for a ride after band practice. She decides to borrow a quarter from her best friend, Julie. Before practice begins, she sits down next to Julie and says _____.*
Sentence imitation	I'm going to say some sentences, and I want you to repeat exactly what I say. Let's try one. *We are going to play ball after school tomorrow.*
Parallel sentence production	Here are two pictures. I'll describe the first one, and then you describe the second one, using the same type of sentence as I use. For example, for this picture I would say, "The girl is riding her bike," and for this one you would say, "The man is driving his car."
Grammatical correctness	I'm going to say a sentence, and I want you to tell if it is correct or incorrect. If it is incorrect, you must correct it. For example, if I say, "Thems is going to the dance," you would respond, "Incorrect. They are going to the dance."

Thought Question 4.4

Did you think initially that testing alone would be sufficient for assessing LI? Can you think of some reasons why testing may not give a total picture of a child's communication?

(Peña et al., 2001). Sometimes called **dynamic assessment**, this probing is invaluable in providing direction for subsequent intervention. Dynamic assessment and techniques that ask children to demonstrate skills that represent realistic learning demands are especially well-suited for children with multicultural or bilingual backgrounds (Peña et al., 2006; Ukrainetz et al., 2000).

Test scores should be interpreted cautiously. For example, the omission of some morphological endings by bilingual children is similar to the error pattern of children with SLI (Paradis, 2005). This can lead to misdiagnosis. In addition, children with language disorders aren't always identified by low scores (Spaulding et al., 2006).

Sampling

Tests do not address all aspects of language. For these reasons, SLPs collect language samples as part of an assessment. Think about how you use language on a daily basis. Most often you use it in conversations. Tests are not good vehicles for assessing conversational skills.

Language is influenced by context. It follows that the context of test taking influences the language a child produces. For some children, test structure decreases performance. This is especially true for young children, children of color, and those with disabilities (Eisenberg et al. 2001).

In sampling, an SLP engages a child in conversation in an attempt to "stretch" language performance and, in the process, reveal possible language difficulties.

For example, the SLP might attempt to get longer, more complex language by asking a child to explain how to do something or to tell about a familiar event. These techniques are especially important for children with ASD who typically do poorly on both standardized tests and less challenging conversational samples (Condouris et al., 2003). Although young children engaged in free play produce more utterances than those telling stories, they produce more complex utterances while telling stories and in conversation (Southwood & Russell, 2004). A variety of language tasks, such as conversation, narration, explanation, and interview, can be included in the sample.

Narratives or stories are especially helpful for exhibiting deficits in school-age children because of the demands on a speaker. In addition, narratives tend to elicit a large number and variety of syntactic structures. The personal narratives of children with LI are often so disordered that these stories negatively impact the social interactions of these children (McCabe & Bliss, 2004–2005). The shorter personal narratives of children with LI often omit key information and violate chronological sequences of events. With adolescents, posing peer-conflict resolution problems or asking for explanations of how to accomplish a task is an effective method for eliciting grammatically complex utterances (Nippold et al., 2007). Figure 4.5 presents two very different types of language samples.

Whenever possible, it is best to collect at least two samples of the child interacting with different partners, locations, and activities or topics (Owens, 2014). For example, parent and teacher perceptions of specific social behaviors in children with ASD do not always agree (Murray et al., 2009). This disparity indicates that specific social behaviors may be context dependent and would suggest collecting data in different communication contexts. Typical performance may also be enhanced if parents or teachers interact with a child in familiar settings. An experienced SLP can also be an excellent conversational or play partner for the child.

Figure 4.5 Examples of different types of language sampling.

Open-Ended	*Structured*
Clinician: I'll play with this farm set, and you can too, or you can pick another toy.	*Clinician:* Well, here's the puppy. What should we say to him?
Child: Want farm.	*Child:* Hi puppy. [GREETING]
Clinician: Oh, you want the farm. We can share. I wonder what we should do first.	*Clinician:* Hi Timmy. I'm hungry. We need to get someone to help us get those cookies.
Child: Open door. Animals come out.	*Child:* You help. Want cookie. [REQUESTING]
Clinician: Okay.	*Clinician:* I wonder how I can reach it.
Child: You be horsie and I man.	*Child:* Get chair. [HYPOTHESIZING]
Clinician: Oh, the farmer.	*Clinician:* Oh, get on the chair. Should I (mumble).
Child: Farmerman chase horsie in barn.	*Child:* Yeah. [DOES NOT REQUEST CLARIFICATION]
Clinician: Oh, he did. I better run fast.	*Clinician:* You want me to (mumble)?
Child: Man go fast in barn.	*Child:* What's that? [REQUESTS CLARIFICATION]
	Clinician: Which do you want, the cookie or the chair?
	Child: Want cookie. No chair. [CHOICE MAKING]

An SLP records the language sample(s) and later carefully transcribes the child's exact words. MP3 players, cell phones, and tablets can be used effectively to collect language samples.

An SLP can analyze a transcript in several quantitative and qualitative ways to determine the extent and nature of a child's language difficulty. Values such as *mean length of utterance (MLU)*, the average number of clauses per sentence, and the number of different words used within a given period of time can be compared to the values for typical children of the same age or developmental level (Johnston, 2001). MLU has been shown to be both a reliable and valid measure of general language development through age 10 for children with SLI (Pavelko & Owens, 2017; Rice et al., 2006). Samples might also provide information on the percentage correct for a language feature, such as past tense *-ed*. More descriptive measures might be the variety of intentions expressed by the child, the conversational styles used, and the types of repair the child uses when the conversation breaks down (Yont et al., 2000). Being as thorough as possible, an SLP attempts to analyze the sample for all aspects of form, content, and use appropriate for the particular assessment. For example, with bilingual clients an SLP might consider **code switching** (the movement between two languages), dialect, English proficiency, and contextual effects in addition to aspects of both languages (Gutierrez-Clellan et al., 2000).

For school-age children experiencing literacy difficulties, an SLP may also want to collect samples of written language. These are discussed in Chapter 6.

 Check Your Understanding 4.3
Click here to check your understanding of the concepts in this section.

INTERVENTION

As you might guess, the complexity of language necessitates using multiple intervention methods. Different intervention approaches target specific aspects of language and employ a variety of procedures. Within limits, we'll explore these diverse approaches to remediation of language impairments.

All aspects of language are interrelated. Changes in one area affect others. For example, learning to use the past tense *-ed* might increase the quality of personal narratives because we usually tell of what happened in the past. In intervention, an SLP should not take such changes for granted and focus solely on one aspect of language. Intervention goals should focus on stimulating the language acquisition process beyond the immediate target (Fey et al., 2003).

Similarly, SLPs should use a variety of intervention techniques. For example, children with ASD can improve social skills better through a combination of peer training and written cues than by either method alone (Thiemann & Goldstein, 2004). The most effective intervention approach for older school-age children and adolescents with deficits in syntax is an integrated one in which naturalistic stimulation approaches are supplemented with deductive teaching procedures. In a deductive method, children are presented with a rule that guides the use of a morphological marker, such as past tense *-ed,* along with models of the inflection (Finestack & Fey, 2009).

Increasingly, SLPs are including other individuals from a child's environment in the training. Without training, day care providers fail to finely tune their language for individual children's needs (Girolametto et al., 2000). In early intervention and in preschool, parents are usually an integral part of their child's language program. Working through parents and other caregivers is different than direct intervention by the SLP with the child, although this is also a program component. Teaching adults to be language facilitators can offer a challenge. Various techniques such as a Teach-Model-Coach-Review instructional approach have been shown to be effective (Roberts, Kaiser, Wolfe, Bryant, & Spidalieri, 2014).

SLPs can help preschool teachers implement intervention both through activities such as dramatic play, art, and storybook reading and through language instruction processes (Pence et al., 2008). Preschool staff being trained to respond to children's initiations, to engage children, to model simplified language, and to encourage peer interactions has a significant effect on children's language production (Girolametto et al., 2003). Even peers can serve as effective tutors or models for children with language impairments (McGregor, 2000).

With the aid of an SLP, these and other care providers, such as parents, may learn how to be better language partners for children. Despite the many demands on and restrictions faced by mothers and children who are homeless, it is possible to teach homeless parents, even those with limited language skills, to use facilitating language strategies during interactions with their preschool children (O'Neil-Pirozzi, 2009).

Target Selection and Sequence of Training

The goal of intervention is the maximally effective use of language to accomplish communication goals within everyday interactions. Although most SLPs would agree on this overall goal, less unanimity exists on the route to achieving it. Decisions on target selection and training vary with each child and each SLP.

> The criteria for target selection will vary with the child, the affected aspects of language, the child's disorder, and the needs of the environment.

Using the same assessment results, SLPs might differ in the targets they select. One SLP might use language acquisition knowledge as a general guide. Another might begin intervention at the point of communication breakdown and frustration for the child. A more classroom-based approach might suggest training for language used within the class. Still another approach might be to begin with language features that are just emerging.

Decisions must also be made about where to begin once the target is selected. Some SLPs prefer to begin with receptive language training and progress to expressive. Others might start with expressive training.

Expressive training may be bottom-up, in which one begins at the symbol level and works toward conversational goals; top-down, in which training is placed within a conversational framework; or a combination of the two. Obviously, the child's abilities are an important determinant of the method selected. To the best extent possible, training should be placed within meaningful communicative contexts.

Evidence-Based Intervention Principles

The needs of children with LI suggest several principles that should guide intervention services. These principles, presented in Figure 4.6, recognize the need to target a child's language abilities in their entirety rather than to focus exclusively on one deficit area. The interrelatedness of all areas of language and the importance of communication context on the form and content of language necessitate a more holistic approach.

Throughout this text, we stress the importance of evidence-based practice (EBP). Although a lack of direct empirical evidence should not automatically rule out a new teaching method, it should be grounds for suspicion (Cirrin & Gillam, 2008, p. 19). Box 4.4 presents recommended practices for language disorders.

Figure 4.6 Principles of language intervention.

1. The goal of intervention should be greater facility of language use in conversation, narration, exposition, and other textual genres in hearing, speaking, reading, and writing.
2. Deficit areas are rarely, if ever, the only areas of language that should be targeted in an intervention program.
3. Select intermediate goals that stimulate a child's language acquisition process rather than goals that focus solely on deficit areas.
4. Select specific goals of intervention based on a child's readiness and need for the targeted goals.
5. Manipulate the context to create more opportunities for the language target to occur.
6. Exploit different genres and modalities to develop appropriate contexts for intervention targets.
7. Manipulate clinical discourse so targeted areas are more noticeable and important in various contexts.
8. Systematically contrast a child's language performance with more mature adult usage by recasting a child's utterances.
9. Provide good models of easily comprehended, well-formed phrases and sentences.
10. Use a variety of verbal and nonverbal strategies to elicit and modify a child's language and to give a child practice in using language to accomplish her or his communication needs.

Note: We are deeply indebted to the fine work of Mark Fey, Steven Long, and Lizbeth Finestack (2003) on which this figure is loosely based. See Fey, M. E., Long, S. H., and Finestack, L. H. (2003). Ten principles of grammar facilitation for children with specific language impairment. *American Journal of Speech-Language Pathology, 12,* 3–15.

BOX 4.4 | **Evidence-Based Practice for Childhood Language Impairments**

General

- More than 200 studies report effectiveness for the vast majority of children.
- Measureable benefits accrue from intervention beginning as early as possible.
- Multiple measures provide the most accurate and valid language assessment.

English Language Learners (ELLs)

- No single measure is adequate for assessment.
- Maintaining the home language enables parents, who may not speak English, to support language development.

Presymbolic Children

- Interactive language intervention in which parents are trained to provide intervention at

home is effective. Long-term and standardized measures have not been applied.

- When compared to SLP-only models, gains for children receiving parent-implemented intervention were significantly higher in both receptive language and expressive syntax.

Children with Autism Spectrum Disorder

- Effective interventions are characterized by early intervention and intensive and individualized instruction.
- Methods used with children with ASD form a continuum from very structured behavioral methods stressing specific cues and reinforcers to more naturalistic play and child-based methods. Both behavioral and naturalistic approaches are

effective in replacing challenging behavior with social interactions, although no method works with all children with ASD.
- Approximately two-thirds of children make significant measureable gains.
- The Picture Exchange Communication System (PECS), in which a picture is used to request items, demonstrates only small to moderate gains in communication and small to negative gains in speech. These gains may be enhanced if others, such as TD peers, are taught to be responsive listeners to preschoolers with ASD.
- Although video-modeling is an effective strategy for teaching some social interactional behaviors, we still need exploration of the efficacy of other methods.

Preschool

- Speech and language intervention are most effective for children with phonological or expressive vocabulary difficulties.
- Parent-implemented language interventions have a significant, positive impact on both receptive language and expressive syntactic skills.
- Intervention of more than 8 weeks results in better outcomes than shorter intervention.
- 70% of preschool children with language impairments make significant measureable gains with intervention.

School-Age and Adolescent

Syntax and Morphology

- Moderately large to large effects follow use of imitation, modeling, or modeling plus evoked production strategies.
- Computerized input strategies alone have not demonstrated extensive benefit as yet.

Semantics and Vocabulary

- A paucity of research exists on effective vocabulary instruction methods for children in early-elementary grades. We do not yet have evidence on the best possible technique.
- Collaborating with teachers on large-group instruction and slowed presentation rate can positively impact vocabulary development.
- Interactive conversational reading strategies may be somewhat helpful for improving receptive and expressive vocabulary.

- There do not seem to be clear differences in outcome between the various methods used to assist children with word finding.

Language Processing (the manner in which children attend to, perceive, discriminate, and recall sounds, syllables, words, and sentences)

- Computer intervention using modified speech stimuli or speech and language games does not improve performance.

Pragmatics and Discourse

- Direct instruction on topic initiation and group entry behaviors can yield moderately large to large effects for students with social communication deficits.
- It is possible to teach social skills to adolescents with ASD. Although several approaches have been used effectively, the data are not sufficient to identify the most effective method of intervention.

Method of Intervention

- Based on very few studies, we can tentatively conclude that preschool and early-elementary children with LI show greater improvement with a collaborative (teacher and SLP) teaching, classroom-based language intervention model than they do in more traditional pull-out intervention.
- Recast sentences are an effective responsive method for grammatical intervention (Cleave, Becker, Curran, Owen Van Horne, & Fey, 2015). In a recast, the SLP modifies the elements in the child's utterance to make it more correct or mature, to change the form of the sentence, or to offer another variation.
- Computer/Internet programs that target cognitive learning rather than specific skills training are effective for working memory and executive function (Peijnenborgh, Hurks et al., 2016).

Source: Based on Bedore (2010); Burgess & Turkstra (2006); Cirrin & Gillam (2008); Cleave, Becker, Curran, Owen Van Horne, & Fey (2015); Dollaghan & Horner (2011); Goldstein & Prelock (2008); Johnson & Yeates (2006); Justice & Pence (2007); Law et al. (2004); McG

Intervention Procedures

Remember that as an SLP, wherever you may work, you are *teaching* communicative skills. SLPs are teachers in the broadest sense. Throwing out questions or cues and hoping for the right response or providing the answer when the child is incorrect is not teaching. Teaching is a systematic analysis of what a child is lacking that results in his or her failure to succeed. As an SLP, you need to break any learning task into the sequential steps required to move from where the child is now to where you want the child to be. Decisions on sequencing should be determined by the complexity of the task, its cognitive and linguistic requirements, and the learning characteristics of the individual child. The SLP enhances teaching by anticipating the types of support that a child is likely to need for success and the types of errors the child is likely to make (Schuele & Boudreau, 2008).

A few basic tenets of good teaching behavior include, but are not limited to, the following:

- *Model the desired behavior for the child*. Modeling may include multiple exposures, called focused stimulation or priming, that occur before the child is required to produce the language feature (Leonard, 2011). In a variation called parallel sentence production, an SLP provides a model of the type of utterance desired. The child is not expected to imitate the model but to provide a similar type of sentence. For example, you might describe a picture by saying "The girl is throwing the ball" and then ask the child to describe a second picture of a boy catching a ball. The need for modeling decreases as the feature is learned. Older elementary school children and adolescents may also benefit from an explanation of the targeted behavior and a rationale for why its correct use is important.

- *Cue the child to respond*. Carefully selected cues, such as the use of the word *yesterday* to signal a past-tense response, serve as aids for the child in conversation. Cues may range from very specific, such as *say*, *imitate*, or *point to*, to more general conversational cues, such as *I wonder what I should say now* to elicit a specific linguistic structure in context or *Maybe Carol can help us if we ask* to elicit a question:

  - Cues may be either verbal or nonverbal. Verbal cues attempt to elicit the language feature by providing a linguistic framework; nonverbal cues use the context of an event to evoke the feature.

  - The SLP should rate each type of cue or prompt from least to most intrusive and supportive (Timler et al., 2007). As intervention proceeds, the SLP works to minimize prompting whenever possible, so the child can become more independent.

- *Respond to the child in the form of reinforcement and/or corrective feedback*. Reinforcement varies from very direct and obvious forms, such as "Good, that was much better," to more conversational responses, such as "That sounds like fun. Tell me more." Conversational responses come in many varieties, including imitating the child, imitating but expanding the child's utterance into a more mature version, replying conversationally, and asking for clarification, to name a few. With some children, especially those with vocabulary deficits, the relationship of the response to the content of the child's utterance has more effect on the child's language than the structural input of the clinician's feedback. In other words, respond to the meaning of what the child said:

SLPs are teachers of language. They must plan their behaviors well to teach without overly relying on less natural strategies, such as drill and the use of edible reinforcers.

- Natural reinforcers flow from the training target. The most obvious example is one in which a child obtains a desired object upon responding to the cue "What do you want?" Conversational responses are natural and reinforcing.

- Corrective feedback may range from a gentle reminder to an instruction. For example, an SLP might recast a sentence. If the child says, "Boy eating cookie," and the target is use of the auxiliary verb *be*, the SLP might recast the sentence as "He *is* eating" or "The boy *is eating* the cookie." Children with SLI and low MLU scores benefit most from responses in which the child is prompted to attempt the structure prior to the adult's recast (Yoder et al., 2011).

- In general, as a language feature is produced more correctly by a child, an SLP relies less on these direct forms. When a language feature is correct most of the time, conversational feedback, such as "What?" or "I don't understand" may be sufficient to cause the child to self-correct the few errors made.

- *Plan for generalization of the learned feature to the everyday use environment of the child.* SLPs can help with generalization by selecting training targets that are highly likely to occur in the child's everyday communication and by including elements of the everyday use environment in the training, such as familiar locations, people, and objects. Parents are often included in the training of young children, whereas teachers may be involved in the intervention of school-age children and adolescents.

Although it may seem counterintuitive, with some intervention targets, such as verb endings, children with LI tend to generalize rules better if they are presented with a wide variety of verbs rather than a restricted set that they hear over and over (Plante, Ogilvie, Vance, Aguilar, Dailey, Meyers, Lieser, & Burton, 2014). In addition, these children produce more utterances that generalize the learning.

Specific examples of each teaching method are presented in Figure 4.7.

 Video Example 4.4

This video shows an example of one technique called "sentence recasts" or reformulating the child's utterance. https://www.youtube.com/watch?v=SNOk2nxBOhl

Effective language intervention should enhance language and social skills in real-life interactions (Timler et al., 2007). Success occurs when the newly taught language feature generalizes to a child's everyday environment.

Children learn to use language through interactions with many individuals and in varying situations.

Figure 4.7 Examples of teaching methods.

Method Modeling	Example
Focused stimulation	I'll pretend to make a cake first. Watch to see if I make a mistake. I'm *putting* the eggs in the bowl and *taking* them to the table. I'm *cracking* the eggs. Now I'm *beating* the eggs. Next, I'm *sifting* the flour. I'm *adding* the flour to the eggs and *mixing* them. Now I'm *measuring* the sugar and *pouring* it into the mix . . . .
Cuing	
Direct Verbal	
Imitation	Say "I want cookie."
Cloze	This is a _____. She should say _____.
Question	What should I say now? What's this? Which one's this?
Indirect Verbal	
Pass it on	I wonder if Joan knows the answer. How could we find the answer? [TARGET IS FORMATION OF QUESTIONS]
Nonverbal	Not giving child all the materials needed to complete a task.
(Inherent in the activity)	Not explaining how to accomplish an assigned task. Playing dumb.
Responding	
Direct Reinforcement	Good, I like the way you said that. Much better than the last time.
Indirect Reinforcement	
Imitation	*Child:* I go horsie. *Clinician:* I go horsie.
Expansion	*Child:* I go horsie. *Clinician:* I'm going to go on the horsie.
Extension	*Child:* I go horsie. *Clinician:* Yes, cowboys go on horses, too.
Corrective Feedback	Remember, when we use a number like two, three, or more, we say /s/ on the word. Listen. One cat. Two cats.

Intervention through the Lifespan

Targets of intervention vary with the age and language skills of a child. An infant in an early intervention program would have different training targets than an adolescent with mild LD. In contrast, an infant may be receiving some of the same training as an adolescent who has profound ID and is functioning below age 1 year.

Early intervention, especially for children with ID and ASD, can have a very positive benefit. Initial training may target presymbolic communicative skills and cognitive abilities, such as physical imitation, gestures, and understanding of object uses. Parents may be trained to treat their child's behaviors as having some communicative value or to interpret consistent behaviors as attempts to communicate. An SLP may attempt to establish an initial communication system by using an augmentative and alternative communication system (AAC) such as gesturing, a communication board, or an electronic device. AAC is discussed in more detail in Chapter 13.

Early symbolic training may focus on receptive understanding, vocabulary acquisition, semantic categories, word combinations, and an array of early intentions. The beneficial effects of treatment for children with delayed language extend beyond the trained targets into other areas of linguistic and overall development. Within a framework of play, shared attention, and naturalistic language teaching, the use of manual signs along with verbal models appears to facilitate development of expressive sign and word communication in some young children with ID (Wright, Kaiser, Reikowsky, & Roberts, 2013).

Children at the preschool language level usually work on language form in both conversations and narratives. Longer utterances, bound morphemes, and early phonological processes may be intervention goals. Vocabulary will continue to be targeted.

Intervention with school-age children may focus on pragmatic skills in conversations and semantic targets, such as figurative language, multiple meanings, abstract terms, and more advanced relational terms, such as conjunctions. Academic skills, including summarizing a reading and different types of writing and note taking, may also be targeted. SLPs may use computerized programs to supplement more face-to-face intervention. Computer use should mesh well with the SLP's overall clinical philosophy and the child's individual needs. Language enhancement can be infused into the curriculum. SLPs may work with the child on both spoken and written language. It is also important for children with LI to learn to navigate the curriculum and understand classroom expectations.

> In schools, SLPs provide individual, group, and classroom language intervention.

Language intervention doesn't end with childhood. Adolescents may continue to exhibit language impairments and be in need of services. Adults with severe ASD or ID will most likely require continued intervention for language and communication deficits and a range of educational and vocational needs. Individuals with LD may require additional support in postsecondary education (Downey & Snyder, 2000; Olivier et al., 2000).

With adolescents, an SLP might focus on multi-clausal or complex sentences, variations in the verb, and expository text which includes persuasive speech and writing, explanations of how to do something, and compare and contrast activities (Scott, 2014). A middle school SLP will need to collaborate with classroom teachers and reading specialists, have knowledge of the Common Core State Standards and the language demands of the classroom, and understand later language development and the reasons for speakers and writers using complex syntax (Nippold, 2014).

 Check Your Understanding 4.4

Click here to check your understanding of the concepts in this section.

SUMMARY

In this chapter, we discussed several types of LI. Although LI is very complex and many-faceted, we have only touched the surface in this chapter. The number of associated disorders, the language features that are affected, and the individual differences among children result in each child's language being very individualistic.

It is very important to remember that each child is a unique case. Given this fact, assessment becomes a search to find and describe a child's individual language abilities. This is accomplished through referral, collection of a case history, interviews, observation, testing, and language sampling.

As a result of the assessment process and through repeated assessment probes during intervention, an SLP attempts to find the most efficient and effective method for teaching new skills. The SLP identifies targets for intervention and trains these through a combination of techniques in various settings with the aid of additional language facilitators.

Obviously, every SLP needs thorough training and extensive experience with LI to serve children with a variety of disabilities. As an SLP, you want to gain a firm foundation of speech and language development, take several courses in LI in both children and adults, and complete practica with both populations.

SUGGESTED READINGS/SOURCES

Nelson, N. W. (2010). *Language and literacy disorders: Infancy through adolescence*. Boston: Pearson.

Owens, R. E. (2018). *Early language intervention for infants, toddlers, and preschoolers*. Boston: Pearson.

Owens, R. E. (2014). *Language disorders: A functional approach to assessment and intervention* (6th ed.). Boston: Pearson.

Reed, V. A. (2018). *An introduction to children with language disorders* (5th ed.). Boston: Pearson.

5

Speech Sound Disorders

LEARNING OUTCOMES

When you have finished this chapter, you should be able to:

- Explain how speech sounds (vowels and consonants) are classified.

- Outline the sequence of normal speech sound acquisition across the lifespan.

- Discuss types of children's speech sound disorders, associated disorders, and related causes.

- Describe the goals and procedures in speech sound assessment.

- Describe approaches and techniques for treatment of articulatory and phonological disorders, including supportive evidence.

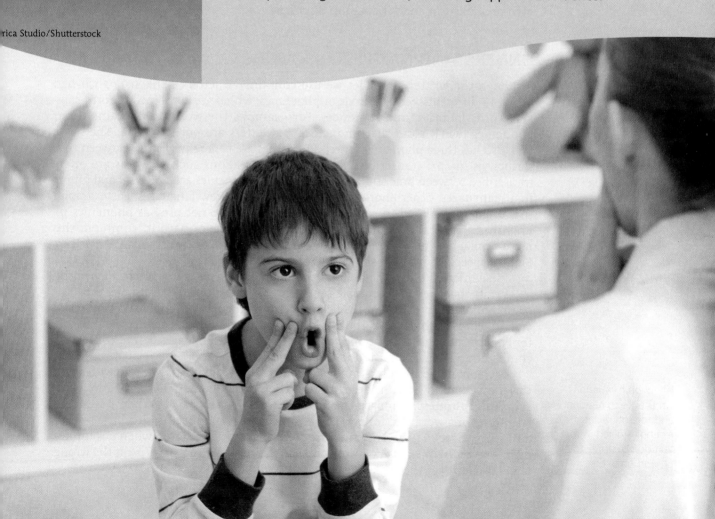

S peech sound disorders in children refer to difficulties related to how speech sounds are used in the language (i.e., phonology), and how sounds of the language are produced (i.e., articulation). Causes of speech sound disorders include impairments in the phonological representation of speech sounds, including knowledge of the rules that govern sound combinations; an inability or difficulty perceiving (i.e., hearing) speech sounds, thereby affecting the ability to acquire and produce those sounds; structural abnormalities (e.g., cleft of the hard and soft palates) that affect the integrity of the speech production mechanism; and/or motor speech disorders such as dysarthria and childhood apraxia of speech that affect motor control pathways governing speech sound production.

Speech sound disorders can be mild in severity, such as when the impairment affects a single sound (e.g., distortion of /r/), to more severe, as when the child deletes all sounds in the final positions of words, making it difficult to understand what the child is saying. To understand speech sound disorders, it is first necessary to have a general understanding of the speech sound system, as well as knowledge of speech sound development. Therefore, our discussion begins here with how speech sounds are produced and classified, followed by a brief overview of normal speech sound acquisition. We'll then distinguish between phonological and articulation impairments, and discuss their potential causes. Finally, we'll describe assessment techniques and evidence-based intervention approaches for children with phonological and articulation disorders.

UNDERSTANDING SPEECH SOUNDS

Although the written alphabet we use contains 26 letters, spoken English has about 43 different speech sounds or phonemes, which are combined to form spoken words, phrases, and sentences. For example, the word *cat* contains three phonemes [kæt]. Note that phonemes and letters are not the same. The word *that* also has three phonemes [ðæt]. Phonemes are generally written between two slashes, as in /p/; transcribed phonemic combinations such as words are often transcribed between brackets, as in [ðæt]. Some phonemes are universal and found in all languages; other phonemes are used in only a few languages. For example, the tongue clicks used in some African languages are not used as phonemes in English. In general, the more phonemes two languages have in common, the more similar the languages sound. The phonemic symbols for standard American English speech sounds are shown in Table 5.1.

In addition to phonemes, which are the building blocks of speech, *phonotactic* rules exist that specify acceptable sequences and locations. For example, the "ks" combination is never used at the beginning of an English word, but it is fine at the end, in words such as *books* [bʊks]. Many Polish and Russian names are difficult for English speakers to pronounce because these Slavic languages permit consonant combinations that are not found in English.

Each phoneme is really a family of related sounds which may be said with some variation but still be considered that particular phoneme. These variations are called **allophones**. Compare the *p* in the words *pot* and *spot*. When *p* is at the beginning of a word and followed by a vowel, it is pronounced with a little puff of air (**aspiration**). However, in most regions of the United States, when *p* is immediately preceded by *s*, it is not aspirated. Still, we recognize both as /p/. If the wrong allophone is used, the spoken words do not sound right.

Allophonic variations contribute to regional and foreign dialects. The examples given in the text do not apply to all English speakers.

TABLE 5.1

Phonemic symbols for standard American English speech sounds

Consonants				Vowels			
Phoneme	Example	Phoneme	Example	Phoneme	Example	Phoneme	Example
/p/	pan	/ʃ/	shed	/i/	eat	/ɔ/	sauce
/b/	boot	/ʒ/	measure	/ɪ/	pit	/ɑ/	father
/t /	t/all	/h/	high	/e/	cake		
/d/	down	/tʃ/	chop	/ɛ/	bed	*Diphthongs*	
/k/	kite	/dʒ/	jump	/æ/	at	*Phoneme*	*Example*
/g/	go	/m/	mat	/ʌ/	cup	/aɪ/	ice
/f/	fan	/n/	noon	/ə/	above	/aʊ/	cow
/v/	vase	/ŋ/	ring	/ɝ/	bird	/ɔɪ/	toy
/e/	thumb	/l/	lamb	/ɚ/	paper		
/ð/	then	/w/	wit	/u/	you		
/s/	sun	/j/	yellow	/ʊ/	would		
/z/	zoo	/r/	rod	/o/	no		

Classification of Speech Sounds

Phonemes are often categorized as either **vowel** or **consonant**. Very generally, vowels are produced with a relatively open or unobstructed vocal tract, and consonants are made with some degree of constriction.

Consonant phonemes may be classified according to which articulators are used (place of articulation), how the sound is made (manner of production), and whether they occur with laryngeal vibration (voicing). Vowels are normally described according to tongue and lip position and relative degree of tension in these articulators. These methods of characterizing phonemes are described next.

> All spoken languages have vowels and consonants. The intelligibility of an utterance is determined largely by the consonants, whereas the sound energy comes primarily from the vowels.

Classification of Consonants by Place, Manner, and Voicing

Consonants are characterized by the degree of constriction or closure somewhere along the vocal tract, referred to as the *manner* of consonant production. The location of this point of closure or constriction refers to the *place* of consonant production. For instance, consonants in which the location or place of constriction occurs at both lips are called **bilabial** sounds, literally meaning "two lips." **Labiodental** consonants are made with the bottom lip and upper teeth in contact. **Interdental** consonants are produced with the tongue between the teeth and are sometimes called **linguadental**. **Alveolar** sounds are made when the tongue tip is touching the alveolar or upper gum ridge. In **palatal** consonants, the center of the tongue is near the hard palate. The rear of the tongue approaches the velum or soft palate in the production of **velar** consonants. When the constriction occurs at the level of the vocal folds, the phonemes produced are called **glottal**.

As previously mentioned, the degree of constriction or closure is used when classifying consonant sounds by *manner*. For instance, complete closure of the vocal tract in which airflow is completely blocked results in the ***stop consonants***

(/p/, /b/; /t/, /d/; /k/, /g/). In the production of stops, air pressure is built up behind the point of constriction, momentarily stopped, and then released, as in the /p/ sound. **Fricatives** (e.g., /s/, /z/; /f/, /v/) are produced with a narrow passageway for the air to pass through, creating a friction-like noise. **Affricates** (e.g., "ch" and "j") begin as stops and then are released as fricatives. The **nasals** (/m/, /n/, /ŋ/) are the only sounds produced with an open velopharyngeal port so that the sound energy comes through the nose as opposed to the mouth. **Glides** (e.g., /w/) occur when the articulatory posture changes gradually from consonant to vowel. **Liquids** include /l/ and /r/ and are produced with an open vocal tract, and are thus considered vowel-like consonants.

Voicing refers to what the vocal folds are doing during consonant sound production. For instance, if the vocal folds are vibrating during sound production, the consonant is said to be voiced. If the folds are not vibrating, the consonant sound is voiceless. The nasals, glides, and liquids are all voiced. The stops, fricatives, and affricates may be voiceless (e.g., /k/, /s/, "ch") or voiced (e.g., /g/, /z/, "j"). Consonants that have the same place and manner (e.g., /p/; /b/) but differ with regard to voicing are called cognate pairs.

Can you describe the place, manner, and voicing features of the consonant sounds in the words "chocolate sundae?"

Classification of Vowels by Tongue and Lip Position and Tension

Vowels are produced when the sound energy produced by the vibrating vocal folds is modified and resonated by the opened vocal tract. The exact sound that is made depends on which part of the tongue is elevated (front, center, or back), its relative height (high, mid, or low), and the amount of tension (tense or lax) in the articulators. Whether the lips are rounded (pursed) or retracted (pulled back into a sort of smile) also influences the sound that is produced. Figure 5.1 is a diagram of American English vowels. In the figure, the higher vowel of the front and back paired vowels and /ɝ/ are relatively tense; all other vowels are lax. High and mid back vowels and the back central vowels are produced with the lips somewhat rounded. All other English vowels are unrounded. All English vowels are normally voiced and not nasal. Exceptions occur when you whisper and when nasal resonance occurs for any number of reasons, including proximity to a nasal phoneme such as /m/ or /n/.

Figure 5.1 Classification of American English vowels by height and frontness/backness of tongue.

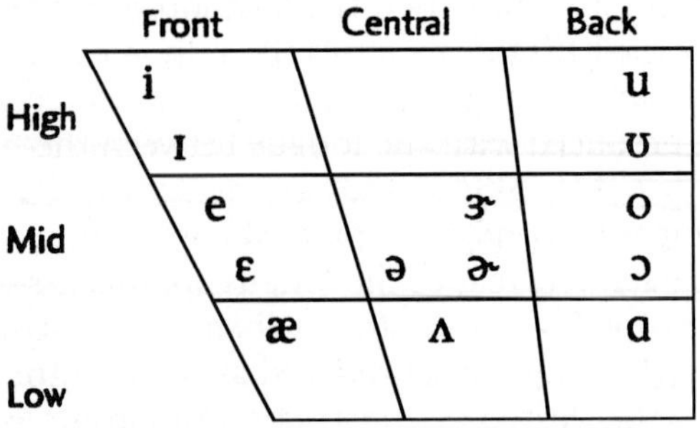

Source: Data from shriberg & Kent (1995) and yavas (1998).

When two vowels are said in close proximity, they produce a special type of phoneme called a **diphthong**. In English, the vowels in the words *sigh*, *now*, and *boy* are diphthongs. *Sigh* contains /aɪ/, *now* contains /aʊ/, and *boy* contains /ɔɪ/. Visit the University of Iowa's interactive phonetics website at http://soundsofspeech.uiowa.edu/ to see how the American English vowels and diphthongs are produced, and to review place, manner, and voicing for the American English consonants. A mobile app is also available for purchase at this website.

 Check Your Understanding 5.1

Click here to check your understanding of the concepts in this section.

NORMAL SPEECH SOUND ACQUISITION THROUGH THE LIFESPAN

Although you gained early control of most of the muscles needed for speech, it took you longer to perfect their movement and to learn to produce all the sounds of American English. Even so, most children can produce all English speech sounds by early elementary school.

CASE STUDY 5.1

Case Study of a Child with a Speech Sound Disorder: Mateo

Mateo, a 4-year-old bright, energetic little boy, was struggling to make friends in preschool. Because his speech was so difficult to understand, he would frequently get frustrated and shut down, preferring not to talk or play with peers. Mateo's preschool teachers also had a difficult time understanding him. He would often use gestures or try to act out what he wanted to say to get his message across to them. They suggested to his mom that he undergo an evaluation by a speech-language pathologist (SLP) to determine if treatment might be helpful in improving his communication abilities.

Case history information collected by the SLP revealed that Mateo had a history of ear infections with intermittent hearing loss. There was also a family history of speech delay on the paternal side. Mateo's uncle received speech therapy for /s/ and /z/ distortions in elementary school. During speech sound assessment, Mateo deleted most sounds in the final positions of words. He also substituted /t/ for /k/ and /f/, and /d/ for /g/ and /v/ in the initial positions of words. Clusters were reduced to singleton sounds (e.g., "spy" became "py"). Three-syllable words were reduced to two syllables (e.g., "banana" became "nana"). Speech

intelligibility in connected speech was less than 30%, even when the topic of conversation was shared. Mateo was determined to have a severe impairment of his speech sound production skills, and speech therapy was recommended. The SLP also made a referral to an Ear, Nose, and Throat (ENT) physician to address Mateo's chronic ear infections.

The ENT recommended bilateral pressure equalization tubes to reduce the risk of future ear infections and hearing loss. After the procedure, Mateo began receiving 1:1 speech-language services twice per week. Within 12 months, Mateo's speech intelligibility improved to 90% in connected speech, although speech sound errors and error patterns continued to persist. By the middle of second grade, Mateo had normalized all speech production errors and was dismissed from therapy.

As you read the chapter, think about:

- Possible explanations for Mateo's speech difficulties
- Phonological patterns (processes) Mateo was exhibiting in his speech
- Specific treatment approaches the SLP might have used with Mateo

Speech Sound Emergence

Although newborns produce predominantly reflexive sounds, such as fussing and crying, and vegetative sounds, such as burping and swallowing, these sounds decrease with maturation. This disappearance is related to the rapid rate of brain growth and to myelination. **Myelination** is the development of a protective myelin sheath or sleeve around the cranial nerves. Myelination is not completed until adulthood.

Initially, newborns cry on both inspiration and expiration. The expiration phase—a more efficient sound production source—gradually increases. Crying helps children to become accustomed to air flow across the vocal folds and to modifying their breathing patterns. Because speech sounds originate at the level of the larynx, this early stimulation is necessary; however, noncrying vocalizations are far more important for speech development.

Noncrying sounds usually accompany feeding or are produced in response to smiling or talking by caregivers. These noncrying vowel-like sounds contain some *phonation* or vibration at the larynx, but the child has insufficient ability to produce full speech sounds.

By 2 months of age, infants develop nondistress sounds called either "gooing" or "cooing." During gooing, infants produce back consonant sounds similar to /g/ and /k/ and middle and back vowel sounds, such as /ʌ/ and /ʊ/, with incomplete resonance.

By 3 months of age, infants vocalize in response to the speech of others. Infants are most responsive if their caregivers respond to them.

Between 4 and 6 months of age, infants begin to imitate the tone and pitch signals of their caregivers. Most infant imitative and nonimitative vocalizations are single-syllable units of consonant-vowel (CV) or vowel-consonant (VC) construction. These sound units that begin around 4 months are called **babbling**. Babbling is random vocal play, and even deaf infants babble. During babbling, infants experiment with sound production.

With maturity, longer sequences and prolonged individual sounds emerge. Children produce increasingly more complex combinations. Sounds are now more like adult speech sounds. As muscle control moves to the front of the oral cavity, we see strong tongue projection in 4- to 6-month-olds. Initially, back consonants predominate in babbling, but by 6 months bilabial sounds, such as /m/ and /p/, are produced more frequently. With age, children's babbling increasingly reflects the syllable structure and intonation of the caregivers' speech.

The consonant-vowel (CV) syllable becomes one of the predominant building blocks in first words.

At about 6 or 7 months, infants' babbling begins to change to **reduplicated babbling**, which contains strings of consonant-vowel syllable repetitions or self-imitations (CV-CV-CV), such as *ma-ma-ma*. Hearing ability appears to be very important. Children with deafness continue to babble, but the range of consonants decreases, and few reduplicated strings are produced.

In contrast to babbling, reduplicated babbling more closely approximates mature speech in its resonant quality and timing. The child is beginning to adapt the speech patterns of the environment. Regardless of the language, infants' vocalizations and later first words have similar phonological patterns. For example, stops (/p, b, t, d, k, g/), nasals (/m, n, ŋ/), and approximants (/w, j/) constitute approximately 80% of the consonants in infant vocalizations and in the first 50 words of Spanish-, Korean-, and English-speaking children.

Between 8 and 12 months, children begin to imitate sounds, but only sounds they have produced spontaneously on their own. Gradually, infants begin to use imitation to expand and modify their repertoire of speech sounds. At about the same time, they begin using gestures, with or without vocalizations, to communicate. Speech during this period is characterized by **variegated babbling**, in which adjacent and successive syllables in the string are purposely nonidentical.

In the second half of the first year, children begin to recognize recurring patterns of sounds in specific situations. The child may even produce sounds in these situations. For example, a child might begin to say *M-m-m* during feeding if this sound is modeled for him or her. In response to caregiver conversations, infants may begin to experiment with **jargon**, or long strings of syllables with adultlike intonation.

Many speech sounds develop sound–meaning relationships. Called **phonetically consistent forms** (PCFs), these sound patterns function as protowords, or "words" for the infant (Dore et al., 1976). The infant notices that adults consistently use certain sound patterns to refer to the same things in the environment.

Word production depends on sound grouping and sound variation. Children adopt a problem-solving or trial-and-error approach to word production. The resultant speech is a complex interaction of the ease of production and perception of the target syllable and its member sounds.

> PCFs are a child's first attempt at consistent use of a sound to represent, or "stand for," something else.

Toddler Speech

At around 12 months of age, you probably produced your first recognizable word. Sometimes a child's word is easily recognizable to others, but some words may be modified by the child for ease of speaking.

When faced with a difficult word, children adopt similar strategies. Armed with the consonant-vowel (CV) structures of babbling and the CV-CV-CV strings of reduplicated babbling, children attempt to pronounce the adult words they encounter. It is therefore not surprising that many words are reduced to variations of a CV structure or another simplification. These adaptations, called phonological patterns (the preferred term) or processes, are presented in Table 5.2.

Toddlers often omit final consonants, resulting in a CVC word being produced as CV, as in *cake* pronounced as *ca*. It is also possible that children will add an additional vowel to form the CV-CV *cake-a*. Multisyllable words may be reduced to one or two syllables, or the syllables may be repeated. For example, *telephone* might become *tephone*, and *baby* might be modified to *bebe*. If the syllables are not duplicated, only the consonants may be, as in *doggie* becoming *goggie*. Consonant blends might be shortened to single consonants, as in *stop* becoming *top*. Finally, one type of sound might be substituted for another. For example, all initial consonants in words might be pronounced as the same consonant, as in, *Go bye-bye* becoming *Bo bye-bye*.

Preschool Speech

Most of the phonological patterns described for toddlers have disappeared by age 4. Consonant blends consisting of two or more adjacent consonants, as in "strong," continue to be difficult for some children, and simplification strategies,

TABLE 5.2

Phonological patterns (processes) of young children

Pattern	Explanation	Example
Final consonant deletion	Reduces CVC structure to more familiar CV	*Cat* becomes *ca*
		Carrot becomes *cara* CVCVC → CVCV
Weak syllable deletion	Reduces number of syllables to conform to the child's ability to produce multisyllable words	*Telephone* becomes *tephone*
		Vacation becomes *cation*
Reduplication	Syllables in multisyllable words repeat	*Baby* becomes *bebe*
		Mommy becomes *mama*
Consonant cluster reduction	Reduces CCV+ structures to the more familiar CV	*Tree* becomes *te Stay* becomes *tay*
Assimilation	One consonant becomes like another, although the vowel is usually not affected	*Doggie* becomes *goggie*
Stopping	Fricatives (/f/, /v/, /s/, /z/, and others) are replaced by stops (/b/, /p/, /d/, /t/, /g/, /k/)	*Face* becomes *pace This* becomes *dis*
Fronting	Velars are replaced with more anteriorly produced sounds	*go* becomes *do ring* becomes *rin*

Development of individual sounds depends on the location in words, frequency of use, and the influence of other speech sounds.

resulting in "tong," may continue into early elementary school. Children who experience continuing phonological difficulties may persist in the use of more immature phonological patterns.

Children continue to master new speech sounds throughout the preschool period. The acquisition process is a gradual one and depends on the individual sound, its location in words, its frequency of use, and its proximity to other speech sounds. A sound may be produced correctly in single words but not in connected speech.

We can make a few generalizations about speech sound acquisition by young children:

- Phoneme acquisition is a gradual process.
- Vowels are easier to master than consonants. Usually, English vowels are acquired by age 3, whereas some consonants may not be mastered until age 7 or 8.
- Many sounds are first acquired in the initial position in words.
- Consonant clusters (e.g., con*sider*; *street*) are not mastered until age 7 or 8, although some clusters appear as early as age 4.
- Some sounds are easier than others to produce and are acquired early by most children. As a group, stops (/p, b, t, d, g, k/), nasals (/m, n, ŋ/), and glides (/w, j/) are acquired first.
- Sounds that are more difficult to produce are acquired later, including fricatives (e.g., /s, /z/), affricates (i.e., "ch"; "j"), and liquids (i.e., /r, l/).
- Much individual difference exists.

Shriberg (1993) examined speech sound mastery in 64 children ages 3–6 years with delayed speech production skills based on spontaneous speech samples, and categorized 24 speech sounds into early-developing, middle-developing, and late-developing groups. This information, referred to as the "Early 8," "Middle 8," and "Late 8," is presented in Figure 5.2. While based on children with speech sound delay, the data were determined to adhere fairly closely to speech sound acquisition data from children without delay (e.g., Sander, 1972; Smit et al., 1990). Additionally, the early, middle, and late speech sound data were more recently replicated in monolingual English-speaking children 3–4 years of age without delay with similar results (Fabiano-Smith & Goldstein, 2010).

Most children can produce all of the English speech sounds correctly by the age of 8. Children with neurological disorders, sensory deficits such as hearing loss, genetic syndromes (e.g., Down syndrome), perceptual problems, or poor learning skills will have difficulty acquiring all the sounds of the language.

School-age Speech

By early elementary school, your phonological system probably resembled that of an adult. A few children will still have difficulty with multiple consonant clusters, such as *str* and *sts*, as in *street* and bea*sts*, respectively.

Other developments, such as **morphophonemic contrasts**—changes in pronunciation as a result of morphological changes—will take several years to master, some extending into adulthood. For example, in the verb *derive* the second vowel is a long *i*, transcribed phonetically as /aɪ/. When we change *derive* to the noun *derivative*, the second vowel is changed to sound like the *i* in *give*, transcribed as /ɪ/. Other contrasts were mentioned in Chapter 2.

Five-year-olds still have difficulty with a few consonant sounds and with consonant clusters. Six-year-olds have acquired most English speech sounds. By age 8, children have acquired consonant clusters, such as *str*, *sl*, and *dr*.

Phonology and Articulation

The correct use of speech sounds in a language requires knowledge of the sounds of the language and the rules that govern their production and combination, called *phonology*. Speech also requires neuromotor coordination to actually say sounds, words, and sentences—termed *articulation*.

To help you understand this distinction, visualize learning a new language such as French. You will be exposed to new words and sound combinations and begin

The distinction between phonology and articulation is often difficult to understand. Articulation refers to the actual production of speech sounds; phonology is knowledge of speech sounds within a language and the ways in which they are combined.

Figure 5.2 Early-, middle-, and late-developing English speech sounds.

The sound ʒ ("zh" in "mea<u>s</u>ure") was excluded from Shriberg's analysis because young children use this sound infrequently in spontaneous conversation.	
Early 8	/m, b, j ("y"), n, w, d, p, h/
Middle 8	/t, ŋ, k, g, f, v, t ʃ ("ch"), dʒ ("j")/
Late 8	/ʃ ("sh"), ð ("th" in "<u>the</u>"), s, z, θ ("th" in "<u>thin</u>"), l, r/

Sources: Based on Shriberg (1993) and Fabiano-Smith & Goldstein (2010)

to grasp the nature of that language's sound system or phonology. But you must also be able to form the words with your lips, tongue, and so on. You might find this very difficult because your neuromotor pathways have been trained to make English words; the inability to coordinate your muscles to produce the words correctly is a problem of articulation.

Phonological impairments are disorders of conceptualization or language rules. Remember that phonology is concerned with classes of sounds and sound patterns within words. For example, English has both open and closed syllables at the ends of words. An **open syllable** is one that ends in a vowel—for example, *hi*; a **closed syllable** ends in a consonant (*hat*). A child who uses only open syllables and deletes all final consonants is likely exhibiting a disorder of phonology. In this example, the child would say *hi* correctly but produce *hat* as *ha*.

Articulation impairments are disorders of production and are therefore motor-based. A child whose only speech error is incorrect production of the /s/ phoneme has a disorder of articulation. Errors typically associated with articulation disorders include:

- Substitutions
- Omissions
- Distortions
- Additions

Substitutions occur when one phoneme is replaced with another. For example, a person who says *shair* for *chair* would be substituting *sh* for *ch*. An omission is the deletion of a phoneme, as in *chai* for *chair*. Distortions occur when a nonstandard form of a phoneme is used. An example of an addition would be *chuh-air* for *chair*.

Distinguishing speech sound disorders as impairments in phonology or articulation can be difficult, especially in young children. For instance, the young child who deletes all final consonants and is said to have a phonological disorder may in fact be unable to motorically produce final sounds. Remember, final sounds are more difficult than initial sounds to produce and acquire. The child's use of only open syllables may in fact be due to an immature or impaired motor system, thus representing a disorder of articulation. It's possible that this same child has an impaired phonological system, along with delayed motor speech skills. In this case, the speech sound disorder represents an impairment in both phonology and articulation.

It's important to remember that young children are learning to acquire the rules of the phonological system at the same time their speech motor abilities are developing. As we talk more about specific patterns and types of errors later in this chapter, think about how such errors could represent impairments in phonology or articulation, especially in young children. In general, however, rule-based errors represent a disorder of phonology, while errors on vowels and prosody, and difficulties with speech production related to weakness, incoordination, or extraneous movements represent motor-based impairments.

 Check Your Understanding 5.2
Click here to check your understanding of the concepts in this section.

ASSOCIATED DISORDERS AND RELATED CAUSES

Speech and language learning is not easy. Words are composed of phonemes that are typically acquired gradually by 8 years of age. When a child is not acquiring speech sounds at the expected rate based on normative data, or when a young child produces errors on later-developing sounds (e.g., distortion of /r/), he or she is said to be *delayed*. However, some researchers argue that these children are actually *disordered* in their speech sound development, since a delay can lead to some aspect of speech or language eventually becoming disordered (Bernthal, Bankson, & Flipsen, 2017). For most children with speech sound disorders, there is no obvious cause or the cause is difficult to determine.

Speech Sound Disorders of Unknown Origin

A classification system proposed by Shriberg and colleagues (2010) to better understand speech sound impairments of unknown etiology considered eight possible subgroups of children. Three subtypes were considered to be forms of speech delay, and were believed to be the result of: 1) a family history of speech or language problems, 2) a history of early and frequent ear infections that involve fluid build-up behind the middle ear, or 3) a personality that makes it more difficult for the child to master speech sound production skills. Children in these subgroups are expected to successfully normalize their speech with treatment.

The next three subtypes of speech disorders of unknown origin are believed to result from motor speech impairments (i.e., childhood apraxia of speech; dysarthria), and are less likely to remediate easily with treatment. The last two subgroups represent children who exhibit distortion errors of later developing sounds (i.e., /s/ and /r/, respectively), perhaps due to the fact that they tried to master these sounds when they were not yet ready. As a result, they habituated and maintained an incorrect production pattern of these sounds through their school-age years, resulting in a persistent speech sound disorder.

Defining subtypes of speech sound disorders of unknown origin in this manner represents only one perspective on the issue, and there is no agreement yet on how best to accomplish this classification. Neither is there agreement on how to differentiate a speech sound delay from a speech sound disorder, given the wide range of behaviors in young children. However, trying to determine a specific cause or causes for the child's speech sound impairment is important in ultimately choosing the most effective treatment approach for the child (Bernthal, Bankson, & Flipsen, 2017).

Lifespan Issues

Approximately 75% of preschool children will normalize their speech sound errors by age 6 with or without treatment (Shriberg, Tomblin, & McSweeny, 1999), and the majority will normalize by age 8. A small percentage, however, will continue to exhibit residual articulation errors past this age despite intervention. These errors can persist into adulthood and usually involve substitution or distortion of /r/, /s/, /z/, or /l/. Such errors may have a negative impact on an individual's academic or professional accomplishments, as well as on personal relationships. Although speech sound production can be modified at any stage of life, speech production patterns become habituated and increasingly difficult to change as we get older.

Correlates of Speech Sound Disorders

As previously stated, the causes of speech sound disorders in most children are not readily identifiable; therefore, researchers have directed their attention to **correlates**, or related factors. Correlation means that two or more things occur together but one does not necessarily cause the other(s).

Nevertheless, correlates may offer some clues to causality that should prompt further research. Figure 5.3 lists some correlates of speech sound disorders in children. In the next few sections, we describe the characteristics associated with a few well-established correlates of phonological and articulation impairments.

Cognitive Impairments

The role intelligence plays in contributing to speech sound disorders has been investigated by researchers for many years. Findings from studies comparing IQ scores within the range of normal (i.e., scores between 85 and 115) in children with and without speech sound disorders indicate a poor relationship between intelligence and speech sound production skill (Bernthal, Bankson, & Flipsen, 2017). On the other hand, findings from studies that have investigated children with impaired intellectual functioning (e.g., Down syndrome) indicate a higher prevalence of speech sound disorders in this population. However, a direct positive correlation between speech sound difficulties and severity of cognitive impairment is still not apparent, particularly in individuals with Down syndrome, indicating the likelihood that other factors (e.g., anatomical differences; impaired motor control processes; poorer short-term memory skills) are contributing to the speech sound disorder (Kent & Vorperian, 2013).

Lifespan Issues

Developmental patterns for babbling in infants with cognitive impairment, such as Down syndrome, are generally similar to that of typically developing infants. However, speech production abilities of cognitively impaired children are

> Most children with disordered articulation and phonology do not exhibit an identifiable physical reason for the problem. The majority of these children will normalize their speech sound errors by age 8.

Figure 5.3 Correlates of speech sound disorders.

History of middle ear infections with fluid build-up
Hearing loss
Diminished speech sound perception and discrimination ability
Impaired oral-motor skills
Motor speech deficits
Feeding difficulties
Tongue thrust swallow pattern after age six
Cognitive impairments
Language impairments
Male sex
Family history of speech or language disorders
Low maternal education
Structural abnormalities of the speech mechanism

noticeably different from typically developing children by about age three (Kent & Vorperian, 2013). For instance, children with cognitive impairment show significant variability in the emergence of speech sounds, where earlier-developing sounds such as /b/ may not be produced for the first time until a much later age (e.g., age 8 versus age 3) (Kumin, Council, & Goodman, 1994). Persistent use of error patterns that are more typical of very young children (e.g., final consonant deletion; weak syllable deletion) is also common, with a general tendency toward deletion errors that negatively impact speech intelligibility, which is observed well into adulthood (Shriberg & Widder, 1990). In children and adults with Down syndrome, vowel errors, inconsistent errors, and prosodic abnormalities have also been noted (Bunton & Leddy, 2011; Kumin, 2006; Shriberg & Widder, 1990); these speech characteristics are consistent with motor planning/programming deficits or *childhood apraxia of speech*, discussed later in this chapter.

Successful communication is a challenge for children and adults with cognitive impairment, such as that associated with Down syndrome; quality of life is negatively affected as a result. Treating speech sound impairments using evidence-based techniques, along with use of alternative and augmentative forms of communication, can help ensure success in all aspects of life.

Language Impairments

In a group of six-year olds with a history of impaired speech production skills, 11–15% were also determined to have a language impairment (Shriberg, Tomblin, & McSweeney, 1999). The areas of language most affected appear to be those related to *morphological* and *syntactic* development. Specifically, difficulties with certain verbs forms (e.g., past tense –*ed* and the verb copula "to be"), and decreased use of complex sentence structures (i.e., embedded clauses) have been observed in children with speech sound disorders (Mortimer & Rvachew, 2010; Rvachew, Gaines, Cloutier, & Blanchet, 2005). Differentiating errors as those associated with impaired expressive language versus impaired speech sound production can be very difficult in some children, especially in those who exhibit final consonant deletion. However, it is important to identify children who have concomitant speech production and language impairments, because these children are at greater risk for later academic difficulties compared to those with a speech sound impairment alone (Lewis, Freebairn, & Taylor, 2000).

Lifespan Issues

Although many individuals with language impairments have normal or nearly normal intelligence, speech sound disorders are likely to affect the acquisition of reading and writing skills. Learning to read requires knowledge and awareness of sounds and how sounds combine to form syllables, words, and sentences (i.e., phonological awareness skills). Children with impaired language and phonological disorders may have poor phonological awareness skills (Larrivee & Catts, 1999; Lewis, Freebairn, & Taylor, 2000; Peterson et al., 2009) and are at greater risk for reading, writing, and spelling difficulties. As a result, they may require academic support and the use of various strategies to achieve their full potential.

Male Sex

Speech sound delay tends to be more common in preschool-aged boys (e.g., Campbell et al., 2003; Everhart, 1960), with a 1.5:1 to 3:1 male-to-female ratio (c.f., Shriberg & Kwiatkowski, 1994 and Shriberg et al., 1999). One possible reason for this is the slower rate of maturation of certain cognitive processes (i.e., attention, planning) in boys compared to girls (Naglieri & Rojahn, 2001). Also, brain areas that control the ability to perform certain fine-motor and tactile tasks have been found to be different in males and females (Rescher & Rappelsberger, 1996). This might explain male-female differences in early speech acquisition skills, given that speech production is a fine-motor skill dependent on tactile feedback. And while males are at greater risk for early speech sound delay, other factors combined with male sex, including family history of speech-language delay and low maternal education (i.e., mother did not graduate from high school), pose an even greater risk for speech sound delay in early childhood (Campbell et al., 2003).

Lifespan Issues

Until about age six, girls tend to acquire speech sounds at a slightly earlier age compared to boys (Smit et al., 1990). Recent studies have also shown that girls use gestures coupled with speech combinations sooner than boys (i.e., approximately 16 months of age for girls versus 19 months of age for boys) (Özçalskan & Goldin-Meadow, 2010). Many tests for articulation and phonology have separate normative data for males and females to account for differences in speech sound acquisition rate in early childhood. However, the differences between boys and girls ultimately disappear as children get older (Bernthal, Bankson, & Flipsen, 2017).

Hearing Loss

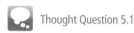

Thought Question 5.1

How does speech differ for someone who has congenital deafness versus someone who became deaf later in life? Why?

Because hearing is the primary way in which we acquire the speech sounds of a language, it is not surprising that children who are hard of hearing or deaf exhibit speech sound disorders. Hearing loss not only impairs a child's ability to hear others, but also affects the ability to monitor his/her own speech production, which is necessary to adequately acquire the sounds of the language. It must be recognized that phonology will not be impaired alone, but all aspects of speech, including voice quality, pitch, rate, and rhythm, will similarly be affected. Although an exact relationship between type and degree of hearing loss and speech cannot be made, certain patterns are frequently observed. Speech sound errors produced by deaf children are described in Table 5.3.

TABLE 5.3

Typical speech sound errors in children who are deaf

Sound Substitution Pattern	Examples
Voiced for voiceless sounds	*see* → *zee* [zi]
	can → *gan* [gæq]
Nasal for oral consonants	*dog* → *nong* [nɔŋ]
Sounds with easy tactile perception for those difficult to perceive	*run* → *wun* [wʌn]
Tense vowels for lax vowels	*sick* → *seek* [sik]
Diphthongs for vowels	*miss* → *mice* [maɪs]
Vowels for diphthongs	*child* → *chilled* [tʃɪld]

Sources: Based on Bernthal, Bankson, & Flipsen (2017) and Calvert (1982).

Lifespan Issues

The age at onset and the degree and type of hearing loss influence the nature of the speech sound disorder. Individuals who are born deaf or with severe hearing impairment typically have poorer speech than those who lose hearing later in life. Speech deteriorates over time, however, for those who are initially hearing and become hard of hearing or deaf later in life. Speech sound production can be enhanced by the use of hearing aids for individuals with some hearing, as well as appropriate training. (See Chapter 12.) Even the best speech of many adults with deafness is nearly unintelligible to others.

Structural Functional Abnormalities

Rapid and accurate movements involving the jaw, lips, tongue, hard and soft palates, and teeth are necessary for articulatory precision; however, usually only gross abnormalities of these structures can negatively impact speech intelligibility. Individuals are remarkably adept at compensating for most structural abnormalities, even partial or complete surgical removal of the tongue. Severe deformity of the hard and soft palates as a result of clefting is far more detrimental to speech production, however, as discussed in Chapter 8.

Lifespan Issues

Many children born with **craniofacial anomalies**, or congenital malformations of the head and face such as a cleft (i.e., abnormal opening) of the lip and palate, struggle not only with speech sound acquisition, but also with feeding and even breathing. Clefts of the lip are typically surgically closed at 3 months of age, while clefts of the hard and soft palates are closed between 9 and 12 months of age. Additional surgeries are usually necessary later to treat continued difficulties with velopharyngeal closure (discussed in more detail in Chapter 8). High-pressure consonants including stops (e.g., /k, g/), fricatives (e.g., /s, z/), and affricates (e.g., "ch") are often problematic for individuals with cleft palate; distortions of these particular sounds can persist into adolescence and even adulthood. Normal articulation can be expected in about 25% of preschoolers with repaired cleft palate who receive care early on from a qualified team of professionals (Peterson-Falzone, Hardin-Jones, & Karnell, 2010). See Chapter 8 for more detail about individuals with cleft palate.

Dysarthria

The dysarthrias are a group of motor speech disorders caused by neuromuscular deficits that result in weakness or paralysis and/or poor coordination of the speech musculature. Dysarthrias typically affect respiration, phonation, resonance, and articulation. They are described in more detail in Chapter 10. A recent study reported that approximately 90% of children with **cerebral palsy (CP)** exhibit some form of motor speech impairment, ranging from very mild dysarthria to having no understandable speech (Mei, Reilly, Reddihough, Mensah, & Morgan, 2014). CP is a neuromotor disorder caused by brain damage that occurred sometime before, during, or soon after birth (Rosenbaum et al., 2007). The location and severity of brain damage predict dysarthria type(s) and degree of communication impairment. Articulatory difficulties and reduced speech intelligibility

CASE STUDY 5.2

Personal Story of a Child with Motor Speech Disorders

Jack was almost 3 years old when we first met him at the University Speech-Language-Hearing Clinic. He was non-verbal, yet his intelligence and receptive language skills were within normal limits. He also had low-tone in his face bilaterally, but range of motion and strength of his oral articulators was deemed adequate for purposes of speech production. Jack cried whenever he came for speech therapy because he was unable to do what the student speech-language clinician wanted him to, whether it was practicing a particular sound in isolation that was not yet his repertoire, or repeating a simple word like "hi." He was assured that all he had to do was try his best. Because he had childhood apraxia of speech, intensive therapy was needed, so he came for speech three times per week for 30 minute sessions, and practiced a small set of functional vocabulary words and phrases such as "eat," "up," "I want," and "I need." He practiced those few words and phrases for over a year until all vowels and consonants were mastered within each target word.

When Jack's speech production began improving due to therapy and maturation, more complex sentence structures and narrative language skills were practiced while focusing on motor speech production skills. Integral stimulation techniques were used to help Jack correctly produce each word in a sentence; then this was practiced over and over again until all sounds were produced correctly in all words. Prosody, including word stress in multisyllable words along with the correct intonation and smooth flow (non-choppy) of speech within sentences, was repeatedly practiced until it was also produced correctly. Jack underwent tongue thrust therapy at age 7, and then was dismissed from treatment due to gains in his speech and language skills. At that point, Jack was 95% intelligible in connected speech, and exhibited expressive language skills that were within normal limits. Jack continued with school-based treatment for another two years to work on inconsistent errors he was still having with "th" and /str/ consonant clusters in connected speech.

After correcting all consonant errors, Jack returned to the University Clinic to participate in intensive treatment using the Lee Silverman Voice Treatment approach; at that point, he was exhibiting some very mild ataxic dysarthria in which reductions in loudness at times caused some of the syllables in lengthy multisyllabic words to sound like they were being dropped. With increased loudness, however, he did not demonstrate this problem. Jack is now 10 and frequently speaks at University events to share his experiences about the speech-language therapy he received, and the immense progress he made over the years. Jack's hard work and his family's support and commitment contributed greatly to his success.

---

are common problems for children with CP (Mei et al., 2014) Cerebral palsy is discussed in greater detail in Chapter 10.

Lifespan Issues

In CP, the general motor and speech signs are present from early childhood onward. Approximately a third of individuals with CP have average to above-average intelligence; the rest exhibit varying degrees of cognitive deficits. Accompanying deficits may include epilepsy, visual processing deficits, and/or hearing impairment (Cummings, 2008). Although the damage to the brain does not progressively worsen, gross motor function, such as walking, deteriorates over time (Haak et al., 2009). The symptoms of dysarthria also appear to change, becoming more severe in some cases with increasing age (Schölderle et al., 2016).

Childhood Apraxia of Speech

Childhood apraxia of speech (CAS) is a neurological speech sound disorder that affects the ability to plan and program the movement sequences necessary for accurate speech production. It is not the result of neuromuscular weakness

(American Speech-Language-Hearing Association [ASHA], 2007). Before speech is produced, the motor plan/program that specifies all the necessary parameters for accurate production of that utterance (e.g., positioning and timing of the articulators; amount of muscle activation) is accessed in the brain. This enables speech to be produced rapidly yet accurately. If we had to think about how each structure needed to move (i.e., lips, tongue, jaw, vocal folds, respiratory muscles) and with how much force every time we spoke, we might need several minutes to produce a sentence rather than the several seconds that is typical.

Because children with apraxia of speech have impaired motor planning and programming capabilities, they are unable to learn the motor plans/programs necessary for rapid, accurate speech production in the same fashion as unimpaired children. As a result, their connected speech is often highly unintelligible, segmented or choppy, disfluent, and lacking in prosodic variation. Children with severe apraxia of speech with normal cognition and receptive language abilities are often aware that speech is difficult and may initially be unwilling to try to talk because they know they will fail. It is therefore important that you as an SLP build a trusting relationship with the child. It is essential that a child at least attempt to imitate words with an SLP to determine if he or she does in fact have CAS. Specific treatment for children with CAS is discussed later in this chapter.

Although there are no definitive neurological or behavioral markers of CAS, ASHA (2007) has proposed the following constellation of speech characteristics to help guide SLPs in properly diagnosing CAS:

- Inconsistent errors on consonants and vowels in repeated productions of syllables or words
- Lengthened and disrupted transitions between sounds and syllables
- Inappropriate prosody, especially in the realization of word or phrasal stress

In addition, children with CAS often have limited consonant and vowel repertoires, may exhibit groping and/or trial-and-error behaviors, frequently omit sounds or inappropriately add sounds, and produce single words better than they produce running speech (Murray, McCabe, & Ballard, 2014). Although most consider CAS to be a motor-speech disorder because speech is necessary to learn language and linguistic sound representations, children with CAS have concomitant expressive language and phonological impairments also.

Lifespan Issues

Children can be diagnosed with CAS as early as 3 or 4 years of age; however, to make this diagnosis correctly the child needs to attend and focus on the clinician and attempt multiple repetitions of word stimuli. Standardized assessments are available, such as the *Verbal Motor Production Assessment for Children* (Hayden & Square, 1999) and the *Kaufman Speech Praxis Test for Children* (Kaufman, 1995); however, no one test has been shown to be completely reliable or valid with regard to diagnosing CAS (McCauley & Strand, 2008). Strand's 10-point checklist (Shriberg, Potter, & Strand, 2011) provides the 10 speech and prosodic features (e.g., distorted substitution errors; syllable segregation; vowel distortions; increased difficulty with multisyllabic words) that are frequently associated with CAS; any combination of at least four out of the 10 features in three speech tasks indicates the presence of motor planning/programming deficits. Children with severe CAS may initially be nonverbal. Therefore, children may need to rely on other means to help communicate effectively (i.e., augmentative or alternative communication) as they are learning to speak.

Children with normal or nearly normal cognition and receptive language abilities have a good prognosis for verbal communication. However, they may continue to have poor intelligibility throughout the school-age years. They will likely also have difficulties with phonological awareness skills, reading, writing, and spelling. Children with CAS continue to exhibit phonological patterns well past the age at which these should have resolved. They may continue to have difficulties with certain classes of sounds and/or production of multisyllabic words (e.g., umbrella) into adolescence and young adulthood. The Apraxia-KIDS website (www.apraxia-kids.org) provides the latest research in the area of CAS for parents and caregivers of children with CAS.

The most readily apparent difficulties in individuals who persist with motor planning/programming difficulties are prosodic abnormalities. Even if speech is intelligible, they may continue to have a segmented (choppy) speech pattern and/or incorrect word and sentential stress. CAS is a speech diagnosis that changes with maturation and with treatment. A child may present early on with a primary diagnosis of CAS, but this may change as he or she gets older. Some children present with a primary diagnosis of phonological impairment, but may also exhibit some mild motor planning/programming difficulties. It is your job as an SLP to correctly differentially diagnose the child to best determine the child's treatment approach and speech targets (Murray et al., 2015; Strand & McCauley, 2008). Table 5.4, which follows, may be helpful for differential diagnosis of speech sound disorders in children.

TABLE 5.4

Differential diagnosis of phonological and motor speech impairments

	Phonological Disorder	**Motor Speech Disorder (apraxia)**	**Motor Speech Disorder (dysarthria)**
Speech Sound Errors	Consonant substitution and omission errors are common. Vowels are not affected.	Consonant substitution, distorted substitutions, omissions, and additions are common; vowel errors are also common.	Consonant distortion errors due to imprecise articulation are common; vowels may also be affected.
Consistency	Errors are generally consistent; patterns can readily be determined (e.g., fronting; stopping). Single word productions may be better than connected speech.	Errors may be inconsistent; patterns are not usually present early on; patterns may be present as child gets older, but are inappropriate for child's age (e.g., use of fronting at age 9). Unusual patterns may be observed (e.g., initial consonant deletion; backing of front sounds). Errors may quickly improve with practice, even during the evaluation session. Single word productions are better than connected speech. Individual sounds may be produced correctly in isolation, but production of those same sounds in words may be very difficult.	Errors are generally consistent, although single word production is often better than connected speech. Improvements with practice will not occur immediately; even with treatment, articulatory imprecision will likely always be present to some degree.

TABLE 5.4
(*Continued*)

	Phonological Disorder	Motor Speech Disorder (apraxia)	Motor Speech Disorder (dysarthria)
Prosody	Normal	Prosodic abnormalities are pervasive, and often persist even after articulation has normalized following intensive treatment. Segmentation (choppy) of speech, equal and excess stress, lengthened intersegment durations, and incorrect word and sentential stress are common.	Prosodic abnormalities are common and may include equal and excess stress, explosive loudness, slow rate, short phrases, or reduced pitch and loudness variability, depending on dysarthria type.
Strength of the oral musculature	Normal	Normal or near normal. Low tone at rest may be observed, but has minimal impact on speech production.	Weakness or paralysis of the oral articulators may be present.
Coordination of the oral musculature	Normal	Coordination difficulties are common, and trial and error groping (articulators searching for correct position) may be present during speech or nonspeech movements.	Discoordination during speech and nonspeech tasks is common in certain types of dysarthria.

Language and Dialectal Variations

If you are a native speaker of American English and go to another country, such as Greece, to live, you will learn Greek to communicate with those around you. When you speak in Greek, your speech will reveal your American background. You will speak Greek with an "American accent." This is not a speech disorder.

Similarly, if you are from Georgia and move to Massachusetts, you will bring your Georgia regionalism with you. Again, this is not a disorder but a dialectal difference to those in your new environment. Many Americans take pride in their regional and linguistic backgrounds and cherish the cultural diversity that characterizes this country.

In assessing phonological skills, an SLP must guard against over- and underdiagnosis, especially with bilingual and minority dialect speakers (Yavas & Goldstein, 1998). The SLP must differentiate between disordered phonology and that which is simply different due to foreign language or dialect influences. This can be accomplished by doing the following:

1. Recognize cultural differences.
2. Evaluate phonological competence in all relevant languages whenever possible.
3. Select appropriate assessment tools (see McLeod & Verdon, 2014).
4. Use nonstandard assessments often, with the help of bilingual assistants.
5. Use dynamic assessments, which involves systematic assessment of stimulability of sounds in a test-teach-test format (Glaspey & Stoel-Gammon, 2007).

> A person whose speech reflects a regional or foreign language influence may also have a speech disorder. However, the regionalism or foreign dialect in itself is not a disorder.

6. Describe phonological patterns (Scarpino & Goldstein, 2012).
7. Diagnose any phonological disorders that exist (Goldstein & Iglesias, 2013; Yavas & Goldstein, 1998).

The SLP then plans and engages in intervention, as appropriate. If dialect differences are targeted, the SLP must assess the client's attitude toward his or her dialect and the individual's motivation for accent reduction. Some generalizations can be made regarding the speech of individuals from various linguistic and regional backgrounds. Table 5.5 highlights just a few of them.

Characteristics of Articulation and Phonology in Dialectal Variation

It is impossible to describe all the variations in articulation and phonology that reflect non-English or dialectal influences. The first language may interfere with languages that are learned later. For example, in Spanish /d/ and /ð/ are allophones, or variations of the same phoneme, whereas in English these are two

TABLE 5.5

Sample phonological characteristics of American English dialects and non-English language influences on spoken English

Rule	Example
African American English	
Final cluster reduction	*presents → presen*
Stopping of interdental initial and medial fricatives	*they → dey*
	nothing → noting
Deletion of *r*	*professor → puhfessuh*
Appalachian and Ozark English	
Addition of *t*	*once → oncet*
Addition of initial *h*	*it → hit*
Addition of vowel within clusters	*black → buhlack*
Portuguese, Italian, Spanish	
Final consonant deletion	*but → buh*
	house → hou
Cantonese	
Confusion of /i/ and /ɪ/	*heat → hit*
	leave → live
	hit → heat
	live → leave
Spanish	
Confusion of /d/ and /ð/	*they → day*
Devoicing of *z*	*lies → lice*
Affrication of /ʃ/	*shoe → chew*

Sources: Based on Goldstein & Iglesias (2013) and Yavas & Goldstein (1998)

separate phonemes, as can be seen in the words *dough* [do] and *though* [ðo]. Native Spanish speakers, however, may confuse the /d/ and /ð/ and pronounce both words the same way (Yavas & Goldstein, 1998). Some first-language interferences are neutral or positive.

Lifespan Issues

Some adults for whom English is a second (or third or fourth) language choose to modify their foreign accent. Often this desire is based on professional considerations. Teachers of English as a second language and SLPs may contribute to the improvement of English expression and comprehension. However, for adolescents and beyond the articulatory patterns of a first language are often firmly established and are difficult to entirely eliminate. The goal, then, is not to make a nonnative speaker sound like a native, but rather to improve intelligibility and thereby the person's communicative effectiveness.

 Check Your Understanding 5.3
Click here to check your understanding of the concepts in this section.

SPEECH SOUND ASSESSMENT

Comprehensive assessment by an SLP is necessary to determine whether treatment is needed, and, if so, what type of treatment is most appropriate (Bernthal et al., 2017). Formal and informal measures specifically designed to assess speech sound impairments are discussed in the following sections. The goals of speech sound assessment are as follows:

- Describe the speech sound system and determine if it deviates from normal to the extent that treatment is necessary.
- Identify phonological patterns if they are present.
- Determine the impact of speech sound errors or error patterns on communicative effectiveness.
- Identify factors that may relate to etiology or maintenance of the speech sound impairment.
- Determine the intervention approach or approaches to be used, and the behaviors to be targeted during therapy.
- Make a prognosis about the likelihood of change with and without treatment.
- Monitor change over time to determine the effectiveness of treatment; update the treatment plan/approach/target behavior as needed, or discharge from treatment if appropriate (Bernthal et al., 2017).

Disorders of articulation and phonology sometimes, but not always, occur with other communication impairments.

In addition, the case history, interview, hearing screening, and structural functional examination may provide insight into the etiology of a disorder and contribute to predictions of improvement. Collection of baseline data from which to measure change over time with or without intervention is an integral part of the initial assessment. Typical assessment procedures are briefly described and explained in the following sections.

Description of Phonological and Articulatory Status

An SLP should obtain data on several aspects of speech sound production.

Speech Sound Inventory

A speech sound inventory and description of word and syllable shapes are highly appropriate for children who are at a very early stage of development and for others whose speech is markedly unintelligible. A recommended system for listing phonemes is by manner of production and syllable and word position (Grunwell, 1987; Klein, 1998). Table 5.6 shows a speech sound inventory for Pablo, a 4-year-old boy who is receiving speech and language therapy.

> If a client has only one or two speech sound errors and all other phonemes are correctly produced, a statement to that effect is sufficient. A listing of all the correct phonemes is not needed.

Syllable and Word Structure

A list of the CV patterns that have been produced in words suggests their complexity. An SLP might list the word and syllable shapes that are most characteristic of a client's speech, as well as the reductions or simplifications that have occurred. Figure 5.4 provides a list of the words in Pablo's language sample, in both standard orthography and phonetic transcription.

Sound Error Inventory

In all cases, an SLP needs to identify phonemes that a client misarticulates. This list is typically compiled on the basis of formal testing of sounds in words. The *Goldman-Fristoe Test of Articulation-3 (GFTA-3)* (Goldman & Fristoe, 2015) and the *Structured Photographic Articulation Test III-Featuring Dudsberry (SPAT-D 3)* (Tattersall & Dawson, 2016) are two commonly used published tests. Sound errors are reported as **substitutions**, **omissions**, **distortions**, and **additions** in syllable/word positions. For example, if 8-year-old Amanda pronounced *lemon* as *wemon*, the SLP might record:

w/l (I) [meaning *w* was substituted for *l* in the initial position; i.e., at the beginning of a word]

Errors can be compared with norms for the child's age.

TABLE 5.6

Phonemes produced in various word positions by Pablo, age 4 years

Manner of Production	Syllable Initial Word Initial	Syllable Initial Word Within	Syllable Final Word Within	Syllable Final Word Final
Nasals	/m/ /n/ *more, no*	/n/ *nana*	/m/ *Sam-uel*	/m/ *drum*
Stops	/p/ /b/ /t/ /d/ *put, ball, top, drum*	/p/ /b/ /d/ *happy, Toby, lady*		
Fricatives	/h/ /f/ /s/ *house, face, see*	/f/ *coffee*		
Glides	/w/ /j/ *wet, you*	/j/ *yo-yo*		

Note: Words were taken from a spontaneous language sample. Italicized words are exemplars of produced phonemes in given word positions. Production accuracy of the entire word is not suggested.

Figure 5.4 Words in Pablo's language sample in standard orthography and phonetic transcription.

more → [mɔə]	*happy* → [hæpi]	*baseball* → [bebɔ]
no → [no]	*Toby* → [tobi]	*ice cream* → [aɪ tim]
banana → [nænə]	*lady* → [ledi]	*face* → [fe]
Samuel → [sæmu]	*house* → [hau]	*wet* → [wɛ]
put → [pʊ]	*face* → [fe]	*you* → [ju]
ball → [bɔ]	*see* → [si]	*yoyo* → [jojo]
top → [tɑ]	*shoe* → [su]	*light* → [jaɪ]
drum → [dʌm]	*coffee* → [tɔfi]	*balloon* → [bʌju]

The word shapes produced include CV ([no]), CVCV ([jojo]), CVC ([dʌm]), and VCVC ([aɪtim])

The word shapes that were reduced are

CVC → CV	(*put* → [pʊ])
CVCVCV → CVCV	(*banana* → [nænə])
CVCCVC → CVCV	(*baseball* → [bebɔ])
VCCCVC → VCVC	(*ice cream* → [aɪtim])

Phonological Pattern Analysis

Many research studies have shown that targeting a pattern rather than an individual phoneme has the advantage of encouraging generalization of learning to similar phonemes and phonological contexts (Gierut, 1998). Therefore, if an individual has numerous errors it is helpful to identify which phonological patterns are apparent. An SLP may analyze phonological pattern information on the basis of transcriptions of a child's conversational or single-word utterances. Often, SLPs use a published test such as the *Khan-Lewis Phonological Analysis–3* (Khan & Lewis, 2015), which analyzes phonological patterns on the basis of the findings of the *Goldman-Fristoe Test of Articulation–3* (Goldman & Fristoe, 2015). Other published tests for determining phonological patterns include the *Hodson Assessment of Phonological Patterns–3 (HAPP-3)* (Hodson, 2004) and the *Bankson-Bernthal Test of Phonology–2* (Bankson & Bernthal, 1990).

Phonological patterns also may be analyzed by using a computerized program. These systems often save time and provide more detailed information than hand-scored procedures. One example of a computerized phonological analysis program is the Computerized Articulation and Phonological Evaluation System (Masterson & Bernhardt, 2001). The *HAPP-3* noted in the previous paragraph is also available in an updated computerized version called *Hodson Computerized Analysis of Phonological Patterns* (4th edition) (Hodson, 2012). The *Khan-Lewis Phonological Analysis–3* mentioned previously also has computer assistive software that can be purchased at an additional cost.

In the case of Amanda above, if her only phoneme error were /l/ → /w/ (I), this would not be indicative of a phonological pattern; it is a *single* sound substitution, an error of articulation. If, however, Amanda produced /l/ → /w/ (I,M) and /r/ → /w/ (I,M), this *pattern* could be described as gliding for liquids, because /l/ and /r/ are liquids and they were produced as the glide /w/.

 Thought Question 5.2

If you had your own clinic or private practice, which standardized articulation or phonological tests (if any) would you purchase, and why?

Although computer analysis of phonological patterns might save time, once the program is learned the SLP must still understand the nature of the patterns in order to work effectively with the client.

Intelligibility

Speech **intelligibility** refers to how easy it is to understand an individual. Poor intelligibility has a negative impact on communicative effectiveness. Intelligibility depends on such factors as the number, type, and consistency of speech sound errors. The person's voice, fluency, rate, rhythm, language, and use of gesture also contribute to ease of comprehension, and these should be noted. Other factors beyond the speaker include the listener's hearing acuity, familiarity with the speaker, and experience listening to disordered speech, as well as environmental noise, message complexity, and environmental cues. Figure 5.5 illustrates a commonly used subjective way of reporting intelligibility.

A more objective measure of intelligibility is percentage of intelligible words. If speech is exceedingly poor, intelligibility may be measured in terms of syllables or consonants (Strand & McCauley, 1997). A recorded sample of continuous speech is transcribed, and the percentage of intelligible words is computed as follows:

$$\text{Percentage of Intelligible Words} = \frac{\text{Number of Intelligible Words}}{\text{Total Number of Words}} \times 100$$

The percentage of intelligible syllables or consonants is computed in a similar fashion. Intelligibility measures are becoming increasingly common in research and clinical use (Shriberg et al., 1997; Wilcox & Morris, 1999). In general, highly unintelligible speech signals a severe disorder, whereas readily intelligible speech suggests that the disorder may be mild.

Prognostic Indicators

Detailed description of a client's speech provide some insight into the prognosis for improvement with and without therapy. The client's age, severity of the disorder, other medical or concomitant problems, and availability of family support also help predict the client's improvement. For adults, the etiology of the speech sound impairment largely impacts prognosis (i.e., stroke vs. neurodegenerative disease). For children, the consistency of speech sound errors, stimulability for correct production of error sounds, and possibly the ability to discriminate error sounds from target sounds may help determine prognosis.

Consistency

Think about your own speech. If you are reading aloud in front of a class, you are likely to be very careful in how you produce all the sounds of the words. In contrast, when you are speaking casually to a friend, your articulation is probably far less precise. Inconsistency is not uncommon, and it may be a clue to the exact nature of an articulation or a phonological error. Let's go back to Amanda. If her misarticulation of /l/ occurs only when she is in conversational speech and then

Figure 5.5 Subjective descriptors of intelligibility.

1. Readily intelligible even when the context is not known
2. Intelligible with careful listening when the context is not known
3. Intelligible with careful listening when the context is known
4. Unintelligible with careful listening even when the context is known

only at the beginning of words, her speech sound error may be more amenable to change. Lack of consistency, in this case, means that Amanda is capable of producing her error sound in some contexts but not in others, which is considered a positive prognostic indicator.

Ironically, an individual with consistent errors may be easier to understand than someone whose error pattern is inconsistent; consistent errors are therefore also considered a positive prognostic indicator. Inconsistent errors, on the other hand, are problematic for a number of reasons. For one, inconsistent errors make it difficult to predict what the child might be saying in connected speech, since there is no error pattern that can be determined. Also, inconsistent errors are often indicative of motor planning/programming deficits, which are more difficult to remediate than speech sound errors associated with a phonological impairment. Therefore, it is important to assess consistency of speech sound errors, which is achieved by evaluating the client's speech during more than one task and in more than one word position and phonemic context (Bernhardt & Holdgrafer, 2001).

Stimulability

Assessment should always include trial therapy. **Stimulability** is the ability of an individual to produce the target phoneme when given focused auditory and visual cues. Typically, an SLP will say, "Look at me. Listen to me. Now say exactly what I say: _____." The SLP will first prompt correct production of the error phoneme or pattern within the word in which it had been misarticulated. If the client does not correctly imitate the SLP, the prompt is moved to the syllable or phoneme level.

Although stimulability is often a positive prognostic indicator, research studies suggest a more complex relationship. Children who are stimulable may respond more quickly to correction of the target phoneme and may also be more likely to self-correct without therapy than those who are not stimulable. Those sounds for which a child is not stimulable are highly unlikely to change without treatment. However, among children in therapy, those with low stimulability scores often make more progress, especially with untreated sounds, than do those who are more stimulable.

> Improvement in non-targeted phonemes, in addition to those that are taught, is often made when the targets are relatively difficult.

Speech Sound Discrimination

Error sound discrimination is often assessed both externally and internally. **External error sound discrimination**, or **interpersonal error sound discrimination**, refers to the ability to perceive differences in another person's speech. For example, in external discrimination the SLP might ask the client, "Are these the same or different: *wemon—lemon?*" Sometimes two words are contrasted, and the client is asked to point to pictures that can be labeled using either the targeted phoneme or the one that was substituted; for example, shown two pictures, the client is told, "Point to awake. Now point to a lake." **Internal error sound discrimination**, sometimes termed **intrapersonal error sound discrimination**, is the ability to judge one's own ongoing speech. The client may be asked to judge the accuracy of her or his phoneme productions.

The relationship of speech sound discrimination to articulation and phonology remains unclear. Perception of a contrast, such as /r/ or /l/ and /w/, usually precedes production in children who are developing typically (Strange & Broen, 1980). In addition, children who are better at internal discrimination have been reported to have more correct articulations (Lapko & Bankson, 1975). From this, we might conclude that error sound discrimination ability signals a more favorable prognosis than the absence of this ability. Two warnings about phoneme discrimination testing are warranted: (1) Only the error phonemes appear to relate to therapeutic prognosis, so only these should be routinely assessed. (2) Many young children do not understand the concept of same vs. different; therefore, their error sound discrimination is difficult to judge.

Check Your Understanding 5.4

Click here to check your understanding of the concepts in this section.

TREATMENT FOR SPEECH SOUND DISORDERS

If the results of an assessment suggest that treatment is appropriate, an SLP must determine how to proceed. Initial questions to be answered include the following:

> Family members may be enlisted to reinforce treatment goals under the guidance of a speech-language pathologist. Carefully structured homework assignments can provide a client with additional beneficial practice.

- Where will therapy occur? (Clinic, school, or home setting?)
- How frequently will the client be seen? (Once or twice a week or three, four, or five times weekly?)
- How long will the sessions be? (The typical range is 20 to 60 minutes.)
- Will therapy be one-to-one or in a group setting?

Answers to these questions will be related to the facilities that are available, as well as to the needs of the client. In addition to such administrative-type decisions, an SLP must determine the following:

- What are the treatment targets?
- What treatment approach appears most suitable?

Target Selection

The major goal of therapy should be to make the client easier to understand and improve communicative effectiveness. One factor is the frequency of a particular misarticulated phoneme within the language: For example, /ʒ/, as in *treasure* ([trɛʒɚ]), does not occur in many American English words, so it would not normally warrant early attention. However, targets that may generalize to correction of phonological patterns would be extremely helpful in improving intelligibility. If a child exhibits the pattern stopping of fricatives, as in saying *zoo* as [du] and *five* as [paɪb], intervention for correct production of /z/ may generalize to other fricatives, including /f/ and /v/.

A second factor in target selection is likelihood of success. An SLP might initially choose targets that a client will probably master relatively quickly. The best predictors of ease of mastery are stimulability and inconsistency. If the client can produce the target phonemes when prompted to imitate with increased visual and auditory stimulation, this is a favorable sign. In addition, if the client does not misarticulate a particular target in all words or situations, this demonstrates that successful intervention is likely (Miccio et al., 1999).

Some research studies have demonstrated that greater generalization to nontarget phonemes occurs when the targets are more difficult—that is, not stimulable, later developing, and more phonetically complex (Gierut, 1998). The complexity approach is discussed later in this chapter. It is up to an SLP to determine whether early success on a few targets or more long-term progress on multiple phonemes is best for an individual client.

Treatment Approaches

A variety of therapy approaches and techniques exist. An SLP might target one or two phonemes or multiple phonemes at a time. Therapy might focus on phonological patterns of errors, emphasize motor speech production, or target the non-segmental aspects of speech such as rate, rhythm, and stress and intonation. Most SLPs adjust their approach to suit each client and combine procedures to provide individually-tailored therapy. Highlights of select therapy approaches are provided in the next few sections (McLeod & Baker, 2017; Kamhi, 2006b for more details), and the evidence in support of specific approaches or techniques is summarized in Box 5.1.

BOX 5.1 | **Evidence-Based Practices for Individuals with Speech Sound Disorders**

General Intervention

- Approximately 70% of preschool children who receive intervention for speech sound disorders exhibit improved intelligibility and communication functioning.
- Approximately 50% of children who are unintelligible to both familiar and unfamiliar listeners progress so that they are intelligible to all listeners.
- More therapy is equated with more improvement.

Specific Behavioral Treatment Approaches or Techniques

- The *traditional motor* and *sensory-motor* approaches are highly effective for children who have only one or a few sounds in error (e.g., /l/, /r/) and for whom language skills are within normal limits.
- *Dynamic Temporal and Tactile Cueing* (DTTC) has been shown to be effective for a small number of children with severe childhood apraxia of speech. This intensive treatment involves speech production practice sessions two times per day (30 minutes each), 5 days per week for a total of 6 weeks. Replication studies examining the effectiveness of DTTC when used fewer times per week (i.e., three times per week for

60 minutes) showed positive results for some but not all research participants. More research is needed to determine the long-term effectiveness of DTTC.

- The *Lee Silverman Voice Treatment* was shown to be effective in four young children with spastic CP. Improvements in loudness and speech intelligibility were maintained at 6 months follow-up.
- The *complexity approach*, based on the work of Judith Gierut and colleagues, has shown that targeting later-acquired sounds and/or consonant clusters leads to increases in treated and in untreated sounds, both within and across sound classes. Also, using phoneme pairs that are maximally contrasted (i.e., differ by major class distinctions) and that compare two new phonemes (vs. including the child's error sound) also results in greater systemwide changes.
- The steps of *whole language/dynamic systems* intervention used during storybook reading improve phonological performance in some children, but more research is needed. This approach is not suitable for children with severe speech sound disorders who require direct, structured therapy.
- The *cycles approach* targets multiple phonological patterns over an extended period of time and is effective for children who are

(continued)

BOX 5.1 *(Continued)*

highly unintelligible. Three to six cycles of phonological intervention involving 30 to 40 hours of instruction are reportedly necessary for a child to become intelligible.

- The *multiple oppositions approach* is best suited for children who substitute one sound for many different sounds. This approach has been shown to be effective for children who are highly unintelligible, particularly during the early stages of treatment.
- The *Metaphon approach* is aimed at developing the child's metaphonological awareness skills in two phases: teaching awareness of sound

differences, and transferring this knowledge through appropriate use of sound contrasts in words when speaking. Limited evidence is available about the effectiveness of this approach, however.

Source: Based on Bernthal, Bankson, & Flipsen (2017); McLeod & Baker (2017); Murray et al. (2014); Fox & Boliek (2012); Gierut (2009); Gierut (2007); Gierut et al. (1996); Hodson & Paden (1991); Hoffman et al. (1990); Howell & Dean (1994); Jarvis (1989); Maas & Farinella (2012); Maas et al. (2012); Strand et al. (2006); Williams (2000).

Bottom-Up Drill Approaches

Bottom-up drill approaches focus on discrete skills, with progression from the simplest to the most complex movements. Some begin with auditory discrimination training, oral-motor exercises, or isolated sound productions and work up to correct production of the error sound in connected speech (Kamhi, 2006b). No evidence supports the use of oral-motor exercises, however, so these are not recommended. The utility of auditory discrimination training is also not well established, and more research is needed.

In bottom-up drill approaches, the error sounds are targeted one at a time. Speech production practice may involve production of an error sound in isolation or in nonsense words, structured phrases, sentences, or conversational speech. Various ways to establish correct production of an error sound may be used, including phonetic placement (e.g., using a tongue blade to push the articulators into position) or sound shaping (i.e., using a sound the child can produce to help produce the new sound).

When a sound is mastered in the therapy setting, speech assignments are provided to allow the client daily practice of his or her new skills and promote generalization outside the therapy setting. Instruction on self-monitoring of correct speech sound production and/or monitoring by others in a child's environment may also be introduced.

The **traditional motor approach** and **sensory-motor approach** are two well-known bottom-up drill approaches. The traditional motor approach begins with auditory discrimination training (i.e., ear training); establishment of the new sound using sound-evoking techniques (e.g., phonetic placement); production practice with the newly established sound in isolation and in nonsense syllables, words, phrases, sentences, and conversation; and generalization and maintenance practice (e.g., homework assignments, practice in other communicative settings or situations) (Van Riper & Emerick, 1984). The sensory-motor approach is similar, but it does not include auditory discrimination training and begins with production at the syllable level rather than the sound in isolation (McDonald, 1964; Pena-Brooks & Hedge, 2007).

Language-Based Approaches

Language-based approaches integrate the learning of error sounds into meaningful, functional contexts either through play or through the reading and retelling of storybooks. The focus is actually on increasing language and/or narrative complexity without explicit instruction on speech-sound production. Rather, instruction is implicit, or within the context of language learning. Such an approach is not suitable for children who exhibit severe speech delays and require more direct, structured speech practice. Language-based approaches have proven effective for promoting generalization of newly learned sounds to spontaneous speech following successful drill-type therapy (Williams, 2000a).

Phonological-Based Approaches

Children who have multiple speech-sound errors and are highly unintelligible may benefit from phonologically-based treatment that focuses on targeting phonological patterned errors (processes) as opposed to individual sounds. By targeting a phonological process, such as final consonant deletion, many sounds can be practiced at one time, thereby increasing the child's speech-sound inventory and improving speech intelligibility more rapidly.

One of the most well-known and widely used phonologically-based approaches is the *cycles approach* (Hodson & Paden, 1991). A cycle can be one 60-minute session, two 30-minute sessions, or three 20-minute sessions. Only one phonological pattern is targeted at a time, and several cycles may be necessary for each target pattern. Therapy begins with the most stimulable phonological pattern and progresses through multiple cycles until all phonological patterns have been addressed.

Cycles training sessions are highly structured. Each session involves review of the previous session, amplified auditory-perceptual training, and production training of selected targets using drill play. Research has shown that children with severe phonological impairments can become intelligible in less than one year using the cycles approach (Hodson, 2007), and the approach can be modified for use with toddlers (Hodson, 2011).

Another well-known and widely used phonologically-based approach is **minimal pair contrasts**, or the contrasting of phonemes in pairs of words. This is accomplished by presenting the child with two pictured words that differ by one phoneme; one pictured word contains the child's error sound/error pattern and the other is the correct form (e.g., *pig–big*). These production exercises involve having the child produce both words in sentences and asking the child if the sentences make sense (e.g., "The *big* lives on the farm"). This approach has been shown to be effective, especially for children with mild to moderate phonological impairment (Williams, 2000a).

In addition to minimal pair contrasts that differ by one or a few phoneme features, treatment approaches may use phoneme contrasts that differ by many different features, including place, manner, and voicing (e.g., *chop–mop*). These phoneme pairs are called **maximal contrasts**. The **multiple oppositions approach** uses maximal contrast word pairs. This approach is effective for children who substitute one sound for multiple sounds, which results in production of the same word for different words (e.g., "dip" is produced for *chip*, *trip*, *ship*, and *kip*). Word pairs are created to contrast all error sounds at the same time.

Other phonologically-based approaches aim to increase the child's **metaphonological skills**, or the ability to analyze, think about, and manipulate speech sounds (Bernthal et al., 2017; Pena-Brooks & Hedge, 2007). One such approach is the **Metaphon approach**, which is designed to increase the child's active cognitive participation in the remediation of his or her speech-sound disorder. Metaphon theorists believe a child must be aware of his or her speech errors, have a desire to modify them, know the relevant speech targets, and have the neuromotor capability to produce the targets correctly with adequate speed in various speech contexts (Hewlett, 1990).

The Metaphon approach consists of two phases. Phase 1 focuses on expanding the child's knowledge of the sound system of the language, thereby preparing him or her to learn how sounds are produced and how they differ from one another. Phase 2 focuses on transferring this knowledge to communicative situations and teaches the child to self-monitor and correct speech output (Howell & Dean, 1994).

Complexity Approach

It has been argued that *what* is treated in therapy is more important than *how* it is treated (Gierut, 2005). Given that no one treatment approach for articulation or phonological impairments has proven more effective than another, eliminating error sound patterns and increasing the child's speech-sound inventory in a shorter time frame may be a better goal in some cases. The complexity approach involves training more difficult sounds (e.g., teaching a 3-year old to produce /v/, which is not mastered until much later), which then leads to generalization of untreated but less complex sounds (e.g., /f/).

This approach is considered more efficient than other phonological approaches (e.g., cycles), because only a few complex targets need to be trained to promote change in the child's overall speech-sound system (e.g., Gierut, 2001, 2007). The caveat, however, is that it may take longer initially to train children to produce more complex speech targets. As a result, these children may remain unintelligible for longer periods at first, thereby becoming frustrated with their continued lack of communicative effectiveness. Therefore, success of this approach depends on the severity of the child's disorder, his or her frustration level, and the overall goal of therapy (i.e., increase speech intelligibility vs. promote significant changes in the child's overall speech-sound system) (Kamhi, 2006; McLeod & Baker, 2017).

Treatment of Motor Speech Disorders

Two evidence-based approaches are gaining in popularity for use with children with neurologically-based motor speech disorders. One was specifically designed for children with childhood apraxia of speech, and the other was adapted from the adult version used with patients with Parkinson disease for children with dysarthria. These specific approaches are discussed in the next section.

Dynamic Temporal and Tactile Cueing

Dynamic Temporal and Tactile Cueing (DTTC) is an intensive motor-based, drill-type treatment designed for children with severe apraxia of speech (Murray et al., 2014; Strand et al., 2006). Unlike in the bottom-up approach, treatment with DTTC targets include a small number of functional words and phrases. Speech production practice of each word or phrase involves use of techniques that are effective for adults with apraxia of speech; specifically, integral stimulation procedures (Rosenbek et al., 1973; Strand & Skinder, 1999). For instance, a clinician says to a client, "Watch me, listen to me, and do what I do" and then provides various levels of cues (e.g., tactile, simultaneous productions), depending on the client's needs.

In DTTC, the client practices the target words slowly and produces them simultaneously with the clinician at first. In addition, this approach incorporates principles that promote motor learning (e.g., daily, repetitive practice, systematic feedback). The clinician may use tactile cues (e.g., physically maneuvering the child's jaw into the correct position) to help the child achieve the correct starting position for the desired utterance. As the child's productions improve, direct imitation, delayed imitation, and spontaneous productions of target utterances are elicited.

The eventual goal is to have the child produce the word correctly spontaneously, both in and out of the clinic. Five to 10 minutes of home practice daily with family members is also recommended. The rationale for practicing only a small set of words is that it will foster neural maturation of motor planning/programming substrates, thus facilitating future speech motor learning (Strand, 2010; Strand et al., 2006).

 Video Exercise 5.1

Speech Errors Associated with Childhood Apraxia of Speech

Click on the link to a watch a video about speech errors associated with childhood apraxia of speech, and complete an exercise.

Lee Silverman Voice Treatment

The Lee Silverman Voice Treatment (LSVT), discussed briefly in Chapter 8, is an intensive treatment provided four sessions per week, 60 minutes per session, for 4 weeks and was originally designed to increase loudness levels of patients with Parkinson disease. This treatment has since been used successfully on children with CP, with only slight modifications (Fox & Boliek, 2012). Note that SLPs must obtain proper training and certification prior to using this approach with clients. Go to the LSVT website (www.lsvtglobal.com) for more information about how to become certified in LSVT.

 Thought Question 5.3

Do you think iPad apps that target speech production are a good way for kids with speech sound disorders to practice at home? Why or why not?

Computer Applications

Computer programs, games, and apps are available that can be used in conjunction with direct treatment provided by an SLP. These programs provide exercises in both perception and production of speech sound targets, as well as nonsegmental targets (i.e., pitch, duration, and loudness). Computer applications provide an opportunity for daily practice of treatment targets, which is essential to the learning of new skills.

Generalization and Maintenance

Once a client has achieved an acceptable level of correct phoneme production, an SLP must ensure that slippage does not occur and that the new speech pattern becomes habitual. Many SLPs introduce self-monitoring exercises from the very beginning of therapy. Doing so helps clients understand that they are ultimately responsible for their own success. Once an SLP believes that a client is ready for dismissal from therapy, follow-up sessions may be scheduled at progressively longer intervals. If the progress has been maintained over time, the remediation has been effective.

Success of treatment is determined by the application of what has been learned in a clinical setting to everyday life.

 Check Your Understanding 5.5
Click here to check your understanding of the concepts in this section.

SUMMARY

Producing the sounds of a language during speech is a complex process. It involves an inner conceptualization of phonemes and phonotactic rules so that in our "mind's ear" we know how the language we are speaking should sound. Speech production also requires the neuromotor ability to move our articulators to form the desired sounds in a smooth, rapid, and automatic fashion. As children develop spoken language, they typically employ phonological patterns that simplify adult forms. If these persist beyond the expected ages, they may present difficulties. Hearing disorders, cognitive-linguistic impairments, motor-based disorders, and structural abnormalities may contribute to speech sound disorders. Foreign language background and regional dialects contribute to variations in speech. Assessment of articulation and phonology includes a detailed description of the individual's speech sound system, as well as investigation of etiology and determination of prognosis. Intervention strategies may include contrasted phonemes in word pairs, speech production drill practice, and use of a core vocabulary for production practice. The general goal is improved intelligibility in spontaneous speech.

SUGGESTED READINGS/SOURCES

Bernthal, J., Bankson, N., & Flipsen, P. (2017). *Articulation and phonological disorders: Speech sound disorders in children* (8th ed.). Boston: Pearson Education.

Kahmi, A. (2006). Treatment decisions for children with speech-sound disorders. *Language, Speech, and Hearing Services in Schools, 37,* 271–279.

McLeod, S., & Baker, E. (2017). Children's speech: An evidence-based approach to assessment and intervention. Boston, MA: Pearson Educational.

Murray, E., McCabe, P., & Ballard, K. (2014). A systematic review of treatment outcomes for children with childhood apraxia of speech. *American Journal of Speech-Language Pathology, 17,* 1–19.

Murray, E., McCabe, P., Heard, R., & Ballard, K. (2015). Differential diagnosis of children with suspected childhood apraxia of speech. *Journal of Speech, Language, and Hearing Research, 58,* 43–60.

Peterson-Falzone, S. J., Trost-Cardamone, J., Karnell, M., & Hardin-Jones, M. (2006). The clinician's guide to treating cleft palate speech. St. Louis, MO: Mosby.

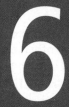

6

Developmental Literacy Impairments

LEARNING OUTCOMES

When you have finished this chapter, you should be able to:

- Explain important aspects of reading and their development
- Characterize reading problems through the lifespan
- Detail assessment and intervention for reading impairment
- Explain important aspects of writing and their development
- Characterize writing problems through the lifespan
- Detail assessment and intervention for writing impairment

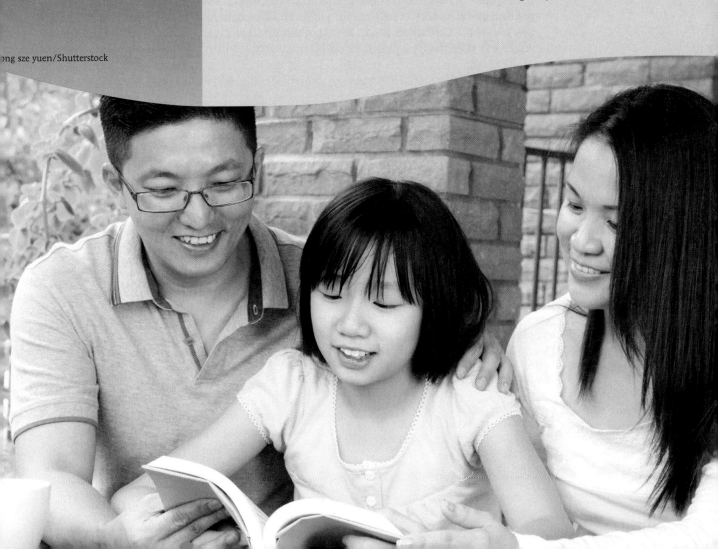

M odern democracy is based on the premise that we are an informed people. In the beginning of the American republic, the best informed were those who were literate. Even in our digital age, being informed means being literate. Using the Internet, texting, and accessing the vast stores of knowledge available requires literacy skills.

Literacy is the use of visual modes of communication, specifically reading and writing. The interrelatedness of aspects of literacy is illustrated by the correlation between reading and spelling ability. Poor readers tend to be poor spellers. But literacy is more than just letters and sounds. Literacy encompasses language; academics; cognitive processes, including thinking, memory, problem solving, planning, and execution; and is related to other forms of communication. Case Study 6.1 presents the narrative of one child with literacy impairment.

Reading and writing are not just speech in print. In addition to the obvious physical difference, reading and writing lack the give-and-take of conversation, are more permanent, lack the paralinguistic features (stress, intonation, fluency, etc.) of speech, have their own vocabulary and grammar, and are processed in the brain in a different manner (Kamhi & Catts, 2005).

The relationship of early oral language difficulties and literacy problems may be more nuanced than a simple transference of problems from one mode of communication to another. There seems to be an interaction between a child's early reading abilities, conversational language abilities, and history of language difficulties (Segebart DeThorne et al., 2010). Conversational language skills contribute a small but significant amount to children's early reading.

CASE STUDY 6.1

Case Study of a Child with Literacy Impairment: Juan

An athletic 7-year-old who loves video games and riding his bike, Juan immigrated to the United States from Colombia when he was 4 years old. With three older sisters, he was the baby of the family and received plenty of attention. His mother reported that his Spanish language development was similar to that of his sisters and that she was not concerned, although her son's speech was sometimes difficult for people outside the family to understand. When the family immigrated, the children began to learn English. As the youngest, Juan learned quickly but experienced some problems with English speech sounds. He received speech and language services in kindergarten, although he was not classified as having a communication disorder.

In first grade, Juan's development of reading was fine initially, but gradually he fell more and more behind his peers. By second grade, he was nearly a year behind his classmates. The speech-language pathologist, reading specialist, and classroom teacher met with the parents to suggest a thorough reading

diagnostic. The evaluation confirmed that Juan was reading below his age, and the reading specialist pledged to redouble her efforts. The speech-language pathologist noted Juan's especially poor performance on phonological awareness (PA) tasks, and with the other team members recommended clinical intervention in this area.

Although she was unsure of the actual factors related to Juan's difficulties, the speech-language pathologist believed that they might be related to his learning of a second language. As if to confirm this hypothesis, Juan quickly excelled in both phonological awareness and reading. As his PA skills improved, his speech sound production also became more accurate.

As you read the chapter, think about:

- Possible explanations for Juan's reading problems
- Possible ways in which the evaluative team could explore different aspects of reading
- Possible explanations for Juan's success

As in other forms of communication, use of literacy presupposes that you can encode and decode, and, more importantly, that you are able to comprehend and compose messages for others. In other words, literacy rests on a language base—and so do literacy impairments.

As you might guess, many of the disorders mentioned under both childhood and adult LI (Chapters 4 and 7) figure prominently in literacy impairments. In fact, as many as 60% of children with LI may experience difficulties with literacy (Wiig et al., 2000). Children with language impairments may be unprepared for literacy learning because they lack emerging literacy skills and a strong oral language base. When compared to children developing typically, preschoolers and kindergarteners with LI may be less able to recognize and copy letters and less likely to pretend to read or write, to engage in daily emerging literacy activities, or to engage adults in question–answer activities during reading and writing.

Academic demands increase as children mature, so literacy impairments don't disappear. You couldn't have read and understood this text as a first grader. As adults, those who experienced literacy deficits in childhood may continue to struggle with reading and writing. One intelligent man in his 50s—known by one of the authors—has continually worked in manual labor positions because his lack of literacy skills has disqualified him from managerial positions.

Literacy deficits vary in complexity and severity. Maybe you are a college student with a literacy problem who has been able to succeed academically by adjusting to, compensating for, or overcoming deficits in your reading or writing. The authors of this text have worked with college students who have had to overcome literacy difficulties.

Although primary responsibility for teaching reading and writing still rests with the teacher and other educational specialists, an SLP is interested in children's language deficits and the ways in which those deficits influence the acquisition of literacy. In recognition of the special skills that SLPs bring to this area, the American Speech-Language-Hearing Association (ASHA, 2001d) recommends that SLPs play a role in literacy intervention.

As a consequence, SLPs are involved in literacy intervention from preschool through adulthood. According to ASHA, SLPs have the following responsibilities:

- Educate both teachers and parents in the relationship between oral language and literacy.
- Identify children who are at risk of having literacy difficulties.
- Make referrals to good literacy-rich programs.
- Recommend assessment and treatment in emerging literacy skills when needed.

> Of necessity, the concerns of SLPs will differ with the maturational level and emerging literacy or literacy abilities of children.

Because children and adolescents with LI are at high risk for literacy disabilities, emerging literacy, reading, and writing assessment should be a portion of any thorough language evaluation, when appropriate. An SLP is concerned with establishing and improving reading and writing skills and helping children and adolescents develop the strong language base needed for both. Assessment and intervention for literacy are also vital parts of any thorough rehabilitative strategy for adults with neurological impairments (see Chapter 7).

As with most other communication impairments mentioned in this text, with literacy impairment SLPs often work as part of a team, collaborating with teachers and reading specialists to design literacy-based programs for vocabulary, language, and thinking skills (Silliman & Wilkinson, 2004). By working with teachers, SLPs

Thought Question 6.1

Many professionals recognize that literacy is not just speech in print form. If this is the case, why is oral language considered so important as a good literacy base?

help children with developmental literacy impairments develop skills needed for meaningful participation in the classroom. Effective collaboration includes curriculum planning, naturalistic language facilitation, and careful teaming of personnel (Hadley et al., 2000). Other members of a literacy intervention team may include a reading specialist, school psychologist, and parent(s).

In the remainder of the chapter, we discuss literacy and associated skills, disorders, assessment, and intervention, first with reading and then with writing. Many language impairments discussed in Chapter 4 also affect literacy acquisition.

READING

Several steps are involved in reading and reading comprehension. Both language and the written context play a role in word recognition and in the ability to construct meaning from print (Gillam & Gorman, 2004).

The first step in reading is **decoding** the printed word, a process that initially consists of breaking or segmenting a word into its component sounds and then blending them together to form a word that is recognizable to the reader. At your level of literacy, visual recognition of a word is generally enough. Individual words take on meaning based on the grammar and context surrounding them. In addition, the reader interprets the print of the page based on her or his linguistic and conceptual knowledge (Whitehurst & Lonigan, 2001). We interpret what we read based on what we know. This is called comprehension. Given these processes, it shouldn't surprise you that a child with an oral language impairment might have reading problems as well. Figure 6.1 is a model of this dynamic process of text interpretation.

Obviously, comprehension requires much more than simply decoding or even interpreting a word in context. As an active reader, you use self-monitoring, semantic organization, summarization, interpretation, mental imagery, connection with prior knowledge, and metacognition or your knowledge about these processes.

In summary, we can say that reading consists of decoding and comprehending text. Although phonological skills are essential for decoding, other areas of language are needed for comprehension (Nation & Norbury, 2005). The reader uses language and experience to interpret the message conveyed by the author. This may give you some idea of why language and literacy go hand in hand. Let's look briefly at three aspects of reading that are of particular interest to SLPs: phonological awareness, morphological awareness, and comprehension.

Phonological Awareness

Yes, it does seem easy to confuse terms. Simply put, phonological awareness is an alertness of phonology; so, yes, it contains the elements of phonology.

Necessary for reading, **phonological awareness (PA)** is knowledge of the sounds and syllables and of the sound structure of words. Phonological awareness includes **phonemic awareness**, which is the specific ability to manipulate sounds, such as blending sounds to create new words or segmenting words into sounds. As you might guess, better phonological awareness, specifically phonemic awareness, is related to better reading skills (Cupples & Iacono, 2000; Hogan & Catts, 2004). In addition, PA skills also are the best predictor of spelling ability in elementary school.

Phonological awareness consists of many skill areas. Not all are required for reading. The auditory ability to determine a word when a phoneme or syllable is deleted (*cart − t = car*), to **blend**, or create a word from individual sounds and syllables, and to compare initial phonemes for likeness and difference are areas of PA that are particularly important for the development of reading.

Figure 6.1 Reading comprehension.

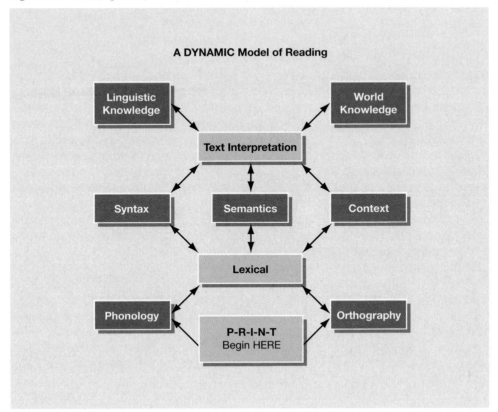

Beginning with print, a reader uses letters and their corresponding speech sounds to decode words that he or she then recognizes based on the reader's lexical or vocabulary memory. The reader combines words with other words and uses syntax, semantics, and context to interpret and comprehend the meaning.

Source: Based on information from "Language and Discourse Contributions to Word Recognition and Text Interpretation," by R. B. Gillam and B. K. Gorman (2004). In E. R. Silliman and L. C. Wilkinson (Eds.), Language and Literacy Learning in Schools (pp. 63–97). New York: Guilford.

 Video Example 6.1

PA provides the basis for reading. Hearing and recognizing sound differences is important. As you watch this video, notice how sound recognition and letter identification, both important prereading skills, are linked.

Morphological Awareness

Although phonological awareness skills are essential for learning to read and write, recent findings suggest that by 10 years of age or even earlier, awareness of and knowledge about the morphological structure of words is a better predictor of decoding ability (Mann & Singson, 2003; Wolter et al., 2009). In fact, morphological awareness is an important factor in literacy performance in early elementary school (Wolter & Pike, 2015). As you moved through the elementary grades and into middle school, morphologically complex words made up an increasing proportion of the words you encountered.

Comprehension

Several levels of text comprehension exist. At the basic level, a reader is primarily concerned with decoding. Meaning is actively constructed from words and sentences and from personal meanings and experiences. Above this level is **critical literacy**, in which a reader actively analyzes and synthesizes information and is able to explain the content. A reader bridges the gaps between what is written and what is meant (Caccamise & Snyder, 2005). At the highest level, **dynamic literacy**, a reader is able to interrelate content to other knowledge through reasoning. Dynamic literacy is comparing and contrasting, integrating, and using ideas to raise problems and solve them (Westby, 2005).

> Each reader must interpret what she or he reads in light of personal experiences and knowledge. In other words, our comprehension will differ based on our own unique self.

A reader's mental representation of meaning is composed of the text and the mental model the reader creates through the comprehension process. Comprehension occurs as a reader combines textual material, text grammar, and his or her own world knowledge and experience.

Reading is a goal directed activity. For example, a reader may be gathering information to be used in a problem-solving task. Knowing what to do and how to do it is called **metacognition**, and two aspects of it are important for reading. One aspect is self-appraisal, or knowledge of one's own cognitive processes. The other is executive function, or self-regulation, and includes the ability to attend; to set reasonable goals; to plan and organize to achieve each goal; to initiate, monitor, and evaluate performance in relation to the goal; and to revise plans and strategies based on feedback. As you read, you form hypotheses about the material, then predict and either confirm or do not confirm your predictions.

Studies with twins indicate that both genetics and the environment are important for reading achievement (Harlaar et al., 2008). In contrast, genetic factors alone seem to play a role in the relationship between early speech and reading (Hayiou-Thomas et al., 2010).

Reading Development through the Lifespan

You may believe that literacy development begins with reading and writing instruction in school. Actually, though, literacy development begins much earlier and continues throughout our lives.

Emerging Literacy

Reading development begins within social interactions between a child and caregiver(s) at around age 1, as parents or others begin to share books with toddlers. Book sharing is usually conversational in tone, with the book serving as the focus of communication. Here's an example:

Adult: This is a book about a . . .
Child: Bear.
Adult: Yeah. And you found him right here. What do bears say?
Child: Grrrrrrrr.
Adult: Um-hm, they growl. Can you find his eye?

Reading the story is secondary to the conversation.

As children mature, some parents engage in **dialogic reading**, an interactive method of reading picture books. When reading, adults encourage their children to become actively involved in the reading process by asking questions and allowing opportunities to become storytellers.

By age 3, most children in the United States are beginning to develop **print awareness**. Early print awareness consists of knowledge of the meaning and function of print, basic concepts concerning the direction print proceeds across a page and through a book, and recognition of some letters. Later-developing skills include recognizing words as discrete units, being able to identify letters, and using terminology, such as *letter*, *word*, and *sentence*. Children with good language skills seem to enjoy reading activities more than children with poor language, and will pretend to read at an early age.

By age 4, children begin to notice phonological similarities and syllable structure in words they hear. This is the beginning of phonological awareness. Four-year-olds also appreciate both sounds and rhymes. Children who have been exposed to a home literacy environment and to print media have better phoneme awareness, letter knowledge, and vocabulary (Foy & Mann, 2003). Children from disadvantaged socioeconomic backgrounds, and those with language impairment and impoverished literacy experiences, may be in danger of not developing these skills (McGinty & Justice, 2009).

Phonological awareness may arise from a child's need to store words in his or her brain with increasingly more detailed representation. This becomes necessary as a child's vocabulary grows, and there are more and more words, some very similar in sound, to store.

Early childhood settings have great potential as sources of emergent literacy experiences for children at risk. Unfortunately, in publicly-funded preschool classrooms serving at-risk children in the United States, the overall quality of literacy instruction is low (Justice et al., 2008). Although many preschool teachers have only limited training in emergent literacy, they can learn to facilitate development of emerging literary skills by using a higher rate of utterances that include print/sound references and decontextualized language (Girolametto et al., 2012).

Although similar language skills contribute to reading across the age span, the relative importance of each changes with literacy stage (Skebo, Lewis, Freebairn, Tag, Avrich Ciesla, & Stein, 2013). The best predictors of kindergarten reading status are oral language, alphabet knowledge, and print concept knowledge, such as how print proceeds across the page and that print stands for words and letters have sounds. These predictors of reading difficulty for children with LI can be estimated in preschool using these predictors (Murphy, Justice, O'Connell, Pentimonti, & Kaderavek, 2016). By middle school, overall language predicts both decoding and reading comprehension at middle school and decoding at high school. Vocabulary predicts reading comprehension at high school. In contrast, among children with speech sound disorders (SSD), vocabulary predicts both decoding and reading comprehension at early elementary school, while among TD children phonological awareness predicts decoding.

By kindergarten additional variables seem to predict reading success by second grade, including rapid automatized naming (RAN) and maternal education level (Catts et al., 2001). RAN is the ability to quickly name a series of items in a category, such as types of clothes or food. Although poor performance on PA tasks is found in children with reading impairments and those with SLI, difficulty with

RAN is more characteristic of children with reading impairments only (De Groot, Van den Bos, Van der Meulen, & Minnaert, 2015).

In general, children develop the skills associated with reading more rapidly at earlier ages than in later ones. Development gradually plateaus and is followed by slow refinement.

In first grade, children are introduced to reading instruction and learn the sound–letter correspondence called **phonics**. A child reads words and links them with meanings stored in memory. Most of the child's effort goes into decoding, leaving little cognitive energy for either comprehension or interpretation. This is one reason we don't assign War and Peace to first-graders.

Phonology (sound) and orthography (letters) are important for early reading, but as reading matures grammar and meaning contribute more. Later, developing knowledge of morphology may aid students in breaking words apart, recombining them, and creating new words (Berninger et al., 2001).

As a child's reading improves, reading becomes more automatic or fluent, especially with familiar words. Fluency is aided by the use of grapheme–phoneme patterns in the child's memory and by analogy, the process of relating unfamiliar words to familiar ones based on similar spelling. For example, *lion* and *lionize* have similar elements.

By third grade, there is a shift from *learning to read* to *reading to learn* (Snow et al., 1999). As language continues to improve, so does comprehension, with a resultant increase in reading fluency.

 Video Exercise 6.1

Emerging Phonological Awareness and Phonics

Click on the link to a watch a video of a young girl who demonstrates phonics and emergent phonological awareness, and complete an exercise.

Mature Literacy

Although all reading begins with the printed word, mature readers like you use very little cognitive energy for determining word pronunciation. At a higher level of processing, a person uses both language and experience to understand text, monitoring automatically to ensure that the information makes sense.

A skilled reader then predicts the next word or phrase and glances at it to confirm the prediction. Printed words are processed quickly, automatically, and below the level of consciousness most of the time. In less than a quarter of a second, your brain retrieves all the information from a word or phrase that it needs to confirm the prediction and form another prediction of the next word or phrase. This process is presented in Figure 6.2.

Rapid and accurate reading is enabled by quick retrieval of orthographic and phonological information along with semantic processes. The reallocation of attention to cognitive and higher language processes is essential for comprehension (Wolf & Katzir-Cohen, 2001).

Mature readers don't simply read the text; they dialogue with it. Reading is an active process in which ideas and concepts are formed and modified, details remembered and recalled, and information checked. Much of this is the unconscious process of the brain partaking of new information.

Establish a habit of reading now. It will serve you well as you mature.

Figure 6.2 Model of mature reading.

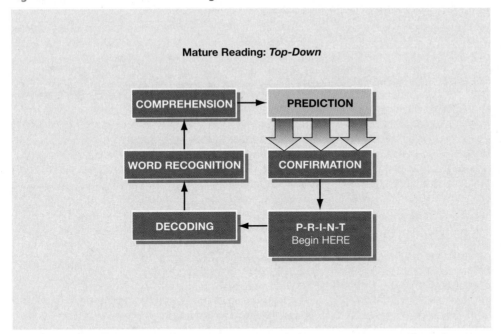

Mature readers use their language skills to predict what words or phrases will appear next in the text, then momentarily glance at the print to confirm their predictions before predicting anew what will follow.

As we mature, the types and purposes of reading change, but we can continue to enjoy the process throughout our lives. Reading skill continues to be strong through adulthood, as long as we exercise our ability and do not experience any neuropathologies, such as those in Chapter 7. Reading is one of the primary ways by which adults increase their vocabulary and knowledge.

 Thought Question 6.2

Why might the child who has not been exposed to books or interactive reading be at a disadvantage?

 Check Your Understanding 6.1

Click here to check your understanding of the concepts in this section.

READING PROBLEMS THROUGH THE LIFESPAN

Risk of reading difficulties is greatest for children with a history of problems in both articulation and receptive and expressive language (Segebart DeThorne et al., 2006). In general, poor reading comprehenders have deficits in oral language comprehension, too, but have normal phonological abilities. In contrast, children who are poor decoders have poor phonological abilities but little or no oral language comprehension difficulties (Catts et al., 2006). The story of a young man with learning disabilities and reading difficulties is presented in Case Study 6.2.

One significant factor in literacy ability and in overall school success is socioeconomic background. As mentioned in Chapter 3, children from low-socioeconomic environments acquire language skills more slowly than those from mid- or high-socioeconomic environments. In addition, these children have

---

CASE STUDY 6.2

Justin, a Young Man with Learning Disabilities

Justin grew up in a midwestern suburb and attended public schools. He's the youngest of four children and the only male. As an adult, he's personable and friendly, works part time, and is attending the local community college. His sisters, especially the next oldest, help him with his homework when possible.

As a preschooler, Justin cared little for books. His language developed more slowly than his sisters', but his parents assumed that he would be fine and that he didn't talk much because his sisters talked for him. Still, his mom enrolled him in preschool to encourage his development. He scored low on his kindergarten readiness test and, although admitted to kindergarten, was later recommended to repeat the experience because of a lack of pre-academic skills needed for first grade. His parents reluctantly agreed.

When he began school, Justin adjusted well, but he quickly began to fall behind other children in both reading and writing. An evaluation at the end of first grade resulted in Justin's being labeled as learning disabled. It was recommended that he remain in a regular classroom and receive additional instruction in literacy. At home, his parents worked closely with him on his reading and written assignments.

Through most of elementary school, Justin saw a reading specialist and a speech-language pathologist several times each week. His speech-language pathologist focused on Justin's language and listening skills and on his reading comprehension.

When Justin entered junior high school, he stopped seeing both the reading specialist and the speech-language pathologist. Instead, his team, including both him and his parents, decided that other measures would be attempted to compensate for his deficits. These included use of a word processor, recording of class lessons, and pre-preparation of lecture notes by his teachers. All through junior and senior high school, Justin met with different teachers after school for extra instruction.

When he graduated, Justin had few plans. He drifted from job to job for nearly a year before his sisters convinced him to apply to community college. Going part-time, he was able to do well in his courses, and he has just been accepted into the physical therapy assistant program. Reading and writing are still difficult, but Justin is determined to do well, and his family members, especially his sisters, are extremely supportive.

---

delayed letter recognition and phonological awareness, and are at risk for reading impairment (Aikens & Barbarin, 2008). They experience less educational success and have the highest drop-out rate, and those who do graduate from high school are 4.3 grade levels behind those of higher SES groups (Palardy, 2008).

The ASHA website (www.asha.org) provides access to many professional articles on reading disorders. For example, click on "Publications" at the top and then click on "The ASHA Leader" in the orange box to the right. Type "Neurobiology" in the search box to access an informative article entitled "The Neurobiology of Reading and Dyslexia" in the September 2007 issue.

Some children have a specific type of learning disability or disorder that is primarily manifested in reading and writing. In the past, this disorder was called *dyslexia*. The fifth edition of the *Diagnostic and Statistical Manual* (DSM-5: APA, 2013), as mentioned in Chapter 4, does away with this term in favor of *specific learning disorder*. Types of specific learning disorders are not labeled but are to be described in a diagnosis. To make this less cumbersome, this book uses the term *SLDL*, for *specific learning disorder in literacy*.

 Video Example 6.2

Watch this video of a short discussion of dyslexia. https://www.youtube.com/watch?v=zafiGBrFkRM

Children with SLDL have poor word recognition or decoding abilities, accompanied by problems with phonological processing. SLDL is a type of learning disability, is neurobiological in origin, and is characterized by difficulties with accurate and/or fluent word recognition and decoding abilities and by poor spelling (Lyon et al., 2003). When we compare children with SLDL to typically developing readers, we find:

- Comparable verbal IQ and/or listening comprehension
- Below-average word reading
- Well-below-average word attack or decoding skills
- Well-below-average phonological processing scores (Sawyer, 2006)

Three distinct types of SLDL have been described, including a language-based disorder that may affect comprehension and/or speech sound discrimination, a speech/motor disorder that may affect speech sound blending and motor coordination, and a visuospatial disorder that may affect letter form discrimination. The language-based disorder is the most common.

Several websites discuss SLDL. The Learning Disabilities Association of America website (www.ldanatl.org) has a brief checklist of symptoms for parents. Simply go to the site and click on "Parents" at the top. Under "Specific Learning Disabilities", click on "Dyslexia" to learn more.

Much more detailed information is available on the MedicineNet website (www.medicinenet.com). Click on "Conditions" at the top, then click on the letter "D," and scroll down to "Dyslexia."

Finally, the website of public service station WETA, LD Online (www.ldonline.org), has a thorough discussion of dyslexia by the International Dyslexia Association titled "Dyslexia Basics." Go to "Getting Started" at the left and click on "Glossary." Once there, scroll down to "Dyslexia," and click on "Dyslexia Basics."

Children with SLI may be similar to those with LD, exhibiting grapheme-phoneme (letter–sound) errors and syntactic, semantic, and pragmatic errors or misinterpretations when reading. Comprehension also may be impaired and may be related to a child's poor vocabulary.

Children with **hyperlexia** have poor comprehension but typical or above average word recognition abilities. Hyperlexia is a near-obsessive interest in letters and words found in some children with ASD. Although these children appear very precocious in their reading ability, they often have poor social skills and extremely limited reading comprehension (Treffert, 2009). Many individuals with ASD have word reading skills that are more advanced than their overall reading comprehension (Church et al., 2000; Diehl et al., 2005; Smith-Myles et al., 2002; Wahlberg & Magliano, 2004).

Causal factors for literacy impairment may be extrinsic or intrinsic to an individual (Catts & Kamhi, 2005). Extrinsic factors may include early exposure to books, reading experience and the manner of instruction. Intrinsic factors may include genetics, vision-based deficits, auditory processing problems, attention deficits, language impairment, and neurological problems. For example, there appear to be differences between the brains of children with SLDL and the brains of typical children (Eckert et al., 2005). Differences have been found in the temporal-parietal region (interior to the ear), in both the left and right linguistic processing areas of the brain, and in the cerebellum (near the brain stem). Neural pathways in the left temporal-parietal area of the brain are important in the development of fluent reading (Deutsch et al., 2005).

Possibly as many as seven chromosomes are involved in various aspects of SLDL (Grigorenko, 2005). Malformations found in the left hemisphere language processing areas and between these areas and the visual processing portions of the brain may be related to these genetic changes (summarized in Galaburda, 2005). Many children at high risk for reading disability have at least one parent with a significantly slower speaking rate than children at low risk for reading disability.

 Video Example 6.3

For a short, 4-minute overview of dyslexia, watch this video. https://www.youtube.com/watch?v=ROPW0R54dgE

As might be expected given their language learning difficulties, many children with ASD have accompanying literacy impairments and uneven development of skills that are predictive of reading. In general, preschool children with ASD are severely delayed in their vocabulary relative to their nonverbal mental ages (Charman et al., 2003). In addition, oral narratives are challenging for these children (Losh & Capps, 2003). As a result, children with ASD and accompanying limited verbal skills often are excluded from standard literacy curricula, under the misguided assumption that they are incapable of learning to read (Koppenhaver & Erickson, 2003).

Similar to what we see in typically developing readers, children with LD acquire reading skills more rapidly in the initial stages and then gradually slow (Skibbe et al., 2008). Even so, these children are substantially below more typical readers by fifth grade.

Phonological awareness is a beginning phase for most readers. Those with phonological disorders, especially perceptual deficits, will find PA challenging. Speech perception seems to be particularly important for the development of PA (Rvachew & Grawburg, 2006).

Most initial reading problems are related to deficiencies in both phonological awareness and processing (Catts & Kamhi, 2005). PA difficulties seem to be related to failure to analyze words into syllables and these, in turn, into smaller phonological units.

In attempting to read, some children with language impairments, especially those with poor phonological skills but average or above-average intelligence, may use memorized word shapes, letter names, or guessing rather than relying on decoding skills. As a result, they are unable to decode unfamiliar words. Without these word attack or decoding skills, by second grade, when formal decoding instruction ends, these children begin to fail.

If a beginning reader has good phonological ability and appears to decode words well, reading comprehension problems may go unnoticed (Nation et al., 2004). Although phonics-based decoding problems often decrease by third grade, comprehension problems may persist (Foster & Miller, 2007). Poor reading comprehension is associated not with PA or phonics (letter-sound matching), but with poor oral language (Nation & Norbury, 2005). If a child isn't comprehending, he or she isn't reading. Some children have difficulty interpreting written narratives because they have poor oral narrative abilities (Naremore, 2001). They may lack the story framework or linguistic skills for telling narratives. The majority of individuals with ASD do not become skilled readers because of their difficulties interpreting both oral and written words (Lanter & Watson, 2008).

Reading comprehension is also dependent on communication, especially conversational skills such as social inferencing and interpersonal reasoning (Donahue & Foster, 2004). Given the low social competence of some children with language impairments, it's easy to see why this aspect of reading might be difficult (Brinton & Fujiki, 2004).

Good readers like you actively guide and control their reading. In contrast, poor readers lack such strategies, reflecting possible deficits in executive function. They may approach reading as a random, unfathomable process. You'll recall that executive function deficit is most evident in children with TBI (traumatic brain injury). In addition, children with ADHD (attention deficit hyperactivity disorder) and LD (learning disability) have been described as inattentive and impulsive, disorganized, unable to inhibit behavior, and ineffective learners, which are characteristics of those with impaired executive function.

As children experience repeated reading failure, they may become frustrated or passive. Lacking persistence and with low self-esteem, they may become apathetic and resigned to failure. In contrast, some poor readers may become aggressive or display acting-out behaviors in the classroom. All these behaviors interfere with further learning and development.

> Competent readers and writers approach the task with a purpose that guides their behavior.

Many children with language impairments are at risk for reading impairment (Hambly & Riddle, 2002; Miller et al., 2001). In general, they:

- Begin with less language and may have difficulty catching up
- Have poor comprehension skills because they lack language knowledge that would enable them to integrate what they read
- Have poor metalinguistic skills
- Possess linguistic processing difficulties

> In case you've forgotten, *metalinguistics* includes the ability to consider language out of context, to make judgments about its correctness, and to understand to some extent the process of using language.

When something goes wrong in the reading process, the result is reading that is less automatic and less fluent. Word decoding or text understanding may be impaired.

As mentioned, reading difficulties do not disappear. They are often related to other language problems. As adolescents, poor readers exhibit vocabulary, grammar, and verbal memory deficits compared to typical readers (Rescorla, 2005).

The more nonmainstream American English (NMAE) dialect a child uses, such as African American English, the poorer that child's reading and overall literacy are likely to be (Charity et al., 2004; Craig & Washington, 2004; Gatlin & Wanzek, 2015; Terry, 2012). Using something other than the majority dialect is a more important factor in reading outcome than socioeconomic background and grade level. Although some dialects may make reading difficult for a child, a dialect is not in and of itself a disorder.

 Check Your Understanding 6.2

Click here to check your understanding of the concepts in this section.

ASSESSMENT AND INTERVENTION FOR READING IMPAIRMENT

As with the speech and language disorders discussed previously, reading impairments require an SLP to thoroughly describe a child's strengths and weaknesses and to determine the appropriate intervention methods. This requires an in-depth understanding of literacy and assessment and intervention techniques.

Assessment of Developmental Reading

In this section we discuss overall assessment, with a more detailed discussion of assessment of phonological awareness, word recognition, comprehension, and executive function. Although SLPs working in preschools do not assess children for emerging reading skills, they may do so if a child fails his or her pre-kindergarten screening. More likely is a scenario in which an SLP assesses an elementary school child for emergent reading skills based on a referral from a classroom teacher or reading specialist.

As mentioned in Chapter 4, assessments begin with an initial data gathering step that may include use of questionnaires, interviews, referrals, and screening. Early literacy questionnaires often ask about the frequency of book reading behaviors, responses to print, language awareness, interest in letters, and early writing. Parental reports of early literacy skills of preschool children with language disorders compare favorably with professional assessments (Boudreau, 2005). Figure 6.3 presents a checklist designed to identify kindergarten and first-grade school children at risk for language-based reading difficulties. No one item on its own indicates a reading problem.

Information can be gathered from interviews with teachers, parents, and the child, and by observation within the classroom. Interview questions should include the child's perceptions of the importance of reading and difficulty with different types of reading, along with the child's self-perceptions. Observation can confirm the child, teacher, and parent responses.

Collaborative reading assessment should include standardized measures, oral language samples including analysis of miscues or mistakes, and written story retelling (Gillam & Gorman, 2004). Formal testing might be accomplished by a school's reading specialist, but an SLP may also wish to give selected tests and to probe specific skills. In a more informal task, a child might be asked to read previously unread curricular materials in an attempt to assess her or his ability to function within the classroom (Nelson & Van Meter, 2002). The child's aloud reading can be recorded for later analysis of the child's miscues. Comprehension can be assessed by using questions, retelling, or paraphrasing.

Phonological Awareness

Phonological awareness assessment is multifaceted and should be accomplished within an overall assessment of reading, spelling, phonological awareness, verbal working memory, and rapid automatized naming (RAN), or the ability to quickly name objects or pictures. In addition to formal testing, an SLP can use informal assessment of rhyming, syllabication, segmentation or breaking words into parts, phoneme isolation, deletion, substitution, and blending or putting word parts together. With school-age children, it is especially important to assess both segmenting and blending.

Word Recognition

Decoding skills, especially knowledge of sound–letter correspondence, is the basis for word recognition. Of interest to an SLP will be decoding of consonant blends, long (*day*) and short (*can*) vowels, different syllable structures, and morphological affixes (*un-, dis-, -ly, -ed*).

Figure 6.3 Checklist for early identification of language-based reading disabilities.

The child . . .

_____ Has difficulty remembering words or names

_____ Has problem with verbal sequences (i.e., alphabet, days of the week)

_____ Has difficulty following instructions and directions, and may respond to a part rather than the whole

_____ Has difficulty remembering the words to songs and poems

_____ Requests multiple repetitions of instructions/directions, with little improvement in comprehension

_____ Relies too much on context to understand what's said

_____ Has difficulty understanding questions

_____ Has difficulty understanding age-appropriate stories and making inferences, predicting outcomes, and drawing conclusions

_____ Frequently mispronounces words and names

_____ Has problems saying common words with difficult sound patterns (i.e., *spaghetti*, *cinnamon*)

_____ Confuses similar-sounding words (i.e., the **Specific** *Ocean*)

_____ Combines sound patterns of similar words (i.e., **nucular** for *nuclear*)

_____ Has speech that is hesitant, contains fillers (i.e., *you know*), or contains words lacking specificity (i.e., *that, stuff, thing, one*)

_____ Has expressive language difficulties, such as short sentences and errors in grammar

_____ Lacks variety in vocabulary and overuses words

_____ Has difficulty giving directions or explanations

_____ Relates stories or events in a disorganized or incomplete manner

_____ Provides little specific detail when relating events

_____ Has difficulty with rules of conversation, such as turn taking, staying on topic, requesting clarification

_____ Doesn't seem to understand or enjoy rhymes

_____ Doesn't easily recognize words that begin with the same sound

_____ Has difficulty recognizing syllables

_____ Demonstrates problems learning sound–letter correspondences

_____ Doesn't engage readily in pretend play

_____ Has a history of language comprehension and/or production problems

_____ Has a family history of spoken or written language problems

_____ Has limited exposure to literacy in the home

_____ Seems to lack interest in books and shared reading activities

Source: Based on information from "The Early Identification of Language-Based Reading Disabilities," by H. W. Catts, 1997, *Language, Speech, and Hearing Services in Schools, 28,* 86–89.

Word recognition assessment should adhere to the following guidelines (Roth, 2004):

- Materials appropriate to the student's age and developmental level
- Various types of tasks to assess different levels of processing
- Use of several measures
- Consideration of a child's cultural and linguistic background
- Demonstration and training of unfamiliar tasks
- Children with emergent literacy skills are not the only ones with reading deficits
- Observation and interpretation of a child's test behaviors

Although traditional assessment procedures stress standardized testing, alternative approaches such as curriculum-based measures and dynamic assessment may be more appropriate for children with LI or from culturally or linguistically diverse backgrounds (Roth, 2004). Dynamic assessment often follows a test–teach–test format, in which a child is assessed for the amount of change she or he can make during the assessment process.

Materials for curriculum-based assessment usually come from the local curriculum and use criterion-referenced scoring, which measures a child against himself or herself over time. In this way, progress is measured without reference to some abstract norm.

Word recognition is more than just the ability to decode a word in isolation. It's important, therefore, that word recognition testing be accomplished with various clues available to the child, such as pictures or different sentence forms, and with words both in isolation and within text. More important than test scores is describing a child's strengths and the strategies used.

When analyzing recorded reading data, an SLP notes all discrepancies in the recorded reading samples. All attempts at word decoding, repetitions, corrections, omitted words and morphemes, extended pauses, and dialectal usages should be noted and analyzed for possible strategies used by the child. Reading errors can be analyzed at the word level by type, such as word order changes, word substitutions, additions, and deletions (Nelson & Van Meter, 2002). The percentage of incorrect but linguistically acceptable words indicates the extent of a child's use of linguistic cues to predict the correct word. In addition, an SLP can note the way in which the child sounds out words (Nelson & Van Meter, 2002).

Morphological Awareness

Textbooks for adolescents and young adults contain a variety of morphologically complex words, such as *regeneration*, *reptilian*, and *strenuous*. Given the importance of derived words for academic success, morphological awareness should be assessed in older children (Nippold & Sun, 2008). At the very least, SLPs should examine adolescent students' understanding of common morphemes such as *-able* (*acceptable*), *-ful* (*powerful*), *-less* (*speechless*), *-tion* (*prediction*), and the like. Actual words can be chosen based on frequency of word use in text and curricular materials.

Text Comprehension

Assessing text comprehension abilities of children is complicated by the many cognitive and linguistic processes involved. At the very least, as an SLP, you or other team members should assess a child's:

- Oral language, with special attention to the child's use of the more elaborate syntactic style used in literature
- Knowledge of narratives and text grammar
- Metacognition (Westby, 2005)

Narrative schemes or the events in a story might be assessed by having a child tell a narrative from pictures or by asking questions about the pictures that relate to the organization of the story. A child's text grammar, consisting of the parts of a story, can be assessed through spontaneous narratives or by retelling previously heard narratives.

Although several norm-referenced tests measure reading comprehension, tests should be supplemented by other measures of a child's ability to identify grammatical units, interpret and analyze text, make inferences, and construct meaning by combining text with personal knowledge and experience (Kamhi, 2003).

Executive Function

Whereas poor readers act as if reading is simply sounding out words rapidly and fluently, good readers expect text to make sense and to be a source for learning information. As a result, good readers read actively and with purpose, constructing mental models and organizing information as they go.

Self-regulation in reading can be assessed in many ways, including (Westby, 2004):

- Interview questions regarding strategies used with different reading tasks
- Verbalizing thoughts called *think-alouds* accompanying reading
- Error or inconsistency detection while a child reads

Errors and inconsistencies can be planted in texts specifically for the assessment.

Intervention for Developmental Reading Impairment

Once the diagnostic data are analyzed and a literacy problem(s) identified, a child and an SLP are ready to begin intervention. Ideally, intervention for developmental literacy impairments is a team effort. The SLP supports the efforts of all the other team members and the explicit instruction of the classroom teacher and reading specialist.

Team members might cooperate in an embedded/explicit model of intervention in which younger children participate both in literacy-rich experiences embedded in the daily curriculum and in explicit, focused therapeutic teaching of reading (Justice & Kaderavek, 2004; Kaderavek & Justice, 2004). The literacy-rich environment might include a message board where children learn to decode an "important" message left daily by the teacher; snack activities in which sounds are embedded in snack names, recipes, music, and print; book and speech sound play; rhyming pictures; and book sharing with the teacher and others (Towey et al.,

Literacy-rich environments are critical for children with literacy impairments.

2004). As little as 8 weeks of one-on-one twice-weekly 15-minute book sharing sessions in which adults read and ask both literal and inferential questions can result in gains in both types of comprehension (van Kleeck et al., 2006).

Effective instruction for reading should include sound and letter processes used in word identification, grammatical processes, and the integration of these with meaning and context (Gillam & Gorman, 2004). Training in phonological (sound) and orthographic (letter) processing together seems to offer a more effective strategy than working on PA skills in isolation (Fuchs et al., 2001; Gillon, 2000).

Beginning in preschool, the SLP can increase a child's print awareness with print-focused reading activities (Justice & Ezell, 2002). Print-focused strategies emphasize word concepts and alphabetic knowledge and include cues such as the following:

Show me how to hold the book so I can read.

Do I read this way or this way?

Where is the last word on the page?

How many words do you see?

Find the letter C. Whose name starts with C?

Such print-focused prompts are easy to teach, and parents have used them successfully at home with only minimal training.

Most integrated approaches to preliteracy and early literacy consider the two semi-independent sets of preliteracy skills presented in Figure 6.4 (van Kleeck & Schuele, 2010):

- *Form foundations* for decoding include learning about the alphabet and becoming aware of phonological units within spoken words
- *Meaning foundations* for reading comprehension include vocabulary and sentence-level semantic-syntactic skills

Figure 6.4 Two-stage intervention.

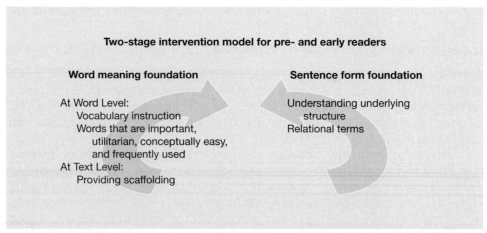

Intervention with young readers should focus on both word meaning and sentence formation.

Source: Based on information from "Emphasizing Form and Meaning Separately in Prereading and Early Reading Instruction," by van Kleeck & Schuele, 2010.

Later, reading intervention might target both linguistic and metalinguistic skills, including recognition of key words, use of all parts of the text such as the glossary and the index, and application of general learning strategies such as graphic organizers containing photos, drawings, and print. Now let's look at intervention for phonological awareness, word recognition, comprehension, and executive function.

Phonological Awareness

As an SLP, you'll have distinct and extensive knowledge related to PA and will play a critical role on educational teams (Cunningham et al., 2004; Moats & Foorman, 2003; Spencer et al., 2008). While classroom instruction focuses on children's achievement of specific curricular outcomes, SLP intervention focuses on the individual learning needs of children who have not achieved these desired classroom goals.

Evidence-based practice (EBP) tells us that children who receive PA training have higher phonemic awareness, word attack, and word identification skills at the end of kindergarten than children who do not receive such training. Even short-term—as little as twice weekly for 6 weeks—high-quality, explicit phonemic instruction with small groups of children can be effective for most children (Koutsoftas et al., 2008). Other EBPs are presented in Box 6.1. In addition to working with individual students, SLPs can offer phonological awareness instruction to teachers, stressing the importance of PA and its integration into the reading curriculum (Hambly & Riddle, 2002). What seems most important is that PA intervention begin before children lag too far behind others, most likely in preschool or kindergarten (Torgesen, 2000).

BOX 6.1 | **Evidence-Based Practice (EBP) for Reading**

General

- Code-focused interventions that included both phonemic awareness and phonics training are the most effective intervention strategies in increasing phonological awareness, alphabet knowledge, oral language, reading, and spelling skills.
- Auditory/language strategies have a greater impact on the reading comprehension of children with LD than visual strategies, demonstrating the underlying spoken-written language link

Phonological Awareness and Metalinguistics

- We can have a moderate degree of confidence in techniques designed to improve phonological awareness in school-age children. Tasks designed to improve rhyming, sound identification, phoneme segmentation, phoneme manipulation,

and grapheme–phoneme correspondence consistently yield moderately large to large effects. Similar effects can be obtained through classroom collaboration and clinician-only approaches.
- Training should be appropriate for the emergent reading or reading level of the child. In deciding whether to provide PA practice to older children, an SLP must consider both the nature of the reading deficit and the level of PA knowledge.
- Little is known about the appropriate length and intensity of intervention.
- Not all phonological skills are of equal importance. Segmenting and blending are critical skills needed for reading. Lower-level skills are important to the extent that they facilitate subsequent development of segmenting and blending. This said, we have not identified the skill level for these two that is needed before word decoding instruction should begin.

(continued)

BOX 6.1 *(Continued)*

- Although the data are limited, it appears that the use of technology/computers can improve PA skills
- Some tasks are easier than others:
  - Consonants are easier to segment than vowels.
  - Initial sounds are easier to segment than final sounds.
  - Shorter words are easier to segment than longer words.
  - It's easier to segment an initial sound in a consonant–vowel–consonant (CVC) word than in a CCV word.

- Highly effective intervention is contingent on adult responses to child errors. In short, adult responses should consider the reason for the child's error and the learning level, and facilitate a correct response.
- Teaching is enhanced when SLPs anticipate the types of errors that a child is likely to make and plan scaffolding or guiding strategies to elicit correct responses.

Sources: Based on Cirrin & Gillam (2008); Lee et al. (2013); Pavelko (2010); Schuele & Boudreau (2008); Sencibaugh (2007).

Phonological awareness training alone is insufficient to increase reading comprehension (Pugh & Klecan-Aker, 2004). Whenever possible with older children, phonological awareness should be taught within meaningful text experiences, such as systematic and explicit classroom instruction, so that the emergent nature of both literacy and PA can support each other (McFadden, 1998).

In general, programs focusing on one or two PA skills yield better results than those that try to teach with a broader focus (National Reading Panel, 2000). It is best to work with one or two sounds at a time. An SLP should teach skills that will directly impact the child's performance of an everyday classroom task.

Intervention can begin with syllable and sound recognition and identification, and can be both receptive and expressive. Next, the SLP can move to syllable segmentation and blending (*stapler* → *stap-ler* → *stapler*) and, finally, to phoneme segmentation and blending (*cat* → *c-a-t* → *cat*). In general, segmentation is easier for most children than blending.

It makes sense to target lower-level PA skills, such a rhyming, to facilitate development of more complex skills, such as segmenting and blending. Once blending and segmenting are established, an SLP can provide a link to classroom decoding and spelling instruction by providing practice that facilitates the application of phoneme awareness to spelling and decoding of words (Blachman et al., 2000).

The concept of syllables can be introduced as naturally occurring "beats" in a word. Multisensory approaches are also helpful and can make the training interesting. Clapping hands or drum beats can be used to help children recognize and identify syllables. Other examples include dropping objects into cans, stacking toys, playing hopscotch, or taking turns in any number of child games during auditory recognition training.

Phoneme intervention might progress from recognition of a target sound in isolation, through identification when paired with other sounds, to sounds in syllables, then words (Gerber & Klein, 2004). Memory can be aided by pairing sounds with real objects or pictures and finally with printed letters and words.

Morphological Awareness

Reading and spelling accuracy can be improved through instruction in morphological awareness together with other forms of linguistic awareness, including knowledge of phonology, orthography, syntax, and semantics (Kirk & Gillon,

2009). Intervention might focus on increasing awareness of the morphological structure of words and the orthographic rules that apply when suffixes, such as -*ly*, are added to a word, changing the *y* in *happy* and *crazy* to an *i* to make *happily* and *crazily*. Apel and Werfel (2014) offer a wonderful tutorial filled with ideas for teaching MA to students with literacy deficits.

Word Recognition

The goals of intervention for word recognition are:

- To teach decoding skills
- To develop a vocabulary of written words
- To improve reading comprehension (Torgesen et al., 2005)

Success in the last two depends on achievement of the first. Teaching decoding skills can result in increases in reading accuracy, fluency, and comprehension (Torgesen, 2005). Support for learning can be provided through encouragement and positive feedback and by breaking tasks into smaller steps or by giving a child as much direction as necessary to complete the task successfully.

Context can be used to help children predict words in text. Intervention might begin with obvious words, such as *I took my umbrella because it looked like _____.* Training can then move to more ambiguous choices and the use of other strategies that include morphological and orthographic cues, such as *Let's have _____ for lunch* followed by *Let's have p_____ for lunch* or *Let's have p_____s for lunch.*

Text Comprehension

Comprehension relies on many different aspects of processing. As mentioned, when we read our knowledge and experience blend with the information on the page to form a mental representation of the meaning. An active reader makes inferences from the text, past knowledge, and experience to bridge these gaps.

Children who lack internalized story frameworks necessary for interpreting narratives might begin intervention with telling stories (Naremore, 2001). Intervention can progress to oral and then written narrative interpretation (Boudreau & Larson, 2004). Storybook reading can be divided into before, during, and after reading activities to aid comprehension. Postreading might include creating story organizers, retelling, and creating variations of the narrative. Narratives can also be divided into story parts and then recombined.

Similarly, comprehension by children who read with difficulty can be improved by also focusing on before, during, and after reading strategies (Vaughn & Klingner, 2004). Through prereading techniques such as establishing the content and setting the scene or context, establishing relationships, and discussing unfamiliar vocabulary and concepts, an SLP or a teacher can assist students in constructing meaning from what they read. Activation of prior knowledge ("What do we know about farms?") can improve comprehension, especially for children with LD.

Comprehension may also be enhanced by teaching children the more explicit and precise language style found in written communication (Westby, 2005). This style can be taught through tasks in which children must follow very explicit oral instructions to be successful or tasks in which contextual cues, such as objects or pictures, are present. Literate vocabularies can be enhanced through prereading activities that focus on the words to be encountered and through use of visual or verbal memory aids. Complex grammar may be taught through books with familiar stories or books in which the grammar becomes increasingly complex.

Thought Question 6.3

As we proceed, is the role of the SLP becoming obvious? What expertise does an SLP possess that a teacher or reading specialist may not have?

Intervention strategies differ according to when they are used in the reading process. For example, prior to reading, semantic strategies, such as giving definitions or synonyms for key words, reduce reading miscues or errors. Graphophonemic strategies are more effective during reading (Kouri et al., 2006). Graphophonemic strategies include encouraging a child to "sound out" a word, calling a child's attention to phonetic regularities, and asking a child to identify initial or final sounds or consonant blends.

During reading, SLPs can facilitate comprehension through instruction, questions, visual and verbal cues, explanations, and comments (Crowe, 2003). Using a conversational style, the SLP provides cues and feedback as oral group reading occurs. It's important that questions reflect the level of comprehension targeted for each child. This semantic strategy should be accompanied by direct vocabulary instruction (Ehren, 2006).

Ideally, students will internalize comprehension strategies and use them as they read actively. Active strategies might include the following:

- Using context to analyze word meaning
- Activating prior knowledge
- Rereading difficult passages
- Self-questioning to help frame key ideas
- Analyzing text structures to determine type of reading
- Visualizing content
- Paraphrasing in one's own words
- Summarizing (Ehren, 2005, 2006; Pressley & Hilden, 2004)

These strategies can be used along with monitoring in which a reader actively decides whether a reading passage makes sense and what to do about it if it does not. Good readers recognize when they have not comprehended a written passage, and they therefore reread it.

When we analyze eye movements of typical readers, we find that their eyes are bounding ahead and back, trying to check the accuracy of words within the surrounding meaning. Children with reading impairments can be taught to use this information to determine individual word meaning (Owens & Kim, 2007).

At another level, comprehension includes a social dialogue with the authors and characters. Comprehension training should also include discussion of the author's goals and the feelings and motivations of characters (Donahue & Foster, 2004). Knowledge of the text can be used to predict a character's behavior within a narrative.

Instruction in multi-strategy approaches to inferencing seems to have a positive effect on the comprehension of struggling middle school readers (Barth & Elleman, 2017). Strategies might include such varied approaches as clarification using text clues, activating and using prior knowledge, understanding character perspectives and author's purpose, and answering inferential questions.

 Video Example 6.4

In this video, a young person discusses having a reading comprehension disability. Watch the first eight minutes or so, and note the other aspects of life affected by the difficulties with reading and the strategies that helped. https://www.youtube.com/watch?v=CcSqq45T7C0

Executive Function

Specific areas of executive function that might be targeted in intervention include working memory, self-directed speech (*How can I figure out the meaning of this word?*), and problem solving (Westby, 2004). Just teaching these strategies is not enough. An SLP and a classroom teacher must help each child achieve independent and appropriate use of these strategies.

Of importance for more advanced readers is *distancing*, or moving away from dependence on the text and toward independent thinking about the text. This can be accomplished by questions that move from answers explicitly stated in the text (*What did she do next?*) to ones in which the question is generated by something in the text but the answer is generated from the student's knowledge (*Could she have solved the problem differently?*).

Hopefully, you're motivated to learn more. Several resources are available online. The Mayo Clinic website (www.mayoclinic.com) covers signs, symptoms, causes, and treatment of reading disability. Just type "dyslexia" in the search box to the right. Then click on "Dyslexia: Symptoms" or "Treatments."

Several commercial sites are available. Please be aware that with these commercial sites, materials that are mentioned do not necessarily represent what we authors would recommend. Just browse the possibilities. The Bright Solutions for Dyslexia website (www.dys-add.com) has several definitions and offers useful teaching tips.

The Scholastic Publications website (www.scholastic.com/home/) offers resources and links. Click on "Teachers" and then type "dyslexia" in the "Search the Teachers Site" box. Scroll down to "Dyslexia: What Teachers Need to Know" and read this interesting article on ideas and teaching methods.

 Check Your Understanding 6.3

Click here to check your understanding of the concepts in this section.

WRITING

Like all other modes of communication, writing is a social act. Just like a speaker, a writer must consider the audience, but because the audience is not present when the writing occurs, writing demands more cognitive resources for planning and execution than does speaking.

In short, writing is using knowledge and new ideas combined with language knowledge to create text. It's a complex process that includes generating ideas, organizing, and planning, along with acting on the plan, revising, and monitoring based on self-feedback. It includes motor, cognitive, linguistic, affective, and executive processes.

Writing is more abstract and **decontextualized** than conversation and requires internal knowledge of different writing forms, such as narratives and expository (explain, compare, contrast, convince) writing. *Decontextualized* means "outside of a conversational context." When you write, the entire context is contained in the writing. You create the context with your language rather than having the context created by your conversational partners.

Several aspects of the writing process are of concern for an SLP. These include (Berninger, 2000):

- Spelling
- Executive function
- Text construction, or going from ideas to writing
- Memory

As mentioned previously, executive function is self-regulation and includes attending, goal setting, planning, and the like. Memory provides ideas for content, language symbols, and rules to guide the formation of that content, and is used for word recognition and storage of ideas as they are worked and reworked. As you can see, writing is a very complicated process. Let's look more closely at spelling and then writing development and impairment, followed by assessment and intervention.

Spelling

Spelling of most words is self-taught using a trial-and-error approach. It is estimated that only 4,000 words are explicitly taught in elementary school. Rather, classroom teachers focus on strategies and regularities that children can use to determine word spelling.

Good spellers use a variety of strategies and actively search words for patterns and consistency. More specifically, mature spellers like you rely on memory; on spelling and reading experience; phonological, semantic, and morphological knowledge; orthographic or letter knowledge and mental grapheme representations; and analogy (Apel & Masterson, 2001). Semantic knowledge is concerned with the interrelationship of spelling and meaning, whereas morphological knowledge is knowing the internal structure of words, affixes (*un-*, *dis-*, *-ly*, *-ment*), and the derivation of words (*happy*, *unhappily*). Mental grapheme representations are best exhibited when you ask yourself "Does that word look right?" Your representations are formed through repeated exposure to words in print. Finally, through analogy a speller tries to spell an unfamiliar word using prior knowledge of words that sound the same.

Spelling competes with other aspects of writing for our limited cognitive energy. Excessive energy expended at this level comes at the cost of higher language functions. As a result, poor spellers generally produce poorer, shorter texts.

Writing Development through the Lifespan

Writing and speaking development are interdependent and parallel, and many aspects of language overlap both modes. In turn, writing development includes development of several previously mentioned interdependent processes. For example, typically developing children and those with Down syndrome (DS) matched for reading level both exhibit oral narratives that are longer and more complex than written narratives. Among the children with DS, vocabulary comprehension is the best predictor of narrative skills (Kay-Raining Bird et al., 2008).

Emerging Literacy

Initially, children treat writing and speaking as two separate systems. Three-year-olds, for example, will "write" in their own way—usually scribbling—but don't yet realize that writing represents sounds. The story may be contained in an

Your brain doesn't store words letter-by-letter; rather, it stores them by more useful units. For example, *stand* is probably stored as *st-and*, which enables you to spell *land*, *band*, *hand*, *bland*, *strand*, and so on.

accompanying drawing. By age 4, some real letters of the parent language may be included.

As with reading, in early writing children expend a great deal of cognitive energy on the mechanics, such as sound–letter associations and letter formation. Gradually, spelling, like reading, becomes more accurate and fluent or automatic.

For a few years, the spoken and written systems converge, and children write in the same manner as they speak, although speech is more complex. Around age 9 or 10, talking and speaking become differentiated as children become increasingly literate. Slowly, writing overtakes speech as written sentences become longer and more complex than speaking. Children display increasing awareness of the audience through their use of syntax, vocabulary, textual themes, and attitude. Some language forms are used almost exclusively in either speech or writing, such as using *and* to begin many sentences in speech but only rarely in writing.

Mature Literacy

In a phase not achieved by all writers, speaking and writing become consciously separate. The syntax and semantics are consciously recognized as somewhat different, and the writer has greater flexibility of style. You may or may not have achieved this phase yet. If you find yourself using an enlarged vocabulary when writing or pondering how sentences flow from one to the next, then you are probably there. As with reading, practice results in improvement that should continue throughout the lifespan. In general, the writing of adults as compared to adolescents contains longer, more complex sentences and uses more abstract nouns, such as *longevity* and *kindness*, and more metalinguistic and metacognitive words, such as *reflect* and *disagree* (Nippold, Ward-Lonergan, & Fanning, 2005).

Writing includes, among other things, spelling; executive function; and text generation, or going from ideas to written text. Let's discuss, in that order, the aspects of particular interest to speech-language pathologists.

Spelling

Spelling development is a long, slow process. As mentioned, initial *preliterate* attempts at spelling consist mostly of scribbling and drawing, with an occasional letter thrown in. Later, children use some phoneme–grapheme knowledge along with letter names. For example, *bee* might be spelled as *B*. Gradually, children become aware of conventional spelling and are able to analyze a word into sounds and letters, although vowels, especially in English, will be difficult for some time.

As knowledge of the alphabetic system emerges, a child slowly connects letters and sounds and devises a system called "invented spelling" in which the names of letters may be used in spelling, as in *SKP* for *escape* or *LFT* for *elephant*. One letter may represent a sound grouping, as in *set* for **street** (*s* for *str*). Because children lack full knowledge of the phoneme–grapheme system, they have difficulty separating words into phonemes.

As spelling becomes more sophisticated, children learn about spacing, sequencing, various ways to represent phonemes, and the morpheme–grapheme relationship. The parallel development of reading aids this process.

Children who possess full knowledge of the alphabetic system of letters and sounds can segment words into phonemes and know the conventional phoneme-grapheme correspondences. As children begin to recognize more regularities and consolidate the alphabetic system, they become more efficient spellers (Ehri, 2000). Increased memory capacity for these regularities is at the heart of spelling ability.

Many vowel representations, phonological variations (such as *later–latter*), and morphophonemic variations (such as *sign–signal*) will take several years to acquire. Gradually, children learn about consonant doubling (la**dd**er), stressed and unstressed syllables (**report–re*port***), and root words and derivations (*add–addition*).

Most spellers shift from a purely phonological strategy to a mixed one between second grade and fifth grade. As words and strategies are stored in long-term memory and access becomes fluent, the load on cognitive capacity is lessened and can be focused on other writing tasks.

Adults spell in several ways: letter-by-letter, by syllable, and by sub-syllable unit, such as *ck*, used for *back*, *stick*, and *rock* but never in *ckar* (car). The method used seems to vary with the task. Next time you're typing words, notice whether your spelling is conscious letter-by-letter or more automatic.

Executive Function

It is not until early adulthood—about where you probably are right now—that writers develop the cognitive processes and executive functions needed for mature writing (Berninger, 2000; Ylvisaker & DeBonis, 2000). It takes this long because of the protracted period of anatomical and physiological development of your brain's frontal lobe, where executive function is housed.

Until adolescence, young writers need adult guidance in planning and revising their writing. By junior high school, teens are capable of revising all aspects of writing. Improved long-term memory results in improved overall compositional quality.

Text Generation

Once children begin to produce true spelling, they begin to generate text. In first grade, text may consist of only a single sentence, as in *My dog is old*. Early compositions often lack cohesion and use structures repeatedly, as in the following:

I like school. I like gym. I like recess. I like art.

In contrast, mature writers use sentence variety for dramatic effect. The facts and events characteristic of early writing evolve into use of judgments and opinions, parenthetical expressions, qualifications, contrasts, and generalizations (Berninger, 2000).

Initially, compositions lack coherence and organization. Later, ideas may relate to a central idea or consist of a list of sequential events.

Written narratives or stories emerge first, followed by expository texts. Expository writing, the writing of the classroom, is of several genres: procedural, as in explaining how to do something; descriptive; opinion; cause-and-effect; and compare-and-contrast.

By adolescence, expository writing has greatly increased in overall length, mean length of utterance, multi-clause production, and use of literate words that transition between thoughts, abstract nouns, and metalinguistic/metacognitive verbs (Nippold, Hesketh, Duthie, & Mansfield, 2005). Literate words include *however*, *finally*, and *personally*; abstract nouns are words such as *kindness*, *loyalty*, and *peace*; and metalinguistic and metacognitive verbs include *think*, *reflect*, and *persuade*.

Thought Question 6.4

We have mentioned a few times that literacy is more than speech in print and that reading and writing are not opposite processes. How do the processes of reading and writing differ?

 Check Your Understanding 6.4

Click here to check your understanding of the concepts in this section.

WRITING PROBLEMS THROUGH THE LIFESPAN

Children with LI often have writing deficits. Unfortunately, their writing difficulties may remain through the lifespan, and the gap between their writing abilities and that of children developing typically widens.

In general, children with language impairment (LI) exhibit reduced written productivity, as measured by total number of words, total number of utterances, or total number of ideas (Puranik et al., 2007; Scott & Windsor, 2000). Similarly, these same children exhibit deficits in writing *complexity* (Fey et al., 2004; Mackie & Dockrell, 2004; Nelson & Van Meter, 2003; Puranik et al., 2007; Scott & Windsor, 2000). Finally, children with LI exhibit reduced *accuracy*, as measured by number of errors (Altmann et al., 2008; Mackie & Dockrell, 2004; Nelson & Van Meter, 2003; Puranik et al., 2007).

Children with LD may have difficulties with all aspects of the writing process (Wong, 2000). A sample of the writing of a child with LD is presented in Figure 6.5. Because they have little knowledge of the writing process, these children fail to plan and to make substantive revisions. They are easily discouraged and may devote very little time to a given writing task. Clarity and organization are forsaken for spelling, handwriting, and punctuation, leaving little cognitive capacity for text generation. In the process, meaning suffers.

Deficits in Spelling

Poor spellers view spelling as arbitrary, random, and seemingly unlearnable. Misspellings are characterized by omission of syllables, morphological markers such as plural *s*, and letters; letter substitutions; and confusion of homonyms such as *to/too/two*. Even adults, especially those with LD, often cite spelling as their primary area of concern.

Usually, deficits in spelling represent poor phonological processing and poor knowledge and use of phoneme–grapheme information. Although most spellers

Figure 6.5 Sample writing of an 11-year-old child with SLDL.

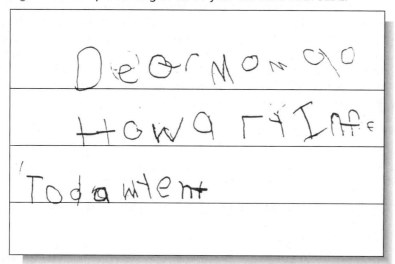

Dear mom and dad, How are you? I am fine. Today we went . . .

shift to greater use of analogy between second grade and fifth grade, poor spellers tend to rely on visual matching skills and phoneme position rules to compensate for their limited knowledge of sound–letter correspondences (Kamhi & Hinton, 2000).

Deficits in Executive Function

When you write, you begin with ideas. You convert your ideas into language. At this point, executive function becomes important.

When executive function or self-regulation is impaired, communication and even problem-solving abilities are diminished, especially in complex linguistic tasks such as writing. Lacking self-regulation, some children with LD follow a writing strategy of putting on paper whatever comes to mind, with little thought to planning. They produce and elaborate little, revise ineffectively and with seeming indifference to their intended audience, detect errors poorly, and experience difficulty executing intended changes. Planning is difficult because of language formulation difficulties.

One adult professional with LD, known to the authors, uses different templates for his reports in which he fills in the blanks. Otherwise, the task of planning, writing, and revising a report would overwhelm his executive abilities. Until he and his spouse devised the templates, he would call from work at the end of each day to have his spouse talk him through the report writing process.

Just as a poor reader expends all his or her energy in decoding, a poor writer becomes bogged down in the mechanics of the writing and spelling process. Both leave the poor reader or writer with little energy for higher cognitive functions such as comprehension or text generation, respectively.

Deficits in Text Generation

In narrative writing, as in storytelling, children with LI may lack mature internalized story models or may be unable to visualize the words even from their own spoken narratives. When compared to the narratives of chronological age-matched peers with typical language, the narratives of children with LD contained shorter, less complex sentences (Scott & Windsor, 2000). As a result, both the oral and written narratives often are shorter and have fewer episodes, contain fewer details, and fail to consider the needs of the listener.

Expository writing tasks follow a format, such as statement of a problem, examination of several factors, and conclusion. Children with LI have difficulty with these writing tasks and approach them with seemingly little thought or planning. The results are often extremely short, poorly organized, and containing numerous errors of grammar, punctuation, and spelling. There is often little revision. In addition, children with LD have substantial difficulty with morphological endings, such as regular past tense and regular plurals, even when they demonstrate accuracy with these units in their speech (Windsor et al., 2000).

 Check Your Understanding 6.5

Click here to check your understanding of the concepts in this section.

ASSESSMENT AND INTERVENTION FOR WRITING IMPAIRMENT

As with the speech and language disorders discussed previously, writing impairments require an SLP to thoroughly describe a child's strengths and weaknesses and to determine the appropriate intervention methods for various aspects of writing. This requires an in-depth understanding of literacy and assessment and intervention techniques.

Assessment of Developmental Writing

One method of assessing writing in the classroom is through the use of portfolios of children's writing (Paratore, 1995). A portfolio is a collection of meaningful writing selected by a child, an SLP, and a teacher that contains samples of the child's writing over time, thus enabling the child to demonstrate progress. The wide variety helps to increase the validity of the sample. Items in a portfolio may include SLP or teacher observation notes, work samples, and first drafts of writing samples, such as journal entries, and projects/papers, final drafts of the same, and peer and teacher evaluations.

Narrative samples are best for young elementary school children. Older elementary school children or adolescents can provide expository writing samples.

Executive function is best measured within actual writing tasks as part of an overall writing assessment rather than separate from functional communication tasks. Samples should be written in ink to allow for analysis of revisions. It's helpful to allow children to plan and to write drafts. All notes and plans should be collected, along with the finished product, and added to the child's portfolio. Price and Jackson (2015) offer a wonderful tutorial based on the professional literature for the collection of writing samples, variables that are useful to assess, and manual and computer-aided techniques for analyzing writing samples.

> Executive function is very difficult to assess without some task to accomplish; thus, the context is very important.

Whenever possible, an SLP, a teacher, or an instructional aide can observe the writing process for evidence of planning and organizing, drafting, writing, revising, and editing. Added information can be obtained if children read their paper aloud while being recorded. This procedure aids the SLP or teacher in interpreting garbled or poorly spelled words.

Writing can be analyzed on several levels, including textual, linguistic, and orthographic (spelling). At a textual level, an SLP can note length, any indication of the amount of effort, overall quality, and structure, or the way in which comments support the topic (Berninger, 2000). Of interest are the total number of words, clauses, and sentences, as well as the structural complexity, as measured in words per clause and clauses per sentence. Writing conventions, such as capitalization and punctuation, plus the use of sentences and paragraphs, should be noted.

Assessment of Spelling

Spelling deficits are very complex and can be difficult to describe. Collection should be of sufficient quantity to allow for a broad-based analysis. Spelling deficits should be assessed through both dictation and connected writing such as that in a child's portfolio (Masterson & Apel, 2000). Standardized tests should also be included, and can be administered by a classroom teacher, writing specialist, or school psychologist. Informal assessments should include several phoneme–grapheme variations, such as single consonants in various positions in words, consonant blends (*str-*), morphological inflections (*-est*, *dis-*), diphthongs, digraphs (two letters for one sound, as in *ch* and *sh*), and complex morphological derivations.

Single-word spelling does not measure a child's ability in a real communicative context. Connected writing, such as that found in a portfolio, can offer samples closer to actual practice.

Descriptive analysis should focus on patterns evident in the child's spelling (Bear et al., 2000). Of interest are the most frequent and the lowest-level patterns. Figure 6.6 presents a possible analysis system that suggests several possible intervention strategies.

Assessment of Text Generation

SLPs and teachers can assess a child's writing using the papers assembled in his or her portfolio. Analysis may include the total number of words and the number of different words. This is an overall measure of a child's vocabulary and flexibility in its use. Other measures might include the maturity of the words used, clause and sentence length, and coherence. Narratives and expository writing can be analyzed for the presence or absence of elements of both forms. For example, does a narrative include a setting statement of *who, what, when, where?*

Figure 6.6 Examples of language-based spelling analysis.

Phonological: Segmenting, blending, and phonemic awareness

Omission of internal and unstressed phonemes and cluster reduction

  Stop → SOP   Sand → SAD

Syllable deletion

  Elephant → ELFANT

Letter reversal (most common with liquids and nasals)

  Sing → SIGN

Orthographic: Sound–symbol relationship (/k/ = k, c, ck, cc, ch, q, x), letter combinations, letter and positional patterns, and grapheme representations

Letter-sound confusion

  Cash → CAS

Nonallowable letter sequences

  Dry → JRIE   Queen → KWEN

Possible spellings that violate location-pattern rules

  Chip → TCHIP   Corn → CKORN

Different spellings on repeated attempts (no cognitive representation or graphemic representation of word)

Morphological: Inflectional (-ed, -ing, -s) and derivational (un-, dis-, -er, -ist, -ment) morphemes, relationship of root word, and inflected or derived form

More difficult if a form has more than one meaning (fast**er**, teach**er**), multiple pronunciations (walk**ed**, jogg**ed**, collid**ed**), and both phonological and orthographic properties are changed when inflected or derived (*ascend* and *ascension*).

Semantic: Effect of spelling on meaning

Homophone confusions

  Won → ONE   They're → THER   Which → WITCH

Intervention for Developmental Writing Impairment

Intervention for writing may involve both general training and more specific and explicit techniques for both narrative and expository forms. To learn to write, you must write, so intervention needs to focus on the actual writing process. Although our evidence is slim, we can make some tentative statements about intervention (see Box 6.2).

The Creative Writing Solutions website (www.creative-writing-solutions.com) has some practical guidelines for teaching writing. Click on "Article Index" at the left and then find the article "Writing with Dyslexia" under "Learning Disabilities."

Spelling

Spelling intervention should be integrated into real writing and reading within the classroom. Words are the vehicles for teaching spelling principles. Ideally, intervention can occur when a child is actually writing and can be reminded of alphabetic and orthographic principles (Scott, 2000). Spelling can be taught within teaching of general executive function in which the child is taught to proofread, correct, and edit.

The way children spell is indicative of the way they read (Templeton, 2004). This would suggest that spelling intervention should also be integrated with reading to enable a child to learn and to use word knowledge.

Words selected for intervention should be individualized for each child and should reflect the curriculum, the child's desires, words attempted but in error, and error patterns (Bear et al., 2004). Spelling strategies can be discussed with a child, using the data from an SLP's analysis. The goal is to learn strategies of spelling and rules rather than specific words. For example, if a child's errors are primarily morphologic (see Figure 6.6), the SLP can target root words and the influence of various morphemes through morpheme-finding and word-building tasks. Intervention

---

BOX 6.2 | **Evidence-Based Practice for Writing**

English Language Learners (ELLs)

- Although there is limited evidence on using writing strategies to improve writing, self-regulation strategies, including explicit instruction, self-review, and peer modeling, show promise.
- Literacy instruction in Spanish while children continue to learn English supports ELLs' literacy development in English.

General

- Data are inconclusive on the beneficial effects of the teaching of phonics on spelling.
- Self-regulated strategy instruction, or teaching students a strategy for approaching a writing task, works well with adolescents.

- Across different writing genres, improvements have been seen using writing process strategies (e.g., planning, writing, and revising); awareness of text structures (e.g., expository vs. narrative text); and guided feedback about the overall quality of writing, missing elements, and strengths.
- Questioning strategies involving self-instruction (executive function), paragraph restatements, and strategies that focus on the text structure work well in combination.

Sources: Based on Brea-Spahn & Dunn Davison (2012); Brooks et al. (2008); Gersten & Baker (2001); Jacobson & Reid (2007); Suggate (2014); Thomason et al. (2007).

An SLP should not be teaching the class's spelling words for the week. An SLP should target spelling strategies, not individual words.

focusing on increasing awareness of the morphological structure of words, with particular attention to the orthographic rules that apply when suffixes are added, can significantly increase both spelling and reading accuracy and can generalize to new words (Kirk & Gillon, 2008). In contrast, if a child's errors are orthographic, the SLP can teach rules through key words, demonstrating alternative spellings, and acceptable and unacceptable sound–letter combinations.

Children with LD benefit from multisensory input such as pictures, objects, or actions. Several multisensory techniques have been proposed in which the child may complete any of several steps, including listening to the SLP say and spell the word, saying the word aloud while looking at it or touching it, writing it while saying it, checking spelling, saying the letters in sequence, tracing the word while saying it, closing his or her eyes and visualizing the word, and rewriting the word and checking or comparing the spelling.

Word analysis and sorting tasks, or placing words into groups, can be used (Scott, 2000). Sorting tasks will differ based on the targeted error patterns found in the child's misspellings. Pairs of words that differ on the bases of these patterns, such as *pint-pit, meant-meat,* and *bunt-but,* can be used to demonstrate the consequences of misspelling. For example, word meaning could be used to help a child note the difference between *head* and *hid.* Other contrasting words might include *dead-did, read-rid,* and *lead-lid.* An SLP should begin with known, frequently used words and gradually introduce less frequently used and unknown words to facilitate generalization. Different spelling/meaning patterns might provide clues to the meaning and spelling of unfamiliar ones (Templeton, 2003). For example, a child might be helped to see the relationship between *evaluate* and *evaluation.* Some principles for word study and spelling intervention are included in Figure 6.7.

Use of computers aids spelling somewhat. Although use of word processing can encourage editing in children, spell checkers, as you know, are not foolproof, and a

Figure 6.7 Principles for guiding spelling intervention.

Focus on what students are "using but confusing" in their spelling rather than beginning with focusing on what a child doesn't know.

Step back and consolidate learning before moving forward.

Use words students know and can read so that one literacy aspect influences another.

Compare words that do have the spelling feature, such as silent *e* with words that don't, as in *dime-dim, tone-ton,* and *cube-cub.*

Help a child look at words in many ways through sorting tasks that include sound, sight, and meaning.

Begin with obvious contrasts first—ones that are easy to hear or clearly demonstrate a rule.

Don't hide exceptions; rather, deal with them because they will enhance generalization.

Avoid rules until a child has learned enough examples to see a rule clearly.

Work for sorting and spelling fluency.

Glean words from a child's writing and reading, and then return to meaningful tasks and texts.

Source: Based on information from Words Their Way: Word Study With Phonics, Vocabulary, and Spelling Instruction (3rd ed.), by D. R. Bear, M. Invernizzi, S. Templeton, and F. Johnston, 2004. Boston: Merrill/Prentice Hall.

child may learn little in the process. In general, spell checkers miss words in which the misspelling has inadvertently produced another word. Suggested spelling may also confuse the child with poor word attack skills. In addition, suggested spellings may be far afield if the original word is seriously misspelled. Spell checkers help less for children with LD than for children developing typically.

If children with literacy impairments are taught to spell phonetically when unsure of the correct spelling, spell checkers generate more correct suggestions, but a child must still select the correct one from the choices offered. Proofing and editing on a hard copy also seems to increase the number of correctly spelled words.

Word prediction programs reduce spelling errors of children with LI by over half, although the user must get the initial letters correct for the program to work effectively. It's important that a word prediction program's vocabulary match the writing task. Several commercial programs incorporate word frequency or various topics.

Thought Question 6.5

Have you gained a new impression of how you spell and learned to spell? If so, what has changed?

Executive Function

Executive function can be targeted within the writing process by using a *goal-plan-do-review* format. An SLP can provide external support to enable children to experience some level of success (Ylvisaker & DeBonis, 2000).

When children are allowed to select their own topics, it increases motivation and shifts the focus to ideas. In the planning phase, an SLP and a child can brainstorm ideas for inclusion in the writing. Drawings and ideational maps, or "spider diagrams," can help. It is also helpful for a child to focus on the potential audience. The SLP can ask questions such as the following:

Why are you writing?

Who will read this paper?

What does the reader know?

What does the reader need to know?

The SLP and child may prefer to use computers as an assistive technology for writing (MacArthur, 2000). Software, such as Inspiration (Inspiration Software, 2017), can aid text generation, and a child or teacher can easily modify the result. Children with LD who receive training in executive function along with word processing make greater gains in the quality of their writing than children instructed only in executive function or word processing alone.

Grammar checkers miss many errors, especially if there are multiple spelling errors. In addition, a child may be unable to figure out just what the error is. Speech recognition software allows a child to compose by dictation. The software cannot overcome oral language difficulties, although these can be moderated with the additional use of grammar checkers.

Narrative Text Generation

For some children, narrative writing intervention may need to begin at the oral narrative level (Naremore, 2001). They may need to learn to tell common event sequences, such as getting ready for school, and they may need help including all the elements of a narrative. Collectively called a **story grammar**, the elements, such as a "setting statement," are common in all Western literate narratives.

Children with LI and writing impairment may not realize that they know a narrative or how to get it started. Story swapping with peers, spin-off stories from reading or real life, draw–tell–write methods, or topic selection from a prepared list can all be used to facilitate this process (Tattershall, 2004). Once a topic is selected, an SLP can encourage a child to write one statement, then another and another ("And then what happened?"). An SLP or a classroom teacher can guide a child by using narrative-enhancing questions and pictures that outline the story events.

During the writing process, an SLP or a classroom teacher can guide a child's writing through the use of brainstorming of ideas, story guides, prompts, and acronyms. Story guides are questions that help a student construct a narrative, and prompts are story beginning and ending phrases. Acronyms, such as SPACE for *setting*, *problem*, *action*, and *consequent events*, can also act as prompts for guiding writing (Harris & Graham, 1996). An SLP or a teacher can also encourage a child to write more with verbal prompts such as "Tell me more." The SLP or teacher can encourage feelings and motivations with pictures and questions such as "How do you think she felt?" (Roth, 2000).

Written narration may require explicit instruction in story grammar or structure. Story maps using pictures that highlight a narrative's main events or story frames may be initially necessary. Story frames are written starters for each main story element. The child completes the sentence and continues with that portion of the narrative. Cards or checklists can also be used to remind the child of story grammar elements.

Expository Text Generation

Procedures for intervention with expository writing may include collaborative planning and guidance by SLP/teacher and peer input; individual, independent writing; conferencing with the SLP/teacher and peers; individual, independent revising; and final editing (Van Meter et al., 2004; Wong, 2000). Collaborative planning is important. Children can think aloud and solicit opinions. Such brainstorming often provides a child with alternative views.

One promising method of teaching expository text writing is called Em-POWER, which treats writing as a problem-solving task involving six steps: **E**valuate, **M**ake a **P**lan, **O**rganize, **W**ork, **E**valuate, and **R**ework (Englert et al., 1988). In addition, research has indicated that certain strategies, presented in Figure 6.8, are especially effective with children with LD (Singer & Bashir, 2004).

Once a topic is selected and discussed in small groups, with a peer and/or with an SLP, the SLP can give the child a planning sheet to help organize her or his thoughts. After the child has completed the sheet, the SLP can help the child organize the information. This is a great time to challenge and help a child clarify views and prepare for independent writing.

Writing, even independent writing, can be fostered through the use of a prompt card containing key words for each major section of the paper. Figure 6.9 presents some sample prompts.

After a child has completed the paper, he or she can conference with peers for feedback while the SLP mediates. The child then revises the paper, based on this feedback.

At each stage in the process, a child can record progress on a checklist that provides a model for the writing process. The checklist can also motivate a child as she or he notes progress.

Figure 6.8 Strategies for teaching expository writing.

Include other students in a supportive environment.

Place training within a literacy-rich environment.

Provide extensive modeling.

Teach:

    Writing explicitly and systematically.

    Various types of writing.

    Planning and organizing strategies

Use:

    Verbal prompts to support self-regulation.

    A variety of strategies to address different needs.

    Graphics for display and as a means of storing test-relevant information such as words, grammar, and ideas.

Move from oral to written forms by integrating the two.

Provide ample opportunity for communication and language to develop.

Collaborate with teachers in mentoring students to write.

Ensure the seamless integration of language intervention and classroom instruction and learning.

Source: Based on information from "EmPOWER, A Strategy of Teaching Students with Language Learning Disabilities How to Write Expository Text" by B. D. Singer and A. S. Bashir (2004). In E. R. Silliman and L. C. Wilkinson (Eds.), Language and Literacy Learning in Schools (pp. 239–272). New York: Guilford.

Figure 6.9 Sample prompts for opinion writing.

Section of Paper	*Examples*
Introduction	*In my opinion . . .*
	I believe . . .
	From my point of view, . . .
	I disagree with . . .
	Supporting words: *first, second, finally, for example, most important is . . . , consider, think about, remember*
Counter opinion	*Although . . .*
	However, . . .
	On the other hand, . . .
	To the contrary, . . .
	Even though . . .
Conclusion	*In conclusion, . . .*
	After considering both sides, . . .
	To summarize, . . .

Sources: Based on Wong (2000); Wong et al. (1996).

Check Your Understanding 6.6
Click here to check your understanding of the concepts in this section.

SUMMARY

Although many aspects of literacy impairment clearly are the domain of the classroom teacher and reading specialist, some justifiably belong in the SLP's realm. Speech sound recognition and production are the domain of the SLP, so phonological awareness and its relationship to reading are areas in which the SLP can help emergent readers and spellers. Language intervention occurs in all forms of communication, including written text. Children with speech and language difficulties often have difficulty moving from spoken to written forms of expression.

Working with a team, including the teachers and reading specialist, an SLP helps a child obtain language-based skills on which literacy is based. This is a natural extension of the SLP's concern for language in all modes of communication.

SUGGESTED READINGS/SOURCES

Catts, H. W., & Kamhi, A. G. (2012). *Language and reading disabilities* (3rd ed.). Boston: Pearson.

Nelson, N. W. (2010). *Language and literacy disorders: Infancy through adolescence.* Boston: Pearson.

The Understood Team. (2017). *Understanding dyslexia.* Accessed at https://www.understood.org/en/learning-attention-issues/child-learning-disabilities/dyslexia/understanding-dyslexia

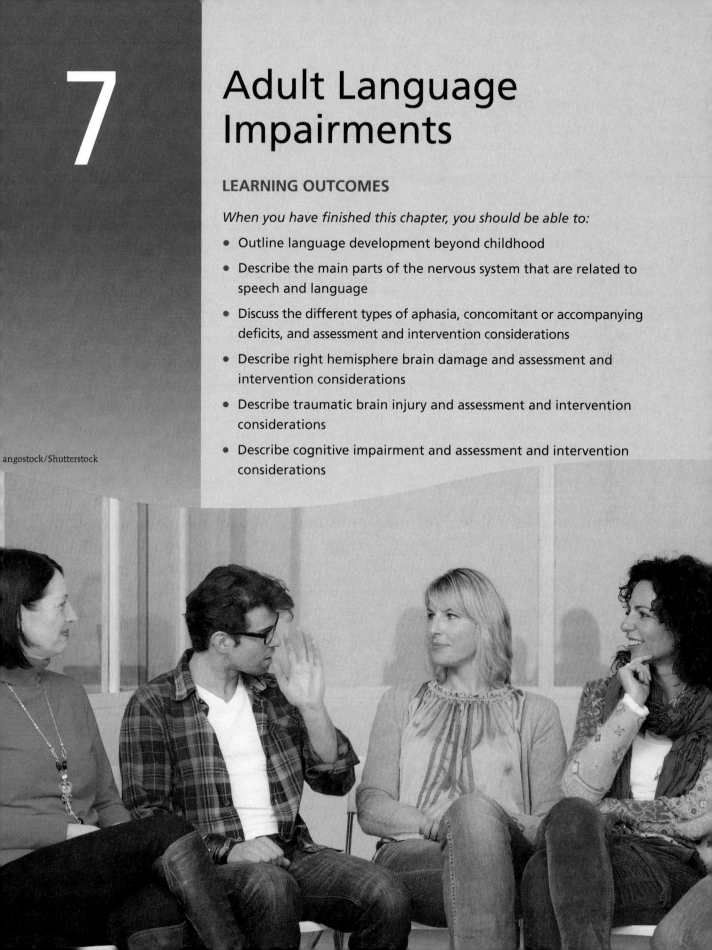

7

Adult Language Impairments

LEARNING OUTCOMES

When you have finished this chapter, you should be able to:

- Outline language development beyond childhood
- Describe the main parts of the nervous system that are related to speech and language
- Discuss the different types of aphasia, concomitant or accompanying deficits, and assessment and intervention considerations
- Describe right hemisphere brain damage and assessment and intervention considerations
- Describe traumatic brain injury and assessment and intervention considerations
- Describe cognitive impairment and assessment and intervention considerations

M any language impairments found in childhood continue into the adult years. Intellectual disability, autism spectrum disorder, and learning disability do not disappear, although they may change or alter with age. Approximately 70% of adults who were initially identified as having a speech or language impairment at age 5 continued to demonstrate less than typical language skills in early adulthood (Johnson et al., 1999). Persistent deficits in adults may entitle them to academic support services or workplace accommodations.

Although the continuation of language disorders of childhood is an important topic, it is not the focus of this chapter. Rather, this chapter focuses on language disorders that occur or develop during adulthood (see Case Study 7.1). Specifically, we discuss aphasia, right hemisphere brain damage, traumatic brain injury, and degenerative neurological conditions. We describe language problems related to interruption of blood supply to the brain, direct destruction of neural tissue, or a pathological process. This will be your introduction, and, of necessity, it will only scratch the surface. Although as an SLP you'll be concerned primarily with communication, the disorders described in this chapter also require an understanding of the medical conditions from which they originate.

In this chapter, we'll discuss adult language, introduce the nervous system, and explore four neurological impairments that affect adult language. For each impairment, we'll discuss characteristics, causes, lifespan issues, and assessment and intervention for language deficits.

CASE STUDY 7.1

Case Study of an Adult with Language Impairment: Marsha

A single mom, Marsha has been the sole breadwinner in her family for several years. Two of her three children are grown, and her youngest is in high school. With no high school diploma, Marsha has had to work in sales or housekeeping jobs to make ends meet. Most recently, she has been a sales associate in the women's fashions section of a large department store.

Nearly a year ago, Marsha awoke one morning with a very strong headache. Although she felt somewhat unsteady on her feet, she determined that she should go to work anyway. Her right leg became weak as she walked to the bus stop, and she collapsed before she had reached her destination.

She awoke in the hospital several hours later, confused and disoriented. She tried to talk with the staff and with her family but seemed unable to comprehend their speech and to form replies. Her medical team, consisting of her physician, a neurologist, a speech-language pathologist, a physical therapist, and an occupational therapist, recommended that Marsha be released from the hospital after 1 week and that she receive services in a rehabilitation center. Both of her older children were eager to help.

The speech-language pathologist worked with Marsha and her family on strengthening Marsha's comprehension and production of language and on her speech. Her intervention services were comprehensive and involved both physical and occupational therapy as well. To date, Marsha has recovered much of her speech and language. Some speech sounds are slightly slurred, and she still has some lingering word retrieval difficulties. She was able to return to her job and is able to communicate well.

As you read the chapter, think about:

- Possible causes of Marsha's stroke
- Possible ways in which the team could coordinate services and work together
- Possible problems Marsha might still experience at work

Space precludes examining all possible neurological disorders. For example, we will not be discussing impairments such as chronic schizophrenia, which typically affects pragmatic aspects of language, such as turn-taking, topic selection, and intentions (Meilijson et al., 2004).

As you might suspect, the ASHA has plenty of good information on adult disorders. The ASHA website (www.asha.org) describes the role of SLPs in these disorders. Go to the website and type "role of SLP" followed by the disorder, as in "role of SLP aphasia" in the search box at the top right. The information the site returns will give you some idea of the scope of practice for SLPs working with these populations.

For easy-to-understand descriptions of some of the adult disorders discussed in this chapter, begin with the ASHA site and scroll down and click on "Public." Click on "Speech and Language Disorders and Diseases" under "Speech, Language and Swallowing." Go to the bottom of the next page and click on "Adult Speech and Language." Now you're free to click on a whole range of adult language impairments, such as aphasia, dementia or cognitive impairment, right hemisphere brain injury, and traumatic brain injury. There's a wealth of information here.

LANGUAGE DEVELOPMENT THROUGH THE LIFESPAN

By adulthood, speech and language have matured, and adults are able to communicate in a variety of modes, using not only speech and language but paralinguistic and nonlinguistic signals effectively. A subtle pause or shift in word emphasis can signal important differences of meaning to a mature speaker. Reading and writing are also essential communication tools.

Unless debilitated in some way through accident, disease, or disorder, adults continue to refine their communication abilities throughout their lives. Writing and speaking abilities continue to improve with use, new words are added to vocabularies, and new styles of talking are acquired.

> Language and communication should continue to develop throughout one's life.

Language development proceeds slowly throughout adulthood. Even individuals with delayed development, such as those with ID, experience continued but slowed language growth.

Use

Through the use of various communication techniques, competent adults can influence others, impart information, and make their needs known. Some adults are even capable of oratory on a par with that of Martin Luther King Jr., which can call up the heroic and the unselfish in others.

> Adult language use is extremely flexible because of the variety of language forms, the large size of the vocabulary, and the breadth of language uses.

Compared to children, adults are very effective communicators and skilled conversationalists who have a variety of styles of talking, from formal to casual. Styles require modification not only in the manner of talking but also in the topics introduced and the vocabulary used. As *The Little Prince* noted when talking with adults (Saint-Exupéry, 1968):

> I would talk . . . about bridge, and golf, and politics, and neckties. And the grown-up would be greatly pleased to have met such a sensible man.

Competent adult communicators quickly sense their role in an interaction and adjust their language and speech accordingly. For example, some people are addressed as *sir* and some as *honey*, and adults do well not to confuse the two. Communication may vary from direct, as in *Turn up the heat*, to indirect, as in *Do you feel a chill?* These two communications share the same goal, but their linguistic methodologies are very different.

The number of communicative intentions increases gradually, so that adults are able to hypothesize, to cajole, to inspire, to entice, to pun, and so on. A skilled speaker knows how to fulfill these intentions and when to use them.

Although adults continue to refine both their writing and reading ability, these changes are not dramatic. In general, the writing of adults as compared to adolescents uses more complex, lengthy sentences (Nippold, Ward-Lonergan, & Fanning, 2005).

Adult narratives improve steadily into middle age and the early senior years (Marini et al., 2005). Abilities decrease some after the late 70s. Those over 75 have less flexibility and ease with word retrieval and make more language form errors.

Content

Adults continue to add to their personal vocabularies, and most use between 30,000 and 60,000 words expressively. Receptive vocabularies are even larger. Specialized vocabularies develop for work, religion, hobbies, and social and interest groups. Some words fade from the language and are used less frequently, such as *dial* a phone number, while new words are added, such as *texting*. Multiple definitions and figurative meanings are also expanded.

Typical seniors experience some deficits in the accuracy and speed of word retrieval and naming. When compared to younger adults, seniors use more indefinite words, such as *thing* and *one*, in place of specific names. These deficits reflect accompanying deficits in working memory and, in turn, they affect ability to produce grammatically complex sentences (Kemper et al., 2001).

Form

Within language form, adults continue to acquire prefixes (*un-*, *pre-*, *dis-*), morphophonemic contrasts (*real*, *reality*), and infrequently used irregular verbs. Conversations become more cohesive through more effective use of linguistic devices, such as pronouns, articles, verb tenses, and aspect (which, for example, allows us to talk about the past from the vantage point of the future, as in *Tomorrow, I'll look back and say, "That was a great picnic"*). In general, the form of written language is more complex than the form of spoken language.

 Thought Question 7.1

Where is the emphasis in adult language development? Does it differ from earlier child development? If so, how?

The length and syntactic complexity of oral sentences increases into early adulthood and stabilizes in middle age (Nippold, Hesketh, et al., 2005). As mentioned previously, older seniors experience a decline in complex sentence production that seems related to word retrieval problems. There is also a decline in oral and written language comprehension, understanding of syntactically complex sentences, and inferencing.

 Check Your Understanding 7.1

Click here to check your understanding of the concepts in this section.

THE NERVOUS SYSTEM

It's difficult to discuss disorders with neurological causes without first understanding your nervous system itself. In this section, we'll briefly describe the major elements of this system, beginning with nerve cells (or neurons) and progressing through the central and peripheral nervous systems.

Your nervous system consists of your brain, spinal cord, and all associated nerves and sense organs. The **neuron** is the basic unit of your nervous system. Each neuron has three parts: the *cell body*, a single long *axon* that transmits impulses away from the cell body to the next neuron, and several branching *dendrites* that receive impulses from other cells and transmit them toward the cell body. A nerve is a collection of neurons. Neurons do not actually touch but are close enough so that electrochemical impulses can "jump" the tiny space, or **synapse**, between the axon of one neuron and the dendrites of the next.

Central Nervous System

Your brain and spinal cord comprise your **central nervous system (CNS)**. The CNS communicates with the rest of your body through the nerves. All incoming stimuli and outgoing signals are processed through the CNS. In this section, we introduce your brain and the areas related to incoming and outgoing language processing.

The Brain

Your brain consists of the cerebrum (or upper brain), cerebellum, and brainstem. The cerebrum, depicted in Figure 7.1, is divided into right and left hemispheres. For the most part, the sensory and motor functions of the cerebrum are *contralateral*,

Figure 7.1 Schematic diagram of the human brain.

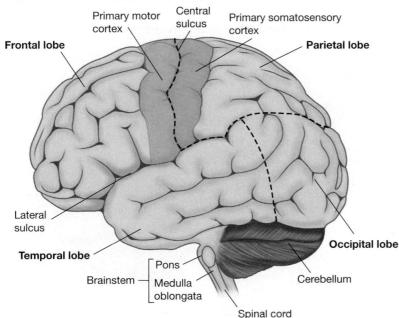

meaning that each hemisphere is concerned with the opposite side of your body. Each hemisphere consists of white fibrous connective tracts running below the surface and covered by a gray cortex of cell bodies approximately 0.25 inch thick. The cortex has a wrinkled appearance caused by little hills called *gyri* and valleys called *fissures*, or *sulci*. Each of your hemispheres is divided into four lobes: *frontal*, *parietal*, *occipital*, and *temporal*.

It is not entirely accurate to conceptualize your brain as having specific, localized areas with unique functions. There is a great deal of redundancy and diffuse organization of function, such that damage to a specific brain region may not completely eliminate the ability to perform that particular function. That said, there are generalized areas that are responsible for particular operations.

Although your cerebral hemispheres are roughly symmetrical, for specialized functions such as language and speech they are asymmetrical. In 98% of individuals, the left hemisphere is dominant for most aspects of receptive and expressive language and motor speech production. In general, all right-handers and 60% of left-handers are left-dominant for language, and the remainder of left-handers are right-dominant. A very small percentage of people have no apparent hemispheric dominance of language function.

The primary anatomical asymmetry in your brain is found in the left temporal lobe, where much language processing occurs. Studies using functional magnetic resonance imaging (fMRI) have shown a strong left hemispheric language dominance of auditory comprehension abilities in children as young as 7 years of age (Balsamo et al., 2002). Other studies have found predominantly bilateral activation of auditory comprehension in younger children. Continued research is needed in this area.

At the base of the brain, your **cerebellum**, or "little brain," consists of right and left cerebellar hemispheres and a central vermis. The cerebellum coordinates the control of fine, complex motor activities, maintains muscle tone, and participates in motor learning. The cerebellum was historically thought to be for motor signals only. Increasing evidence suggests its involvement in language as well. See Figure 7.2 for the cerebellum and other subcortical and lower brain structures.

Figure 7.2 Subcortical and lower brain structures.

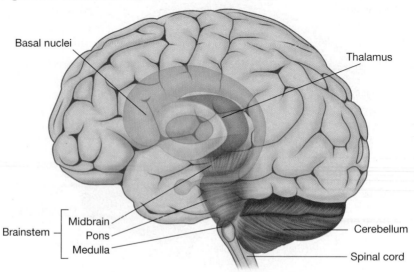

Neuroimaging studies indicate that the cerebellum also has considerable influence on language processing and on higher-level cognitive and affective or emotional functions (Highnam & Bleile, 2011). The cerebellum's posterior lobe has been shown to modulate nonmotor processing. This may include:

- Executive functioning, or the ability to manage several cognitive tasks to reach a particular objective.
- Working memory, which is critical for storage and manipulation of information during processing. The cerebellum is actively involved in verbal working memory.
- Divided attention or paying attention to more than one stimulus or to a stimulus presented in more than one modality.
- Modulation of affect or emotion.

Information flows from the cortex to the cerebellum and back again in the form of feedback on the progress of the communication process. However, the precise role of the cerebellum is somewhat unknown.

Language Processing

Let's discuss language processing very briefly so you will have some idea of how various disorders affect this endeavor. In most individuals, linguistic information is processed in the left hemisphere (see Figure 7.1). Nonlinguistic and paralinguistic information are primarily processed on the right. Studies of split brain patients reveal that the right hemisphere also has a role in language processing, perhaps in storage of multiple meanings and language use. More subtle inferencing and body language may also be influenced by the right hemisphere. In addition, regions on the right are activated during speech production (Shuster & Lemieux, 2005; Shuster, 2009).

Your brain is a complex, interconnected organ, so these are gross overgeneralizations at best. Although several areas have been identified specific to language processing, it's very important to remember that brain functions are broadly distributed across the brain. There are multiple interconnected aspects of language processing. In general, the key regions for language processing are the inferior frontal lobe, the temporal lobe, and occipito-temporal areas. With neuroimaging, researchers are able to map areas of the cerebral cortex important for language processing. Using functional MRI, they measure changes in blood flow throughout the brain while people listen to or produce language.

Incoming auditory information is held in working memory in **Broca's area** in the frontal lobe while it is processed. Broca's area is relatively diffuse. Although it exists on both sides, higher cell density exists in the left hemisphere, indicating increased workings on this side of the brain.

Most incoming linguistic processing occurs in **Wernicke's area** in the left temporal lobe, assisted by the angular gyrus for words and the supramarginal gyrus for grammar, although information is coming from storage areas throughout the brain. For outgoing information, the process occurs somewhat in reverse. Concepts are formed, and the angular and supramarginal gyri contribute to the overall message formation that occurs in Wernicke's area while held in working memory in Broca's area. In addition, Broca's area sends programming information to the

Thought Question 7.2

Pick one of the areas of the brain important for language processing. What would happen if that area was damaged in some way?

motor cortex (see Figure 7.1), which in turn sends signals to the motor neurons for speech. The cranial nerves responsible for transmitting information to and from the brain are presented in Figure 7.3. Although the process is much more complex, you should have enough understanding to comprehend why, for example, Wernicke's aphasia can be so devastating for an individual. Wernicke's area is an interface between the motor cortex for speech and temporal cortex, and is important in sensory integration (Hickok et al., 2008; Wise et al., 2001). The superior or upper portion of the temporal lobe is important for phonological processing and perception of words and for long term memory of words (Belin et al., 2000; Hickok et al., 2008; Wise et al., 2001)

Figure 7.3 Cranial nerves that are important in speech and hearing.

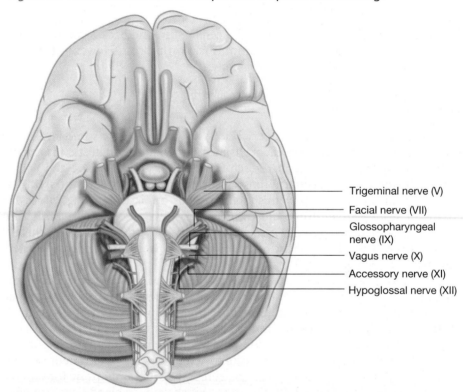

Trigeminal (V): A mixed nerve with both sensory and motor functions for the jaw and tongue for speech and chewing.

Facial (VII): A mixed nerve for sensation of taste and motor control of the facial muscles important in facial expression, such as smiling, tearing, and salivation.

Glossopharyngeal (IX): A mixed nerve with sensory input from the tongue for taste and motor control of the pharynx for salivation and swallowing.

Vagus (X): A mixed nerve serving the heart, lungs, and digestive system. A sensory nerve to the larynx and throat. A motor nerve to the larynx for phonation, the soft palate for lifting, and the pharynx for swallowing.

Accessory (XI): A motor nerve controlling muscles of the pharynx, soft palate, head, and shoulders.

Hypoglossal (XII): A motor nerve controlling the muscles of tongue movement.

Check Your Understanding 7.2

Click here to check your understanding of the concepts in this section.

APHASIA

Language is a complex process performed by many different areas. Brain-imaging techniques have identified several regions of the brain that are active during speech sound processing. The number and location of activated regions differs across individuals and with the task, the type of input and output, the amount and kind of memory required, the relative difficulty, the attention level, and other simultaneous tasks.

Although there is little evidence of a unitary language processing area, some areas do seem to be more important than others, especially the frontal and temporal regions of the left hemisphere. These areas are more active than other regions in both perception and production.

Aphasia means literally "without language," a feature that describes the most severe varieties of this impairment. The population with aphasia is extremely diverse. Although aphasia results from localized brain damage, the exact locations and the resultant severity and type of aphasia are not a perfect match. Although individuals with mild aphasia may have language that is similar to that of typical elderly persons, individuals with aphasia usually exhibit greater deficits in expressive language and overall efficiency of communication (Ross & Wertz, 2003).

It is estimated that more than 1 million Americans have aphasia. More than 200 individuals—primarily adults—acquire aphasia in the United States each day. For these people, language has suddenly become a jumble of strange and seemingly unfamiliar words that they are unable to comprehend and/or produce. Many of you are likely to have had some experience with aphasia through a relative, friend, neighbor, or possibly firsthand.

Many severities and varieties of aphasia exist. Problems in two areas, auditory comprehension and word retrieval, seem to be common to varying degrees in all. Word retrieval difficulties suggest that memory may also be impaired in some way.

Aphasia may affect listening, speaking, reading, and/or writing as well as specific language functions, such as naming. In general, individuals with aphasia experience more difficulty with reading than with listening, especially for infrequently used words (DeDe, 2012). Related language functions such as doing arithmetic, gesturing, telling time, counting money, or interpreting environmental noises such as a dog's bark may also be difficult. The relationship between deficits in gesturing and in verbal language suggest that at some level, though separate, the two are cognitively linked. (Mol, Krahmer, & van de Sandt-Koenderman, 2013). Given the great variation possible, it may be better to think of aphasia as a general term that represents several syndromes.

Expressive deficits may include reduced vocabulary, either omission or addition of words, stereotypic utterances, either delayed and reduced output of speech or hyperfluent speech, and word substitutions. Each of these characteristics is a symptom of a deeper language-processing problem. **Hyperfluent speech**, very rapid speech with few pauses, may also be incoherent, inefficient, and pragmatically inappropriate.

Language comprehension deficits, whether spoken or written, involve the impaired interpretation of incoming linguistic information. Although individuals with aphasia may have normal hearing and vision, difficulty comes in the

It is rare that brain injury is so precise as to affect only language. Other related areas of cognitive function and motor behaviors may also suffer damage.

interpretation or the ability to make sense of the incoming signal. In general, those with aphasia and typical adults both demonstrate more similar processing of complex sentences in reading than in speech (DeDe, 2013). In either case, more complex sentences are more difficult than simpler ones.

Severity may range from individuals with a few intelligible words and little comprehension to those with very high-level subtle linguistic deficits that are barely discernible in normal conversation. Severity is related to several variables, including the cause of the disorder, the location and extent of the brain injury, the age of the injury, and the age and general health of the individual. Differences in individual brains may account for different aphasic characteristics and for the lack of similar characteristics when similar areas of the brain are injured.

Although those with aphasia differ from one another greatly, several patterns of behavior exist that enable us to categorize the disorder into numerous types, or *syndromes*. Although categories of the disorder describe certain similarities among individuals with aphasia, they do not adequately characterize any one individual. SLPs and other professionals, such as neurologists and psychiatrists, must thoroughly assess each individual and describe individual strengths and weaknesses.

Not all brain damage results in aphasia. Aphasia is not a result of a motor speech impairment, cognitive impairment or dementia, or deterioration of intelligence. Damage to the brain may result in loss of motor or sensory function, impaired memory, and poor judgment while leaving language intact.

Other neurogenic disorders—those that affect the central nervous system—such as apraxia or dysarthria often exist along with aphasia, and these complicate classification. Apraxia and dysarthria are discussed in Chapter 10. Individuals with aphasia may also experience seizures and depression. Depression is also a common condition in neurological disorders. Most individuals with aphasia also have a variety of attention and other cognitive deficits, indicating an association between attention, language, and other cognitive domains (Murray, 2012).

Hemi means "half," as in "hemisphere."

This is an appropriate place to stress that it is extremely difficult to identify the exact spot where language and speech reside in the brain. As best as we can, we'll try to identify the areas of the brain affected by the disorders being discussed. These are presented in Figure 7.4. You'll want to refer back to this figure as we proceed.

Figure 7.4 Brain schematic showing probable locations of selected aphasias.

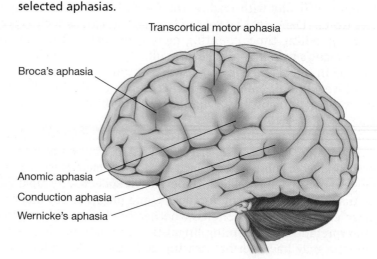

Transcortical motor aphasia

Broca's aphasia

Anomic aphasia

Conduction aphasia

Wernicke's aphasia

Concomitant or Accompanying Deficits

Physical and psychosocial problems may accompany aphasia, and may be traced to the same cause. Physical impairments may include hemiparesis, hemiplegia, and hemisensory impairment. **Hemiparesis** is a weakness on one side of the body in which strength and control are greatly reduced. In contrast, **hemiplegia** is paralysis on one side. Finally, **hemisensory impairment** may accompany either, and is a loss of the ability to perceive sensory information. The client may complain of cold, numbness, or tingling on the affected side and may be unable to sense pain or touch.

Visual processing deficits may affect communication. Individuals with deep lesions in the left hemisphere interior to the ear and across the top of the brain may experience blindness in the right visual field of each eye. Called **hemianopsia**, this condition will affect the individual's ability to read.

When paresis, paralysis, and/or sensory impairment involve the neck and face, the client may have difficulty chewing or swallowing. There may be accompanying drooling or gagging. This condition, known as **dysphagia**, is also a concern of SLPs and is addressed in Chapter 11.

In addition, brain damage may result in seizure disorder seen in approximately 20% of adults with aphasia. Seizures may be of the tonic-clonic type, which result in periods of unconsciousness, or the *petit mal* and psychomotor types, in which the client may lose motor control but remain conscious.

The discussion of aphasia is complicated and uses terminology that might be unfamiliar to you. As we discuss each characteristic related to aphasia, try to think of it as an extreme form of some behaviors that you already manifest. For example, occasionally we all have difficulty recalling a name or remembering a word. In its extreme form, we call this *anomia*. Some of the most common terms follow, with brief descriptions. Examples of written expressive deficits of adults with aphasia are presented in Figure 7.5.

Figure 7.5 Examples of the expressive language deficits in the writing of adults with aphasia.

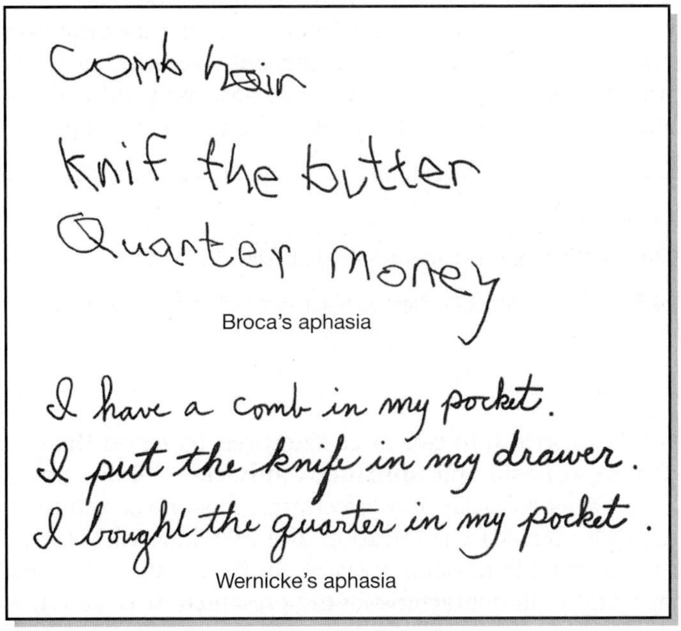

Comb hair
knif the butter
Quarter money
Broca's aphasia

I have a comb in my pocket.
I put the knife in my drawer.
I bought the quarter in my pocket.
Wernicke's aphasia

Agnosia: A sensory deficit accompanying some aphasias that makes it difficult for the client to understand incoming sensory information. The disorder may be specific to auditory or visual information.

Agrammatism: Omission of grammatical elements. Individuals with aphasia may omit short, unstressed words, such as articles or prepositions. They may also omit morphological endings, such as the plural *-s* or past-tense *-ed*.

Agraphia: Difficulty writing. Writing may be full of mistakes and poorly formed. Clients may be unable to write what they are able to say. Agrammatism, jargon, and neologisms may be present in written language as well as in spoken.

Alexia: Reading problems. Clients may be unable to recognize even common words they use in their speech and writing. Paraphasia and neologisms may also be present.

Anomia: Difficulty naming entities. Clients may struggle greatly. Individuals who have recovered from aphasia report that they knew what they wanted to say but could not locate the appropriate word. An incorrect response may continue to be produced even when the client recognizes that it is incorrect.

Jargon: Meaningless or irrelevant speech with typical intonational patterns. Responses are often long and syntactically correct although containing nonsense. Jargon may contain neologisms.

Neologism: A novel word. Some individuals with aphasia may create novel words that do not exist in their language, using those words quite confidently.

Paraphasia: Word substitutions in clients who may talk fluently and grammatically. Associations to the intended word may be based on meaning, such as saying *truck* for *car*; on similar sound, such as *tar* for *car*; or on some other relationship.

Verbal stereotype: An expression repeated over and over. One young man responded to every question with "I know," occasionally stringing it together to form "I know I know I know." Sometimes the expression is an obscene word or expletive or a neologism. One Mother Superior, seen in the clinic, continually uttered the same obscene word with great gusto, to her total embarrassment, but seemed to be unable to stop.

 Video Exercise 7.1

Identifying Naming Difficulties in Patients with Aphasia

Click on the link to a watch a video of a client with aphasia, and complete an exercise.

Types of Aphasia

Aphasias can be classified into two large categories based on the ease of producing speech: **fluent aphasia** and **nonfluent aphasia**. Not all aphasias can be so neatly classified. Other aphasias may affect primarily one communication modality, such as writing. Aphasia classification and its relationship to the location of lesions are controversial issues and areas of continued study. The most common types of aphasia and their characteristics are presented in Table 7.1.

TABLE 7.1

Characteristics of fluent and nonfluent aphasias

Aphasia Type	Speech Production	Speech Comprehension	Speech Characteristics	Reading Comprehension	Naming	Speech Repetition
Wernicke's	Fluent or hyperfluent	Impaired to poor	Verbal paraphasia, jargon	Impaired	Impaired to poor	Impaired to poor
Anomic	Fluent	Mild to moderately impaired	Word retrieval and misnaming, good syntax, and articulation	Good	Severely impaired in both speech and writing	Good
Conduction	Fluent	Mildly impaired to good	Paraphasia and incorrect ordering with frequent self-correction attempts, good articulation, and syntax	Good	Usually impaired	Poor
Transcortical sensory	Fluent	Poor	Paraphasia, possible perseveration	Impaired to poor	Severely impaired	Unimpaired
Broca's	Nonfluent	Relatively good	Short sentences, agrammatism; slow, labored, with articulation and phonological errors	Unimpaired to poor	Poor	Poor
Transcortical	Nonfluent	Mildly impaired	Impaired, labored, difficulty initiating, syntactic errors	Unimpaired to poor	Impaired	Good
Global	Nonfluent	Poor, limited to single words or short phrases	Limited spontaneous ability of a few words or stereotypes	Poor	Poor	Poor, limited to single words or short phrases

Fluent Aphasias

The fluent aphasias are characterized by word substitutions, neologisms, and often verbose verbal output. Lesions in fluent aphasia tend to be found in the posterior portions of the left hemisphere of the brain. Let's briefly mention the most common fluent aphasias.

> Adults with fluent aphasia have typical rate, intonation, pauses, and stress patterns.

As a fluent aphasia, **Wernicke's aphasia** is characterized by rapid-fire strings of sentences with little pause for acknowledgment or turn-taking. Individuals are often unaware of their difficulties. Content may seem to be a jumble, and may be incoherent or incomprehensible although fluent and well articulated. The following is an example of the speech of a client with Wernicke's aphasia:

I love to go for rides in the car. Cars are expensive these days. Everything's expensive. Even groceries. When I was a child you could spend five dollars and get a whole wagon full. I had a little red wagon. My brother and I would ride down the hill by our house. My brother served in World War II. He moved away after the war. There was so little housing available. My house is a split-level.

 Video Example 7.1

Watch and listen to an example of Wernicke's fluent aphasia in this video. https://www.youtube.com/watch?v=3oef68YabD0

As the name suggests, **anomic aphasia** is characterized by naming difficulties. Most aspects of speech are normal, with the exception of word retrieval. The following is an example of the speech of a client with anomic aphasia:

It was very good. We had a bird . . . a big thing with feathers and . . . a bird . . . a turkey stuffed . . . turkey with stuffing and that stuff . . . you know . . . and that stuff, that berry stuff . . . that stuff . . . berries, berries . . . cranberry stuffing . . . stuffing and cranberries . . . and gravy on things . . . smashed things . . . Oh, darn, smashed potatoes.

Like the other fluent aphasias, **conduction aphasia** is characterized by conversation that is abundant and quick, although filled with paraphasia. Paraphasia may be severe enough to make the speech of an individual with conduction aphasia incomprehensible. The following is an example of the speech of a client with conduction aphasia:

We went to me girl, my girl . . . oh, a little girl's palace . . . no, daughter's palace, not a castle, but a pal . . . place . . . home for a sivit . . . and he . . . visit and she made a cook, cook a made . . . a cake.

The rarest of the fluent aphasias, **transcortical sensory aphasia**, is characterized by conversation and spontaneous speech as fluent as in Wernicke's aphasia, but filled with word errors.

Nonfluent Aphasias

Nonfluent aphasia is characterized by slow, labored speech and struggle to retrieve words and form sentences. In general, the site of the lesion is in or near the frontal lobe.

Broca's aphasia is associated with damage to the anterior or forward parts of the frontal lobe of the left cerebral hemisphere, which is responsible for both motor planning and working memory. The most common traits are short sentences with agrammatism; slow, labored speech and writing; and articulation and phonological errors. The following is an example of the speech of a client with Broca's aphasia:

Foam, foam, phone, damn, phone . . . not ude . . . phone not ude . . . ude . . . ude . . . use . . . can't ude . . . no foam can ude.

Adults with nonfluent aphasia have slow rate, less intonation, inappropriately placed and abnormally long pauses, and less varied stress patterns than typical speakers.

> **Video Example 7.2**
>
> You can sense the frustration in the speaker with Broca's aphasia in this video. https://www.youtube.com/watch?v=khOP2a1zL9s&list=PLmSOr2uF4WXbGpbKJ4acpUL4Zbvd6oKR

A nonfluent counterpart of transcortical sensory aphasia, **transcortical motor aphasia** is characterized by difficulty initiating speech or writing. Severely impaired speech is characteristic of damage to the motor cortex, although the areas that are affected may go well below the surface of the brain.

As the name implies, **global, or mixed, aphasia** is characterized by profound language impairment in all modalities. It is considered the most severely debilitating form of aphasia. Global aphasia has both the auditory comprehension problems found in some fluent aphasias and the labored speech of nonfluent aphasias. These symptoms are associated with a large, deep lesion in an area below the brain's surface.

Causes of Aphasia

The onset of aphasia is rapid. Usually, it occurs in people who have no former history of speech and language difficulties. The lesion or injury leaves an area of the brain unable to function as it had functioned just moments before.

The most common cause of aphasia is a **stroke**, or **cerebrovascular accident**, the third leading cause of death in the United States. Strokes affect half a million Americans annually. Seventy percent of these are over 65 years of age (Internet Stroke Center, 2005). Although strokes are rare in children, infants suffer strokes at a rate similar to elderly adults (Lee et al., 2005). The National Aphasia Association estimates that as a result of strokes, approximately 100,000 people acquire aphasia each year.

Strokes are of two basic types: ischemic and hemorrhagic. **Ischemic stroke**, which is the more common type of stroke, results from a complete or partial blockage (occlusion) of the arteries transporting blood to the brain, as in cerebral arteriosclerosis, embolism, and thrombosis. **Cerebral arteriosclerosis** is a thickening of the walls of cerebral arteries in which elasticity is lost or reduced, the walls become weakened, and blood flow is restricted. The resulting ischemia, or reduction of oxygen, may be temporary or may cause permanent damage through the death of brain tissue. An **embolism** is an obstruction to blood flow caused by a blood clot, fatty materials, or an air bubble. The obstruction may travel through the circulatory system until it blocks the flow of blood in a small artery. For example, a clot may form in the heart or the large arteries of the chest, break off, and become an embolus. As in cerebral arteriosclerosis, blockage results in a lack of oxygen-carrying blood, depriving brain cells of needed oxygen. Similarly, a **thrombosis** also blocks blood flow. In this case, plaque buildup or a blood clot is formed on site and does not travel. The result is the same.

Some individuals experience a **transient ischemic attack (TIA)**, sometimes called a mini-stroke, a temporary condition whose symptoms mirror those of a stroke. A TIA occurs when blood flow to some portion of the brain is blocked or reduced. After a short interval, the symptoms decrease as blood flow returns. TIAs should be taken seriously, because they can be a warning sign of increased likelihood of a stroke occurring in the future.

Stroke is caused by an interruption of the blood supply to the brain.

A **hemorrhagic stroke** is one in which the weakened arterial walls burst under pressure, as occurs with an aneurysm or arteriovenous malformation. An **aneurysm** is a saclike bulging in a weakened artery wall. The thin wall may rupture, causing a cerebral hemorrhage. Most aneurysms occur in the meninges, the layered membranes surrounding the brain, and blood flowing into this space can damage the brain or, in serious cases, cause death.

Arteriovenous malformation is rare and consists of a poorly formed tangle of arteries and veins that may occur in a highly viscous organ such as the brain. Malformed arterial walls may be weak and give way under pressure.

Patterns of recovery differ with the type of stroke. Often, with ischemic stroke there is a noticeable improvement within the first weeks after the injury. Recovery slows after 3 months. In contrast, the results of hemorrhagic strokes are usually more severe after injury. The period of most rapid recovery is at the end of the first month and into the second, as swelling lessens and injured neurons regain functioning.

Damage from stroke may occur in any part of your brain. In all right-handed individuals and in some left-handed ones, injury to left hemisphere language areas produces aphasia. Injury to the right hemisphere results in aphasia in only a small percentage of cases, usually left-handed individuals whose right hemisphere is more important for language.

Aphasia-like symptoms also may be noted with head injury, neural infections, degenerative neurological disorders, and tumors. In most of these cases, however, other cortical areas are also affected, resulting in clinically different disorders.

One syndrome, **primary progressive aphasia**, should be mentioned here. Primary progressive aphasia is a degenerative disorder of language, with preservation of other mental functions and of activities of daily living. The disorder, which takes at least 2 years to develop, is not a loss of cognitive functioning, and many individuals with primary progressive aphasia can take care of themselves, some even remaining employed. Over its course, the disorder progresses from primarily a motor speech disorder to a near-total inability to speak, although comprehension remains relatively preserved.

The human brain is extremely complex. Categorizing the types of aphasias that we have discussed helps bring some understanding to the subject of brain disorders but may have little practical clinical value. Each client presents unique characteristics. It is all the more important, therefore, that SLPs describe each client's abilities and disabilities carefully and clearly.

> The results of a stroke are further complicated by the prestroke storage patterns for language.

Lifespan Issues

Although children and adolescents can experience aphasia, especially accompanying brain tumors, most victims are adults in middle age and beyond who previously lived healthy, productive lives. The risk of stroke is increased in an individual who has a history of smoking, alcohol use, poor diet, lack of exercise, high blood pressure, high cholesterol, diabetes, obesity, and TIAs or previous strokes. Usually, the onset of symptoms is rapid when the cause is vascular, but it can take months or years to become evident with a tumor or degenerative disease. These patterns are presented in Figure 7.6.

In the most common situation, an individual suffers an ischemic stroke, depriving the brain of a needed supply of oxygenated blood. First indications may be loss

Figure 7.6 Severity of symptoms by neurological condition. Individuals differ in severity and path of the disorder.

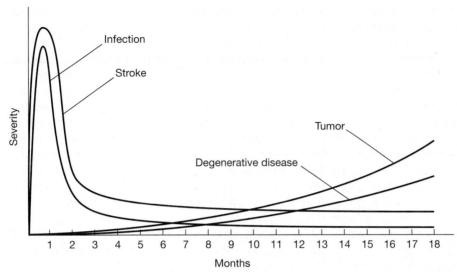

of consciousness, headache, weak or immobile limbs, and/or slurred speech. This condition *may* be either temporary, in which case function returns quickly, or more permanent. Some individuals may experience a series of TIAs spaced over a period of years before they become alarmed. Some TIAs go undetected by the individual.

Usually, at the onset of aphasia, regardless of the cause, the person is rushed to the hospital. Approximately a third of individuals die from the stroke or shortly thereafter. For those who survive, there may be a period of unconsciousness, followed by disorientation. Deep long-lasting periods of unconsciousness or coma are associated with poorer eventual recovery.

For an individual who has experienced a stroke, language is probably not his or her immediate or central concern. Initial reaction may be fear or anxiety. The patient and the family are focused on survival and may be fearful of another stroke. For most individuals this is a novel situation, and they are unaware of how possible limitations will affect their future. As chronic effects settle in, an individual begins to focus on the physical and language complications. This can lead to frustration and depression; indeed, the mother of one of the authors refused to participate in physical therapy in this stage. A newly aphasic patient may not be ready to receive factual information about his or her condition or structured intervention.

Likewise, families of individuals with aphasia are often frightened and confused. Because no one prepares in advance for stroke, families are usually ill informed. In other words, the patient and family are in crisis.

Most individuals remain in acute care for only a few days until their condition stabilizes. Following this, an individual may receive a variety of types of care, depending on the severity of the stroke. These include rehabilitative hospitalization, outpatient rehabilitation, or nursing home care. Most return home, but with some impairment and need for support.

Although intervention services can continue for years, most individuals receive services for at least the first several months. In addition to neuromuscular deficits and seizures, an individual with aphasia may exhibit behavior changes, including perseveration, disinhibition, and emotional problems, depending on the site of the lesion. *Perseveration* is the repetition of inappropriate responses in which the client may become fixed on a single task or behavior and repeat it. *Disinhibition* is a seeming inability to inhibit certain asocial or inappropriate behaviors, such as touching others. Finally, brain damage may contribute to exaggerated swings in emotion.

Emotional behavior must be considered in light of the extreme frustration experienced by some individuals with aphasia. Depression is also common.

Speech and language services are part of a team approach to intervention for individuals who have experienced a stroke.

Immediately after an incident, neurological functioning is most severely affected. Within days, the body's natural recovery process begins. As swelling is reduced, injured cells may recover and begin to function normally. Adjacent areas of the brain that shared brain functions with the injured area may begin to play a larger role. The course and extent of this recovery process are difficult to predict, but the rate is fastest during the first few weeks and months after the stroke, and then it slows, usually ceasing after 6 months. During this process, the entire syndrome that the client presents may change, and most certainly will lessen in severity. The most frequent linguistic gains are in auditory comprehension. In general, less severely affected individuals and those who are younger, in general good health, and left-handed recover from aphasia better and faster than those who are more severe, older, in poor health, and right-handed.

Most individuals experience some type of **spontaneous recovery**, a natural restorative process. In general, individuals who experience ischemic strokes begin spontaneous recovery earlier but improve less rapidly than those who experience intracerebral hemorrhage. Although the anatomical and physiological basis for the spontaneous recovery of language is not well understood, maximum improvement is seen in the first 3 months. This immediate physiological restitution may be complemented by reorganization of brain function in the later stages of recovery. Neuroimaging studies show use of left hemisphere structures that were previously involved in language function and use of similar regions in the right hemisphere with a corresponding shift in some language functioning to the right (Pataraia et al., 2004; Thompson, 2004).

Approximately 4% of the population are either right-hemisphere dominant for language or have bilateral language processing. If these individuals become aphasic as a result of left-hemisphere brain damage, they usually experience milder impairment and quicker recovery than those who are left-hemisphere dominant. The role of the right hemisphere is unclear in the recovery of left-dominant individuals with aphasia.

Communication is so entwined in our social interactions and in our very definition of who we are that the effects of aphasia reach well beyond speech and language.

With or without spontaneous recovery, assessment and intervention begin as soon as an individual's condition permits. Clients who are most responsive are probably the best candidates for intervention services. A general rule is that the earlier the treatment, the better the rate of recovery, but clients do not all recover similarly. An SLP's first goal is to determine the feasibility of clinical intervention. Although it is not possible to predict accurately how much gain will result from spontaneous recovery and how much will result from intervention, an SLP attempts to determine which clients will benefit most from clinical intervention.

Loss of the ability to use language efficiently changes the social role of each individual with aphasia, and can result in social isolation. This situation is complicated by the often incorrect assumption that cognitive abilities are also damaged. In addition, inability to communicate may cause an affected individual to become dependent on others for the simplest of daily tasks. Family roles and responsibilities may also change. Wives, husbands, and children may have to take on new responsibilities. If an individual supported his or her family prior to the incident that caused aphasia, there may be economic problems in addition to medical ones. Case Study 7.2 presents the story of one individual with aphasia.

Before we move on to a discussion of assessment and intervention, you might want to check a few web sources. The National Aphasia Association website (www. aphasia.org) has links to several useful sites. Scroll down and click on "I am a professional." Scroll down again and click on "Resources" to locate therapy guides and videos. The National Institute of Deafness and Other Communication Disorders website (www.nidcd.nih.gov/Pages/default.aspx) has an in-depth description of

Thought Question 7.3

How is recovery influenced by the type of stroke? Why do you think the patterns of recovery differ?

CASE STUDY 7.2

Personal Story of an Adult with Aphasia

When Mr. W. was 55 years of age, he looked fitter than most men 10 years his junior. Having earned a master's degree in labor relations from Cornell University, Mr. W. was employed for many years as a labor mediator by the small city in which he lived. Mr. W. was viewed as cheerful by his circle of friends, primarily fellow hikers with whom he explored mountain trails almost every Saturday.

Although Mr. W. had been rugged and capable of vigorous outdoor activity, he knew that he had high blood pressure, and he was taking medication under a doctor's care. Mr. W. was rarely ill, and he had been hospitalized only once, for acute appendicitis, before his stroke.

One Sunday afternoon, Mr. W. decided to lie down after a 4-hour cross-country ski outing. He had a bad headache, and he hoped that a short rest would relieve it before a dinner date with skiing buddies. When he awoke from his nap, he got up to go to the bathroom but collapsed. His friends were concerned when he failed to meet them. They phoned and got no answer, so someone went to his home. Mr. W. was found on the floor, breathing but unconscious. He had suffered a cerebrovascular accident (CVA), or stroke.

Mr. W. was taken to the emergency room of the local hospital. When he became conscious, he was disoriented, did not seem to understand what was said to him, and was unable to speak. The right side of his body was partially paralyzed. The medical report stated that he had "sustained a left CVA that resulted in right hemiplegia and aphasia." He remained hospitalized for 6 weeks. In addition to the attending neurologist and family physician, Mr. W. was seen by a SLP and a physical therapist. The SLP performed an initial bedside assessment and counseled family members and friends.

The SLP's initial report stated that "Mr. W. presented with severe expressive/receptive aphasia characterized by severe oral motor apraxia and a severe auditory comprehension deficit with moderate to severe reading comprehension deficits for single words."

When Mr. W. was discharged from the hospital, he moved in with his sister and her family. He was cared for largely by family and friends, and he was taken for medical appointments and twice-weekly physical and speech-language therapy. Early goals were simple auditory comprehension requiring yes/no head nods as responses, and the expression of needs such as "eat."

Two years after the stroke, Mr. W. was able to walk with a walker. Family members reported that they could understand approximately 85% of his intentional speech. Strangers could understand only about 20%. He used gestures and largely unintelligible sounds to express himself. Mr. W.'s ability to comprehend language had improved dramatically, and he was now able to follow directions that contained three critical elements ("put the pencil on top of the card and then put it back"). Friends reported that he often seemed agitated, but he apparently liked their visits. Because Mr. W. had always enjoyed being outdoors, his friends frequently took him for short walks. Family members said that they tried to sing together on a regular basis and that Mr. W. joined in to the extent that he was able.

Recently, Mr. W. was evaluated for augmentative/alternative communication. He has received an electronic voice output system and is being taught how to use it. He will never be able to speak normally, but this device should greatly facilitate his ability to communicate.

aphasia. Click on "Health Info" at the top, click on "Voice, Speech, and Language," and find "Aphasia" at the top of the list.

Assessment for Aphasia

Assessment and intervention may begin in the hospital and continue as outpatient service. Successful intervention is a team effort. A person who has had a stroke will most likely receive services from a team of professionals. Team members may include a neurologist, a physical therapist, an occupational therapist, a nutritionist, a speech-language pathologist, and an audiologist. Life changes and family concerns may necessitate the services of a counseling social worker, psychologist, psychiatrist, and/or pastoral counselor. The relative importance of each specialist will change as the client recovers. In addition, a spouse, another family member, or a close friend may be a critical participant in the recuperative process.

Counseling with the family by team members will be ongoing. The family and client may need professional counseling to cope with the enormous changes that have occurred in their lives.

Before beginning any intervention, it is necessary to complete a thorough assessment of each client's abilities and deficits. This process may continue in several stages as the client stabilizes and experiences spontaneous recovery.

Especially important are the person's medical history, the interview with the client and family, examination of the peripheral speech mechanism, hearing testing, and direct speech and language testing. The medical history can reveal information about general health and previous cerebrovascular incidents. In addition, current neurological reports and medical progress notes provide valuable information on present and changing status.

In addition to collecting data during the interview, it will be necessary for an SLP to provide information. The client may be disoriented and need reassurance. Family members will have many questions regarding recovery, family dynamics, income, medical expenses, and the like. Often a social worker will address these issues also. It is important for families to know the extent of the injuries and to have a realistic appraisal of recovery with and without professional assistance.

Careful observation is essential, especially shortly after the incident when more formal testing is not possible. It is important to observe the individual's general speech and language behavior, and to listen to and observe what is communicated and how. Observing spontaneous language use can give an SLP important information on the nature and extent of the disorder.

A thorough examination of the peripheral speech mechanism is important because of the potential for either neuromuscular paralysis or weakness. Speech disorders such as apraxia and dysarthria frequently are associated with aphasia and should be described or ruled out. See Chapter 10 for a fuller discussion.

Possible hearing loss must also be ascertained, especially given the older age of most individuals with aphasia. It is important in an assessment to distinguish hearing loss from comprehension deficits.

Initial speech and language testing often occurs at the patient's bedside and can be confounded by spontaneous recovery that decreases the need for extensive formal testing at this stage. Therefore, an SLP administers informal probes of the patient's language strengths and weaknesses. More formal testing is usually postponed until the patient has maintained a stable level on simple language tasks

Comprehensive testing of clients with aphasia should include at least the two input modalities vision and audition and the three output modalities speech, writing, and gestures.

for at least several days. Simple tasks are administered at least once daily in a short 15-minute time frame (Holland & Fridriksson, 2001). The SLP notes subtle changes in the patient's behavior. It's important not to tire the patient, because fatigue can have a negative effect on communicative ability. Figure 7.7 presents a sample of some of the tasks involved in a bedside assessment.

SLPs can expect some improvement in some areas over just a few days. Positive changes should be reinforced and pointed out to the patient and family members.

Later, more formal speech and language testing and sampling should assess overall communication skills as well as receptive and expressive language in all modalities (reading, writing, auditory comprehension, expressive language, and gestures and nonlinguistic communication) and across all five aspects of language (pragmatics, semantics, syntax, morphology, and phonology). With higher-functioning clients, an SLP will want to assess higher language skills such as verbal reasoning and analogies, figurative language, categorization, and explanations of complex tasks. Table 7.2 is an overview of the areas that ASHA recommends to be evaluated in a functional assessment of communication abilities.

Several standardized tests are available for assessing specific language skills. Formal tests must be selected carefully. Most tests include picture or object naming, pointing to pictures named, automatic language, repeating sentences, describing pictures and answering questions, reading and answering questions and/or drawing conclusions, and writing. It is important for an SLP to remain flexible and to continue to probe a client's behavior for the duration of intervention, especially as behaviors change. In this way, assessment is an important part of intervention.

Figure 7.7 Possible components of an informal bedside evaluation.

Memory: Once introduced, names can be used to assess verbal memory on subsequent visits.

Reading: Ask the patient to read get-well cards.

Writing: Observe patient studying and filling in a hospital menu.

Word retrieval and writing: Provide writing implements and ask the patient to write a few words, such as the names of his or her children.

Memory and more complex language: Ask the patient to identify the person who sent each greeting card.

Naming: Ask patient to name a few common objects around the room.

Auditory comprehension: Note how the client responds during conversation.

Auditory comprehension and working memory: Have the patient follow a few simple commands.

Automatic language: Ask the patient to count or say the alphabet or days of the week.

Pragmatics: Note greeting and leave-taking; make a few simple mistakes, such as calling the patient by the wrong name, and observe the response; ask absurd questions (e.g., "Do helicopters eat their young?"); and take careful note of the conversational repairs, turn-taking behavior, and general appropriateness of the conversation structure.

TABLE 7.2

ASHA recommendations for a functional assessment of communicative abilities with adults with aphasia

Assessment Domain	Behaviors
Social communication	Use names of familiar people
	Express agreement and disagreement
	Request information
	Exchange information on the telephone
	Answer yes/no questions
	Follow directions
	Understand facial expressions and tone of voice
	Understand nonliteral meaning and intent
	Understand conversations in noisy surroundings
	Understand TV and radio
	Participate in conversations
	Recognize and correct communication errors
Communication of basic needs	Recognize familiar faces and voices
	Make strong likes and dislikes known
	Express feelings
	Request help
	Make needs and wants known
	Respond in an emergency
Reading, writing, and number concepts	Understand simple signs
	Use reference materials
	Follow written directions
	Understand printed material
	Print, write, and type name
	Complete forms
	Write messages
	Understand signs with numbers
	Make money transactions
	Understand units of measure
Daily planning	Tell time
	Use a phone
	Keep scheduled appointments
	Use a calendar
	Follow a map

Source: Data from American Speech-Language-Hearing Association. (1994). *Functional assessment of communicative skills for adults (FACS).* Washington, DC: Author.

Interpretation of client behavior during testing is critical. For example, the SLP will want to determine whether the client failed to respond because she or he could not retrieve the answer or because she or he did not comprehend the verbal cue.

Most test tasks involve decision making or problem solving, the endpoints of several cognitive and linguistic processes. Subcomponents of the process are not assessed individually. *Online* assessment, which measures effects at various points within the process, may be more sensitive to individual strengths and weaknesses. To date, most online analysis is limited to research, but such procedures are slowly being adapted for clinical use.

> Because most individuals with aphasia have some residual communication impairment, the goal of intervention is to maximize communication effectiveness in the face of this impairment.

Intervention

The overall goal of intervention is to aid in the recovery of language and to provide strategies to compensate for persistent language deficits. Individual intervention goals are determined by the results of the assessment and by the desires of both the client and family. Goals will be individualized according to the type and severity of the aphasia and upon the individual needs of each client. It cannot be stressed enough that intervention that is effective for one person may be less so for another who differs in the type of aphasia and the severity (Edmonds & Babb, 2011)

Ideally, the goals are mutually acceptable to the client, family, and SLP. All members of the team coordinate their efforts to strengthen treatment received from others. Some guidelines for working with individuals with aphasia are presented in Figure 7.8.

Intervention approaches reflect an SLP's theoretical position on aphasia plus a strong dose of practical knowledge regarding the most effective techniques. Each clinician must decide whether to work on underlying skills, such as memory and auditory comprehension, or to begin with specific skill deficits, such as naming.

Figure 7.8 Guidelines for intervention with individuals with aphasia.

Treat the client in an age-appropriate manner.

Keep your own language simple, clear, and unambiguous, and control for length and complexity.

Adjust your language and the speed of production for the processing capabilities of the client.

Use everyday items and tasks, and involve the family.

Use repetition and familiar routines, situations, and responses to facilitate learning.

Structure tasks to improve performance, and adjust the amount of structure just enough to support the client's efforts but not foster dependency.

Provide a context to support the client's language processing.

Gradually increase the demands made on the client based on the client's abilities.

Teach the client to use his or her strengths to compensate for weaknesses.

If an SLP decides that a client's brain needs help to reorganize, he or she may choose cross-modality training, such as reading aloud while tracing the letters with one's finger.

An SLP can also take advantage of cross-modality generalization, in which skills trained in one modality generalize to another. For example, some individuals with agrammatism benefit from comprehension training more than production training (Jacobs & Thompson, 2000). Comprehension training seems to generalize to comprehension and production. Similarly, generalization occurs across linguistically-related structures and from more complex structures to less complex ones (Thompson et al., 2003).

There is very little data on the effects of treatment during the early phases of recovery. Although the focus of early aphasia management often consists of providing support, prevention, and education rather than structured language therapy, many individuals benefit from less directive, more counseling-oriented treatment (Holland & Fridriksson, 2001).

In adults, words are storied by association with other words. These then form interconnected webs of words which facilitate word memory and word retrieval. For example, word associations might include synonyms (e.g., *rich – wealthy*), antonyms (e.g., *short – tall*), or function (e.g., *bike – ride*), themes (e.g., *kitchen – sink*), category membership (e.g., *horse – cow*), category name (e.g., *dog – pet*), rhyming, and alliteration. Use of such semantic associative increases naming accuracy in patients with anomic aphasia (Hashimoto, 2016). Intervention for anomia using production of sounds and sound sequences relative to word-retrieval also shows promise (Kendall, Oelke, Brookshire, & Nadeau, 2015).

In both initial and follow-up intervention, conversational techniques can provide language therapy and therapeutic support, especially in the early stages of intervention (Holland & Fridriksson, 2001). Within a therapeutic conversation, the client carries as much of the "communication burden" as possible. Mindful of small improvements by the client, the SLP revises the demands made of the client. In short sessions using conversation, the SLP reassures, explains what's happening to the client, and points out positive changes. As an individual progresses, the SLP provides less support and provides a variety of communication contexts and experiences.

Another method of intervention is to have the client attempt to access the language in the left hemisphere by "bridging" from the right. This might be attempted by teaching the client to gesture or sign and simultaneously attempt to say the names of familiar objects. It is reasoned that gestures or signs, being visuospatial in nature, are processed in the right hemisphere. Reportedly, the use of both gestures and pantomime have a positive effect on noun retrieval, although more data is needed on generalization and long-term effects (Ferguson et al., 2012). Other methods use the client's usually intact right hemisphere ability to produce intonational patterns or rhythms. The signs or intonational patterns are gradually faded as the client begins spontaneously to produce the targeted words and phrases without their aid.

As in many other areas of language intervention, unanimity on cross-hemispheric treatment methods does not exist. Many SLPs prefer to remediate language deficits by more direct multimodality stimulation of the affected cognitive processes (Peach, 2001). The goal is reactivation of speech areas in the dominant hemisphere.

Sign, gesture, or some other form of augmentative/alternative communication may become the primary communicative modality for clients who possess profoundly impaired language and/or speech disorders. Communication boards or electronic forms of communication, such as use of an iPad, may be appropriate for those who also have neuromuscular impairments. Amerind, or American Indian signs, may also be useful because many require only one hand and are easily guessable by others. See Chapter 13.

Intervention might also focus on cognitive abilities, such as memory and attention, in addition to more linguistic targets. Clinician-assisted training may also be supplemented by more minimally assisted training, such as computer-provided reading tasks, including visual matching and reading comprehension.

The adaptive capacity of the central nervous system, called *plasticity*, holds promise. Data strongly suggest that neurons and other brain cells have the ability to alter their structure and function in response to a variety of pressures, including training. Plasticity may be the key to helping damaged brains either access or relearn lost behavior through intervention. Much more research is needed to translate from clinical research and practice (Kleim & Jones, 2008).

If a client's family is amenable, it is usually beneficial to involve them in the communication training program under the SLP's guidance. The familiar atmosphere of the home and the objects, actions, and people in it can provide a context that can facilitate a client's recovery and strengthen his or her relearned communicative behaviors.

It is important for professionals to remember that the beneficial involvement of the family must not be at their emotional expense. Family members must not be made to feel guilt if the client shows little progress.

Volunteers can also be trained to support the conversational attempts of individuals with aphasia (Kagan et al., 2001). These individuals need to acknowledge and respond to a client's interactive behaviors. This feedback can affect motivation and performance, and is an essential part of intervention.

> Augmentative/alternative communication may become the primary mode of communication or may be used as a facilitative tool to access verbal language.

 Thought Question 7.4

Why might it be better to work on language processes in a communication framework rather than separately or individually?

Evidence-Based Practice

Although we can conclude from the myriad studies on intervention with individuals with aphasia that intervention promotes recovery, we cannot definitively say which intervention methods are best for the various forms of aphasia (Raymer et al., 2008). What we can say is that failure to participate in intervention has an adverse effect on recovery. Other evidence-based practice (EBP) findings are presented in Box 7.1.

Conclusion

Aphasia is a complex impairment that varies in scope and extent across individuals. In addition, clients may have other impairments, such as paralysis, as a result of their injury. Only a careful description of individual abilities and deficits in each specific modality of communication will enable an SLP to plan and carry out effective intervention. The individual variation in symptoms and severity, the team approach to intervention, and the possibility of spontaneous recovery complicate our efforts to measure intervention effectiveness, and offer opportunities for those of you interested in research.

BOX 7.1 | Evidence-Based Practice for Individuals with Aphasia

Overall Methods of Intervention

- Individuals with aphasia significantly benefit from the services of SLPs over those who receive no intervention. At least 80% make measurable progress affecting both the quantity and quality of language.
- Behavioral intervention promotes language recovery. In general, aphasia treatment is more effective than spontaneous recovery alone.
- The most effective forms of intervention for different forms of aphasia and different language behaviors have not been thoroughly evaluated. Most evaluative studies use test performance rather than investigate the effect of aphasia treatment for functional use of communication. More research is needed on how stroke recovery factors, such as lesion size and location, age, and type of language deficit, influence treatment, especially neural reorganization.

Specific Techniques

- Although timing of intervention after an injury is critical, the optimal interval before beginning intense intervention is unknown. In general, we can say that treatment within the first 3 months is maximally beneficial but that later treatment can also improve language ability and use.
- Repetition is important for maintaining changes in brain function and physiology.
- Although more intense intervention (9 or more hours/week) yields better results, the optimal amount is unknown. In chronic aphasia, there is modest evidence for more intensive treatment. Of particular interest is *constraint-induced language therapy (CILT)* (Pulvermuller et al., 2001). CILT involves (1) requiring the patient to use verbal language while limiting or constraining all other use channels and (2) massed practice or a high-intensity treatment schedule of 3 to 4 hours daily for 2 weeks. The effects are similar to those of other intensive treatments that do not employ the use of constraint (Cherny et al., 2008).

- Training complex language results in improvements in less complex, untrained language when the trained and untrained material are linguistically related. Training simple language has little effect on learning of more complex material.
- The results on the use of augmentative and alternative methods of communication (see Chapter 13) are inconclusive.
- Although word finding treatments using semantic, phonological, or mixed treatment approaches result in positive change, no one intervention approach is better than another.
- Computer-based cognitive rehabilitation interventions can have significant positive effects on the cognitive function of stroke patients in both the acute and chronic phases.

Generalization

- Research results on the generalization of treatment effects to untrained language behaviors are mixed.
- Generalization is most likely to occur to a language feature that is similar to one that is trained, such as generalization to untrained sentences that are syntactically related to trained sentences.

Source: Based on Cha & Kim, 2013; DeRuyter et al. (2008); Koul & Corwin (2010); Raymer et al. (2008); Wisenburn & Mahoney, 2009.

✔ Check Your Understanding 7.3
Click here to check your understanding of the concepts in this section.

RIGHT HEMISPHERE BRAIN DAMAGE

SLPs in health care settings are increasingly involved in the assessment and management of cognitive-communication disorders in individuals with **right hemisphere brain damage (RHBD)**. The term RHBD refers to a group of deficits that result from injury to the right hemisphere of the brain, the nondominant hemisphere for nearly all language functions. RHBD has been found to result in impairments as varied as visuospatial neglect and other attention deficits; difficulties with memory and components of executive function, such as problem solving, reasoning, organization, planning, and self-awareness; and a wide range of communication impairments (ASHA, 2000; Blake, 2006; Lehman & Tompkins, 2000; Myers, 2001; Tompkins et al., 2013). Although it is estimated that 50% to 78% of individuals with RHBD exhibit one or more communication impairments, many do not receive treatment for these difficulties (Blake et al., 2002; Côté et al., 2007; Ferré et al., 2009).

Less information exists on RHBD than on damage to the left hemisphere, although approximately half the individuals who have suffered stroke have right hemisphere involvement. The communication disorders that individuals with RHBD experience do not seem to be strictly language-based. Rather, a combination of cognitive deficits results in the communication problem. As a result, the efficiency, effectiveness, and accuracy of communication are affected.

Although there is greater activation in the left hemisphere during both reception and production, some right hemisphere involvement also occurs (Fridriksson et al., 2009). The role of the right hemisphere in language processing has not been explored as much as that of the left. Linguistic information is processed on the left, and nonlinguistic and paralinguistic information are processed on the right. In general, the right plays a role in some aspects of pragmatics, including the perception and expression of emotion; understanding of jokes, irony, and figurative language; and production and comprehension of coherent discourse. The right hemisphere also plays a greater role in processing emotion in nonverbal contexts.

The right hemisphere is involved in semantic processing. Let's take a look at sentence processing for a moment. In the sentence "Ann bumped into Kathy, and she fell over," the person who fell is in doubt. We don't know who fell. If we measure brain activity using event-related potentials (ERPs), a measure of the electrical activity generated by the brain, we find that the right hemisphere is much more involved in processing sentences such as this as the brain attempts to clarify the meaning (Streb et al., 2004).

Characteristics

Deficits in RHBD are not as obvious as those that result from left hemisphere brain damage. Deficits may be very subtle, but can have a great effect on everyday life. Although these deficits may seem nonlinguistic in nature, they can have a great effect on communication. The most common characteristics include the following:

- Neglect of all information from the left side
- Unrealistic denial of illness or limb involvement

- Impaired judgment and self-monitoring
- Lack of motivation
- Inattention

Disturbances can be grouped into attentional, visuospatial, and communicative. Attentional disturbances are characterized by a client's lack of response to information coming from the left side of the body. This phenomenon is exhibited in the drawings of individuals with mild RHBD who may omit all or provide few left-side details. Figure 7.9 shows an example of left-side neglect in a drawing. More severely impaired individuals may even refuse to look to the left side (in front of themselves).

Visuospatial deficits may include poor visual discrimination and poor scanning and tracking. The client may have difficulty recognizing familiar faces, remembering familiar routes, and reading maps. Some clients fail to recognize family members.

Data from ASHA's National Outcomes Measurement System (NOMS) reveal that individuals with RHBD resulting from stroke are treated for difficulties in swallowing (52%), memory (41%), and problem solving (40%). Intervention for disorders of expression (22%), comprehension (23%), and pragmatics (5%) occurs far less frequently (ASHA, 2008). These low percentages of treatment may be due, in part, to the difficulty in identifying right hemisphere communication impairments, to the few available assessment tools available, and to lack of clarity regarding the types of communication intervention available (Lehman Blake et al., 2013).

The communication deficits associated with RHBD affect the exchange of communicative intent through nonlinguistic and paralinguistic as well as linguistic means. Facial expression, body language, and *prosody* (intonation) are all nonverbal

Figure 7.9 Drawings of an individual with mild RHBD that demonstrate left-side neglect.

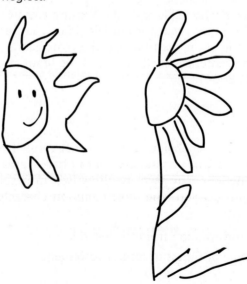

means of conveying intent. Intent can also be conveyed by words, sentences, and *discourse*, which is two or more sentences organized to convey information.

Individuals with RHBD may exhibit poor auditory and visual comprehension of complex information and limited word discrimination and visual word recognition. When we interpret a word or sentence, we activate a web of meanings and categories, some closely related to the word and others more distant. The word *banana* might activate closely-related terms such as *tropical fruit*, but less closely relates to ones such as *slippery*. The right hemisphere is important for activation of distant word and sentence meanings. It is believed that those with RHBD have reduced activation that affects their conversation (Tompkins et al., 2008, 2013).

Many words have multiple meanings. It's believed that all the multiple meanings of a word are activated when that word is heard or read, but that the brain quickly inhibits meanings that do not fit the context (Blake, 2009; Blake & Lesniewicz, 2005; Tompkins et al., 2000, 2001, 2004). A listener's failure to suppress irrelevant or inappropriate information affects comprehension (Tompkins et al., 2000). When we hear about a *bride's train*, we suppress meanings related to railroads. An individual with RHBD is slower in suppressing those meanings, making him or her less inefficient in interpreting conversations (Tompkins et al., 2000, 2013).

Of the various aspects of language, pragmatics, or the functional use of language in context, seems to be the most impaired (Myers, 2001). For example, topic maintenance, appreciation of the communication situation, and determination of listener needs are affected. In general, the expressive language of individuals with RHBD is characterized as tangential to the topic and more egocentric. There are also extremes of verbosity or paucity of speech (Lehman Blake, 2006). Contextual cues such as familiarity with the communication partner, social status of speaker and partner, or use of a specific speaking style, may be missed or ignored (Blake, 2007; Ferré et al., 2011).

Sentence and discourse deficits can affect efficiency and effectiveness of both comprehension and production (Myers, 2001). Discourse is frequently described as disorganized, tangential, and overpersonalized (Blake, 2006; Myers, 2001).

Comprehension deficits include misinterpretation of intended meaning, which is related to difficulties using contextual cues and generation of inferences or links between sentences. This can also include deficits in comprehension of nonliteral language, including metaphors, idioms such as *hit the roof*, humor, sarcasm, and indirect requests such as "Is it chilly in here?" It is unclear whether such a difficulty is due to an underlying deficit in nonliteral language processing or a deficit in the use of nonlinguistic and contextual cues.

Individuals with RHBD exhibit poor judgment in determining which incoming information is important and which is not. A similar pattern of difficulty with selectivity is noted in expressive use of language. Clients may include unnecessary, irrelevant, repetitious, and unrelated information, seemingly unable to organize their language in meaningful ways or to present it efficiently. Other problem areas include naming, repetition, and writing, especially letter substitutions and omissions.

Paralinguistic deficits include difficulty comprehending and producing emotional language. The speech of individuals with RHBD may lack normal rhythm or prosody and the emphasis used to express joy or sadness, anger or delight. Called *aprosodia*, it is the reduced ability or inability to produce or comprehend affective aspects of language (Baum & Dwivedi, 2003; Pell, 2006). Speech production may sound "flat," or monotone.

Thought Question 7.5

Why are the symptoms of RHBD different from those for aphasia?

For a succinct and well-informed list of the characteristics of RHBD, go to Professor Patrick McCaffrey's page at the California State University at Chico website (www.csuchico.edu/~pmccaffrey/). Click on "CMSD 636" and then scroll down to "Chapters 13 and 14," which offers a detailed description of the characteristics and diagnosis of RHBD.

 Video Example 7.3

You'll find an interview with a client with RHBD and an explanation of associated behaviors in this video. https://www.youtube.com/watch?v=YgfSgn0Brmc&list=PLX_PzwBeQwbKDX5T0XeKnW-RqfBqHcREP

Assessment

As with aphasia, the assessment of individuals with RHBD is a team effort involving many of the same professionals and diagnostic tasks. An SLP is interested in visual scanning and tracking, auditory and visual comprehension of words and sentences, direction following, response to emotion, naming and describing pictures, and writing. For example, an SLP may ask a client to re-create patterns with blocks or to find two objects or pictures that are the same; to recall words or sentences heard, seen in print, or both; and to describe a picture accurately enough for the SLP to re-create it. Sampling and observational data are essential in assessing pragmatic abilities in conversational contexts.

Because of the diffuse effects on behavior seen in RHBD, we know less about the treatment of these patients.

Portions of aphasia batteries, standardized tests for RHBD, and nonstandardized procedures may be used in the assessment. Nonstandard procedures include interviewing, observation, and ratings of the client's behavior, along with testing of communication.

Intervention

Intervention often begins with visual and auditory recognition. These skills are essential before progressing to more complex tasks such as naming, describing, reading, and writing. Self-monitoring and paralinguistics are introduced, and the complexity of the content is gradually increased. Despite increasing knowledge about the deficits of individuals with RHBD, knowledge about how to treat them is limited (Lehman Blake, 2007). What we do know is presented in Box 7.2.

For individuals with expressive aprosodia, SLPs may use several methods. In imitative treatment, a client repeats a sentence in unison with the SLP in response to a question. Another approach, called cognitive-linguistic treatment, uses various cues to modify the client's prosody, or the rhythm, stress, and intonation of speech. These include use of an emotion label such as happy or angry, a description of the prosodic characteristics for conveying that emotion, and a facial picture depicting the emotion. When the client is successful, the cues are systematically removed.

In order to interpret nonliteral or figurative language, such as "home is where the heart is," an individual must be able to combine the literal meaning of the words *home* and *heart* with the metaphorical sense of these words. For example, *heart* is used to signify a warm, comforting feeling, as is *home*. In a semantic intervention approach, word meanings and connotations are mapped using spider diagrams and the two words connected in this way (Lundgren et al., 2011).

BOX 7.2 | **Evidence-Based Practice for Individuals with Right Hemisphere Brain Damage**

General

- Cognitive rehabilitation intervention has positive effects on attention, functional communication, memory, and problem solving.
- Approximately 70% to 80% of clients who receive SLP intervention services make significant measurable improvements in communication.
- Communication intervention services as part of a broader interdisciplinary approach including physical, emotional, vocational, and communication, plus family education and support, resulted in greater independence in daily living and return to modified work programs.
- Despite promise, treatment studies have been few and have included a relatively small number of participants.

Specific Interventions at the Sentence and Conversational Level

- In interventions for aprosodia or difficulty expressing emotion through intonation, both imitation and cognitive-linguistic treatment show promise.

- In interventions for receptive language, techniques that provide pre-stimulation of word meanings prior to interpretation show promise, although generalization data are still lacking.
- The use of narratives to improve organization of conversations has mixed results on very limited data.
- Pragmatic intervention, whether a social skills–based treatment using a combination of videotaped feedback, modeling, coaching, and rehearsal strategies or an auditory stimulation approach to enhance attending and attentional control, has mixed results.

Source: Based on Lehman Blake et al. (2013) and Lehman Blake & Tompkins (2008).

Intervention for activating meanings and for suppression of noncontextual ones can be accomplished through a technique called *contextual pre-stimulation*. In this method, still in its infancy, a client is given sentences to activate different meanings prior to being given a word. For example, the client might hear "He slipped and fell on the floor" before being asked to connect *banana* with *slippery* (Tompkins et al., 2011).

Clients are helped to respond appropriately to common communicative initiations and to track increasingly complex information in conversations. Beginning with questions from the SLP that require precise information, the client learns to make responses that come to the point. These questions become more open-ended as the client learns to make off-topic responses less frequently. Similarly, time restraints may limit conversational turns to keep the client from rambling.

Sequencing tasks and explanations of common multistep actions, such as making coffee, will be introduced to help the client organize linguistic content and make relevant contributions. Cues such as objects or pictures may be used initially to aid organization.

Finally, within conversations, an SLP will help a client synthesize these many skills. Visual and verbal cues may aid in turn-taking. Important nonlinguistic markers such as eye contact, body language, and gestures may be targeted. Topic maintenance and relevant conversational contributions are stressed.

Check Your Understanding 7.4

Click here to check your understanding of the concepts in this section.

TRAUMATIC BRAIN INJURY (TBI)

A traumatic brain injury (TBI) is a disruption of normal functioning caused by a blow or jolt to the head or a penetrating head injury. The leading causes of TBI are falls (28%); motor vehicle/traffic crashes (20%); blows to the head, often from sports (19%); and assaults (11%) (National Center for Injury Prevention and Control, 2009). Falls mostly affect the very young and the very old. The two age groups at highest risk for TBI are 0- to 4-year-olds and 15- to 19-year-olds. The increase in use of motor vehicles, motorcycles, and off-road vehicles is directly related to the increase in TBI among teens and young adults. Another disturbing increase is the rise in attempted homicides and gun-related injuries, especially in urban areas. The authors have seen adult clients with TBI resulting from automobile, motorcycle, and bicycle collisions; falls; violent crime; and failed suicide attempts involving firearms.

Annually, approximately 1.5 million people sustain TBI in the United States (National Center for Injury Prevention and Control, 2009). Most are treated in emergency rooms and released, but 50,000 die, and 235,000 require longer hospitalization. Motor vehicle accidents result in the greatest number of hospitalizations. The number of people with TBI who do not seek medical treatment or care is unknown. It's estimated that as a result of TBI, at least 5.3 million Americans—approximately 2% of the U.S. population—currently have a long-term or lifelong need for help performing daily living activities. Males are about twice as likely as females to sustain a TBI.

The statistics tell a chilling story, but do not begin to explain the pain and suffering or the long struggle to recover.

Case Study 7.3 presents the personal story of one young man with TBI. For further information, it is suggested that you check the National Institute of Neurological Disorders and Stroke website.

You will recall from our discussion of language disorders in children that, unlike stroke, which usually injures a specific area of the brain, TBI can include diffuse injury to the entire brain. Diffuse injury comes from the blow and counter blow resulting from the brain shifting within the skull due to acceleration forces. In general, closed head injuries that include swelling of the brain result in diffuse injury. In contrast, open head injury may accommodate swelling, resulting in less damage that is more focused. For this reason neurosurgeons may elect to open the skull to allow for brain swelling. In either case, damage may result from:

- Bruising and laceration of the brain caused by forceful contact with the relatively rough inner surfaces of the skull
- Secondary **edema**, or swelling due to increased fluid, which can lead to increased pressure
- Infection
- Hypoxia (oxygen deprivation)
- Intracranial pressure from tissue swelling
- **Infarction**, or death of tissue deprived of blood supply
- **Hematoma**, or focal bleeding

CASE STUDY 7.3

Personal Story of a Young Man with TBI

His family called him Felipe, but he preferred to use the more Americanized nickname "Chip" that his friends had given him. He was excited to be leaving home for college. Thoughts of being on his own thrilled him with endless possibilities. Even though he was only a freshman, he planned to live with some older friends in their off-campus apartment.

A few weeks after school began, Felipe decided to hitchhike home to surprise his mother, who missed him a great deal. He stuck out his thumb early on Friday afternoon, but never made it home. After his first ride, he bought a soda and began to thumb anew. Shortly afterward, he was struck in the head by the mirror on a pickup truck. Luckily, Felipe was carrying identification in his backpack, and his family was alerted shortly after he was admitted to the hospital.

When he regained consciousness, a few hours after the accident, Felipe was extremely disoriented. He made no attempt to speak and was very lethargic. Although he seemed to recognize his family, he made no attempt to communicate with them. Over the next few weeks, his condition slowly stabilized. Physicians were initially concerned about swelling in the area

of the injury. There was evidence of some internal bleeding, but it was not a major problem.

Once the swelling began to recede, Felipe's abilities slowly returned. He began to recall the names of family members and common objects. Walking was extremely difficult because of paralysis on the right side of his body. He dropped out of college and remained at home, where he received intervention services. As an outpatient, he was seen by a speech-language pathologist, a physical therapist, and an occupational therapist.

After a year's absence from school, Felipe returned and was able to be successful with some adaptations, such as the use of a tape recorder and extra time for completing written tests. He retains a slight limp in his right leg and some minimal weakness in his right arm. His language and speech skills have returned, although he has some mild word-finding difficulties. His cognitive abilities are more concrete than those he had before the accident, and problem-solving tasks require greater effort. All indications are that he will be successful in his academic pursuits, although his physical and cognitive limitations will continue to affect him.

Aphasia-like symptoms are rare, but linguistic impairments related to cognitive damage are not. In addition, an individual with TBI may have sensory, motor, behavioral, and affective disabilities. Neuromuscular impairments may include seizures, hemisensory impairment, and hemiparesis or hemiplegia. The symptoms and the life changes that result can be profound.

Characteristics

Adults with TBI are a heterogeneous group with a diverse collection of physical, cognitive, communicative, and psychosocial deficits. Usually, the most devastating aspect is an inability to resume interests and daily living tasks to the level that existed before the injury. Some clients exhibit nearly total dependence on others. Cognitive difficulties may be evident in orientation, memory, attention, reasoning and problem solving, and executive function, which is the planning, execution, and self-monitoring of goal-directed behavior.

Language is affected in three of four individuals with TBI. The two most commonly reported symptoms for TBI are anomia and impaired comprehension.

As with children, the most disturbed language area and that with the most pervasive problems is pragmatics. Most published tests target language form and content, and may miss pragmatic deficits that are evident in conversation.

Pragmatic impairments result from the inability to inhibit behavior and from errors of judgment. The result may be rambling speech and incoherence, as manifested by off-topic and irrelevant comments and inability to maintain a topic, as well as by poor turn-taking skills, such as frequent interruption of others. In addition, communication may be marked by poor affective or emotional language abilities and inappropriate laughter and swearing.

Deficits are not limited to language, and may include speech, voice, and swallowing difficulties. Approximately a third of all individuals with TBI exhibit dysarthria, a disorder resulting from weakness or incoordination of the muscles that control speech production (see Chapter 10). Language deficits reflect underlying disruptions in information-processing, problem-solving, and reasoning abilities. In addition, psychosocial and personality changes may include disinhibition or impulsivity, poor organization and social judgment, and either withdrawal or aggressiveness. Physical signs may include difficulty walking, poor coordination, and vision problems. A more complete list of the possible outcomes of TBI is presented in Figure 7.10.

Severity seems to be related to initial levels of consciousness and posttraumatic amnesia. Consciousness levels can be classified along a continuum from extended states of unconsciousness or coma, in which the body responds only minimally to external stimuli, to consciousness with disorientation, stupor, and lethargy. Amnesia, or memory loss, is a frequent result of TBI. The duration of both coma and amnesia has been used successfully, but not infallibly, to predict severity and prognosis. In general, the shorter both are, the less severe the resultant deficits of TBI and the better the potential outcome.

One overall measure of brain damage in TBI, such as brain volume loss, may be predictive of general cognitive functioning but not conversational narrative ability

Figure 7.10 Possible outcomes of TBI.

Cognition	Emotion/Personality
Inattentive	Aggression/withdrawal
Disoriented	Apathy and indifference
Poor memory	Denial
Poor problem-solving abilities	Depression
Language, Speech, and Oral Mechanism	Disinhibition and impulsivity
Dysphagia	Impatience
Dysarthria	Phobias
Possible mutism	Socially inappropriate behavior and comments
Pragmatic difficulties (talks better than can communicate)	Suspiciousness and anxiety
Confused language—irrelevance, confabulation or casual unfocused chatting, circumlocution, off-topic comments, lack of logical sequencing, and misnaming	

(Lê, Coelho, Mozeiko, Krueger, & Grafman, 2014). Measures of atrophy in specific regions of the brain may be more informative about specific language functions.

Lifespan Issues

Most adults with TBI are young and have experienced an auto or motorcycle accident. Imagine that you, a college student, are riding in a friend's car. The next thing you remember is waking in the hospital, dazed, disoriented, and unaware of your surroundings. You may have language or other impairments that will change your life forever, or at least for the immediate future.

Several phases of recovery exist, and clinical intervention varies with each. Most individuals will not reach full recovery, and some residual deficits will most likely remain. Initially, the individual may be nonresponsive to stimuli and may need total assistance in a hospital setting.

When the individual does begin to respond, his or her behavior may not reflect the varying nature of the stimuli. In other words, the patient may persist with a response although the situation has changed. Responses may be delayed. Vocalizations may seem purposeless.

Gradually, the individual begins to respond differently to different stimuli and to recognize familiar individuals. Response to commands is still often inconsistent.

As the individual becomes more alert, he or she may seem confused or agitated. Short-term memory and goal-directed behaviors may be poor. Although the client is able to sit and walk, these behaviors are performed without purpose. The client may be subject to mood swings and may have incoherent, inappropriate, or emotional language. Although the individual still needs rehabilitative hospital care, he or she has recovered enough to move from intensive care.

As agitation fades and language continues to return, the individual can remain alert for short periods of time and hold brief conversations if strong external cues, such as pictures or objects, are used. There are still periods of nonpurposeful behavior. Short-term memory is still severely impaired. With structure, the patient can perform learned tasks but is still unable to learn new behaviors.

As the individual continues to improve, he or she needs less assistance. Able to attend for up to 30 minutes with redirection, the individual is aware of the appropriate responses to self, family, and basic needs, which become more goal-directed. Relearned tasks exhibit some carryover to other situations, although new learning does not. Language is used appropriately only in highly familiar contexts.

Gradually, the individual becomes oriented to persons and place. Time is still confusing, and the individual demonstrates only superficial understanding of his or her condition. Usually in outpatient status, the individual is able to learn and carry over this learning to other tasks and to monitor his or her own behavior with minimal assistance. Still unable to recognize inappropriate social behavior, the client is often uncooperative, unrealistic in his or her expectations, and unaware of the needs and feelings of others.

As the individual gains more of an understanding of his or her condition and is able to plan and initiate routine tasks, frustration may build, and he or she may become depressed, argumentative, irritable, or overly dependent or independent. Living at home and possibly having returned to work, the individual may be able to concentrate for an hour even with distractions, to recall past and present events, and to learn new tasks with only minimal assistance.

Increasing abilities may not reduce the individual's low tolerance for frustration, although behavioral responses may be less. In the later stages of recovery, the individual can shift between tasks for up to 2 hours and initiate and carry out familiar tasks. Able to acknowledge his or her impairment, the client is able to consider the consequences of his or her actions and to recognize the needs and feeling of others.

Finally, the individual may be able to consistently act in a socially appropriate manner, to respond appropriately to others, and to plan, initiate, and complete both familiar and unfamiliar tasks. Periodic depression may occur, and irritability may reappear with illness, inability to perform a task, and in emotional situations.

An individual with TBI may face a long period of rehabilitation. Even those who have made a nearly full recovery will have some lingering deficits, especially in pragmatics. The authors have worked with college students with TBI who were able to gain their degrees with only minimal adaptations.

Before we move to a discussion of assessment and intervention, you might want to check out the National Institute of Neurological Disorders and Stroke website (www.ninds.nih.gov/index.htm) for a description of traumatic brain injury and links to several other useful sites. Click on "Disorders" at the top, then click "T," and then scroll down to and select "Traumatic Brain Injury Information Page."

Assessment

An SLP is a member of an interdisciplinary team of rehabilitation specialists who collaborate in assessment of and intervention with persons with TBI. As such, the SLP is responsible for assessing all aspects of communication, cognitive-communicative functioning, and swallowing.

Unlike individuals with aphasia, those with TBI progress through recognizable stages of recovery. Assessment must be ongoing, and varies with each stage. Neurological, psychiatric, and psychological reports will aid in the planning of both assessment and intervention. Observation can aid the SLP in deciding which areas to probe, especially in determining pragmatic deficits that may be missed in formal testing.

To date, few comprehensive tools exist for assessment of language skills in individuals with TBI. Many SLPs working with this population have compiled a series of individual tests for aspects of both language and cognition. These tests are often portions of larger test batteries. Language testing must be comprehensive. Tests that emphasize language form and content may fail to adequately assess pragmatics, thus underestimating the extent of the language impairment.

Sampling is essential because pragmatic behavior that varies across communicative contexts cannot be adequately assessed in a testing context alone. Sampling contexts should include functional activities, such as talking on the phone or grocery shopping, in natural environments, such as the home. Sampling should occur within a discourse unit, a series of related linguistic units that convey a message.

Intervention

With or without intervention, the pattern of recovery for individuals with TBI is predictable. Unlike those with focal damage such as a stroke, who progress smoothly, those with TBI usually recover in a plateau fashion characterized by periods of little or no change interspersed with periods of rapid improvement. After a period of unconsciousness, the person often responds indiscriminately and seemingly without purpose. Attention may be fleeting, and overall level of arousal may fluctuate. The client is often hyper-responsive to stimuli and easily irritated and agitated. Clients may become very emotional and exhibit shouting, emotional language, and, in some cases, repetitive, stereotypic movements such as rocking. With recovery, a client's behavior becomes more purposeful, although restlessness and irritability may persist.

As the client becomes more oriented in place and time, he or she is better able to respond to simple requests, although attention span is short and distractibility high. Memory and abstract reasoning may continue to be a problem even as the client becomes better able to manage daily living and to begin to function independently.

> Cognitive rehabilitation promotes independent functioning in daily life by focusing on specific cognitive processes such as memory and language processing.

Intervention for cognitive-communicative deficits with individuals with TBI is called **cognitive rehabilitation**, a treatment regimen designed to increase functional abilities for everyday life by improving the capacity to process incoming information. The two primary approaches are restorative and compensatory. The restorative approach attempts to rebuild neural circuitry and function through repetitive activities, while the compensatory approach concedes that some functions will not be recovered and develops alternatives. Restorative techniques might include classification tasks and word associations. In contrast, compensatory strategies to improve memory might include focused attending and rehearsal of new information. Traditionally, restorative strategies are attempted first and may include rehearsal and encoding strategies and the use of memory aids. Compensatory methods are typically used when restorative attempts have failed. Slowly, professionals are recognizing that compensatory strategies aid in restorative development, and both methods are being used simultaneously.

An SLP is responsible for designing and implementing treatment programs to decrease the effects of impairment. Evidence-based practices are presented in Box 7.3. In addition to providing direct intervention, an SLP helps to identify functional supports, such as memory logs, and work adjustments that aid in successful independent living.

BOX 7.3 | Evidence-Based Practice for Individuals with Traumatic Brain Injury

General

- The most effective interventions are those that are tailored to the individual client's unique needs and situation. Those receiving communication intervention make gains in cognitive communication, activities, and social participation.
- Those receiving communication services are discharged with higher levels of cognitive functioning and in greater percentages to home versus long-term care.
- More than 80% of clients with TBI make significant measureable gains in memory, attention, and pragmatics.

Source: Based on Coelho et al. (2008).

Intervention programs vary depending on the stage of recovery. During the early stages, intervention focuses on orientation, sensorimotor stimulation, and recognition of familiar people and common objects and events. Early intervention results in shorter rehabilitation and higher levels of cognitive functioning.

In the middle stages, training becomes more structured and formal. The goals are to reduce confusion and improve memory and goal-directed behavior. Much of the training involves increasing the client's orientation to the everyday world. Consistency and routines are important in orientation training. An SLP may target active listening and auditory comprehension and following directions with increasingly more complex information. Word definitions, descriptions of entities and events, and classification of objects and words are also targeted. Conversational speech training is also attempted. For example, one SLP, recognizing that the act of taking a conversational turn is too difficult for some clients, begins by using an object that is passed back and forth to signal turn changes. Over time, the object is replaced with subtle nonverbal signals, such as eye contact.

During the late stages of recovery, the goal is client independence. Targets include comprehension of complex information and directions and conversational and social skills. An SLP helps a client to explore alternative strategies for word recall, memory, and problem solving. Conversational problem-solving tasks are also targeted, along with self-inhibition and self-monitoring. Real-world contexts are emphasized, especially those that are potentially confusing or emotional.

 Check Your Understanding 7.5
Click here to check your understanding of the concepts in this section.

COGNITIVE IMPAIRMENT

We live in a youth-oriented culture. Commercial images lead to the stereotype of older people with deteriorated bodies and minds. Although physical decline with age is inevitable, intellectual capacity is frequently unimpaired. Fewer than 15% of elderly people experience dementia or cognitive impairment, and as many as 20% of these respond positively to treatment (Shekim, 1990). The incidence of cognitive impairment is increasing rapidly as the percentage of the U.S. population over age 65 increases. It is estimated that as many as 48% of new admissions to long-term care facilities have a diagnosis of cognitive impairment (Magaziner et al., 2000).

Cognitive impairment is an umbrella term for a group of both pathological conditions and syndromes that result in the decline of memory and at least one other cognitive ability that is significant enough to interfere with daily life activities (American Psychiatric Association [DSM-5], 2013). It is acquired and is characterized by intellectual decline due to neurogenic causes. Memory, as mentioned, is the most obvious function affected. Additional deficits include poor reasoning or judgment, impaired abstract thinking, inability to attend to relevant information, impaired communication, and personality changes. Irreversible cognitive impairment is most frequently caused by Alzheimer's disease (AD), vascular cognitive impairment (VCI) or multi-infarct dementia, or a combination of both, referred to as mixed cognitive impairment (Ritchie & Lovenstone, 2002).

Cognitive impairment can be divided into cortical and subcortical types, based on patterns of neurophysiological impairment. The characteristics of cortical

> Cognitive impairment or dementia is an impairment of intellect and cognition.

cognitive impairments, such as Alzheimer's and Pick's diseases, resemble those of focal impairments such as aphasia and RHBD. These include visuospatial deficits, memory problems, judgment and abstract thinking disturbances, and language deficits in naming, reading and writing, and auditory comprehension. Alzheimer's disease accounts for 60% to 80% of all cognitive impairment cases, or 5.5 million adults in the United States (Alzheimer's Association, 2017).

Subcortical cognitive impairments may accompany multiple sclerosis, AIDS-related encephalopathy, and Parkinson's and Huntington's diseases. A slow, progressive deterioration of cognitive functioning occurs with deficits in memory, problem solving, language, and neuromuscular control. Disorders that involve neuromuscular functioning, such as Parkinson's, will be discussed in Chapter 9 and Chapter 10.

Differences in the brain location of cognitive impairment affect behavior in different ways. Individuals with Parkinson's disease produce fewer formulaic expressions than those with AD. *Formulaic language* consists of fixed, unitary expressions, such as "You betcha," "You've got to be kidding," "That's the way the cookie crumbles," and "When it rains, it pours"; it is used as a compensation strategy that enables individuals to participate in conversations. In comprehension, those with AD perform significantly worse than participants with Parkinson's (Van Lancker Sidtis, Choi, Alken, & Sidtis, 2015).

The language functions that most depend on memory seem to be primarily affected by cognitive impairment. Communication disorders associated with cognitive impairment progress over time and include anomia, discourse production and comprehension deficits, and, eventually, the inability to express oneself via speech and language (Bourgeois & Hickey, 2009).

A significant decline is noted in naming and word retrieval. Language form—phonology, morphology, and syntax—is generally less disordered, although syntax may be less coherent than before as the client struggles with anomia. As a result, conversations may lack coherence and may be filled with repetitions, stereotypic utterances, false starts, verbal repairs, jargon, neologisms, and the use of phrases such as *that one* and *you know*. One client would repeat "I know" several times.

For an SLP working in a health care setting, a large proportion of the caseload is individuals with cognitive impairment. Only individuals with dysphagia and aphasia are a larger portions of the caseload (ASHA, 2008).

Alzheimer's Disease

Alzheimer's disease (AD) is a cortical pathology that affects approximately 13% of individuals over age 65 and possibly as many as 50% of those over age 85, or approximately 4.1 million individuals in the United States (Alzheimer's Association, 2017). Given the aging U.S. population, the prevalence of Alzheimer's disease will increase 50% by 2030 unless science finds a way to slow the progression of the disease or prevent it. Although cancer and heart disease result in more direct deaths, Alzheimer's is the most expensive disease in the United States, costing families and society around $200 billion annually, most of this total spent on long-term care (Associated Press, 2013). Individuals with AD are a heterogeneous population and may be primarily impaired in memory, language, or visuospatial skills. AD is twice as common in women as in men, primarily because women tend to live longer.

Alzheimer's is characterized by microscopic changes in the neurons of the cerebral cortex.

The cause of AD is unknown, but may be a combination of genetic and environmental factors. The neuropathology is characterized by the presence of twisted neurofilaments in the cytoplasm of neurons that deteriorate cell functioning. These tangles are most pronounced in the temporal lobe and in associational areas of the brain (see Figure 7.11). Nerve fibers degenerate, resulting in brain atrophy that may decrease brain weight as much as 20%, especially in the temporal, frontal, and parietal lobes. Other physical changes include extensive damage to the hippocampus, located on the interior portion of the temporal lobes (interior to the ears), and formation of senile plaques within the cortex that affect nerve cell interactive functioning. A variation of the APOE gene found in all humans greatly increases the likelihood of developing AD. Environmental risk factors include head trauma, heart and circulatory problems, poor overall health, and diabetes.

Mild cognitive impairment may be characterized by name recall difficulties, occasional disorientation, and memory loss. Memory problems are the most obvious changes. Retention of newly learned information is most impaired. Long-term memory is unimpaired initially but deteriorates as the disease progresses.

It's important to realize that memory affects multiple aspects of daily living. In addition, there may be accompanying problems.

Language is not affected in all individuals initially. Early problems involve word finding, off-topic comments, and comprehension. At these early stages, deficits are mostly pragmatic and semantic-conceptual in nature, and syntax is relatively unaffected compared to that of elderly individuals not affected by AD (Kavé & Levy, 2003).

Later characteristics include paraphasia (word substitution) and delayed responding. In more severe stages, expressive and receptive vocabulary and complex sentence production become reduced; pronoun confusion, topic digression, and inability to return to and to shift topic are more pronounced; and writing and reading errors occur. In the most severe form of AD, the language of individuals is characterized by naming errors and the use of generic words (*this*, *that*), syntactic errors, minimal comprehension, jargon, echolalia, or mutism. As might be expected, increased severity results in more conversational breakdowns.

Figure 7.11 Alzheimer's disease.

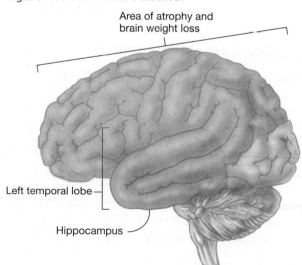

Area of atrophy and brain weight loss

Left temporal lobe

Hippocampus

All areas of communication, including writing, are affected. Writing impairment may arise at several different steps in the process, including planning, sequencing, and organization at the letter, word, sentence, and narrative levels (Neils-Strunjas et al., 2006). Deficits may include misspelling, poor narrative organization, content word errors, perseveration (or repetition of words or ideas), grammatical errors, and reduced syntactic complexity. Problems with writing reflect general language deficits as well as deficits in working memory, attention, and motor control.

 Video Example 7.4

In this video, you'll get an idea of what it's like to have Alzheimer's disease. https://www.youtube.com/watch?v=LL_Gq7Shc-Y

Lifespan Issues

AD is a genetic disorder that lies in hiding, although early screening is possible in some cases. Often the person who will be afflicted with the disease is unaware and/or ignores early signs. At present there are no cures, but some early drug therapies seem to lessen the effects.

In the early stages of AD, the individual experiences memory loss, especially of new information. The individual experiences word retrieval problems and some difficulty with higher language functions, such as humor and analogies. The individual may seem indifferent and may initiate little communication. Able to live at home, the individual can become an increasing burden on an elderly spouse or on adult children who may have families of their own.

As the disease progresses, memory loss increases, resulting in a decrease in vocabulary. Comprehension is reduced. Language production may be reduced to ritualistic or high-usage phrases accompanied by poor topic maintenance and repair of errors, frequent repetition and word retrieval problems, and insensitivity to conversational partners. Irritability and restlessness may increase. The individual may be able to live at home with visiting nurse care to help with daily living routines.

In the most advanced stages of the disease, all intellectual functions including memory are severely impaired, and almost all individuals reside in nursing homes. Language may be meaningless, or the individual may be mute or echolalic. Most clients cannot recall the names of loved ones and may undergo radical personality changes. Motor function is also severely impaired, and the individual needs total care.

 Thought Question 7.6

Try to visualize the four cognitive disorders discussed. Begin with causes. How do they differ? Which are progressive? Which are not? How is language affected?

Assessment

Definitive diagnosis of AD is difficult in the early stages of the disease. Use of neuroimaging techniques may help in early identification, especially for specific protein buildup in the brain (DeKosky, 2008). Pupil dilation tests may also indicate the presence of the disease in the early stages. Finally, computer-based assessments, such as the Computerized Assessment of Mild Cognitive Impairment (CAMCI), are being developed and tested. These measures usually test attention, recognition, and recall of both words and pictures.

Working as a member of a diagnostic team, an SLP usually helps identify changes in language performance that may signal intellectual deterioration and aspects of behavior amenable to change (Hopper, 2005). The results of this assessment may help differentiate AD from other neuropathologies.

Genetic history and general and neurological health data are important elements in the assessment process. Observation of the individual in different communication environments is also important. In the early stages, cognitive impairment may be confused with other disorders such as depression. The progressive nature of the disorder makes it imperative that the SLP remain current on the changing condition and learning ability of a client.

Few language tests for this population exist. Of importance are assessment of retrieval, perceptual, and linguistic deficits and the client's ability to participate in the give-and-take of daily communication in a number of areas.

Writing assessment is important because decline in written language may precede other cognitive and spoken language deficits (Kavrie & Neils-Strunjas, 2002). Functional writing tasks, such as writing a letter, are one of the earliest affected areas of linguistic performance.

> With cognitive impairment, language is affected by deficits in memory.

Several scales exist for rating the severity of a client's loss. Of particular importance are memory deficits. In addition, many assessment batteries that are used with individuals with aphasia can be helpful in evaluating the communication skills of persons with cognitive impairment. Detailed understanding of a client's strengths and weaknesses is essential for helping family members choose the most effective communicative strategies.

Intervention

Intervention with those with progressive disorders can sometimes feel like trying to hold back the tide. Decline is inevitable, given the present state of our knowledge. However, this does not mean that we do nothing. Quite the contrary: Clinical intervention by an SLP can help maintain the client at her or his highest level of performance and help others maximize the client's participation in conversational interactions. It is imperative, therefore, that an SLP emphasize the use of intact cognitive abilities to compensate for deficient ones (Hopper, 2005). The ASHA website defines the role of the SLP with clients with cognitive impairment (go to ASHA's website and type "cognitive impairment" into the search box).

Professionals use three general approaches with individuals with cognitive impairment. In *cognitive rehabilitation*, the client, health professionals, and families develop individualized goals and implement strategies based on those goals. Goals may be very basic, such as appropriately recalling a family member's name, or, in less impaired clients, reading a book to grandchildren. A second approach, *cognitive training*, is used to denote structured practice to improve specific cognitive functions, such as attention, memory, and executive functions. Tasks might include memorizing a grocery list or attending to a prerecorded conversation for a short period. Finally, a third intervention method, called *cognitive stimulation*, is less direct. Usually conducted in groups, cognitive stimulation is concerned with general enhancement of cognitive and social functioning and might involve relaxation exercises or music therapy.

With no cure for cognitive impairment on the immediate horizon, much research and intervention has focused on nonpharmacological therapies to lessen the symptoms of cognitive impairment and to improve the quality of life for individuals with cognitive impairment and for their caregivers. A wide range of nonpharmacological therapies are used to treat cognitive impairment or mild cognitive impairment (MCI). These include direct interventions focused on the person with cognitive impairment, such as computer-assisted cognitive interventions, reminiscence or recall therapy, errorless learning (EL), simulated presence therapy, Spaced-Retrieval (SR), and vanishing cues (VC), as well as indirect interventions for use with caregivers, such as caregiver-administered cognitive stimulation and caregiver education in communication strategies (Olazarán et al., 2010). While it isn't possible to discuss all these methods in detail, we'll try to give you a taste of many of them. Today's best evidence on effectiveness is presented in Box 7.4.

Many intervention methods involve the use of cues or prompts to elicit the correct behavior, such as a request for a desired item or for assistance, names, and events. In errorless learning (EL), a memory intervention technique, SLPs use cues or instructions to prevent or reduce the likelihood of individuals making mistakes (Clare & Jones, 2008). In this way, desired information is accessed and, presumably, the neural pathway to that information is enhanced. As a client progresses, the SLP may use vanishing cues (VC), a technique in which cues or prompts are gradually decreased one at a time, following each successful recall trial. In a variation of VC, cues may be withheld and then added one at a time following an incorrect response. When a correct response is achieved, the cues are faded (Sohlberg et al., 2005). Finally, with spaced-retrieval (SR) the prompted recall of a response occurs at spaced or delayed intervals.

BOX 7.4 | **Evidence-Based Practice for Individuals with Cognitive impairment**

Guidelines

- Although evidence is limited for individuals with moderately severe and severe cognitive impairment, those with mild and mildly moderate to moderate cognitive decline may be able to learn and relearn facts and procedures using specific cognitive intervention strategies.
- Spaced Retrieval, errorless learning, vanishing cues, and specific cueing are promising techniques, although more research is needed.
- Intervention tasks should be as functional as possible and should include ecologically valid facts and procedures.
- Although improvement on trained items may be expected, carryover and long-term maintenance of facts and procedures may be limited unless there is additional intervention.

- Improvement in general cognitive functioning should not be expected from intervention on specific cognitive tasks and information.
- SLPs should consider ethnic, cultural, linguistic, and educational factors when making prognostic statements about learning outcomes.
- Patients with AD have more positive outcomes in individual treatment than in group therapy.
- Restorative strategies are most effective at improving cognitive and functional abilities. These include general cognitive stimulation, such as practicing conversation skills, prompting recall of remote memories, reading, problem solving and participating in creative activities; computerized visuospatial drills; and memory drills that emphasize repetition.

Source: Data from Hopper et al. (2013); Sitzer, Twamley et al. (2006).

Intervention is not undertaken in isolation. As in the other disorders discussed in this chapter, an SLP is a member of a team. Professionals consult with one another and with the client and family on the best course of action.

An SLP may target memory or word retrieval by working on word associations and categories; auditory attending and comprehension in conversational contexts; coherent verbal responses; and formation of longer, more complex utterances with the help of memory aids. Family members can help to keep conversations focused on the present, to validate the client's comments, to reduce distractions and limit the number of participants, and to foster comprehension and participation by slowing the rate and decreasing the complexity of their utterances, using nonlinguistic cues and yes/no response questions (Small & Perry, 2005). Interactive strategies that result in the least communication breakdown include eliminating distractions, speaking in simple sentences, and using yes/no questions. Relatively intact reading and visual memory can be used to facilitate verbal memory (Hopper, 2005).

New drug and gene therapies and bioengineering techniques hold the promise that many of the diseases that cause cognitive impairment may one day be controllable. At present, intervention that stimulates cognitive processes combined with pharmacological approaches that increase certain neural chemicals important for memory is best. Stem cells may also be used to someday regenerate brain tissue.

> Appropriate and effective intervention requires that the SLP understand what the family of the client is experiencing.

Check Your Understanding 7.6

Click here to check your understanding of the concepts in this section.

SUMMARY

Aphasia, right hemisphere brain damage (RHBD), traumatic brain damage (TBI), and cognitive impairment result in very different types of language impairment. Aphasia, which results from a focal brain injury, most likely a stroke, may result in a wide variety of impairments that may affect one or more modalities of communication; comprehension, speech, and naming are usually impaired. Stroke is also the primary cause of RHBD. Comprehension and production of paralinguistics and complex linguistic structures are affected. Pragmatics is the most affected aspect of language. This is also true for traumatic brain injury, which, in contrast to aphasia and RHBD, is a diffuse injury rather than a focal injury. Finally, cognitive impairment, particularly Alzheimer's disease, is a degenerative disease. Word-finding difficulties, off-topic comments, and comprehension deficits are the most common characteristics.

In the adult language impairments discussed, an SLP functions as a member of a multidisciplinary collaborative team. The role of the SLP includes assessment of communicative abilities and the implications of other cognitive deficits, swallowing, and associated neurological disorders. SLP responsibilities include treatment planning and programming, direct intervention services, interdisciplinary consultation, and family training and counseling. Intervention usually focuses on retrieval of language skills and on compensatory strategies.

SUGGESTED READINGS/SOURCES

Brookshire, R. H., & McNeil, M. R. (2014). *Introduction to neurogenic communication disorders* (8th ed.). Boston: Elsevier.

Davis, G. B. (2007). *Aphasiology: Disorders and clinical practice* (2nd ed.). Boston: Pearson.

Martin, N., Thompson, C., & Worrall, L. (2007). *Aphasia rehabilitation: The impairment and its consequences*. San Diego: Plural.

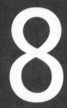

8

Fluency Disorders

LEARNING OUTCOMES

When you have finished this chapter, you should be able to:

- Describe the differences between fluent speech and stuttering.

- Outline and describe the onset and development of stuttering through the lifespan.

- Describe the major etiological theories and conceptual models of stuttering.

- Describe the stuttering evaluation.

- Describe efficacious treatment approaches for children and adults who stutter.

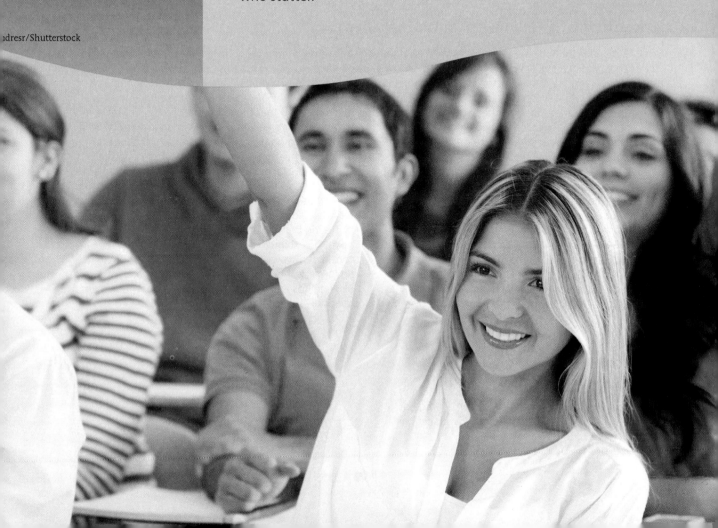

F luent speech is the consistent ability to move the speech production apparatus in an effortless, smooth, and rapid manner, resulting in a continuous, uninterrupted forward flow of speech. Several conditions that adversely affect speech and language production can also disrupt the fluency of speech. Dysarthria, apraxia, and some forms of aphasia affect the fluency of speech. These disorders and their effects on speech and language production are discussed in Chapters 7 and 10 of this book. The focus of this chapter is on a disorder of speech called *developmental stuttering*. Developmental stuttering, or simply *stuttering*, primarily influences the speaker's ability to produce fluent speech. Stuttered speech is characterized by involuntary repetitions of sounds and syllables (e.g., *b-b-b-ball*), sound prolongations (e.g., *mmmmm-mommy*), and blocks (e.g., *b—oy*). All three of these interruptions are considered to be stuttering behaviors, and they have a negative impact on a speaker's ability to produce fluent speech. Case Study 8.1 provides an example of a preschool child with developmental stuttering.

In this chapter, we define stuttering and discuss how stuttering begins and develops as a disorder, paying particular attention to how stuttered speech differs

---

CASE STUDY 8.1

Case Study of a Child with Stuttering: Diego

Mrs. Hernandez brought her 4-year-old son, Diego, to the speech and hearing clinic at a nearby university. In an interview with the clinic director, Mrs. Hernandez explained that when Diego was about $3\frac{1}{2}$ years old, he had trouble starting to speak because he repeated the first sounds and syllables at the beginning of each utterance, like *C-c-c-can I have some ice cream?* or *Ba-ba-ba-baseball is fun*. This difficulty lasted about 3 weeks, and then it went away as abruptly as it had begun. Diego's speech was free of such disruptions for the next 6 months. Mrs. Hernandez further explained that about 2 weeks prior to their visit to the clinic, Diego's speech interruptions reappeared, but they seemed to be worse. She showed great concern when she told the clinic director that in addition to repeating sounds and syllables at the beginning of utterances, he was holding or prolonging sounds at numerous places in his utterances, like *I-I-I-I want to sssssssssssit over there*.

The clinic director observed Mrs. Hernandez and her son interacting with one another in an adjoining room via a one-way mirror. The clinic director observed Diego's repetitions of sounds in words to be rapid, with occasional eye blinking. A formal evaluation of his speech revealed that he produced an average of 15 instances of stuttering per 100 words spoken, and

frequently turned away from the examiner, losing eye contact. His stuttering was determined to be mild to moderate based on his scores on the *Stuttering Severity Instrument – 4 (SSI-4)*. Based on these findings, it was recommended that Diego be seen for direct treatment two times per week, and Mrs. Hernandez would be instructed on how to administer a home-based behavioral treatment program for stuttering, as well as learn how to monitor Diego's feelings about this speech to ensure he did not develop negative attitudes or frustration about speaking because of his stuttering.

After four months of direct intervention, Diego's stuttering behaviors were markedly reduced; at this point, he exhibited normal disfluencies that were considered typical for his age. Additionally, he was no longer exhibiting secondary behaviors (i.e., eye blinking; losing eye contact), and no negative feelings about his speech were noted by his mother.

As you read this chapter, think about:

- The nature of the speech interruptions Diego had developed
- The developmental course of Diego's disfluent behaviors
- Why the clinic director recommended direct intervention for Diego

from fluent speech. Consideration is given to some of the major theories regarding stuttering, the clinical diagnosis of stuttering, and, finally, evidence-based treatment practices.

The cause of stuttering remains elusive, and our understanding of stuttering is incomplete despite its long and diverse history. Stuttering has been part of the human condition for all recorded time. Clay tablets found in Mesopotamia dating from centuries before the birth of Christ record the disorder, hieroglyphics from the 20th century B.C. depict stuttering, and poems written in China more than 2,500 years ago allude to stuttering (Van Riper, 1992). Stuttering occurs all over the world and affects people regardless of age, sex, race, or intellectual level.

The *incidence* of stuttering or number of adults who report that they have stuttered at some time in their life is 5% (Andrews et al., 1983; Conture & Guitar, 1993). Relatively new information, however, indicates that the lifetime incidence of stuttering may be as high as 8% (Yairi & Ambrose, 2013). How stuttering is defined and differences in data collection procedures among researchers seem to contribute to discrepancies in incidence rates for stuttering (Guitar, 2014). The fact that a high percentage of children who begin to stutter will recover without treatment also contributes to difficulties in accurately determining stuttering incidence. Yairi & Ambrose (1999) reported a natural recovery rate of 74% after a minimum of four years post-onset of stuttering in 84 children. In 51 preschool children, Mansson (2000) reported that 71% naturally recovered within two years after starting to stutter, and 85% recovered over the next few years, at around 8 or 9 years of age.

It is not well understood why some children naturally recover from stuttering and others do not. However, certain factors seem to contribute to the persistence of stuttering in some children. For example, females appear to recover from stuttering more frequently and more quickly than males. A family history of stuttering increases the risk that stuttering will persist. A child with a later onset of stuttering (after 3.5 years of age), or a child who continues to stutter more than a year post-onset, is at greater risk for persistent stuttering also (Guitar, 2014). The prevalence of stuttering is determined by ascertaining the number of cases in a given population (usually school-age children) during a given period of time. Research findings of many studies conducted in the United States, Europe, Africa, Australia, and the West Indies suggest an average prevalence rate of 1% for school-age children (Bloodstein & Ratner, 2008). Prevalence data are higher for preschool-aged children (around 2% according to some estimates); this makes sense given that natural recovery with or without treatment will occur a little later (Yairi & Ambrose, 2013).

Stuttering affects more males than females; however, reported sex ratio differences are age-dependent. In very young children (age 3 and under), there is no statistically significant difference between boys and girls who stutter (Yairi & Ambrose, 2013). By first grade, however, the sex ratio difference has been found to be about 3.0 to 1 (Bloodstein & Ratner, 2008). This difference has been attributed to differences in the physical maturation rates of boys and girls, and to differences in speech and language development. However, genetic factors are more likely responsible for the sex difference (Ambrose, Cox, & Yairi, 1997).

Stuttering has a high degree of familial incidence; approximately 30 to 60 percent of people who stutter report that they have a relative who stuttered at some time in his or her life (Yairi, Ambrose, & Cox, 1996). Persistent stuttering also runs in families; children who do not naturally recover from stuttering are likely to have a relative whose stuttering persisted. On the other hand, children who do recover tend to come from a family where a relative who stuttered eventually recovered

(Ambrose, Cox, & Yairi, 1997). In addition, if one twin stutters, there is a high probability that the other twin will stutter, and the rate of concordance (both twins exhibiting the disorder) is higher for monozygotic twins (genetically identical) than for dizygotic (fraternal) twins. Because there isn't a 100% concordance of stuttering in twins, environmental factors must also play a role in the onset and persistence or recovery of stuttering, in addition to genetic factors (Ambrose, Cox, & Yairi, 1997).

DIFFERENCES BETWEEN FLUENT SPEECH AND STUTTERING

Anyone who has listened carefully to a young child speak can attest to the fact that the flow of most children's speech is not continuously forward and uninterrupted. Children exhibit many hesitations, revisions, and interruptions in their utterances. Children are not born as fluent speakers. Fluency requires some degree of physical maturation and language experience, but it does not develop linearly as the child matures. Longitudinal research indicates that children around 25 months of age are more fluent than they will be at 29 months and at 37 months of age (Yairi, 1981, 1982). There is a gradual increase in disfluent speech behaviors beginning around 2 years of age that peaks around the third birthday. Fluency then improves after age 3, and the types of disfluency change.

Normal Disfluencies

The type of disfluency exhibited by a normally developing child changes between the ages of 25 and 37 months. At approximately 2 years of age, typical disfluencies are whole-word repetitions (*I-I-I want a cookie*), interjections (*Can we-uhm-go now?*), and syllable repetitions (*I like ba-baseball*). Revisions such as *He can't-he won't play baseball* are the dominant disfluency type when the child is approximately 3 years old (Yairi, 1982). Normal disfluencies persist throughout the course of one's life, but they do not tend to adversely affect the continuous forward flow of speech. Normally fluent speakers frequently interrupt the forward flow of speech by repeating whole multisyllablic words (*I really-really like hockey*), interjecting a word or phrase (*He will, uhhhhh, you know, not like that idea*), repeating a phrase (*Will you, will you please stop that*), or revising a sentence (*She can't-She didn't do that*).

Stuttering

What is stuttering? How is it different from normally fluent and normally disfluent speech? These are not simple questions, and there are no simple answers. The issue of what stuttering is and how to define it lies at the center of some unresolved issues (Ingham & Cordes, 1997). Can clinicians determine reliably whether and when stuttering has occurred? Do normal disfluencies and moments of stuttering lie along the same continuum, or are they categorically different behavioral events? There are no absolute answers to these questions. At present, no universally accepted definition of stuttering exists. However, a reasonable framework from which one can begin to distinguish between normal disfluencies and those that are likely to be regarded as stuttering has been proposed.

Specifically, stuttering or stuttered speech involves certain core behaviors, including repetitions of sounds, syllables, or one-syllable words, prolongations of sounds, or blocks, where an inappropriate stop in the flow of air or voice occurs during speech production (Guitar, 2014). Part-word repetitions and single-syllable word repetitions are the most frequently observed stuttering behaviors reported by parents when their child is just beginning to stutter. In addition, children who stutter exhibit more repeats of a word or syllable (more than two), and repetitions are three times faster than the repetitions produced by normally disfluent children (Guitar, 2014; Yairi & Ambrose, 2013). Children who stutter generally do not exhibit repetitions of multisyllabic words. Repetitions, revisions, and pauses that frequently occur in children with typical speech and language development are not considered to be stuttering behaviors (Guitar, 2014).

In young children, there continues to be some debate about when speech disfluencies constitute stuttering behaviors. Some studies have shown that children who are considered to be stuttering produce many more within-word disfluencies, including part-word repetitions and prolongations, than do children who are exhibiting normal disfluencies. Other studies have found that the amount of disfluency is important when differentiating stuttering from normal disfluencies, regardless of the type of disfluency produced. For instance, young preschool children who are normally disfluent tend to produce fewer than 10 disfluencies per 100 words, and these disfluencies may be within-in word disfluencies (e.g., syllable repetitions) or between-word disfluencies (e.g., whole-word repetitions). However, stuttering frequency by itself is not a definitive clinical measure for stuttering because some normally disfluent children may exhibit more than 10 disfluencies per 100 words on occasion (Guitar, 2014).

Stuttering behaviors are also differentiated from normal disfluencies by the number of repetition units. As previously stated, more than two repetitions of a sound or word is considered a stuttering moment, but one extra repetition (e.g., "I-I want more juice"; "I li-like ice cream") is believed to be a normal disfluency (Guitar, 2014). Similarly, one or two repetitions of an interjection (e.g., "um") is generally considered a normal disfluency, but more than two repeats of

TABLE 8.1

Examples of stuttering behaviors and normal disfluencies

Type of Disfluency	Stuttering Behavior	Normal Disfluency	Examples
Sound/syllable repetitions (more than two repeats)	X		*He's a b-b-b-boy.* *G-g-g-g-go away.* *Yes, puh-puh-puh please.*
Sound prolongation	X		*Ssssssee me swing!* *My name is Tiiiiiiiimmy.*
Block	X		*Base-(pause)-ball.*
Monosyllabic whole-word repetitions	X		*I-I-I-hit the ball.* *It's my-my-my-turn.*
Multisyllabic whole-word repetitions		X	*I'm going-going home.*
Phrase repetition/interjection		X	*She hit–she hit me.* *I like, uh, ya know, big boats.*
Revisions		X	*He went, he came back.*

Source: Based on Guitar (2014) and Yairi & Ambrose (2013); Guitar, B. (2014). Stuttering: An integrated approach to its nature and treatment (4th ed). Baltimore, MD: Lippincott Williams & Wilkins.; Yairi, E., & Ambrose, N. (2013). Epidemiology of stuttering: 21st century advances. Journal of Fluency Disorders, 38(2), 66–87.

an interjection is equated with stuttering. Table 8.1 provides specific examples of stuttering behaviors and normal disfluencies.

You can visit the Stuttering Foundation website (www.stutteringhelp.org) to listen to the personal stories of children and adolescents who stutter; type "videos" into the search engine at the bottom of the webpage to access the videos titled "Stuttering: Straight Talk for Teens" and "Stuttering: For Kids, by Kids." You'll see firsthand examples of the core stuttering behaviors discussed in this section (i.e., repetitions, prolongations, and blocks) in each video clip.

More than one type of within-word disfluency may be present in a given disruption that interferes with the forward flow of speech. Consider the following disfluent production of the word *mommy* that contains elements of both sound repetition and a prolongation: *m-m-m-mmmommy* (Yaruss, 1997). Such productions, called "clustered disfluencies," are quite common in the speech of young children who stutter. Some researchers have suggested that the presence of clustered disfluencies may also indicate incipient stuttering (stuttering that is just beginning).

> Some parenthetical interjections or asides that are common interruptions in adult speech are devices that help to maintain listener interest. An example of a parenthetical interjection is "When John slipped on the stairs—like Mary slipped in the same spot last week—he broke his ankle."

Other behaviors may accompany instances of speech disfluency. Such behaviors that occur concomitantly with stuttered disfluencies are called *secondary behaviors* or *accessory characteristics*, and are widely varied and idiosyncratic. Some common secondary behaviors include blinking of the eyes, facial grimacing, facial tension, and exaggerated movements of the head, shoulders, and arms. Children who are normally disfluent generally do not exhibit secondary behaviors, although occasionally tense pauses may be observed (Guitar, 2014). In older individuals, interjected speech fragments that are superfluous to the utterance are also considered to be secondary behaviors, particularly when they occur in conjunction with a moment of disfluency. An example of an interjected speech fragment is the superfluous phrase *that is to say* in the utterance *I met her in T-T-T-T, that is to say, I met her in Toronto.*

Secondary behaviors are adopted in an effort to reduce instances of stuttering (Bloodstein, 1995). The person who stutters discovers through trial and error that some action (e.g., bodily movements) momentarily distracts from the act of speaking and that action appears to help terminate or avoid an instance of stuttering. Behaviors such as eye blinking, however, soon lose their apparent power to reduce stuttering, and the individual is forced to replace the ineffective behavior with a new behavior, such as shrugging the shoulders, to reduce stuttering. Unfortunately, the eye blinking behavior may have become so strongly habituated that it will remain permanently associated with a person's stuttering. How do these cardinal stuttering behaviors and secondary behaviors develop, and how do they change over the course of an individual's life?

 Check Your Understanding 8.1
Click here to check your understanding of the concepts in this section.

THE ONSET AND DEVELOPMENT OF STUTTERING THROUGH THE LIFESPAN

Although stuttering can develop at any age, the most common form of stuttering begins in the preschool years and is called *developmental stuttering*. Developmental stuttering is contrasted with another form of stuttering, called

neurogenic stuttering, which is typically associated with neurological disease or trauma, and is acquired after childhood. Neurogenic stuttering differs from the more common developmental stuttering in several ways.

Disfluencies associated with developmental stuttering usually occur on content words (e.g., nouns, verbs), whereas disfluencies associated with neurogenic stuttering occur on function words (e.g., conjunctions, prepositions) and content words. People who have developmental stuttering frequently exhibit secondary behaviors and fear and anxiety about speaking, whereas individuals with neurogenic stuttering do not. Also, developmental stuttering tends to occur on the initial syllables of words, whereas neurogenic stuttering can be more widely dispersed throughout an utterance (Ringo & Dietrich, 1995). Unlike with developmental stuttering, with neurogenic stuttering there are no clear differences in stuttering frequency across speaking tasks (i.e., word imitation vs. connected speech); finally, neurogenic stuttering does not improve (i.e., adapt) with repeated readings or singing, as it does with developmental stuttering (Duffy, 2013). We will focus primarily on developmental stuttering at this point.

It is generally accepted that the onset of developmental stuttering occurs between the ages of 2 and 5, and that 75% of the risk of developing stuttering occurs before the child is $3^1/_2$ years old (Yairi, 1983, 2004; Yairi & Ambrose, 1992a, 1992b, 2004). The onset of stuttering is gradual for the majority of children who develop the condition, with stuttering severity increasing as the child grows older. When stuttering develops in a gradual manner, some general trends regarding stuttering behaviors, reactions to stuttering, and conditions that seem to promote stuttering can be observed. We will outline some of these developmental trends in the following sections (Bloodstein, 1995; Guitar, 2014). Not all children exactly follow this developmental framework of stuttering, but it generally does capture the onset and progression of the disorder. This developmental framework is divided into four specific age-groups that are sequentially related: younger preschool, older preschool, school-age, and adolescents and adults (Guitar, 2014). The development and progression of stuttering by age-group is summarized in Table 8.2.

In the younger preschool years, roughly between two and three years of age, periods of stuttering are followed by periods of relative fluency. The episodic nature of stuttering is an indication that stuttering is in its most rudimentary form. The child may be said to be exhibiting borderline stuttering (Guitar, 2014), and may stutter for weeks at a time between long periods of normally fluent speech. The child tends to stutter most when he or she is upset or excited, and in conditions of communicative pressure, such as when a parent forces a child to recite in front of friends or relatives. Sound and syllable repetitions are the dominant feature, along with monosyllabic whole-word repetitions, compared to multisyllabic word and phrase repetitions (Yairi & Ambrose, 2013). Stuttering tends to occur at the beginnings of sentences, clauses, and phrases on both content words (e.g., nouns, verbs) and function words (e.g., articles, prepositions, etc.), unlike with more advanced forms of stuttering, in which disfluencies are generally confined to content words. Finally, most children at this age are unaware of the interruptions in their speech or are not bothered by them. They generally do not exhibit secondary behaviors, although there may at times be a slight degree of tension during stuttering moments (Guitar, 2014).

In older preschoolers between about four and six years of age, a progression of the disorder occurs; stuttering repetitions may begin to sound rapid and irregular. Blocks, or the inappropriate stoppage of the flow of air or voice may begin to appear, and increased tension of the speech mechanism may be observed (Guitar, 2014).

TABLE 8.2

Summary of the development and progression of stuttering

Developmental Age-Group	Approximate Age	Highlights
Younger preschool	2–3 years	Stuttering is episodic.
		Most stuttering occurs when the child is upset or excited. Sound/syllable repetitions and monosyllabic word repetitions are the dominant speech features. Child seems unaware of the stuttering.
Older preschool	4–6 years	Stuttering is still episodic, but the child is aware of his/her stuttering and may become frustrated when speaking.
		Stuttering is more dispersed throughout the utterance. Stuttering repetitions begin to sound rapid and irregular; blocks and muscular tension begin to appear. Secondary behaviors such as eye blinking may appear.
School-age	6–13 years	Fear of stuttering and attempts to avoid certain speaking situations are common. Certain words are regarded as more difficult than others.
		Circumlocutions and word substitutions are frequent. Blocks with increased muscular tension are the most frequent type of stuttering behavior, although repetitions and prolongations still occur.
Adolescence and Adulthood	14+ years	Stuttering is at its apex of development.
		There is fearful anticipation of stuttering. Longer, more tense blocks mixed with repetitions and prolongations are frequent. Certain sounds, words, and speaking situations are carefully avoided. Circumlocutions, word substitutions, and interjections are used extensively as avoidance strategies.

Source: Based on Bloodstein (1995) and Guitar (2014), Bloodstein, O. (1995). A handbook on stuttering. San Diego, CA: Singular.; Guitar, B. (2014). Stuttering: An integrated approach to its nature and treatment (4th ed). Baltimore, MD: Lippincott Williams & Wilkins.

Stuttering is more widely dispersed throughout the child's utterances. Secondary behaviors such as eye blinking may begin to appear; the child has a conscious awareness of his/her stuttering and may become frustrated at times. At this point, the child is exhibiting incipient (or beginning) stuttering (Guitar, 2014).

By school-age, fear and avoidance of stuttering begin to emerge; stuttering seems to be in response to specific situations such as speaking to strangers or speaking in front of groups. The individual who stutters will approach these situations with dread, and will later try to avoid these situations at all costs (Guitar, 2014). In addition, certain words are regarded as more difficult than others, and the person who stutters attempts to avoid such words by using word substitutions and circumlocutions. An example of a word substitution is *I want a ni-ni-ni-five cents*; the individual substitutes *five cents* for the originally intended word *nickel*. Circumlocutions are roundabout or indirect ways of speaking. A circumlocution used to avoid the term *fire truck* in a child's request for a toy might take on the following form *I want a-ya know-red thing-sirens and ladders-truck for my birthday*. Blocks are now more common than repetitions and prolongations, and characterized by excessive muscular tension; the increased tension is believed to result from negative feelings of fear, embarrassment, and helplessness about the anticipation of stuttering (Guitar, 2014).

In older teens and adults, stuttering is in its most advanced form; the individual has developed a self-concept as a person who stutters and will often refer to himself or herself in this way. A primary characteristic of this age-group is vivid and fearful anticipation of stuttering; the person who stutters tries to control the environment so that situations in which stuttering might occur are avoided (Guitar, 2014). Certain sounds and words are carefully avoided also; the person with advanced stuttering may plan the verbal message ahead of time to ensure he/she avoids sounds and or words believed to be more difficult. Longer, tense blocks are the most frequent core stuttering behavior; repetitions still occur but they are more rapid and irregular and may co-occur with tense blocks (Guitar, 2014). Secondary behaviors such as word substitutions, interjections (e.g., "um"), and circumlocutions continue to be common avoidance strategies. Feelings of embarrassment, helplessness, fear, and shame are common in individuals with advanced stuttering. See Case Study 8.2 for the personal story of a man whose fear of what people might think about of his stuttering almost interfered with his career aspirations.

Stuttering does not always develop gradually. For some individuals, when stuttering is first diagnosed in young children, the symptoms appear to be very advanced, and secondary characteristics may be present (Van Riper, 1982; Yairi, 2004; Yairi & Ambrose, 1992a, 1992b, 2004; Yairi et al., 1993). The onset may be a distinct and sudden event for as many as 36% of children, and the stuttering behaviors may be considered to be moderate to severe (Yairi & Ambrose, 1992a).

CASE STUDY 8.2

Personal Story of a Man with Stuttering

Philippe Bodine was 34 years old when he decided to go back to college to get his master's degree in education. For the past 8 years, he had worked as a grant writer for the large public school district in his hometown. Philippe always wanted to be a history teacher working with high school students, but as a person who stuttered he feared he would be perceived as inadequate and unintelligent; as such, he believed it wasn't possible for him to achieve his career goal. He became a grant writer after he graduated with his bachelor's degree because it required minimal communicative interactions with others, and he didn't need to worry about what people thought about his stuttering. After enrolling in the master's degree program, he sought treatment for his stuttering at the University's speech-language-hearing clinic. Formal assessments conducted by the SLP indicated his stuttering was severe; secondary behaviors included head nodding and slapping his leg. Frequent attempts to avoid difficult words, including his name, resulted in frequent repetitions of the interjection "um."

In addition to working towards increased fluency, treatment included encouraging Philippe to use the strategy of "self-disclosure," which involved having him tell new communication partners in certain speaking situations that he is a person who stutters. During Philippe's student-teaching experience, he self-disclosed his stuttering to school personnel and his high school students by stating, "Hi, my name is Mr. Bodine and I am a person who stutters. You might hear me repeat words or prolong sounds when I speak, but if at any time you don't understand me, please let me know and I'll be happy to say it again." This strategy eased his anxiety about speaking in front of his class, and eliminated his avoidance behaviors.

Philippe completed his student-teaching experience successfully, and was subsequently hired by the school as a history teacher. His dream of becoming a high school teacher came to fruition, something Philippe never thought possible.

Thought Question 8.1

What kinds of jobs require a great deal of speaking? Do you think people who stutter avoid such jobs?

More research is needed about the onset and development of stuttering and the factors that underlie persistence and natural recovery.

 Check Your Understanding 8.2

Click here to check your understanding of the concepts in this section.

THEORIES AND CONCEPTUAL MODELS OF STUTTERING

An examination of some of the most prominent etiological theories of stuttering will provide you with an appreciation of the various models that have influenced stuttering research and treatment for over 80 years. In addition, various aspects of some of the theories we consider are implicitly present in contemporary stuttering research and treatment. Etiological theories of stuttering can be classified into three categories: organic, behavioral, and psychological.

Organic Theory

Organic theories propose an actual physical cause for stuttering. Speculations about a physical cause for stuttering date back to the writings of Aristotle, who suggested that stuttering is a disconnection between the mind and the body and that the muscles of the tongue cannot follow the commands of the brain (Rieber & Wollock, 1977). Many organic theories have been proposed since Aristotle's writings, but they have all failed in one manner or another to explain stuttering satisfactorily. For example, the *theory of cerebral dominance*, or the "handedness theory," proposed by Samuel Orton and Lee Travis in the 1930s (Guitar, 2014), assumed that when neither cerebral hemisphere is dominant, both send competing neural impulses to their respective muscles of speech, resulting in a discoordination between the right and left halves of the speech musculature. Orton and Travis believed that this discoordination resulted in stuttering. A renewed interest in this theory has come about due to recent findings from brain-imaging studies that have revealed structural and functional differences in the brains of adults with chronic developmental stuttering.

Current brain-imaging research may facilitate the development of a comprehensive neurophysiological model for both fluent and stuttered speech that could lead to new stuttering prevention and treatment methods (Brown et al., 2005; Chang et al., 2017; Ingham et al., 2003).

Behavioral Theory

Behavioral theories assert that stuttering is a learned response to conditions external to the individual. Wendell Johnson developed a prominent behavioral theory, the *diagnosogenic* theory, during the 1940s and 1950s. According to this theory, stuttering began in the parent's ear, not in the child's mouth. Overly concerned parents would react to the child's normal speech hesitations and repetitions with negative statements, admonishing the child to speak more slowly and not to stutter. Such parental behaviors made the child anxious about speaking, and the child's anxiety fostered further hesitations and repetitions.

Not only is there no evidence to support this theory, there is evidence to the contrary. Studies have shown that the process of natural recovery may actually be due in part to parents explicitly telling their child to slow down, stop, and start again, or think before speaking when their child is stuttering (e.g., Ambrose & Yairi, 2002; Langford & Cooper, 1974; Martin & Lindamood, 1986).

Psychological Theory

Psychological theory contends that stuttering is a neurotic symptom with ties to unconscious needs and internal conflicts, treated most appropriately by psychotherapy. Some psychological theories regard people who stutter as individuals with neuroses; other theories regard stuttering as a phobic manifestation. Some people who stutter may indeed have neuroses, but psychological theory has yet to provide a satisfactory explanation for the underlying cause of stuttering or its onset and development.

Current Conceptual Models of Stuttering

The *covert repair hypothesis*, based on a language production model, assumes that stuttering is a reaction to some flaw in the speech production plan (Postma & Kolk, 1993). Speakers have the capability of monitoring their speech as it is being formulated and detecting errors in the speech plan. People who stutter have poorly developed phonological encoding skills that cause them to introduce errors into their speech plan. If there are more errors in the speech plan, there will be more occasions for error correction. Stuttering is not the error. Rather, stuttering is a "normal" repair reaction to an abnormal phonetic plan.

Another conceptualization of stuttering is the *demands and capacities model (DCM)* (Starkweather, 1987, 1997). This model asserts that stuttering develops when the environmental demands placed on a child to produce fluent speech exceed the child's physical and learned capacities. The child's capacity for fluent speech depends on a balance of motor skills, language production skills, emotional maturity, and cognitive development. Children who stutter presumably lack one or more of these capacities for fluent speech. Parents of a child who lacks the required motor skills for fluency might talk rapidly; rapid rates of speech may put time pressure on the child that exceeds his or her motoric ability to respond. Other parents might insist on the use of advanced language structures that are in excess of the child's language development. In every case of stuttering within the DCM, there is an imbalance between the environmental demands that are placed on the child and the child's capacity for fluent speech.

The DCM is not a theory of stuttering, and it does not suggest a cause for stuttering. Rather, the DCM is a useful tool that helps clinicians understand the dynamics of forces that contribute to the development of stuttering. Therapeutically, the DCM provides useful guidelines for understanding what capacities a child may lack for fluent speech production and the elements of the child's environment that may be challenging those capacities.

A recent model of stuttering that takes the DCM theory a step further, referred to as the Packman and Attanasio 3–factor model (or P & A model), suggests that there are three factors that cause moments of stuttering: 1) a deficit in the neural processing of language and inherent instability of the speech production system, 2) triggers, or certain features of spoken language that are associated with greater speech motor demands that negatively affect an already unstable speech production system, and 3) modulating factors, such as physiological arousal in an individual that can alter the threshold at which a stuttering moment occurs (Packman, 2012).

In other words, in individuals who stutter there exists an impairment in brain function that affects speech motor stability, such that attempts to produce longer or more linguistically complex utterances result in an increased probability for stuttering moments to occur. Fear and anxiety about speaking, influenced by an individual's past experiences (e.g., bullying in childhood), contributes to the variability of stuttering in the individual in different speaking situations (Packman, 2012; Smith et al., 2010). The P & A model of stuttering is an attempt to take into account the complex, multifactorial nature of stuttering, including an individual's perceptions and/or reactions to stuttering, which must be addressed in stuttering treatment discussed later in this chapter.

Computer simulation models of speech production have been programmed to simulate stuttering, providing further evidence for a disruption in neural processing in individuals who stutter (e.g., Civier, Tasko, & Guenther, 2010). These scientifically sophisticated models may further our understanding of the basic nature of stuttering and help advance treatment of stuttering.

 Check Your Understanding 8.3

Click here to check your understanding of the concepts in this section.

EVALUATION OF STUTTERING

When parents are concerned that a child is stuttering, it is an SLP's responsibility to determine whether there should be concern and, if so, to plan an appropriate course of action. Two important components of the evaluation of a child suspected of stuttering are observations of the child speaking and a detailed parental interview (see Figure 8.1 for some common questions for parents with a disfluent child).

The primary component of a stuttering evaluation is a detailed analysis of the child's speech behaviors. The SLP determines the average number of each type of disfluency the child produces (e.g., within-word repetitions, sound prolongations, interjections). More than 10 disfluencies per 100 words spoken may indicate that the child has a fluency problem (Guitar, 2014). The presence of interjections, revisions, and whole-word repetitions tend to be more common in nonstutterers, whereas sound prolongations and part-word repetitions may be more indicative of stuttering. The SLP will also measure the number of units that occur in each repetition or interjection; recall that more than two repetitions is likely to represent stuttering versus normal disfluency.

Standardized tests such as the *Stuttering Severity Instrument-Fourth Edition (SSI-4)* (Riley, 2009) may also be used in a stuttering evaluation. The SSI-4 may be used with children or adults. This test determines frequency of stuttering measured in percent of syllables stuttered, duration of stuttering moments, and secondary behaviors. An SLP will also record the types of secondary behaviors. A wide assortment of secondary behaviors may indicate a progression of the disorder.

Determining the child's or adult's feelings and attitudes about his/her stuttering is an essential component of the stuttering evaluation. Informal assessment tools are available for young children through to adulthood for this intended purpose. One such tool for children is the *KiddyCAT Communication Attitude Test for Preschool and Kindergarten Children Who Stutter* (Vanryckeghem & Brutten, 2006), which consists of 12 yes/no questions that the SLP asks the child. An example question is "Is talking hard for you?" Research has shown that this questionnaire effectively taps into children's awareness and attitudes about stuttering, and

Figure 8.1 Common questions for parents of a disfluent child.

Introduction

Why are you here today?

Tell us (me) about your child's problem.

Medical/Health History

Were there any problems with your pregnancy or with the birth of your child?

Does your child have any medical or health concerns? Does he/she take any medications?

Was your child ever hospitalized?

Family History

Do any other family members have speech, language, or hearing problems?

Did they receive speech therapy?

Does anyone in the family currently stutter, or previously stuttered at some point in their life?

Speech/Language and Motor Development

When did your child say his or her first words?

When did your child say his or her first phrases and sentences?

Describe your child's motor development.

How does your child's speech-language and motor development compare with his or her siblings?

History/Description of the Problem

Describe your child's speaking problems.

When did the problem start?

Can you describe your child's disfluencies when they were first noticed?

Have they changed over time?

Is your child aware of his/her disfluencies?

Does he/she avoid certain words or avoid talking in certain situations?

Does your child have any excessive body movements when talking?

Have you done anything about your child's disfluency problem?

Have you seen a doctor or other specialist for your child's disfluency problem?

Family Interactions

How does your child get along with his/her siblings?

What is a typical day like for you and your child?

What kinds of things do you do as a family?

Source: Based on Guitar (2014) and Shipley & McAfee (2016). Guitar, B. (2014). Stuttering: An integrated approach to its nature and treatment (4th ed). Baltimore, MD: Lippincott Williams & Wilkins.; Shipley, K., & McAfee, J. (2016). Assessment in speech-language pathology: A resource manual (5th ed). Boston, MA: Cengage Learning.

can help differentiate children who stutter from their typically fluent peers (e.g., Vanryckeghem, Brutten, & Hernandez, 2005).

Similar informal assessment questionnaires are available for adolescents and adults also; one such questionnaire is the *Overall Assessment of the Speaker's Experience of Stuttering (OASES)* (Yaruss & Quesal, 2006). This assessment tool is for individuals who are 18 years and older, and includes four sections: I. General Information, II. Reactions to Stuttering, III. Communication in Daily Situations, and IV. Quality of Life. Its purpose is to determine the overall impact the stuttering impairment has on an individual's life, as well as document changes in more functional communication outcome measures, such as the speaker's difficulties communicating in daily situations, before and after treatment (Yaruss & Quesal, 2006).

An SLP's decision to recommend treatment is not based on any single behavior or test result. Certain risk factors associated with persistent stuttering (e.g., family history of persistent stuttering) will play a role in determining the need for immediate treatment. For children exhibiting borderline stuttering (i.e., more than 10 disfluencies per 100 words with no tension or hurry during the first 12 months after onset) with no significant family history, immediate treatment may not be necessary. Rather, following these children and monitoring their disfluencies to ensure stuttering behaviors decrease during that first year may be all that is needed. The following factors are generally associated with natural recovery of stuttering without treatment:

- There is a decrease in stuttering behaviors during the 12 months after initial onset
- The child is female
- There is no family history of stuttering, or relatives who stuttered at some point in their lives recovered completely from stuttering
- Receptive and expressive language, and phonological skills, are typical for the child's age
- Cognitive abilities are within the typical range for the child's age
- The child has an outgoing, carefree personality and therefore is less sensitive to potential stressors in his/her environment (e.g., possible negative reactions by family members to his/her stuttering) (Guitar, 2014).

 Check Your Understanding 8.4
Click here to check your understanding of the concepts in this section.

TREATMENT FOR STUTTERING

If an SLP determines that a child has a stuttering problem or a high probability of developing stuttering, therapeutic intervention is indicated. In general, two broad intervention strategies can be used with young children who stutter: indirect treatment and direct treatment. Indirect approaches are considered viable for children who are just beginning to stutter and whose stuttering is fairly mild. Direct approaches are typically reserved for children who have been stuttering for at least a year and who exhibit moderate to severe stuttering.

Indirect Treatment

An indirect approach does not explicitly try to modify or change a child's speech fluency; it focuses instead on the child, the child's parents, and the child's environment. Important aspects of indirect treatment are sharing information and teaching parents to provide a slow, relaxed speech model for the child. Play-oriented activities that encourage slow and relaxed speech are the central component of such intervention. There is no explicit discussion about the child's fluent or stuttering speaking behaviors. The goal of indirect treatment is to facilitate fluency through environmental manipulation This approach is often effective for younger preschool children over a period of one to two months; however, if stuttering does not decrease within six weeks, direct treatment approaches may be recommended (Guitar, 2014).

Direct Treatment

Direct approaches involve explicit and direct attempts to modify the child's speech and speech-related behaviors. In direct treatment, for instance, concepts such as "hard" and "easy" speech may be introduced. Hard speech is rapid and relatively tense (such as a tense sound prolongation of /s/ in *sssssssssss-snake*), whereas easy speech is slow and relaxed. The terms "hard" and "easy" are simple and carry little negative connotation for the child. Children are taught to identify both types of speech, indirectly at first, while the clinician models "hard" and "easy" speech during play interactions, and comments about it to the child, later having the child identify these types of speech in his/her own ongoing productions. Once the child is able to identify hard and easy speech segments accurately and reliably, the SLP teaches the child strategies that will help him or her increase easy speech and change from hard speech to easy speech when required. The therapeutic sequence of identification followed by identification/modification forms the core elements of many strategies for children and adults.

Treatment of Stuttering in Preschool-Age Children

A direct treatment approach shown in randomized clinical trials to be effective in reducing stuttering to zero or near-zero levels in children younger than 6 years of age is the *Lidcombe Program* (Packman et al., 2015). The *Lidcombe Program* involves parent-administered verbal contingencies for stutter-free speech (e.g., "that was nice and smooth") and stuttering (e.g., "oops, that was bumpy"), as well as requests for self-correction (e.g., can you say that more smoothly?). Verbal contingencies are first administered each day to the child by the parent during structured play interactions, and then during unstructured, daily interactions (e.g., during meals or riding in the car). Weekly clinic visits with the SLP involve direct measurement of the child's stuttering, and also involve checking to ensure the program is being implemented correctly by the parent. Parents also provide a weekly stuttering severity rating to the SLP so that frequency of stuttering outside of the clinic setting can be monitored. While this approach has been shown to be highly successful in eliminating stuttering in young children, it is uncertain which aspects of the program are responsible for its positive effects. Therefore, it is important that parents are taught to administer the program in the way it is described in the treatment manual found here: https://sydney.edu.au/health-sciences/asrc/docs/lp_treatment_guide_2015.pdf

Treatment of Stuttering in Older Children and Adults

Individuals who continue to stutter into their teenage years and beyond will likely have many negative reactions to speaking situations that may affect their social lives and vocational goals. Many of these individuals will have had previous unsuccessful speech treatment and perhaps other forms of remediation to combat the fluency problem. An adult who stutters experiences many psychosocial stresses which have a negative impact on his/her well-being and on overall quality of life (e.g., poor self-esteem). In addition to treating stuttering behaviors, the psychosocial variables related to quality of life must also be addressed to maximize the effectiveness of stuttering treatments (Boyle, 2015).

Recent research shows that adults who stutter who have more helpful social support networks and higher levels of social functioning and activity, including involvement in self-help support groups, have a higher quality of life. Therefore, involving family members and significant others in the treatment process, and encouraging the individual who stutters to increase social connection with others may prove more beneficial in the treatment of stuttering than just teaching the individual to modify his/her speech (Blumgart et al., 2014; Boyle, 2015).

Similarly, working with older children to combat the fear, embarrassment, and feelings of shame frequently associated with stuttering will be necessary for intervention to be successful. Teaching older children to be more open about their stuttering, and acknowledging their stuttering in a casual manner can be an effective strategy (Guitar, 2014). For instance, the older child who stutters during a class presentation might say "Gee, I really got stuck there for a moment," or he can use the strategy of "self-disclosure" discussed in Case Study 7.1, in which he can say "I might stutter during my presentation; if you have trouble understanding me during those times, I'll be happy to repeat myself" (Byrd et al., 2017; Byrd et al., 2016; Guitar, 2014). Regardless of the particular strategy used, it's important for the child to come up with his own comments when he feels ready to be more open about his stuttering (Guitar, 2014).

Thought Question 8.2

If you were a person who stutters, would you feel comfortable using "self-disclosure" as a treatment strategy? Why or why not?

Direct Therapeutic Techniques

In the next section, we'll discuss specific therapeutic techniques used to manage stuttering in older children and adults. In particular, we explore direct techniques that are used to establish fluency. Changing certain aspects of one's speaking behavior is of fundamental importance in stuttering intervention, and is often a source of confusion among clinicians who treat older children and adults who stutter (e.g., Yaruss et al., 2017).

Therapeutic techniques designed to modify stuttering behaviors are classified generally into two broad categories: *fluency-shaping techniques* and *stuttering modification techniques*. When used properly, both techniques have a powerful effect in reducing stuttering. Fluency-shaping techniques involve changing the overall speech timing patterns of the individual in an effort to reduce or eliminate stuttering. This is typically accomplished by lengthening the duration of sounds and words and greatly slowing down the overall rate of speech. Stuttering modification techniques involve changing only the stuttering behaviors. This is typically accomplished by lengthening the duration of or in some way modifying only the speech segment on which the stuttering is occurring. Treatment programs for stuttering often combine these two approaches (Guitar, 2014). See Prins and Ingham (2009) for a historical, evidence-based perspective of fluency-shaping and stuttering modification treatments.

Fluency-Shaping Techniques

Reducing speech rate, known as **prolonged speech**, is one of the most powerful ways to reduce or eliminate stuttering. Prolonged speech may be a specific therapeutic goal, or it may involve use of various techniques that serve to reduce speaking rate and increase fluency. The term *prolonged speech* arose from research conducted in the 1960s regarding the effects of delayed auditory feedback (DAF) on speech production. DAF is a condition in which a speaker hears his or her own speech after an instrumental delay of some finite period of time, such as 250 or 500 milliseconds. When a person speaks under DAF, his or her speech is slowed involuntarily because the duration of syllables is prolonged. For example, when people who stutter speak under conditions of DAF, speaking rates decrease dramatically; the longer the delay, the slower the speech. This slowing of speech rate under DAF conditions is accompanied by a substantial decrease in stuttering.

Delayed auditory feedback systems use a microphone and earphones. A person wearing the earphones speaks into the microphone, which transmits the speech to a device that electronically delays sending the speech to the earphones. If the delay were set at 250 milliseconds (or ¼ second), the speaker would hear his or her utterance ¼ of a second after it was uttered. Delaying the auditory feedback causes the speaker to reduce the rate of speaking.

When DAF is used clinically to prolong speech, the feedback delay is set to promote speaking rates of about 30 to 60 syllables per minute. During this initial phase, the person who stutters is taught to prolong the duration of each syllable but not to increase the duration of pauses between syllables (Boburg & Kully, 1995; Max & Caruso, 1997). This prolonged speech pattern is systematically altered over the course of intervention by adjusting the DAF times to reduce the magnitude of syllable prolongation while maintaining fluent speech. Speech rates ranging from 120 to 200 syllables per minute are typical targets for the termination of treatment.

Behavioral techniques that serve not only to reduce speech rate but also reduce physical tension in the speech musculature before and during occurrences of stuttering, promoting smooth speech, are *light articulatory contacts* and *gentle voicing onsets (GVOs)*. The therapeutic use of light articulatory contacts involves instructing the speaker to use less tension in the articulators, particularly during production of stop consonants (/p/, /b/, /t/, /d/, /k/, and /g/) that involve a complete constriction of the vocal tract (Max & Caruso, 1997).

People who stutter frequently use excessive articulator pressure when producing sounds. They may, for example, press the tongue very hard on the roof of the mouth during the production of /t/ and /d/ sounds. Teaching the individual to reduce such pressure, or make light articulatory contacts, promotes fluency.

Reducing articulatory tension is believed to prevent occurrence of prolonged articulatory postures that interfere with smooth articulatory transitions from sound to sound. Light touches promote continuity and ease of articulation by preventing excessive pressure and tension in the articulators (Boburg & Kully, 1995).

Gentle voicing onsets (GVOs) are a cardinal feature of many treatment programs, and they are known by many different names, such as Fluency Initiation of Gestures (FIGS) (Cooper, 1984). The basic characteristic of GVOs is a tension-free onset of voicing that gradually builds in intensity. One can appreciate the dynamics of this technique by initiating production of the vowel /a/ in a whisper, gradually engaging the vocal folds such that the vowel is produced with a breathy voice quality, and finally increasing the vowel's intensity. GVOs are typically learned in a hierarchical fashion beginning with vowel production, followed by syllable productions, and then word productions.

Another clinical rate reduction technique that has an ameliorative effect on stuttering is called *pausing/phrasing*, and it is designed to lengthen naturally occurring pauses (clause and sentence boundaries) and to add pauses between other words or phrases. In addition, pausing/phrasing techniques may attempt to limit utterance length to two to five syllables. A formal stuttering treatment known as the *Gradual Increase in Length and Complexity of Utterance (GILCO)* program (Ryan, 1974) capitalizes on the underlying principles of pausing/phrasing techniques, and has been found to be effective in reducing or eliminating stuttering, particularly in school-age children. Another powerful fluency-shaping therapeutic intervention consistently found to reduce or eliminate stuttering is response-contingent stimulation (RCS). RCS procedures have their origins in learning theory, and are based on B. F. Skinner's behavioral (operant) conditioning paradigm. Operant conditioning results in the association between a behavior (response) and the stimulus that follows (consequence), and thus determines the future occurrence of that behavior.

Skinner's system of behavioral modification is the basis for response-contingent time-out from speaking (RCTO), which requires the individual to pause briefly from speaking after a stuttering behavior has occurred. This pause or cessation from speaking serves as the consequence for stuttering. Research has consistently shown its positive effects on reducing stuttering frequency to zero or nearly zero levels. Adolescents and adults who stutter have also been taught to self-administer a time-out from speaking immediately after a self-identified instance of stuttering

Well-controlled experimental investigations over the past 30 years have consistently demonstrated the robust and immediate effects of behavioral modification techniques such as rewarding fluent speech and correcting stuttered speech.

Dr. Charles Van Riper was a distinguished professor of SLP for many years at Western Michigan University. Dr. Van Riper learned to control his stuttering and spent most of his life searching for the cause and cure of stuttering. Intervention techniques that he developed are still in use today.

(Hewat et al., 2006; James, 1981b). The mechanism underlying the success of RCTO remains elusive, however. Response-contingent procedures form the basis of the *Lidcombe Program*, discussed previously.

Stuttering Modification Techniques

Unlike the fluency-shaping approach that seeks to reduce or eliminate stuttering by teaching the individual who stutters to speak in a way that prevents stuttering, the stuttering modification approach teaches the person who stutters to react to his or her stuttering calmly, without unnecessary effort or struggle (Prins & Ingham, 2009). Stuttering modification procedures were born out of Charles Van Riper's conceptualization of stuttering as a disruption in speech timing, causing fluency breakdowns, as well as the triggering of negative reactions to such breakdowns.

As such, three techniques developed by Van Riper work to not only modify speech timing but also to modify abnormal reactions to stuttering (Prins & Ingham, 2009). They are known as *cancellations*, *pull-outs*, and *preparatory sets*.

These three techniques are introduced therapeutically in sequential order, beginning with stuttering cancellation. During the cancellation phase of treatment, an individual is required to complete the word that was stuttered and pause deliberately following the production of that stuttered word. The individual pauses for a minimum of 3 seconds, and then reproduces the stuttered word in slow motion. This ostensibly provides practice with the motoric integration and speech timing movements that are required for a fluent production of that word. When the individual reaches a criterion level of cancellation proficiency, he or she will move to the second technique, known as pull-outs.

During the pull-out phase of treatment, the individual does not wait until after the stuttered word is completed to correct the inappropriate behavior. Rather, the individual modifies the stuttered word during the actual occurrence of the stuttering. This modification involves slowing down the sequential movements of the syllable or word when stuttering occurs, in a fashion similar to the slowed and exaggerated movements used in the cancellation phase of treatment. In essence, the individual is modifying the stuttering online, "pulling out" of the stuttering behavior and completing it with a more fluent production of the intended word. Once again, when the individual reaches a criterion level of proficiency, he or she will move to the last stage, known as preparatory sets.

The preparatory sets stage involves using the slow-motion speech strategies that were learned during the first two phases of treatment, not as a response to an occurrence of stuttering, but in anticipation of stuttering. A person who stutters typically knows when and on what word a stuttering moment will occur. When an individual anticipates stuttering, he or she starts preparing to use the newly learned fluency-producing strategies before the word is attempted. The goal of this phase of treatment is to initiate the word in a more fluent manner, even though the individual is producing consecutive speech movements and transitions in a slowed manner.

Selecting Intervention Techniques

An SLP's selection of a specific management technique depends on many factors, including the individual's age, severity of the stuttering problem, the motivation and specific needs of the person who stutters including psychosocial variables, and the SLP's knowledge of the specific techniques available. Careful and detailed observation of an individual's stuttering behaviors before initiating treatment and during the treatment process is essential to successful clinical management of stuttering.

 Audio Exercise 8.1

Examining a Four-Year-Old Boy Who Stutters

Click on the link to listen to a speech sample of a child who stutters, and complete an exercise.

Effectiveness of Stuttering Intervention through the Lifespan

Determining the effectiveness of stuttering treatment depends largely on how *effectiveness* is defined. This is a complex issue. However, a "treatment for stuttering might be considered *effective* if it resulted in the individual's being able to speak with disfluencies within normal limits whenever and to whomever he or she chose, without undue concern or worry about speaking" (Conture, 1996, p. S20). The treatment of stuttering differs across an individual's life-span in terms of frequency and nature, as well as rates of recovery. Therefore, the review of treatment efficacy is best considered relative to age group: preschool, school-age children, teenagers, and adults. Review of the published research in stuttering intervention provides support for use of several treatment approaches and/or techniques. These are briefly reviewed in Box 8.1.

BOX 8.1 | **Evidence-Based Practices for Individuals with Stuttering**

General

- Individuals who stutter can benefit from intervention by an SLP at any time during their life.
- Treatments with the greatest efficacy for reducing stuttering in older children and adults include those that change the rate of speech and tension during speaking.
- Comprehensive approaches focusing on the individual's attitude toward speaking and on addressing the negative impact of stuttering on one's life are reported by clients as being of more benefit than approaches that focus on speech alone.
- Between 60% and 80% of clients who participate in stuttering treatment make significant improvement.

Specific Behavioral Treatment Approaches or Techniques

- Indirect treatment approaches that teach parents to reduce their conversational speaking rate have been shown to facilitate fluent speech in preschool children.

- The long-term effectiveness of the parent-administered behavioral intervention, the *Lidcombe Program*, is well established, particularly for preschool children. Parents are taught to provide positive praise for their child's fluent speech by saying, "Good job, that was nice and smooth" and to acknowledge or correct stuttered speech by saying, "Oops, that was bumpy, can you say _____ again." The program recommends far more verbal contingencies for stutter-free speech than stuttered speech.
- A program of gradual increase in length and complexity of utterances, called GILCO, in which a child progresses from one-word stutter-free responses to 5 minutes of stutter-free speech during reading, monologue speaking, and conversation has been found to be highly effective with older children.
- Prolonged speech techniques (e.g., prolonging syllable durations; use of light articulatory contacts, or gentle voicing onsets) have been found to be highly effective with older children and adults, particularly when taught in the context of a structured program with opportunities for

BOX 8.1 *(Continued)*

daily practice. No one technique has been found to be effective on its own, however.

- Smooth speech, a derivative of prolonged speech, uses multiple strategies (i.e., pausing/phrasing, gentle voicing onsets, light articulatory contacts) to first slow speech rate and prolong syllables, and then increase speech rate to normal levels. This approach has been shown to be effective with older children and adolescents who stutter, and tends to result in more natural sounding speech; therefore, it may be preferred over other prolonged speech treatments.
- RCTO from speaking is based on behavioral (operant) conditioning and involves the individual pausing briefly from speaking immediately after a stuttering event. This procedure is highly effective in reducing stuttering in adolescents

and adults. Usually, the SLP tells the individual to stop speaking after an instance of stuttering; however, individuals can be taught to self-deliver a time-out from speaking following a self-identified stuttering moment.

- Cognitive-behavior therapy strategies, widely used in clinical psychology, can be learned and applied by speech-language pathologists. These strategies have been shown to effectively decrease social anxiety and reduce avoidance in adults who stutter.

Source: Based on Bothe et al. (2006); Conture & Yaruss (2009); Craig et al. (1996); Ellis & Beltyukova (2012); Guitar (2014); Hewat et al. (2006); James (1981b); Menzies et al. (2009); Nye et al. (2013); Packman et al. (2015); Sawyer et al. (2017); Ryan (1974); Ryan & Van Kirk Ryan (1995).

Efficacy of Intervention with Preschool-Age Children

In general, the findings of most recent studies are quite encouraging and indicate the potential benefits of early diagnosis and treatment of stuttering. Indirect and direct treatment approaches for preschool children have both been found to be effective (Franken et al., 2005), and may be even more effective when combined (Gottwald, 2010). Among preschool-age children enrolled in a parent-conducted intervention program, all maintained their fluent speech in long-term clinical follow-up studies after dismissal from treatment (e.g., Jones et al., 2008; Lincoln & Onslow, 1997).

Efficacy of Intervention with School-Age Children

Thought Question 8.3

What might be the advantages and disadvantages of social media for school-age children who stutter?

Research has shown that the various treatment approaches and techniques available for school-age children who stutter are effective in establishing fluent speech; however, the child's ability to use these techniques in different settings and maintain improvements in fluent speech over time appears to be problematic (Yaruss & Pelczarski, 2007). With school-age children, it is important to address the psychosocial aspects of stuttering, namely the fear, anxiety, avoidance, and other negative reactions commonly associated with stuttering, for treatment to be effective in the long-term (Yaruss, Coleman, & Quesal, 2012).

Efficacy of Intervention with Adolescents and Adults

Teenagers who stutter can be difficult to manage clinically; establishing a collaborative relationship based in trust and mutual respect is essential to success with this population (Zebrowski & Wolf, 2011). Similarly, a positive client-clinician relationship has also been shown to contribute to successful treatment outcomes in adults who stutter (e.g., Plexico et al., 2010). In addition, a wide variety of adult stuttering treatment techniques have been investigated, ranging from behavioral conditioning techniques to participation in self-help support groups. Collectively, these studies suggest a 60% to 80% improvement rate, regardless of the therapeutic technique used. Treatment that addresses negative feelings and attitudes, in addition to establishing fluency, is more effective than treatment that just focuses on speech alone.

In summary, stuttering intervention across all age groups results in an average improvement for about 70% of all cases, with preschool-age children improving more quickly and easily than people who have a longer history with stuttering. The clinical research that we have considered indicates that effective treatment of stuttering involves a comprehensive approach that considers the broader consequences of stuttering, in addition to the observable stuttering behaviors.

The Effects of Stuttering through the Lifespan

Current evidence suggests that stuttering affects the ability to communicate and participate in life situations from an early age (Millard & Davis, 2016). More than 50% of disfluent preschool children are aware of their stuttering, and develop negative feelings about their speech. As a result, they may use more gestures to communicate, or withdraw from play interactions with peers (Boey et al., 2009; Langevin et al., 2009). School-age children who stutter are more likely to be bullied, teased, viewed negatively by peers, and less likely to be nominated as leaders (Davis, Howell, & Cooke, 2002). Reduced classroom participation and poorer academic achievement are also more common in children who stutter compared to their non-stuttering peers (e.g., Daniels, Gabel, & Hughes, 2012).

The educational and personal disadvantages stuttering may impose on a young person do not end when the child leaves school. Stuttering can also have a negative impact in the workplace, and is a vocationally disabling condition because employers view it as a disorder that decreases employability and opportunities for promotion (Hurst & Cooper, 1983; Palasik et al., 2012). Despite this view, when an employee who stutters seeks treatment, there is an attendant improvement in the employer's perception of the employee (Craig & Calvert, 1991). This enhanced perception is reflected by increased numbers of job promotions among employees who sought treatment and were successful in maintaining fluency following treatment.

Stuttering has a potentially negative effect on an individual's emotional well-being and overall quality of life (Boyle, 2015). Individuals who stutter tend to withdraw from people and social situations due to their fear and embarrassment about their stuttering, thereby causing social isolation and reduced social support networks. There is also a high rate of social anxiety among individuals who stutter (Iverach & Rapee, 2014). Consequently, individuals who stutter are more prone to anxiety, depression, and negative affect. Encouraging individuals who stutter to engage in social activity, and helping them accept who they are, is integral to the treatment process.

 Check Your Understanding 8.5

Click here to check your understanding of the concepts in this section.

SUMMARY

Stuttering is a disabling condition primarily characterized by sound and syllable repetitions and sound prolongations that interrupt the smooth forward flow of speech. Stuttering is a universal problem that affects males more than females. In most cases, stuttering appears between the ages of 2 to 4 years, and as the disorder progresses it increases in severity. Stuttering can adversely affect an individual's school performance, employment, and social interactions. The treatment of stuttering is most effective when it is initiated in early childhood, although treatment at any age can reduce stuttering.

A number of theories—organic, behavioral, and psychological—attempt to account for the onset and development of stuttering, but its cause is unknown. Pinpointing the cause of stuttering will undoubtedly require expertise from many specialists, including speech-language pathologists, neurolinguists, geneticists, and medical specialists.

SUGGESTED READINGS/SOURCES

Bothe, A., Davidow, J., Bramlett, R., & Ingham, R. (2006). Stuttering treatment research 1970–2005: I. Systematic review incorporating trial quality assessment of behavioral, cognitive, and related approaches. *American Journal of Speech-Language Pathology, 15*, 321–341.

Guitar, B. (2014). *Stuttering: An integrated approach to its nature and treatment* (4th ed). Baltimore, MD: Lippincott Williams & Wilkins.

Prins, D., & Ingham, R. (2009). Evidence-based treatment and stuttering—Historical perspective. *Journal of Speech, Language, and Hearing Research, 52*, 254–263.

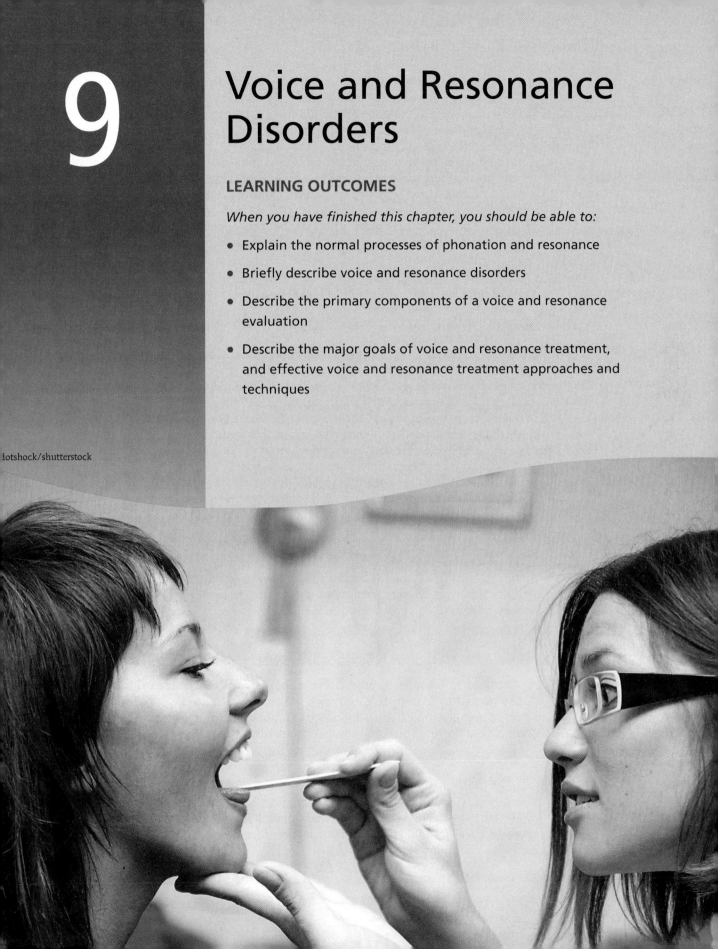

9

Voice and Resonance Disorders

LEARNING OUTCOMES

When you have finished this chapter, you should be able to:

- Explain the normal processes of phonation and resonance

- Briefly describe voice and resonance disorders

- Describe the primary components of a voice and resonance evaluation

- Describe the major goals of voice and resonance treatment, and effective voice and resonance treatment approaches and techniques

V oice is our primary means of emotional and linguistic expression, and is an essential feature of the uniquely human attribute known as speech (Boone, McFarlane, Von Berg, & Zraick, 2010; Titze, 1994). Your voice reflects gender, personality, personal habits, age, and the general condition of your health. Research has shown that certain characteristics of the voice reflect various personality dimensions, and these vocal characteristics correlate well with standardized tests of personality (Colton & Casper, 1990; Markel et al., 1964). Your voice is an emotional outlet that mirrors your moods, attitudes, and general feelings. You can express anger by shouting and express affection by speaking softly; these types of vocal expression have great potential to evoke emotional responses from a listener.

Resonance refers to the quality of the voice that is produced from sound vibrations in the pharyngeal, oral, and nasal cavities. Recall from Chapter 3 that sound energy produced by the vibrating vocal folds travels through the vocal tract, an acoustic resonator that serves to enhance or reduce particular frequencies of that sound. Thus, the size and shape of the pharynx, oral cavity, and nasal cavity will directly affect the perceived sound, or quality, of your voice. In addition, the velopharyngeal mechanism, responsible for coupling and decoupling the oral and nasal cavities during speech and swallowing, regulates sound energy and air pressure in the oral and nasal cavities (Kummer, 2011a; Kummer & Lee, 1996). Recall that the production of most speech sounds requires the velum to be elevated to prevent air from escaping through the nose and also to ensure adequate air pressure buildup in the oral cavity to produce high-pressure consonants (e.g., /p/, b/, /s/). Failure of the velopharyngeal mechanism to separate the oral and nasal cavities during speech production and swallowing is called **velopharyngeal dysfunction (VPD)**. VPD is a frequent result of malformations of the hard and soft palate early in embryonic development.

In this chapter, we will extend some of the basic concepts related to normal voice and resonance, as well as discuss disorders of voice associated with structural pathologies, neurological disorders, and psychological and stress conditions. We will also discuss disorders of resonance related to *craniofacial anomalies*, or congenital malformations involving the head and face (i.e., cleft palate). Finally, we will discuss assessment, treatment, treatment efficacy issues, and evidence-based practices as they pertain to voice and resonance.

NORMAL VOICE AND RESONANCE PRODUCTION

As discussed in Chapter 3, production of normal voice depends on the integrity of the phonatory system (e.g., larynx), while normal resonance depends on the opening and closing of the velopharyngeal port. The physiologic and perceptual correlates of normal voice and resonance are discussed in the following section.

Vocal Pitch

Recall from Chapter 3 that speech production begins with phonation, or sound produced by vocal fold vibration. Fundamental frequency is associated with the speed of vocal fold vibration and is measured in **hertz (Hz)**, or the number of complete vibrations per second.

During one complete vibratory cycle of vocal fold vibration, the vocal folds move from a closed or adducted position to an open or abducted position and back to the closed position. Figure 9.1 depicts the normal vocal folds in the abducted position during endotracheal intubation.

Figure 9.1 Normal, healthy vocal folds in abducted (open) position during endotracheal intubation.

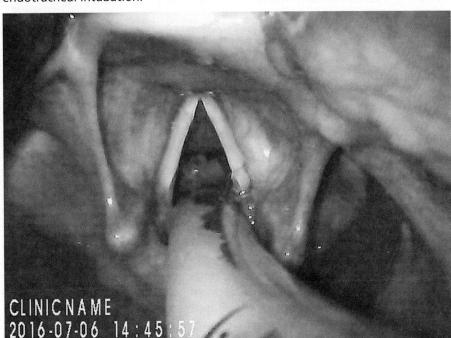

(Photograph courtesy of Steven R. Knight)

The perceptual correlate of fundamental frequency is *pitch*. For example, on average, adult men have fundamental frequencies of around 125 Hz (the vocal folds open and close 125 times per second), whereas adult women have fundamental frequencies around 250 Hz. Therefore, the perceived pitch of male voices is, on average, lower than the perceived pitch of female voices. The fundamental frequency of young children's voices can be as high as 500 Hz, resulting in a very high-pitched voice. The difference in vocal fundamental frequency (and resulting vocal pitch) among men, women, and children is due largely to the structure of the vocal folds themselves. The structural changes of the vocal folds and the relationship to vocal fundamental frequency through the lifespan are summarized in Table 9.1.

Although individuals have a habitual speaking frequency (average pitch), the frequency of the voice constantly varies during speech production. A monotonous or **monopitch** voice is the result of not varying the habitual speaking frequency during speech production. People who use a monotone voice are not terribly interesting to listen to, and listeners quickly lose interest in what is being said. Varying the pitch of the voice also has linguistic significance. Consider these two sentences:

Tom has a dog.

Tom has a dog?

TABLE 9.1

Summary of laryngeal development and fundamental frequency characteristics through the lifespan

Time	Structural Development	Fundamental Frequency
Birth	Larynx positioned high in the neck; vocal fold length is 2.5–3 mm	Average is about 400 Hz; unstable
6 years	Vocal fold length is about 8 or 9 mm; minimal sex difference in vocal fold length until about 10 years	About 200 to 300 Hz; stable until about 10 years of age with minimal sex-related difference
Puberty	Increases to about 12–17 mm in girls, and 15–25 mm in boys	One octave decrease for males to about 130 Hz; a much less downward change in females
Adulthood	Vocal fold length is about 17–29 mm in men, and 12.5–21 mm in women	Males' average is 125 Hz; females' average is 250 Hz

Source: Based on Hixon, Weismer, & Hoit (2014); Kent (1997).

The words in these two sentences are identical, but the sentences' meanings are quite different. "Tom has a dog" is a statement of fact (a declarative), whereas "Tom has a dog?" is a question (an interrogative). Say those two sentences out loud, paying particular attention to what happens to your pitch at the end of each sentence. For the declarative, the pitch of your voice will decrease or fall off as you are saying the word *dog*. In contrast, for the interrogative, the pitch of your voice will increase when you are saying the word *dog*. How does one change the pitch of the voice? Modifications in the length and tension of the vocal folds are necessary to produce pitch change.

Vocal Loudness

Like changing the pitch of the voice, changing vocal loudness is also necessary for adequate communication. **Monoloudness**, or a voice that lacks normal variations of loudness that occur during speech, may reflect an inability to change loudness voluntarily due to neurological impairment or psychiatric disability, or it may be merely a habit associated with the person's personality.

Vocal loudness is the perceptual correlate of intensity, which is measured in **decibels (dB)**. In general, as vocal intensity increases, the perceived loudness of the voice increases. The loudness of normal conversational speech, such as conversations at the dinner table, averages around 60 dB. Changes in vocal intensity require the vocal folds to stay together longer during the closed phase of vibration, but alveolar pressure is the major determinant of vocal intensity (Hixon et al., 2014; Zemlin, 1998). As discussed in Chapter 3, alveolar pressure is the pressure placed on the vocal folds by the lungs. Every time alveolar pressure doubles, there is an 8 to 12 dB increase in vocal intensity. The *Guinness Book of World Records* reports that the loudest scream ever recorded was produced at 123.2 dB, and a man named Anthony Fieldhouse won the World Shouting Contest with a yell that was registered at 112.4 dB (Kent, 1997). Unless you are a record seeker, this kind of behavior is not recommended, as we see later in this chapter. Check out the National Center for Voice & Speech website www.ncvs.org and type "tutorials" into the search bar for an in-depth look at pitch and loudness control.

Voice Quality

Voice quality is a perceptual attribute related to the sound of the voice that is difficult to quantify like fundamental frequency or vocal intensity (Behrman, 2007; Titze, 1994). The unique traits of an individual's voice quality are derived from the anatomy of the larynx, the shape of the vocal tract and its resonant characteristics, and suprasegmental aspects of speech such as rate and rhythm, which can alter the way the vocal folds vibrate. Therefore, voice quality is based on genetics (e.g., laryngeal anatomy is partially determined at birth) and learned behaviors (e.g., how fast or slow you talk) (Titze, 1994).

Lifespan Issues

After the structure and function of the larynx reach full maturity in early adulthood, it continues to change with age, causing functional changes in the voice. For instance, beginning in the third decade for men, and the fourth decade for women, some of the laryngeal cartilages and joints begin to ossify, or turn to bone, while others calcify, or turn to salt, causing the larynx to become stiff and brittle (Hixon et al., 2014). This can result in reduced movement of laryngeal structures in older individuals, and interfere with the ability of the vocal folds to fully come together during phonation (Kahane, 1988). Age-related changes to the larynx can lead to **presbyphonia**, a voice disorder characterized by perceptual changes in pitch, pitch range, loudness, and voice quality in the voice of older individuals (Roy et al., 2007).

As mentioned in Chapter 3, fundamental frequency gets lower in women and higher in men with advancing age. Menopause and hormone-related factors causing increased *edema*, or swelling due to an accumulation of fluid, may be responsible for the change in women. For men, age-related changes to laryngeal muscle due to **atrophy**, or loss of tissue resulting in a decrease in the overall mass of the vocal folds, may be responsible for the increased fundamental frequency in older men (Hixon et al., 2014; Hirano, Kurita, & Sakaguchi, 1989).

 Thought Question 9.1

Do you think there is such a thing as a "voiceprint" similar to a person's fingerprint?

Resonance

The sound produced by the vibrating vocal folds would not result in a rich, full, or loud enough voice without the additional component of resonance (Boone et al., 2010). Normal resonance is largely determined by the velopharyngeal structures and the adequacy of their function. Structures of the velopharyngeal mechanism include the velum (soft palate), the lateral pharyngeal walls, and the posterior pharyngeal wall. Velopharyngeal closure is achieved by the combined action of velar elevation in a flap-like fashion and movement of the lateral pharyngeal walls and posterior pharyngeal wall in a sphincter-like fashion. The velopharyngeal port remains open most of the time to allow for nasal breathing. It is also open for production of the nasal consonants (i.e., *m, n, ng*), but must achieve complete or nearly complete closure for production of oral speech sounds (Hixon et al., 2014).

Lifespan Issues

Velopharyngeal closure patterns vary among individuals, and can change over time with age. For instance, young children with enlarged adenoids may achieve velopharyngeal closure via elevation of the velum against the adenoid mass. If an adenoidectomy is performed, the child may experience hypernasal-sounding speech, or speech that sounds like it is resonating through the nasal cavity, following the surgery. Luckily, most children undergo a natural reorganization of their systems during development such that velopharyngeal closure patterns slowly begin to involve movement of the pharyngeal walls to accommodate for the lack of adenoid tissue (Hixon et al., 2014). From young adulthood through to advanced age, velopharyngeal function during speech production remains intact and unchanged (Hoit et al., 1994).

 Check Your Understanding 9.1

Click here to check your understanding of the concepts in this section.

DISORDERS OF VOICE AND RESONANCE

Voice disorders are characterized by deviations in voice quality, pitch, and/or loudness resulting from disordered laryngeal, respiratory, and/or vocal tract functioning. It is estimated that 3% to 9% of adults in the United States have a voice disorder (Ramig & Verdolini, 1998), with women more commonly affected than men at a reported ratio of 1.5 to 1.0 (Martins et al., 2016; Roy, Merrill, Gray, & Smith, 2005). In children 3–10 years of age, the prevalence of voice disorders is estimated at about 6%, with boys affected more often than girls (Black, Vahratian, & Hoffman, 2015; Carding et al., 2006).

Specific vocal behaviors such as loud talking, coughing, or throat clearing may predispose some individuals to voice disorders (Titze, 1994). Certain occupational groups like teachers and singers, who regularly engage in vocally intense activities, are also more prone to voice disorders (Thibeault et al., 2004). For instance, teachers of primary and secondary education were found to have a higher prevalence of voice disorders than nonteachers in the general population (11.0% vs. 6.2%), although their voice problems were reportedly short-lived (i.e., less than 4 weeks in duration) (Roy et al., 2004). On the other hand, music teachers were found to experience more chronic voice problems, suggesting that regular singing poses a greater risk of injury to the vocal folds than other vocal activities (Thibeault et al., 2004).

Unlike voice disorders in children, which are usually related to vocal misuse or abuse (e.g., yelling, loud talking) and in most cases are temporary, adult voice disorders are quite varied and can be associated with vocal misuse/abuse behaviors, neurological disorders, psychological conditions, or some combination of these factors. Perceptual signs of a voice disorder are related to specific characteristics of a person's voice and can be evaluated by the speech-language pathologist (SLP). Clinically, perceptual signs in conjunction with a person's case history serve as the initial benchmarks in the differential diagnosis of a voice disorder. When one or more perceptual aspects of voice such as pitch, loudness, or voice quality are outside the range of normal for an individual's age, sex, cultural background, or geographic location, we say a voice disorder exists (Boone et al., 2010).

Classification of Voice Disorders

A number of different classification schemes exist to characterize voice disorders (cf., Stemple, 2007; Verdolini, Rosen, & Branski, 2006); here we will classify voice disorders into two distinct categories: *organic*, which have an underlying physical or neurological basis, and *functional*, which manifest as the result of vocal misuse or abuse and/or psychological factors (e.g., stress), but do not result in changes in structure. Voice disorders can overlap, however. For instance, vocal misuse or abuse (functional etiology) can lead to structural abnormalities such as vocal fold lesions (organic consequence). For our purposes here, we will discuss structural abnormalities at the level of the larynx as "organic" disorders, and voice disturbances that do not alter laryngeal structure as "functional" disorders.

Organic Voice Disorders

Two types of organic voice disorders can occur; those associated with structural changes or abnormalities of the laryngeal mechanism, and those associated with neurological disorders. As mentioned previously, physical changes to the larynx can result from aging (e.g., laryngeal muscle atrophy; cartilage ossification) or structural abnormalities (e.g., vocal fold lesions), both of which negatively impact voice. Neurological disorders, on the other hand, interfere with normal vocal fold vibration as the result of damage to central or peripheral nervous system substrates that control laryngeal functioning. The following sections will describe some of the more common structural abnormalities of the larynx, along with neurological disorders that result in deviations in voice quality, pitch, and loudness.

Structural Abnormalities Resulting in Voice Disorders

As stated, structural abnormalities of the laryngeal mechanism result in disordered voice, or **dysphonia**. In the following sections, we'll discuss a few of the more common structural abnormalities of the phonatory system, their etiologies, and their primary voice symptoms.

Vocal Nodules. **Vocal nodules** are a common vocal fold pathology that is secondary to vocal misuse/abuse. Nodules are localized growths on the vocal folds that result from frequent, forceful adduction of the vocal folds that occurs, for example, during yelling or shouting (Stemple, Roy, & Klaben, 2014). They are generally bilateral (appearing on both vocal folds), although they can appear on only one vocal fold (see Figure 9.2). Nodules are soft and pliable early in their formation. Over time, however, they become hard and fibrous, interfering significantly with vocal fold vibration. Nodules usually appear at the juncture of the anterior one third and posterior two thirds of the vocal folds where contact is greatest. Nodules occur most frequently in adult women, particularly those between 20 and 50 years of age; nodules are rarely present in adult males. In contrast, male and female children who engage in excessive loud talking or screaming can develop vocal nodules (Stemple, Roy, & Klaben, 2014).

The primary perceptual voice symptoms of vocal nodules are *hoarseness*, or a rough, raspy sounding voice, and **breathiness**, or the perception of audible air escaping through the glottis during phonation due to inadequate glottal closure during vocal fold vibration. People who have vocal nodules may complain of soreness in the throat and an inability to use the upper third of their pitch range.

Newly formed nodules are often treated with vocal rest (no talking). To prevent their return, however, individuals with vocal nodules must alter the vocal behaviors that produced the nodules. Consulting an SLP for voice intervention and education is usually recommended. Longstanding nodules may require surgical removal followed by voice intervention designed to eliminate vocally abusive behaviors.

Some research suggests that typical female voices are perceived to be more breathy than typical male voices. Research also suggests that young women use more air than young men to produce a syllable.

Figure 9.2 Unilateral vocal fold nodule.

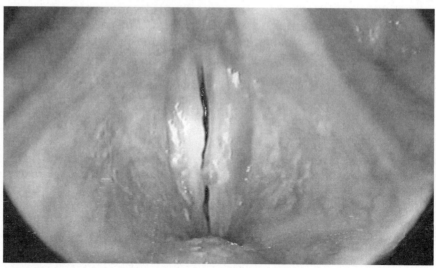

(Photograph courtesy of Robert Orlikoff)

See Case Study 9.1 for the personal story of a college music student with nodules that were effectively treated with intervention and vocal rest.

Vocal Polyps. **Vocal polyps**, like vocal nodules, are caused by trauma to the vocal folds associated with vocal misuse or abuse. Polyps develop when blood vessels in the vocal folds rupture and swell, developing fluid-filled lesions. Polyps tend to be unilateral, larger than nodules, vascular, and prone to hemorrhage. Unlike vocal nodules, polyps can result from a single traumatic incident such as yelling at a sporting event (Colton, Casper, & Leonard, 2011).

Two general types of polyps have been identified: sessile and pedunculated (Colton, Casper, & Leonard, 2011). A **sessile polyp**, closely adhering or attaching to vocal fold tissue (see Figures 9.3 and 9.4), can cover up to two thirds of the vocal fold. A **pedunculated polyp** appears to be attached to the vocal fold by means of a stalk, and can be found on the free margins of the vocal folds as well as on the upper and lower surfaces of the folds.

Hoarseness, breathiness, and **diplophonia**, or the perception of two different pitches during phonation, are the primary vocal symptoms. Diplophonia occurs because of the increase in mass of one vocal fold as a result of the polyp. Individuals who have a vocal polyp may also report the sensation of something in the throat. The combination of surgical removal of the polyp and voice intervention to eliminate vocal misuse or abuse is effective in treating this condition. Voice therapy alone can sometimes effectively improve the voice for some individuals, but not fully eliminate the polyp (Boone et al., 2010; Cohen & Garrett, 2007).

Contact Ulcers and Granulomas. **Contact ulcers** are small, reddened ulcerations that develop on the posterior surface of the vocal folds in the region of the arytenoid cartilages. Contact ulcers, like vocal nodules, are usually bilateral, but unlike nodules they can be painful. Pain is either unilateral or bilateral, and it may radiate into the ear. As contact ulcers heal, they are replaced by granulated tissue, referred to as a **granuloma** (see Figure 9.5). It was once believed that

CASE STUDY 9.1

Personal Story of a College Woman with Vocal Nodules

Bianca, a voice major, decided to pledge a sorority in the fall semester of her sophomore year. A talented vocal performer, Bianca had aspirations to teach singing and to perform professionally. During the fall semester, her course work was demanding, requiring several vocal performances and long hours of rehearsal. Pledging turned out to be vocally demanding also. Bianca was talking excessively all day long and well into the night, in addition to shouting loudly at sorority events.

During the fifth week of the semester, Bianca noted that her voice fatigued easily, she sounded hoarse, and she could not reach some of the high notes required in her singing. Her voice teacher suggested that she be evaluated at the university's speech-language-hearing clinic, in an effort to determine the cause of her diminished vocal capacity. A perceptual and instrumental evaluation of Bianca's voice was performed by two graduate students enrolled in the university's communication sciences and disorders program. The findings of this evaluation suggested the possibility of vocal nodules. During the consultation after the evaluation, the supervising professor and the two graduate students explained their findings to Bianca and told her that she needed to be examined by an otolaryngologist before they could proceed further. Otolaryngologic examination is required to confirm or disconfirm the presence of nodules, and

SLPs are ethically required to ensure that such an examination has been performed before they initiate treatment.

The otolaryngologic examination confirmed the presence of newly formed bilateral vocal nodules. Her physician prescribed complete vocal rest for a week, followed by voice intervention. Bianca enrolled in voice treatment at the university for six weeks. Vocal hygiene was stressed during treatment sessions. Bianca was examined by her otolaryngologist at the end of week six of treatment. Her vocal nodules were significantly reduced in size and were no longer adversely affecting her voice.

Bianca completed her academic semester and sorority pledging successfully, graduated two years later, and went on to graduate school at the Juilliard School of Music in New York City. She maintains contact with the university's speech-language-hearing clinic and reports that she continues to practice good vocal hygiene.

As you read the chapter, think about:

- What factors are present that put Bianca at risk for developing a voice disorder?
- What assessment tasks were administered to Bianca by the SLP?
- What other types of voice intervention in addition to vocal rest may have been used?

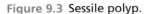

Figure 9.3 Sessile polyp.

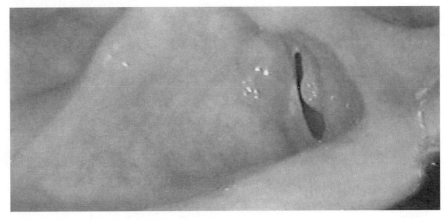

(Photograph courtesy of Robert Orlikoff)

Figure 9.4 Two sessile polyps stacked on top of each other on the right vocal fold.

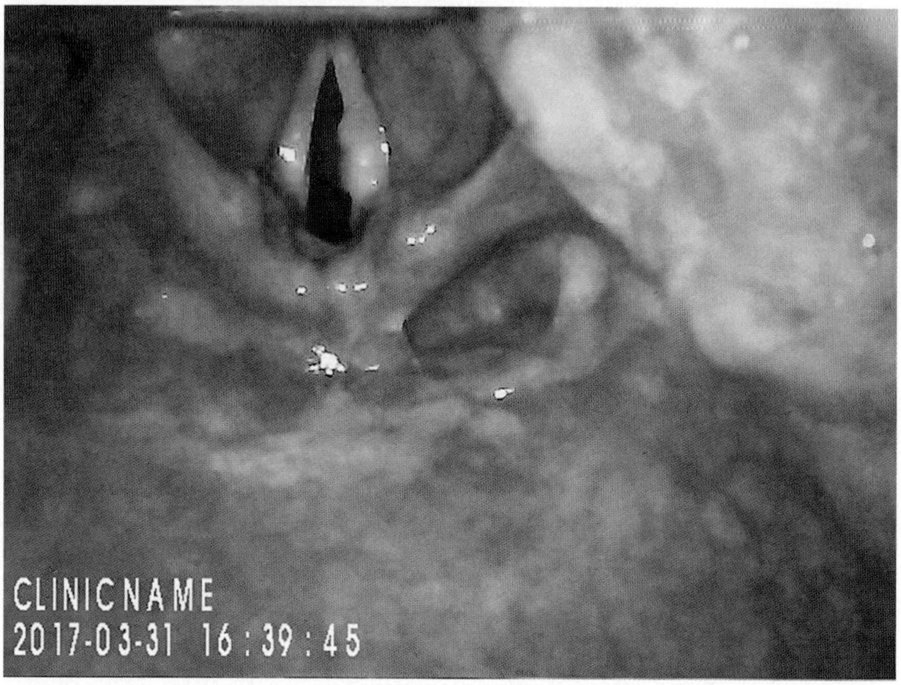

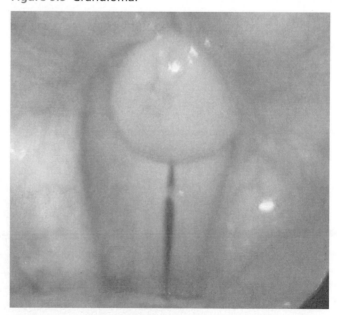

(Photograph courtesy of Steven R. Knight)

Figure 9.5 Granuloma.

(Photograph courtesy of Robert Orlikoff)

contact ulcers, which occur predominantly in men older than 40 years, resulted primarily from forceful and aggressive speaking behaviors (Colton, Casper, & Leonard, 2011). Contemporary thought, however, suggests that gastroesophageal reflux disease (GERD) is a significant contributing factor; stomach acids irritate vocal fold tissue and promote excessive throat clearing, which is also abusive to tissue, thereby causing the ulcerations (Colton, Casper, & Leonard, 2011). The condition is complicated by regurgitation of stomach acids into the esophagus and throat during sleep, causing further irritation of the ulcer (Deem & Miller, 2000).

In rare cases, contact ulcers and granulomas can develop as the result of trauma induced during surgical intubation of the larynx (respiratory tube placed between the vocal folds); the risk is greater in women and children who have smaller airways (Boone et al., 2010).

The primary voice symptoms of contact ulcers are vocal hoarseness and breathiness. Throat clearing and vocal fatigue accompany the disorder. Although some individuals claim that contact ulcers can be treated effectively with voice intervention (e.g., Boone & McFarlane, 2000), others suggest that successful treatment is questionable and not well documented. Quite frequently, contact ulcers reappear after surgical removal; therefore, managing gastroesophageal reflux with medication prior to surgical intervention has been suggested (Catten et al., 1998).

Laryngitis. Acute laryngitis and **chronic laryngitis** are inflammation of the vocal folds that can result from exposure to noxious agents (tobacco smoke, alcohol, etc.), allergies, GERD, or vocal abuse (Colton, Casper, & Leonard, 2011). Acute laryngitis is a temporary swelling of the vocal folds that can result in vocal hoarseness.

Chronic laryngitis is a result of vocal abuse during periods of acute laryngitis, and it can lead to serious deterioration of vocal fold tissue. The vocal folds appear thickened, swollen, and reddened because of excessive fluid retention and dilated blood vessels in the vocal folds. If chronic laryngitis persists, a marked atrophy (wasting away of tissue) of the vocal folds will occur. The vocal folds become dry and sticky, resulting in a persistent cough, and the individual reports frequent throat aches (Stemple, Roy, & Klaben, 2014). The voice symptoms of chronic laryngitis range from mild hoarseness to near-aphonia, lowered pitch, and complaints of vocal fatigue. Voice treatment, including a period of vocal rest and modification of vocally abusive behaviors (Boone et al., 2010), along with lifestyle changes (e.g., diet changes to manage GERD; avoiding smoking and alcohol), are necessary to treat chronic laryngitis effectively.

Papillomas. Laryngeal papillomas are small wart-like growths that cover the vocal folds and the interior aspects of the larynx. These lesions are caused by the human papillomavirus (HPV), and are the most common abnormal laryngeal pathology in children younger than 6 years (Boone et al., 2010). Papillomas are noncancerous, but they can obstruct the airway, hindering breathing. Children with the disorder exhibit inspiratory **stridor**, or noisy breathing during inhalation, indicative of a narrowing in the airway (Stemple, Roy, & Klaben, 2014). Papillomas must be surgically removed, but they have a strong tendency to reappear, requiring multiple operations that may damage vocal fold tissue.

Webs. Laryngeal webs are the result of connective tissue growing between the vocal folds; they can be congenital (present at birth), or acquired as the result of trauma or prolonged infection (Boone et al., 2010). Congenital laryngeal webs typically form on the anterior aspects of the vocal folds and can interfere with breathing, causing inspiratory stridor and shortness of breath. Laryngeal webbing must be removed surgically. Webs may produce a high-pitched, hoarse voice quality, **aphonia**, or complete absence of voice depending on the severity of the web (Boone et al., 2010; Deem & Miller, 2000).

Cancer. Laryngeal cancer is the most serious organic disorder of the voice; it has been linked to cigarette smoking and excessive use of alcohol, although other risk factors have been identified (e.g., HPV infection, poor nutrition, age, race, family history, GERD) (American Cancer Society, 2016). Figure 9.6 is a photo of laryngeal cancer that is obstructing view of the vocal folds in a chronic smoker and heavy alcohol user.

One of the early signs of laryngeal cancer is persistent hoarseness in the absence of colds or allergies (Stemple, Roy, & Klaben, 2014). Once cancer is diagnosed, it is frequently necessary to remove the entire larynx to prevent the spread of the cancer to other parts of the body. When the larynx is removed surgically, the trachea is repositioned to form a stoma (mouthlike opening) on the anterior aspect of the throat for breathing purposes.

Removal of the larynx requires alternate methods of producing voice. Some alaryngeal (without larynx) speakers use a technique called **esophageal speech**, which uses the esophagus as a vibratory source. Essentially, these individuals

> More than 75% of people who are diagnosed with cancer of the larynx are or were heavy cigarette smokers. Particles in tobacco smoke are a major irritant to vocal fold tissue. Figure 9.7 depicts the thickened and pre-cancerous vocal folds of a heavy smoker.

Figure 9.6 Laryngeal cancer.

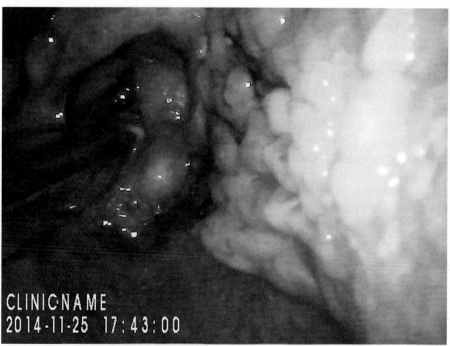

(Photograph courtesy of Steven R. Knight)

Figure 9.7 Hypertrophic (thickened) and pre-cancerous vocal folds of a heavy smoker.

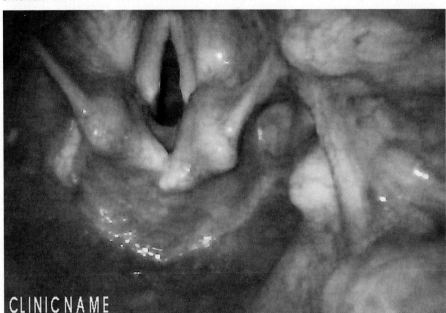

CLINICNAME
2017-03-28 20:47:24

(Photograph courtesy of Steven R. Knight)

learn to speak using "burps" as a substitute for actual voice production. Some individuals are incapable of producing esophageal speech. Several prosthetic devices are available to produce an alternative form of voicing for these alaryngeal speakers. One such device is a battery-powered **electrolarynx**. The electrolarynx has a vibrating diaphragm that is placed on the lateral aspects of the neck. This vibration excites the air in the vocal tract and thus serves as an alternate form of voicing. Some alaryngeal speakers may be candidates for devices that are inserted through a surgical opening in the throat. A device called a **tracheoesophageal puncture (TEP) or tracheoesophageal shunt** directs air from the trachea into the esophagus, allowing the speaker to use respiratory air and a muscle of the esophagus, the cricopharyngeous muscle, for voice production (Stemple, Roy, & Klaben, 2014). This device enhances esophageal speech. Other augmentative and alternative communication systems are available (see Chapter 13).

 Video Exercise 9.1

Examining a Vocal Fold Lesion

Click on the link to watch a video of a laryngoscopic examination of a 40-year-old male with a voice disorder, and complete an exercise.

Neurologic Voice Disorders

The second major group of organic voice disorders is that caused by damage to the central nervous system (CNS) or peripheral nervous system (PNS). Recall from Chapter 7 that the CNS comprises the brain and spinal cord, and areas of the brain such as the primary motor cortex in the frontal lobe control activation of muscles that initiate speech and voice production via connections with the PNS. The PNS consists of the 12 cranial nerves that activate the muscles responsible for speech and voice after receiving signals from the CNS; cranial nerve X (vagus) innervates the muscles of the larynx and is primarily responsible for voice production.

Disorders of the CNS or PNS can result in speech and voice disorders that are characterized by muscle weakness, paralysis, discoordination, or involuntary movements. Most of these disorders, generally called *dysarthrias* (discussed further in Chapter 10), involve generalized neurological damage resulting in complex patterns of speech and voice symptoms. In the next few sections, we'll focus primarily on the voice characteristics associated with neurological disease or damage, and the treatment options available. We will discuss damage to the PNS first.

The recurrent laryngeal nerve branch of the vagus nerve was frequently severed in the early days of open heart surgery, resulting in postoperative aphonia. Improved surgical procedures have minimized this problem, although the risk still exists.

Damage to Cranial Nerve X (Vagus). Unilateral and bilateral **vocal fold paralysis** result from damage to the 10th cranial nerve, or the vagus nerve, which controls the laryngeal muscles for phonation. Specifically, the **recurrent laryngeal nerve (RLN)** of the vagus is the nerve supply for most of the laryngeal muscles associated with voice production. The left recurrent laryngeal nerve leaves the brain stem and travels down into the chest cavity, loops around the heart's aorta, and then courses upward, inserting into the larynx from below. Damage to the left RLN can occur through injuries to the head, neck, or chest, from viral infections, or sometimes during neck or chest surgery. Unilateral vocal fold paralysis results in these cases since the nerve is only damaged on one side.

The voice symptoms of unilateral vocal fold paralysis include a hoarse and breathy voice quality, reduced loudness, monoloudness, and **pitch breaks**, or sudden uncontrolled upward or downward changes in pitch. Since the paralyzed vocal fold is flaccid (limp or weak) in comparison to the nonparalyzed vocal fold, the two vocal folds vibrate at different speeds, resulting in *diplophonia*.

When both recurrent laryngeal nerves are damaged, the result is bilateral vocal fold paralysis. In these cases, the voice is very breathy, weak, or totally absent (aphonic). Bilateral vocal fold paralysis can be a life-threatening situation; airway blockage results when the folds are paralyzed in the *adducted*, or midline position, usually requiring a tracheostomy. The risk of **aspiration** during swallowing increases when the folds are paralyzed in the *abducted*, or open position (Boone et al., 2010).

If nerve regeneration and improved function are not observed within 9 to 12 months after the injury, surgical treatment may be required to facilitate vocal fold closure. Soft tissue fillers such as fat can sometimes be injected surgically into a paralyzed vocal fold to build up its mass; surgical procedures to move the paralyzed fold into the midline position can also promote vocal fold contact (Boone et al., 2010). Voice treatment following surgery aims to increase vocal fold closure and vocal loudness.

Parkinson Disease. Turning our attention now to diseases of the CNS, **Parkinson disease** results from degeneration of dopaminergic neurons in the substantia nigra (located in the midbrain of the brain stem), interfering with the function of *basal ganglia* circuitry. Muscle rigidity, reduced range of movement, tremor at rest, and an overall slowness of movement, or **hypokinesia**, are characteristics of Parkinson disease. Facial appearance is unemotional, and is sometimes referred to as masklike. The voice symptoms associated with Parkinson disease include reduced loudness, monopitch, monoloudness, hoarseness, harshness, and breathiness (Duffy, 2013). Go to www.lsvtglobal.com to watch the pre-/post-treatment video of Shirley, a woman with Parkinson disease; note her complaints about her voice before treatment.

Parkinson disease is a serious medical condition that is typically treated aggressively with a variety of drugs, and in some cases surgical procedures such as *Deep Brain Stimulation (DBS)*. Although such neuropharmacological and surgical treatments have a positive effect on limb movement, speech and voice symptoms are not consistently improved. Intensive voice treatment (e.g., Lee Silverman Voice Treatment) aimed at increasing vocal fold adduction has been successful in improving vocal loudness and speech intelligibility (e.g., Fox et al., 2002).

> Deep Brain Stimulation is a surgical procedure that involves implantation of electrodes into the brain to alter neural activity in structures of the brain implicated in Parkinson disease; namely, the basal ganglia.

Amyotrophic Lateral Sclerosis (ALS). **Amyotrophic lateral sclerosis (ALS)**, also known as Lou Gehrig's disease, is a neurodegenerative disease caused by damage to multiple areas of the CNS. ALS is a motor neuron disease characterized by degeneration of both the upper and lower motor neurons causing flaccid and spastic weakness, and ultimately paralysis. Voice symptoms can vary, and may include breathiness, harshness and/or a strained/strangled voice quality, reduced loudness, monoloudness, inspiratory stridor, and abnormally high or low pitch (Duffy, 2013). Early on, reduced loudness can be a prominent feature, and assistive devices, such as a voice amplifier, are often helpful. However, given the degenerative nature of the disease, direct voice treatment is not recommended; rather, compensatory strategies such as use of gestures or an alphabet board, a communication tool in which the individual points to the first letter of every word he/she produces, are beneficial. An AAC device (see Chapter 13) is eventually needed for the individual with ALS to effectively communicate and maintain quality of life as the disease progresses.

Spasmodic Dysphonia. **Spasmodic dysphonia (SD)** is a neurological voice disorder reflecting damage to basal ganglia and cerebellar control circuits; it involves abnormal, involuntary movements of the larynx, with adductor-type SD occurring in the majority of cases. The average age of onset is 45 to 50 years of age, with more women affected than men (Duffy, 2013). For years, SD was believed to be a psychological voice disturbance resulting from stress, anxiety, or emotional trauma. We know now that SD can be neurological, psychological, or idiopathic (of unknown etiology). Psychological, or **psychogenic**, voice disturbances are discussed later in this chapter. SD of neurological origin results from an abnormal adductor laryngospasm that causes a strained, effortful, tight voice and intermittent voice stoppages. SD can be associated with **voice tremor** that is best heard during prolongation of the /a/ vowel. Botulinum toxin (Botox) injection into specific laryngeal muscles to cause incomplete paralysis is the preferred method of treatment for neurological or idiopathic SD (Duffy, 2013).

> Botulinum toxin (Botox) is one of the most poisonous substances known. It is produced by bacteria found in contaminated meat products. When ingested, it causes paralysis of muscles in the body, including the respiratory muscles that regulate breathing, and can lead to death. However, in small doses injected into localized areas, Botox has been found to be a safe and effective way to weaken or paralyze selected muscles temporarily for medical and cosmetic reasons, including reducing abnormal muscle contractions, managing pain, and reducing the appearance of wrinkles.

Functional Voice Disorders

As mentioned previously, functional voice disorders can result from misuse, abuse, or overuse of the voice, or psychological or stress factors, without causing physical changes to the larynx. We'll begin our discussion with one of the more common functional voice disorders, *muscle tension dysphonia*, followed by voice disorders associated with psychological or stress conditions.

Muscle Tension Dysphonia

Generally associated with hyperfunction of laryngeal muscles, **muscle tension dysphonia (MTD)**, or more specifically, *primary* MTD, refers to a voice disturbance caused by abnormal muscle activity in the absence of structural or neurological abnormalities; the underlying cause of this abnormal muscle activation is not well understood, however (Roy, 2008; Verdolini, Rosen, & Branski, 2006). Certain factors may contribute to the development of abnormal laryngeal tension, including significant emotional stress, excessive use or misuse of the voice, GERD, or learned compensatory behaviors following an upper respiratory infection (Boone et al., 2010; Roy, 2008); women are more affected than men. Voice symptoms overlap with other voice disorders, making differential diagnosis difficult. Hoarseness is a common voice symptom, although others can include strained-harshness, strained-breathiness, aphonia, and intermittent pitch breaks (Duffy, 2013; Roy, 2004). Voice treatments that address laryngeal **hyperadduction** are generally used to manage individuals with MTD, although the evidence is limited regarding the effectiveness of these treatment approaches with this population (Roy, 2008).

Visit the Johns Hopkins Medicine Otolaryngology–Head and Neck Surgery website at http://www.hopkinsmedicine.org and click "Patient Education Videos" in the Voice and Laryngeal Disorders section to see videos of voice disorders just discussed in the previous sections.

Conversion Aphonia

Your voice involuntarily responds to emotional changes. Strong emotional reactions such as extreme sadness, fear, anger, or happiness are reflected by your voice. When experiencing strong emotions, you might not be able to control your voice.

Strong emotions, when they are suppressed, can cause *psychogenic* voice disorders. Psychogenic voice disorders that result from psychological suppression of emotion are called **conversion disorders** because the person is converting emotional conflicts into physical symptoms. In these cases, the vocal folds are structurally normal, and they function normally for nonspeech behaviors. One type of vocal conversion disorder is called **conversion aphonia**. People who suffer from conversion aphonia whisper to produce voice. Although these individuals are capable of coughing and clearing the throat, indicating the capability of glottal closure, they do not approximate the vocal folds for speech production. In many cases, people with conversion aphonia believe they have a physical condition that prevents them from using their voice (Aronson, 1990a; Duffy, 2013).

It is believed that conversion aphonias develop out of a desire to avoid some type of personal conflict or unpleasant situation in the person's life (Aronson, 1990a; Duffy, 2013). Conversion aphonia is not a common condition, and it will likely persist until the person is willing to resolve the emotional conflict. People with deeply rooted psychological problems may require psychotherapy or psychiatric treatment.

Mutational Falsetto

Also known as *puberphonia* or juvenile voice, **mutational falsetto** is the continual use of a high-pitched voice by adolescent or adult males who have completed the maturational changes associated with puberty (Boone et al., 2010). While mutational falsetto can occur in females, it is more common in males between the ages of 11 and 15 (Dagli et al., 2008). Mutational falsetto is usually the result of the individual trying to avoid transition from childhood to adulthood, along with the responsibilities and feelings associated with becoming an adult (Boone et al., 2010). Psychological counseling is sometimes necessary, but most individuals with mutational falsetto benefit from behavioral voice treatment focused on lowering pitch (Boone et al., 2010; Stemple, Roy, & Klaben, 2014).

Resonance Disorders

Resonance disorders can accompany voice disorders, particularly in cases when the CNS or PNS are damaged or disordered; they result when there is any disruption to the normal balance of oral and nasal resonance. They can also be caused by a number of structural abnormalities, including clefts of the palate. A cleft is an abnormal opening in an anatomical structure (Shprintzen, 1995) caused by failure of structures to fuse or merge correctly early in embryonic development. Alternatively, a resonance disorder may develop when there is a blockage in the nasopharynx that impedes sound energy from traveling through the nose for production of nasal sounds (Kummer & Lee, 1996).

 Thought Question 9.2

What impact might a cleft palate have on family-infant bonding?

When the velopharyngeal mechanism fails to decouple the oral and nasal cavities, **hypernasality** secondary to *velopharyngeal dysfunction (VPD)* occurs. VPD is a frequent result of palatal clefts, and is associated with velar soft tissue and muscle tissue deficiencies. VPD also occurs in neurodegenerative diseases like ALS that result in damage to the motor neurons that control the velopharyngeal mechanism. People with VPD are said to have a hypernasal voice quality; however, hypernasality is not a problem associated with phonation. Rather, it is a result of not partitioning the oral and nasal cavities by actions of the velopharyngeal mechanism. Hypernasality is a resonance problem created by the nasal cavity acting inappropriately as a second "filter," coupled to the oral cavity. Addition of this second filter alters the vocal tract's output in such a way that it sounds as though the individual is talking through the nose.

VPD can also result in **audible nasal emission**, particularly during production of high-pressure consonants (e.g., /p/, /b/, /s/, *sh*, *ch*, *j*). When an individual with VPD attempts to build up the necessary air pressure in the oral cavity for production of high-pressure sounds, the air pressure subsequently escapes through the nasal cavity. This may be heard as a very loud, turbulent sound called a *nasal rustle*, or *nasal turbulence*, believed to be a friction noise caused by a large amount of air moving through a small velopharyngeal opening (Kummer & Lee, 1996; Peterson-Falzone et al., 2006). When there is an insufficient amount of nasal resonance as is needed during production of the nasal sounds /m/, /n/, and *ng*, speech may sound hyponasal. Your voice may have a hyponasal quality when you experience a bad head cold. **Hyponasality** occurs when there is a partial blockage somewhere in the nasopharynx or nasal cavity. When there is a complete blockage, denasality occurs, resulting in a more severe resonance disorder where nasal sounds are imperceptible from oral consonants produced with the same place of articulation (Peterson-Falzone et al., 2006).

Check Your Understanding 9.2

Click here to check your understanding of the concepts in this section.

EVALUATION OF VOICE AND RESONANCE DISORDERS

Evaluation of voice and resonance disorders requires a multidisciplinary team approach. The specific nature and cause of a disorder determines the precise composition of the team. At a minimum, a voice evaluation requires an otolaryngologist (or Ear, Nose, and Throat doctor) and an SLP. For evaluation of resonance disorders, particularly of VPD secondary to cleft palate, a cleft palate or craniofacial team comprising but not limited to surgeons, SLPs, dental specialists, audiologists, and social workers is necessary for effective clinical management of this population.

The Voice Evaluation

Optical fibers are specially constructed flexible, tubular-shaped rods of glass that conduct light in only one direction. In an endoscope, small optical fibers transmit light from a source to illuminate an object, and a larger optical fiber transmits light from the illuminated object to a camera lens or viewing instrument.

The primary objectives of the clinical voice evaluation are to: 1) determine the presence or absence of a voice disorder, 2) determine the nature of the voice disorder, and 3) determine the severity of the voice disorder (Barkmeier-Kramer, 2016). It is necessary for the individual presenting with a suspected voice disorder to have an examination performed by an otolaryngologist. The otolaryngologic examination provides information about vocal fold tissue damage, presence of nodules, polyps, or other abnormal growths, including more serious conditions like laryngeal cancer. A direct examination of the vocal folds and other laryngeal structures is essential to determine whether the voice disorder has an organic basis. Direct observation of the laryngeal structures can be achieved using laryngeal mirrors (similar to the mirror used by a dentist) or with an **endoscope**. An endoscope (see Figure 9.8) is basically a lens coupled with a light source. The light source[1] illuminates the larynx, and laryngeal structures are viewed through the lens. Biopsies of vocal fold tissue may be taken if laryngeal cancer is suspected.

The SLP involved in the voice evaluation typically begins by obtaining a thorough case history. A description of the voice problem, when it started, the duration of the disorder, what the client believes might be causing it, how it affects daily life activities, the person's social and vocational use of the voice, and his or her overall physical and psychological condition are important areas of interest when taking a case history (Boone et al., 2010).

The SLP also conducts an auditory-perceptual evaluation to describe the pitch, loudness, and voice quality characteristics of the voice. The *Consensus Auditory-Perceptual Evaluation of Voice (CAPE-V)* is a tool that was developed to help SLPs standardize the way in which these parameters of voice are evaluated and judged (Barkmeier-Kramer, 2016); data are used to determine what additional voice assessments are needed to accurately diagnose the voice disorder. Speech tasks to perceptually judge voice include sustained vowel prolongation of /a/ and /i/, sentence repetition, and elicitation of a 20-second spontaneous speech sample. A copy of this assessment tool can be requested for noncommercial purposes at http://www.asha.org/Form/CAPE-V/.

---

[1]The light source can be a stroboscopic light that flashes light rapidly in synchrony with vocal fold vibration.

Figure 9.8 An endoscope.

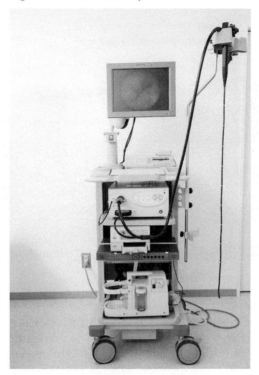

(KPG Payless/Shutterstock)

In addition to auditory-perceptual assessment, the clinical voice evaluation may also involve detailed acoustic and physiological measurements regarding vocal function that can be compared to normative data. Quantitative acoustic measurements of voice are easily made by using specially designed computer hardware and software. Kay Elemetrics, for example, manufactures a computer-based instrument called the VisiPitch (see Figure 9.9). It is a user-friendly instrument that permits numerous objective assessments of the physical correlates of voice, such as average fundamental frequency, frequency variability, and average vocal intensity. Similar measures can be made using a free software program called PRAAT, which you can download to your computer (download at http://www.fon. hum.uva.nl/praat/). *Spectrograms*, or graphic representations of frequency and intensity of sound as a function of time, can also be generated with the Visipitch or PRAAT software; these graphs can also provide useful visual feedback during voice treatment. Quantitative measurements of voice are not necessary to accurately diagnose a voice disorder, however, and should only be used to supplement the auditory-perceptual evaluation.

Instruments are also available that measure airflow and air volume exchanges during phonation that can be used to objectively assess vocal breathiness. These instruments can be interfaced with specially designed computer hardware and software for vocal assessment. Normative data exist for many objective correlates that are related to the perceptual signs of voice disorders (see, e.g., Baken & Orlikoff, 2000). Objective assessments are valuable for diagnostic purposes as well as for monitoring improvements during voice intervention.

Figure 9.9 Kay Elemetrics VisiPitch.

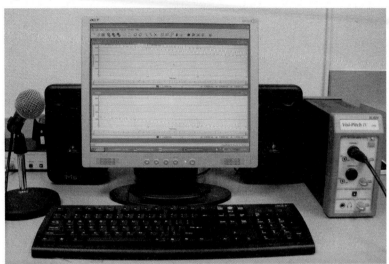

(Photograph courtesy of Kim Farinella)

Following auditory-perceptual and instrumental assessment of voice, obtaining information about the client's perception regarding how the disorder may be impacting his/her quality of life is also important. The *Voice Handicap Index* (VHI: Jacobson et al., 1997) is a 30-item questionnaire that can help determine the psychosocial handicapping effects of a voice disorder; patients respond to questions such as "My voice makes me feel incompetent" and "I use a great deal of effort to speak" using a 5-point scale where "0" indicates "never" to "5" which indicates "always." Similar instruments include the *Voice-Related Quality of Life (V-RQOL)* (Hogikyan & Sethuraman, 1999) and the *Voice Outcome Survey (VOS)* (Glicklich, Glovsky, & Montgomery, 1999); each instrument can be accessed online. These instruments can also be used as patient-reported outcome (PRO) measures pre- and post-treatment to determine the patient's perspective on treatment effectiveness (see Francis et al., 2017).

The voice evaluation would not be complete without perceptual judgments of resonance, since abnormalities of resonance can affect the perception of voice quality or can lead to hyperfunction of the voice as a compensatory response. Behavioral and instrumental techniques for assessing resonance are discussed in the next section.

The Resonance Evaluation

Before making clinical judgments about resonance, it's important to obtain case history information about velopharyngeal function. Interviewing the client or client's caregiver about the history of the presenting problem is essential to the evaluation process. If the client has a cleft, obtaining information about medical and surgical history is necessary for appropriate treatment planning.

Auditory-perceptual evaluation of resonance is still the "gold standard" with regard to determining whether or not a resonance disorder is present. There are a number of standardized rating scales for assessing resonance. Rating scales permit the assignment of numbers to express increasing severity of the disorder. In general, such rating scales are reliable and valid. Two such rating scales are presented in Figure 9.10.

Figure 9.10 Two examples of scales used to rate the degree of resonance disorders: (a) a 7-point scale emphasizing hypernasality and (b) an 8-point scale for rating nasal resonance.

(a)

		Hypernasality				
Normal		Mild		Moderate		Severe
1	2	3	4	5	6	7

(b)

		Hypernasality					
Hyponasality	Normal		Mild		Moderate		Severe
−1	0	1	2	3	4	5	6

Source: Based on Peterson-Falzone, S., Hardin-Jones, M., & Karnell, M. (2010). Cleft palate speech (4th ed.). St. Louis, MO: Mosby.

To determine the presence or absence of hypernasality and rate its severity during speech production, you might ask the client to repeat sentences containing voiced, oral sounds with few high-pressure consonants (i.e., "How are you"); if you were rating hyponasality, you might ask the client to repeat sentences that contain mostly nasal sounds (e.g., "Mom made lemonade") (Kummer 2011b; 2014a; 2014b). The presence of *audible nasal emission*, or air escaping from the nose during production of oral sounds, can best be determined by having the client repeat sentences loaded with high-pressure consonants (e.g., "Sissy sees the sun in the sky") (Kummer 2011b; 2014c). Additional speech tasks for assessing resonance include counting, syllable repetition (e.g., "pa, pa, pa, pa"), and connected speech (Kummer, 2014a). Listening samples are available to download and practice rating hypernasality in children and adults at http://www.acpa-cpf.org/education/educational_resources/speech_samples/.

Specially designed instruments are also available to assess resonance disorders. Direct and indirect instrumental assessments are sometimes necessary to confirm what the SLP is hearing during the auditory-perceptual evaluation; instrumental procedures are not to be used as substitutes for clinical judgments of resonance, however (Peterson-Falzone et al., 2010).

An indirect technique to quantitatively evaluate resonance requires use of an instrument called a **nasometer**. A nasometer measures simultaneously the relative amplitude of acoustic energy being emitted through the nose and mouth during speech production. A numerical value, the **nasalance score**, is computed to reflect the magnitude of hypernasality. Nasalance scores have been determined to correlate well with perceptual ratings of hypernasality in some studies, but other studies have observed a poor correlation with clinical judgments of hypernasality (cf., Dalston, Warren, & Dalston, 1991; Keuning et al., 2002). Nasometry can also be used as an effective therapeutic feedback technique, especially with young children, since it includes virtual games and animated graphics (Perry & Schenck, 2013).

A direct imaging technique used to dynamically assess velopharyngeal function is **multiview videofluoroscopy**. Videofluoroscopy involves real-time viewing and dynamic X-rays recorded digitally during speech production (Perry & Schenck, 2013). Multiview videofluoroscopy permits the imaging of velopharyngeal function from three different perspectives: from the front (frontal), from the side (lateral), and from beneath (base). These images provide a complete picture of the velopharyngeal mechanism, and can even be useful in confirming the presence of **apraxia of speech** since velar movements can be viewed during production of complex speech tasks (Perry & Schenck, 2013). Disadvantages of videofluoroscopy include exposure to radiation and cost; generally speaking, only SLPs working in hospitals will have the opportunity to use this form of instrumentation.

A less costly, yet more invasive instrumental procedure to directly visualize velopharyngeal function during speech production is **videonasendoscopy** (also known as fiberoptic nasendoscopy). The components of the nasal endoscope are essentially the same as previously discussed for endoscopic observation of the vocal folds (see Figure 9.8), and includes a lens, fiberoptic light cable, insertion tube, camera, and connection to a monitor for recording and display (Perry & Schenck, 2013). Videonasendoscopy does not expose the client to radiation, and therefore can be also used as a visual feedback tool during treatment.

 Check Your Understanding 9.3

Click here to check your understanding of the concepts in this section.

MANAGEMENT OF VOICE AND RESONANCE DISORDERS

Treatment of any voice disorder may involve surgical, medical, or behavioral interventions, or some combination of these by the multidisciplinary team, depending on the specific needs of the individual (Colton, Casper, & Leonard, 2011). Speech-language pathologists manage voice disorders using behavioral interventions with the goal of restoring the best voice possible, and ensuring the individual's voice is functional for employment and general communication purposes (Colton, Casper, & Leonard, 2011).

In the next few sections, we'll discuss how behavioral voice treatments are classified, and then describe general treatment approaches used by SLPs to treat voice disorders associated with benign structural abnormalities (e.g., nodules, polyps, chronic laryngitis), neurological conditions (e.g., Parkinson disease), and those associated with psychological or stress conditions (e.g., conversion aphonia). Specific therapeutic approaches and techniques are described in Box 9.1.

Classification of Behavioral Treatment Approaches for Voice Disorders

Behavioral treatment approaches for voice disorders are frequently categorized as either direct or indirect (e.g., Behrman et al., 2008); direct treatments are those that modify vocal behavior in some manner, either by changing pitch or loudness, or directing the client's attention to feel the reduced effort of vocal fold vibration when working to eliminate laryngeal hyperadduction. Direct voice treatments are classified as either *physiologic*, in which the intervention serves to balance the respiratory, laryngeal, and articulatory/resonatory systems to achieve normal

BOX 9.1 | Evidence-Based Practices for Individuals with Voice and Resonance Disorders

General Intervention for Voice Disorders

- SLP-administered voice intervention is effective when medical intervention, such as surgery, is not warranted.
- For some types of laryngeal pathology, SLP voice intervention may be as effective or more effective than medical intervention.
- In general, voice treatment before and after surgery results in better outcomes than surgery alone.

Direct Physiologic Voice Treatment Approaches

- Vocal function exercises (VFEs), which include sustained vowels, pitch glides, and sustained low and high pitches practiced twice per day, are effective in treating psychogenic voice disorders, as well as voice disorders associated with vocal hyperfunction, by strengthening and balancing the laryngeal mechanism and facilitating production of a more relaxed voice.
- Resonant voice therapy focuses on production of voice through the hearing and feeling of vibratory sensations produced with a "forward focus" in the oral cavity, particularly in the palate, tongue, and lips. It is based on techniques that improve voice production in actors and singers; the goal is production of a strong, clear voice accomplished with minimal impact of the vocal folds. It has been shown to be effective for individuals with hyperfunctional voice disorders.
- Confidential voice therapy or use of breathy phonation is effective in reducing laryngeal hyperfunction by facilitating a continuous, relaxed voice with increased airflow. After several weeks, the client gradually increases voicing and reduces airflow, while maintaining relaxed laryngeal muscles.
- An intensive treatment focused on increasing loudness, the *Lee Silverman Voice Treatment* (*LSVT*) has been repeatedly shown to improve voice production in both children and adults with neurological diseases (e.g., cerebral palsy, Parkinson disease, multiple sclerosis). Treatment entails practicing using a louder voice while saying /a/, producing functional sentences, and producing utterances of increasing complexity four times per week for 4 weeks.

Direct Symptomatic Treatment Techniques

- The *Yawn–Sigh* technique, or instructing the client to simulate a real yawn completed with a sign, effectively lowers the larynx and opens the glottis, thereby decreasing laryngeal tension and facilitating ease of phonation. This technique is suggested for individuals with laryngeal pathology associated with vocal hyperfunction (e.g., vocal nodules).
- Semi-occluded vocal tract phonation (SOVT) involves having the client phonate through a straw to partially close the mouth, thereby increasing air pressure above the vocal folds. The increased air pressure maintains the folds in a slightly abducted position during phonation, allowing vocal fold vibration to occur more easily and with less muscular effort; the straw is eventually eliminated. This technique is useful in achieving a more "resonant" voice.

Surgical Intervention for Cleft Palate

- Although about 90% of children with nonsyndromic clefts are expected to have good velopharyngeal function after the first surgery, speech treatment may still be needed. As structures of the head and face grow, velopharyngeal function may deteriorate.
- The type of secondary surgical procedure used in some children (i.e., secondary palatal surgery and/or pharyngeal flap surgery) depends on the severity of velopharyngeal inadequacy. Following secondary surgery, speech treatment is often needed to eliminate habituated compensatory misarticulations and nasal air emission during production of pressure consonants.

Specific Behavioral Treatment Approaches or Techniques for Resonance Disorders

- *CPAP* treatment is best suited for individuals with a small velopharyngeal gap (less than 2 mm) and a movable velum, and it has been found to be effective in some patients with mild to moderate hypernasality.

(continued)

BOX 9.1   *(Continued)*

- *Electropalatography* (*EPG*) provides visual feedback on the location and timing of tongue–palate contacts, and continues to show promise for remediation of speech-sound disorders in the cleft palate population. EPG is effective in teaching correct production of /s/ in preschool children with cleft palate.
- Bottom-up articulation drill procedures that focus on phonetic placement and sound shaping are recommended for children with repaired clefts, and they may be effective for sounds that are often difficult for this population. For instance, to teach the production of /s/ without nasal emission, have a child produce /t/ with the teeth closed. Then have the child prolong this sound, which should result in the correct production

of /s/. The technique can be applied to other fricative or affricate sounds as well.
- *Enhanced milieu training* (*EMT*) is a naturalistic method of stimulating speech and language development in young children that parents can do at home. This child-led approach involves organizing the environment such that a child must request or comment on objects to receive them.

Source: Based on Colton, Casper, & Leonard (2011); Fox et al. (2002, 2006); Hardin-Jones et al. (2006); Kuehn et al. (2002); Kuehn & Henne (2003); Kummer (2014a); Peterson-Falzone et al. (2006); Pindzola (1993); Ramig & Verdolini (2009); Roy et al. (2001); Stemple, Roy, & Klaben (2014); and van der Merwe (2004).

---

voice production, or *symptomatic*, in which the intervention modifies the deviant aspect of voice (e.g., too high a pitch) (Stemple, Roy, & Klaben, 2014).

Indirect treatments, on the other hand, modify the cognitive, behavioral, psychological, or physical environment in which voicing occurs (Roy et al., 2001; Thomas & Stemple, 2007). Educating the client about **vocal hygiene** or counseling the client to identify psychosocial factors that negatively impact the voice are examples of indirect voice interventions (Van Stan et al., 2015). A combination of indirect and direct treatments is necessary for effective treatment of most voice disorders. Recall that prior to initiation of behavioral voice treatment by the speech-language pathologist, the client must first be evaluated by an appropriate medical professional, usually an otolaryngologist (i.e., ENT doctor), to rule out or determine an etiology for the voice disorder that may require immediate medical management (e.g., laryngeal cancer).

Treatment of Voice Disorders Associated with Benign Structural Abnormalities

Voice therapy is frequently the clinical method of choice for voice disorders associated with benign structural abnormalities (e.g., vocal nodules) that typically result from and are maintained by vocal misuse or abuse (Boone et al., 2010; Colton, Casper, & Leonard, 2011). In such cases, identifying the behaviors that contributed to the laryngeal pathology (e.g., frequent yelling, throat clearing, coughing) is an important first step in the treatment process. Once identified, clients are taught to modify vocally abusive behaviors in a number of ways. As previously mentioned, an indirect treatment approach involves educating the client about *vocal hygiene*. Figure 9.11 lists some suggestions for good vocal hygiene that

Figure 9.11 Behaviors that promote good vocal hygiene.

Drink plenty of fluids, especially water.

Limit the intake of caffeine.

Limit the intake of alcoholic beverages.

Avoid tobacco products.

Avoid yelling and screaming.

Speak at a comfortable loudness level; don't "push" your voice.

Avoid loud, dry, or smoky environments.

Do not use "unnatural" voices, such as imitating cartoon characters.

Practice vocal rest.

Avoid excessive throat clearing and coughing.

the SLP might recommend to the client with a voice disorder. In addition, patients are educated about how forceful adduction of the vocal folds can result in trauma to tissue mucosa that can subsequently lead to laryngeal pathology. Using graphic pictures and descriptions of voice anatomy and physiology during therapy sessions can effectively increase the client's awareness of the negative consequences of laryngeal hyperadduction and poor vocal hygiene on vocal fold tissue (Stemple, Roy, & Klaben, 2014).

Direct treatment approaches and techniques that modify the physiology of the voice mechanism are also taught to the client with benign laryngeal pathology secondary to vocal misuse and abuse (i.e., laryngeal hyperfunction). The goal of these interventions is to teach the client to eliminate the vocally abnormal or abusive behavior (e.g., talking too loudly or too forcefully) by producing a voice that balances the three speech production subsystems; respiratory, laryngeal, and articulatory/resonatory (Stemple, Roy, & Klaben, 2014). There are a number of physiologic voice approaches and therapeutic techniques that are effective in reducing or eliminating hyperfunctional vocal patterns; several of these are described in Box 9.1.

 Thought Question 9.3

If you were prescribed a specified period of vocal rest, how would your daily life activities be affected? Could you comply with this treatment approach?

Intervention for Voice Disorders Associated with Neurological Diseases

Treatment of voice disorders associated with neurological disease processes do not focus on elimination of the disorder (e.g., reducing the size of a nodule) or on precipitating conditions (e.g., frequent yelling at sporting events). Because voice disorders associated with neurological problems are often not the primary disability, treatment may instead focus on increasing overall speech intelligibility, or may involve identifying assistive or alternative means of communication. In some cases, however, direct treatment of the voice is warranted.

When voice intervention is indicated, the overriding therapeutic goal is to assist the individual to produce the best voice possible to remain communicatively functional in vocational and social settings. In addition, the SLP can be helpful in assessing the effects of medications or surgery on voice production. Some of the specific techniques that the SLP uses to establish the best voice possible include increasing respiratory and/or laryngeal function for speech, changing speaking rate, and changing the overall prosody of speech. It is essential that the SLP recognize the limitations of voice intervention for certain medical or physical conditions and help the individual to achieve the best possible means of communication (Colton, Casper, & Leonard, 2011).

Intervention for Voice Disorders Associated with Psychological or Stress Conditions

Treatment of voice disorders associated with psychological or stress conditions can be effective if an SLP succeeds in convincing the individual that there is nothing wrong physically with his or her voice. Individuals who have identifiable conditions of stress or emotional conflict in their lives (e.g., recent divorce) and can recognize the relationship of that stress to their voice problem are the best candidates for voice intervention. These individuals want the ability to use their voice again, and the SLP can help them see how their psychosocial history may have contributed to the voice problem (Duffy, 2013).

A recommended therapeutic technique for voice disorders associated with psychological or stress conditions (conversion aphonia) begins by having the individual initiate the voice from a grunt to a sigh to a prolonged sound, then to a syllable or word (e.g., *uh-huh*). Such techniques provide solid evidence to the individual that he or she is physically capable of normal voice production (Boone & McFarlane, 2000; Duffy, 2013).

For many individuals with conversion aphonia or dysphonia, the voice can return to normal in minutes or over several sessions with the help of an SLP. For these individuals, in fact, psychiatric referral is often not needed after successful treatment by an SLP (Aronson, 1990b; Duffy, 2013).

Elective Voice Intervention for Transgender/Transsexual Clients

Some individuals will seek the help of an SLP to assist in changing various aspects of their voice and communication style following transgender reassignment. This is most typical in male-to-female transgender individuals. For females transitioning to males, hormone replacement often serves to lower pitch to an appropriate level, and thus these individuals do not often seek voice intervention (Van Borsel et al., 2000). On the other hand, individuals transitioning from male to female often need assistance in raising vocal pitch to be perceived as female. Recall that women have a fundamental frequency of about 250 Hz, while men have a fundamental frequency of about 125 Hz. Research has shown that for biological males to be perceived as females, they must raise their fundamental frequency to 155–165 Hz (Gelfer & Schofield, 2000) and, in some cases, as high as 180 Hz (Gorham-Rowan & Morris, 2006).

In addition to raising fundamental frequency, it is also necessary to alter vocal tract resonance in order to achieve a perceptually feminine voice. SLPs can work to train individuals to place their tongue more anteriorly in their mouth when speaking, thereby achieving a more "forward" resonance believed to be characteristic of the female voice (Hancock & Helenius, 2012). More research is needed on transgender clients' self-perceptions and satisfaction with voice therapy. More research is also needed to determine how unfamiliar listeners perceive speaker gender to examine the social validity of voice and communication treatment for transgender clients (Hancock & Garabedian, 2013).

Treatment of Resonance Disorders

Similarly to voice disorders, effective treatment of resonance disorders requires a multidisciplinary team approach, and often involves medical/surgical interventions, prosthetic management, and behavioral treatment. Because clefts of the lip and/or palate are the most frequent craniofacial defects in the world, with an estimated incidence of 1 in 700 births (Murray & Schutte, 2004), the focus of our discussion will be on resonance disorders associated with cleft palate, specifically, hypernasality due to VPD. However, some of the prosthetic and behavioral approaches have been found to be useful with individuals with hypernasality associated with neuromotor speech disorders; these are mentioned in Chapter 10. Specific evidence-based treatments for VPD in the cleft palate population are further described in Box 9.1.

Medical Management

Treatment of hypernasality secondary to VPD in individuals with cleft palate typically begins with surgical intervention. Normal velopharyngeal function cannot be achieved without structural integrity of the velopharyngeal mechanism. Therefore, children born with palatal clefts undergo surgical closure of the cleft between 9 and 18 months of age (Perry & Schenck, 2013). If a child also has a cleft of the lip, surgery to repair the cleft lip frequently occurs before 3 months of age (Kuehn & Henne, 2003).

Prosthetic Management

Following early surgical repair of a cleft palate, it is possible for a *fistula*, or an open hole between the nasal and oral cavities, to open spontaneously (Peterson-Falzone et al., 2010). A **palatal obturator**, which is a prosthetic device similar to a dental retainer, can be used to cover a defect until further surgery is warranted. Obturators are made of acrylic material and are custom built to conform to the general configuration of an individual's oral cavity. An obturator is held in place by clasps that anchor it to the teeth.

Prosthetic devices can also be considered when other anatomical limitations exist, such as when the velum is too short to contact the posterior pharyngeal wall, or for a velum that is completely immobile due to neurological disease. For a velum that is too short, a **speech bulb obturator** can be used. The bulb serves to fill the space between the velum and pharyngeal walls, and thus reduces perceived hypernasality during speech (Kummer & Lee, 1996). For a velum that is immobile due to paralysis secondary to neurological disease, a **palatal lift** can be considered. A palatal lift works to either elevate the velum into full contact with the posterior pharyngeal wall or positions the velum such that pharyngeal wall movement is sufficient to achieve closure (Peterson-Falzone et al., 2006).

Behavioral Management

While surgery is effective in improving the structure of the velopharyngeal mechanism in individuals with cleft palate, it does not serve to improve function. As such, speech-language treatment is typically warranted (Kummer & Lee, 1996). In individuals with VPD resulting in a mild degree of hypernasality following surgical repair of a cleft palate, the cleft palate team may determine that behavioral management is appropriate.

One approach that an SLP may use to treat VPD is a resistance exercise treatment program called continuous positive airway pressure (CPAP). CPAP treatment is an 8-week muscle resistance home-training program designed to strengthen the muscles of the soft palate. A CPAP device, like the one used for patients with obstructive sleep apnea, generates continuous positive air pressure that is delivered through a nose mask. Treatment involves production of 50 specified words and 6 sentences while pressure is delivered through the nose. The amount of pressure delivered and the amount of practice time each week progressively increases (Kuehn, 1991; Peterson-Falzone et al., 2010).

CPAP treatment is based on the exercise physiology principle of progressive resistance training. Progressive resistance training asserts that when muscles are subjected systematically to weights greater than those to which they are accustomed, they adapt by adding muscle tissue, and strength is increased. To continue building muscle tissue, weights are increased systematically until the desired muscle strength is achieved.

The CPAP procedure attempts to strengthen the muscles of the velopharyngeal mechanism by having the velar musculature work against systematic increases of weight. Because it would be quite impractical and probably impossible to use miniature free weights, CPAP uses air pressure in the nasal cavity as a substitute. Heightened air pressure in the nasal cavity is the "weight" that the velopharyngeal mechanism works against (Tomes et al., 1997).

During treatment, the velum works against the increased air pressure in the nasal cavity while producing syllables that contain nasal consonants such as /n/ or /m/, vowels, and nonnasal consonants. The velum is lowered during production of a nasal consonant and elevated during vowel and nonnasal consonant productions. Nasal air pressure is increased systematically during velar elevation associated with production of the nonnasal consonant.

Treatment of Articulation Disorders Secondary to VPD

Individuals with clefts are also at high risk for disordered articulation. Direct intervention by an SLP for speech-sound development should begin prior to the first palatal surgery, and as early as 5 to 6 months of age, just before the onset of babbling (Peterson-Falzone et al., 2006). Early speech-language intervention should focus on increasing the child's consonant inventory, especially pressure consonants, and on increasing oral airflow (Hardin-Jones et al., 2006). The behavioral treatment approaches and techniques described in Chapter 5 for children with speech sound disorders also apply to the treatment of the cleft population. The procedures and techniques used in bottom-up drill approaches may be particularly useful for treating habituated, compensatory misarticulations.

Teaching the difference between nasal and oral sounds, as well as how to direct the air stream through the mouth, might also be useful. This can be accomplished using swimmers' nose clips to prevent nasal air escape and helping the child learn how airflow feels when it is directed through the mouth during speech production (Peterson-Falzone et al., 2006).

For children who continue to substitute glottal stops (i.e., production of a grunt-like sound in the glottis or throat) for high-pressure consonants such as stops, fricatives, or affricates even after surgical correction of the cleft, direct speech treatment should begin as soon as possible. Glottal stops are far easier to eliminate early on than later, and specific treatment procedures are available (see Kuehn & Henne, 2003; Peterson-Falzone et al., 2006).

A promising technique for speech sound production training is **electropalatography (EPG)**. This technique uses an artificial palatal plate containing electrodes that are connected to a computer. The palatal plate is fitted in the client's mouth, and when the tongue contacts these electrodes during speech production, the articulatory patterns can be seen on the computer screen. Children with cleft palate can learn correct placement of the articulators for speech-sound production using EPG.

Efficacy of Voice and Resonance Treatment

Assessing the efficacy of treatment for voice and resonance disorders is complex because of the variety of conditions that produce voice and resonance disorders, the varying severity levels of the specific types of these disorders, the variety and combinations of behavioral and medical treatments available, and the manner in which treatment efficacy is defined. Despite these complexities, clinical and experimental data suggest general clinical effectiveness. For voice disorders, particularly those associated with vocal misuse and abuse (such as disorders with structural tissue damage), neurological conditions like Parkinson disease, and psychological or stress conditions, treatment has shown to be reasonably effective. Similarly, individuals born with cleft palate who receive medical and behavioral treatment earlier in their life generally speak normally by the time they are adolescents (Peterson-Falzone et al., 2010). Box 9.1 briefly summarizes specific approaches and techniques that have been shown to be effective in treating voice and resonance disorders.

In addition, it's important for an SLP to help clients who have voice or resonance disorders comply with specific treatment techniques by being patient and encouraging during treatment sessions. Changing habituated behaviors that contribute to vocal misuse or abuse is hard work and takes time. As an SLP, your dedication to your clients through your hard work and your enthusiasm about even small gains in progress can be overwhelmingly motivating to clients.

SLPs specialize in *communicating*, which we often equate with *talking*, but it is sometimes more important to compassionately listen to our clients and their caregivers. This is particularly the case for parents who have children with cleft palate, which can cause significant anxiety for caregivers about their child's future. While you as an SLP will probably not have specific answers or be able to make any reliable inferences about prognoses for speech and language development, you can listen attentively, acknowledge caregivers' concerns and fears, and act in a caring and empathetic fashion at all times. Your success as an SLP will depend on your ability to build trusting relationships with clients and caregivers, and these relationships will not only contribute to your effectiveness as a clinician but also serve to add genuine meaningfulness to your career and to your overall life.

Check Your Understanding 9.4
Click here to check your understanding of the concepts in this section.

SUMMARY

The human larynx is a versatile instrument that, in addition to its primary biological function of protecting the lower airways from invasion of foreign substances, serves as the primary sound generator for spoken communication. The human voice reflects one's personality, general state of health and age, and emotional condition. The human vocal tract, made up of the pharyngeal, oral, and nasal cavities, acts as a filter, changing in size and shape to alter the sound generated by the larynx, thus contributing to the resonance, or quality, of the voice. Closure of the velopharyngeal mechanism is necessary to produce the majority of speech sounds in the English language, and inadequate closure due to structural abnormalities such as cleft palate results in the perception of hypernasality, or sound energy inappropriately resonating through the nasal cavity.

Disorders of voice and resonance affect a substantial number of people, and vary in both etiology and severity. Voice and resonance disorders can range from relatively uncomplicated abnormalities such as vocal hoarseness resulting from yelling excessively at a sporting event, or hyponasal-sounding speech due to an upper respiratory infection, to cancer of the larynx or bilateral cleft of the lip and palate. The specific method of treatment is largely dictated by the etiology and severity of the disorder.

SLPs play a pivotal role in the treatment of voice and resonance disorders, but effective and ethical management requires a team approach. In many instances, surgical intervention followed by behavioral treatment is the standard protocol. In other instances, medical intervention alone, as in the case of a nasal blockage, or behavioral treatment alone, as is sometimes the case for individuals with vocal nodules, is sufficient. Dealing effectively with individuals with voice and resonance disorders requires detailed and specific knowledge about normal and abnormal function of the laryngeal and velopharyngeal mechanisms. Many voice and resonance disorders respond well to techniques used by SLPs, and working with such disorders can be a rewarding and exciting clinical endeavor.

SUGGESTED READINGS/SOURCES

Hollien, H. (2002). *Forensic voice identification*. San Diego, CA: Academic Press.

Language, Speech, and Hearing Services in Schools, 35(4) (2004)—The entire issue is devoted to the assessment and treatment of children with voice disorders.

Peterson-Falzone, S., Hardin-Jones, M., & Karnell, M. (2010). *Cleft palate speech* (4th ed.). St. Louis, MO: Mosby.

Peterson-Falzone, S., Trost-Cardamone, J., Karnell, M., & Hardin-Jones, M. (2006). *The clinician's guide to treating cleft palate speech*. St. Louis, MO: Mosby.

Shprintzen, R. (2000). *Syndrome identification for speech-language pathology: An illustrated pocket guide*. San Diego, CA: Singular.

Titze, I. R. (2000). *Principles of voice production* (2nd printing). Iowa City, IA: National Center for Voice and Speech.

10 Motor Speech Disorders

LEARNING OUTCOMES

When you have finished this chapter, you should be able to:

- Describe the structures of the brain which are important for motor speech control

- Describe the types and etiologies of dysarthria and apraxia in adults and children

- Discuss assessment techniques for motor speech disorders

- Discuss evidence-based treatments for dysarthria and apraxia in adults and children

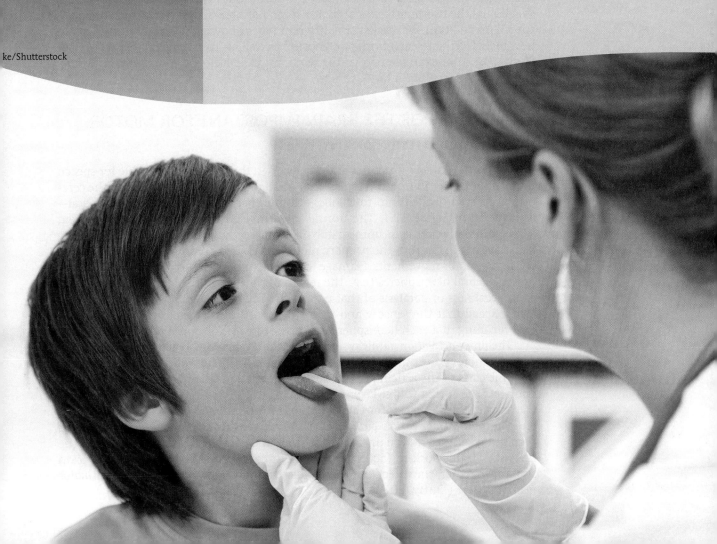

Neurons are the basic unit of the nervous system. Each neuron has three parts: the *cell body*, a single long *axon* that transmits impulses away from the cell body to the next neuron, and several branching *dendrites* that receive impulses from other cells and transmit them toward the cell body. *Lower motor neurons* are responsible for muscle activation. A muscle is innervated by several hundred lower motor neurons. When lower motor neurons degenerate or die, as is the case in diseases such as amyotrophic lateral sclerosis (i.e., Lou Gehrig's disease), muscles become weak and eventually atrophy, or waste away.

Motor speech disorders are difficulties related to problems of movement resulting from neurological disorder or injury. They are a heterogeneous group of neurological impairments that affect motor planning, programming, coordination, timing, and execution of movement patterns used for speech production in both children and adults. Any or all of the processes of respiration, phonation, resonation, and articulation described in previous chapters may be affected. Although voice and fluency may also be involved, these are addressed in other chapters. Language disorders often co-occur with motor speech disorders; these are described in Chapter 7.

This brief explanation does not begin to hint at the complexity of the disorders that fall within the boundaries of motor speech disorders. So finite and particular are the movements needed for speech that more area in the brain is devoted to control of vocal folds, tongue, lips, and other articulators than to any other bodily movement, even walking. Given this complexity, it is amazing that the process of speech production becomes so automatic that we give little thought to it when speaking. In fact, we rarely consider the process unless something goes wrong.

As with language, there does not seem to be a specific area of the brain devoted to speech motor control. Even those areas of the frontal lobe that are important for speech are not solely devoted to speech-specific tasks. They also participate in nonspeech motor tasks. In this chapter, we limit our discussion to motor speech. We discuss the two main types of motor speech disorders: dysarthria and apraxia of speech. In addition, we discuss five different types of dysarthria and briefly explain how to differentiate each from one another as well as from apraxia of speech. Case Study 10.1 is an example of a young woman who developed motor speech disturbances as the result of a brain tumor.

STRUCTURES OF THE BRAIN IMPORTANT FOR MOTOR SPEECH CONTROL

A complex network of structures and pathways in the brain is responsible for speech motor control. Recall from Chapter 7 that the right and left hemispheres of the cerebrum are each divided into four lobes—frontal, parietal, occipital, and temporal—as depicted in Figure 10.1. The frontal lobes house the **primary motor cortex**, a 2-centimeter-wide strip immediately in front of the central sulcus. Descending pathways originate from the primary motor cortex and are important for initiating voluntary motor movements. Damage to an area of the primary motor cortex in one of the cerebral hemispheres (e.g., the region of the arm in the left hemisphere) will cause weakness or paralysis of that part of the body on the opposite side (i.e., right arm). Recall that the sensory and motor functions of the cerebrum are contralateral, meaning that each hemisphere is concerned with the opposite side of the body.

The *direct activation pathway*, known as the **pyramidal tract**, originates in the primary motor cortex and is responsible for rapid, discrete, volitional movement of the limbs and of the articulators for speech production. The pyramidal tract directly connects the cortex (outer layer of the brain) to the neurons that directly control the activation of muscles for the initiation of movement.

The *indirect activation pathway*, or **extrapyramidal tract**, is important for regulating reflexes and maintaining posture and muscle tone, thus providing the necessary framework to facilitate movement carried out by the direct activation system. Together, the direct and indirect activation pathways form the *upper motor neuron system* (Duffy, 2013).

CASE STUDY 10.1

Case Study of a Teen with a Motor Speech Disorder: Sofia

Sofia, a 16-year-old cheerleader and member of the high school drama club, came home early from school because she believed she had the flu. She went to school the next day, but noticed difficulty with her speech and writing. That evening, her parents noted that Sofia's speech was slurred and difficult to understand. They asked her to talk more slowly, but Sofia continued to make speech errors each time she tried to correct herself. She started to get very frustrated, and her parents became worried. The next morning, Sofia began complaining of a severe headache, so her parents rushed her to the emergency room, where she underwent a neurological evaluation, including a brain imaging scan. It was determined that Sofia had a tumor in the left frontal lobe of her brain, causing increased pressure inside her skull; she was scheduled for neurosurgery the following morning.

Although the surgery was successful, Sofia was still experiencing speech difficulties and was referred for a speech-language pathology consult. A comprehensive evaluation of Sofia's motor speech production skills was completed, and the speech-language pathologist (SLP) recommended treatment to improve her speech so that her friends, family, and teachers would be able to understand her. The school-based SLP collaborated with the hospital SLP so that similar services could be provided to Sofia at school.

Sofia received outpatient services at the hospital one time per week; she learned various strategies (e.g., over-articulating; using gestures) to improve the understandability of her speech. The school-based SLP saw Sofia two times per week and worked on the same strategies at school, ensuring that she was using them when participating in class discussions. Her parents participated in her treatment too and helped by reminding her to use her strategies at home. After 8 months, Sofia returned to her normal, pre-trauma levels of speech performance.

As you read this chapter, think about:

- Possible explanations for Sofia's pre- and post-neurosurgery speech difficulties
- Examination tasks the SLP might have used to assess Sofia's motor speech production
- Other treatment techniques that might have been useful for Sofia after her surgery to help her to be better understood

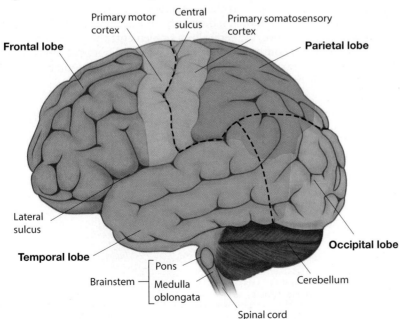

Figure 10.1 Schematic diagram of the human brain.

The **basal ganglia** are large subcortical nuclei that regulate motor functioning and maintain posture and muscle tone; thus, they are part of the brain's extrapyramidal system. The basal ganglia modulate the activity of the primary motor cortex and indirectly influence movement. This is accomplished by direct and indirect control loops that have opposing functions, both of which are regulated by the neurotransmitter dopamine. The direct pathway serves to increase or facilitate movement, while the indirect pathway serves to decrease or inhibit movement; the balance of activity in these two pathways determines the quality of movement. Damage to the basal ganglia will either result in reduced and/or slowed movement, as seen in Parkinson disease, or will result in abnormal, involuntary movements as seen in Huntington's chorea. Chorea involves quick, continuous, and purposeless movements of the head, face, tongue, and/or limbs, discussed a little later in this chapter (Duffy, 2013).

The cerebellum, or "little brain," consists of right and left cerebellar hemispheres and a central vermis. The cerebellum is connected to many other parts of the brain, and has access to much of the brain's information. The cerebellum and its connections coordinate the control of fine, complex motor activities, maintain muscle tone, and participate in motor learning. Figure 10.2 summarizes the areas of the brain important to motor control. Visit http://sciencenetlinks.com to download the free three-dimensional (3D) brain application (type "3D brain" into the search bar on this website) for your computer, Apple, or Android device.

Motor Speech Production Process

In the process of motor speech production, first the movement plan/program, which is an organized set of motor commands that specifies all of the necessary parameters of movement, is retrieved from memory. Next, it is sent to the motor

Figure 10.2 Areas of the brain important for motor function.

Signals to the muscles originate in the motor cortex and are sent deep into the brain to begin their descent. The cerebellum sets the overall tone and posture that gives the motor cortex the ability to execute intentional movements. In addition, although the motor cortex determines where to move, the cerebellum implements the proper timing and force. Motor nerve impulses continue through the pyramidal tract that relays intentional movement and the extrapyramidal tract that relays automatic, involuntary movement.

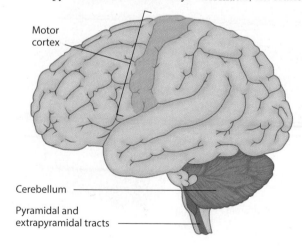

control areas (e.g., primary motor cortex); then it is transmitted with precise timing along the nerves to muscles and structures of the speech mechanism, resulting in sequences of acoustic signals that are recognized as speech sounds. Along the way, these nerve impulses are modified to ensure precise, smooth muscle movement.

Typical movement patterns are purposeful and efficient and are under the control of the individual, who can therefore change or modify the movement. Motor responses are initiated, changed, and coordinated on the basis of both external and internal sensory information. External sensory mechanisms detect and analyze the external environment. Internal movement feedback from muscles (proprioceptive feedback) and nerves helps us know the position and movement of body structures in space. For speech production, auditory and proprioceptive feedback help ensure proper coordination of the speech mechanism. For a comprehensive review of the motor speech production process, see Maas et al., 2008.

Cranial Nerves Important for Speech Production

Whereas the central nervous system (CNS) comprises the brain and spinal cord, the **peripheral nervous system (PNS)** consists of 12 pairs of cranial nerves, most of which originate in the brain stem, and 31 pairs of spinal nerves that exit the vertebral column and travel to and from muscles of the body. By transmitting messages to muscles and receiving sensory information, the PNS helps the CNS communicate with the body.

The **cranial nerves** (Figure 10.3) are especially important for speech production. Because they are arranged vertically along the brain stem, they are referred to by Roman numerals corresponding to their vertical order. Thus, number VII, the facial nerve, is seventh from the top. The majority of the **spinal nerves**—22 of the 31 pairs of these nerves—are important for breathing for purposes of speech production. In contrast, special control centers in the brain stem govern breathing for sustaining life.

 Check Your Understanding 10.1
Click here to check your understanding of the concepts in this section.

MOTOR SPEECH DISORDERS

Damage to any structure or pathway involved in the speech production process can cause a motor speech disorder. As mentioned previously, motor speech disorders are a heterogeneous group of neurological impairments that reflect a disturbance in the motor planning, programming, coordination, timing, and execution of movement patterns used for speech production. Motor speech disorders, therefore, include the dysarthrias and apraxia of speech (Duffy, 2013).

Dysarthria

Dysarthria is a general diagnostic term for a group of speech disorders resulting from disturbances in the central and peripheral nervous systems that control the muscles of speech production. Dysarthria can affect the speed, range, direction,

Figure 10.3 Cranial nerves important in speech production.

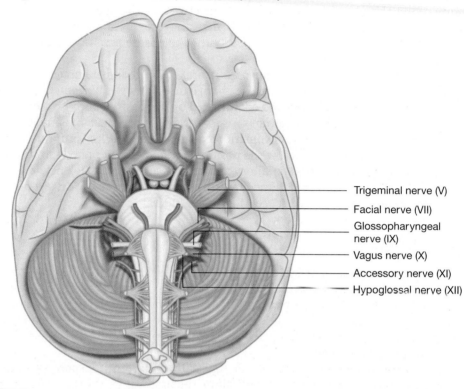

Trigeminal (V): A mixed nerve, with both sensory and motor functions for the jaw and tongue for speech and chewing.

Facial (VII): A mixed nerve for sensation of taste and motor control of the facial muscles important in facial expression, such as smiling, tearing, and salivation.

Glossopharyngeal (IX): A mixed nerve, with sensory input from the tongue for taste and motor control of the pharynx for salivation and swallowing.

Vagus (X): A mixed nerve serving the heart, lungs, and digestive system. A sensory nerve to the larynx and throat. A motor nerve to the larynx for phonation, to the soft palate for lifting, and to the pharynx for swallowing.

Accessory (XI): A motor nerve controlling muscles of the pharynx, soft palate, head, and shoulders.

Hypoglossal (XII): A motor nerve controlling the muscles of tongue movement.

strength, and timing of motor movements for respiration, phonation, resonance, and articulation, and it is a result of weakness, spasticity, discoordination, or involuntary movements. Motor movements that were previously established may have been lost or modified in some way, though the pattern for that movement still exists.

It is important to note that dysarthria is not a language disorder. An individual can present with dysarthria alone and thus exhibit good language structure and vocabulary, good reading comprehension skills, and effectively participate in the give and take of conversation as well as his or her physical limitations permit. An individual with dysarthria can convey by other means, such as a computer device, sentences that he or she may be unable to produce freely through speech.

The muscular disorders that cause dysarthria represent a variety of neurological diseases. Although individuals with dysarthria share some common symptoms, distinct clusters of neurological and speech characteristics exist that describe specific types of the disorder.

Different types of dysarthria result from lesions to different parts of the CNS and/or PNS. Certain commonalities exist across these types, as shown in Table 10.1, including inadequate respiratory drive; voice disturbances such as pitch and loudness problems; prosodic abnormalities such as excessive stress patterns; rate difficulties such as slow, rapid, or varying speeds; hypernasality; and imprecise articulation.

Five distinct types of dysarthria can be identified by their speech characteristics and the impaired neuromuscular processes, including **flaccid**, **spastic**, **ataxic**, **hypokinetic**, and **hyperkinetic** dysarthria (Duffy, 2013). When multiple motor systems are involved, a mixed dysarthria may occur, as in the case of individuals

TABLE 10.1

Characteristics of the dysarthrias

Type of Dysarthria	Lesion Location	Speech Characteristics
Flaccid dysarthria: Muscles are weak and reduced in tone; decreased reflexes; flaccid paralysis; eventual atrophy of muscles	Damage to lower motor neurons (i.e., cranial and spinal nerves) or to the muscle unit itself	Continuous breathiness; monopitch; hypernasal; short phrases; imprecise articulation
Spastic dysarthria: Weak, spastic muscles; hyperactive reflexes; increased muscle tone	Damage to upper motor neurons (i.e., direct and indirect activation pathways)	Slow rate; strain-strangled voice quality; hypernasal; imprecise articulation; excess and equal stress
Ataxic dysarthria: Incoordination; reduced muscle tone; poor accuracy and timing of movements	Damage to the cerebellum or cerebellar control circuitry	Irregular breakdowns in articulation; imprecise consonants; vowel distortions; prosodic abnormalities (e.g., excess and equal stress; prolonged pauses)
Hypokinetic dysarthria: Reduced movement; muscle rigidity and stiffness; difficulties starting and stopping movements	Damage to basal ganglia and basal ganglia circuitry	Accelerated speech rate; imprecise articulation due to reduced range of motion of the articulators; breathy/harsh/hoarse voice quality; reduced loudness; disfluencies
Hyperkinetic dysarthria: Involuntary movements	Damage to basal ganglia and basal ganglia circuitry	Irregular breakdowns in articulation; prosodic abnormalities; variable speech rate
Mixed dysarthrias: Combination of two or more dysarthrias	Damage to multiple brain structures or circuits.	Imprecise articulation; slow rate; harsh voice; monopitch/monoloudness; hypernasality; excess and equal stress

Source: Based on Duffy, J. (2013). Motor speech disorders: Substrates, differential diagnosis, and management (3rd ed.). St. Louis, MO: Elsevier, Mosby.

with amyotrophic lateral sclerosis (ALS), multiple sclerosis (MS), and Wilson's disease, to name a few. Each type of dysarthria is briefly discussed here, along with the neurological impairment that may be associated with a particular dysarthria type.

Flaccid Dysarthrias

Muscles that exhibit flaccid paralysis are weak and soft, exhibit low tone (i.e., hypotonia), and fatigue quickly. Flaccid dysarthria frequently results from lesions of the cranial and spinal nerves, collectively known as the *lower motor neurons*, or damage to the muscle unit itself. Affected muscles may cause reduced respiratory drive for speech breathing, continuously breathy voice quality, reduced pitch and loudness levels, monopitch, hypernasality, and imprecise articulation. Etiologies of flaccid dysarthria include Bell's palsy, a facial nerve (CN VII) disorder, progressive bulbar palsy, myasthenia gravis, and **muscular dystrophy**.

Bell's Palsy

Your body's immune system is a network of cells, tissues, and organs that work to prevent foreign substances that cause infection from entering your body and to destroy invading microorganisms once they have entered. Autoimmune diseases occur when the immune system mistakes healthy cells and tissues as infected and attacks and destroys them. The reason the immune system responds in this way toward healthy body tissues is unclear.

Bell's palsy is an idiopathic condition of underdetermined cause that results in unilateral (i.e., one side) damage to the facial nerve (i.e., cranial nerve VII). It is a fairly common condition that occurs suddenly and resolves spontaneously in the majority of cases. Unilateral damage of the facial nerve affects the muscles of the upper and lower face, and, in some cases, the ability to close the eyelid on the affected side (Duffy, 2013). Flaccid dysarthria associated with Bell's palsy tends to be very mild, with mild articulatory imprecision as its primary speech characteristic.

Progressive Bulbar Palsy

Progressive bulbar palsy is a neurological disease that causes degeneration of lower motor neurons, resulting in flaccid paralysis of muscles and eventual muscle atrophy. Damage to lower motor neurons in progressive bulbar palsy also results in **fasciculations**, or visible, isolated twitches in resting muscle due to spontaneous firing of nerve impulses in response to nerve degeneration (Duffy, 2013). Individuals with progressive bulbar palsy have described fasciculations as feeling like a bubbling under the skin. In flaccid dysarthria secondary to progressive bulbar palsy, fasciculations are often seen on the tongue or in the chin region, and speech sounds weak, hypernasal, and monopitched, along with imprecise articulation.

Myasthenia Gravis

Myasthenia gravis is an autoimmune disease that affects the neuromuscular junction (i.e., the area between the motor nerve axon and the muscle). The disorder is characterized by rapid weakening of muscles due to the inadequate transmission of nerve impulses to the muscles. With repeated use such as during speech production, muscles become progressively weak, but regain their strength with a short period of rest. The flaccid dysarthria that results is characterized by imprecise articulation and hypernasality that rapidly gets worse with prolonged speaking, but dramatically improves following 1 to 2 minutes of rest.

Spastic Dysarthria

Spastic paralysis of muscles reflects the combined effects of weakness and loss of inhibitory motor control. As a result, reflexes become hyperactive, muscle tone is increased at rest, and individuals exhibit *spasticity* or increased resistance to passive stretch. Spasticity of the speech mechanism is the hallmark of spastic dysarthria, causing movements of the articulators to become slowed and reduced in force and range of motion. Spasticity at the level of the larynx causes the vocal folds to inappropriately adduct (close) during speech production, resulting in a strain-strangled voice quality. Spastic dysarthria typically results from bilateral upper motor neuron lesions (due to strokes) in the cerebral hemispheres or from a single lesion in the brain stem, where direct and indirect activation pathways are in close proximity (Duffy, 2013).

 Video Exercise 10.1

Identifying Spastic Dysarthria

Click on the link to watch a video of a 58-year-old man with spastic dysarthria, and complete an exercise.

Ataxic Dysarthria

Damage to the cerebellum or cerebellar control circuitry results in incoordination and reduced muscle tone, called *ataxia*. Ataxic dysarthria reflects the effects of incoordination and the improper timing of movements, causing irregular breakdowns in articulation and abnormalities of prosody. Ataxia and ataxic dysarthria are not caused by weakness. Muscles are not reduced in strength; rather, they are poorly timed and improperly coordinated during movement. Movements are inaccurate, jerky, and lacking smoothness. Too much alcohol consumption can result in temporary ataxia. In fact, individuals who have had a stroke in the cerebellum, or who have a neurological disease that causes degeneration of the cerebellum, often complain that they look and sound drunk.

Hypokinetic Dysarthria

Hypokinetic movements are slow and reduced in range of motion due to the effects of rigidity or increased resistance to passive stretch in all directions. Individuals with **hypokinesia** (i.e., reduced movement) feel stiff and find it difficult to get movements started. Once started, they then struggle to stop. The most common cause of hypokinesia is Parkinson disease, where a degeneration of dopaminergic neurons (i.e., neurons that make dopamine, a neurotransmitter important in motor control) in the brain stem prevents proper functioning of the basal ganglia, the subcortical structure that indirectly influences the quality of movement. Reduced range of motion is the hallmark of hypokinetic dysarthria. The articulators appear to be barely moving during speech production, and as a result speech rate becomes very fast. Disfluencies are common, and loudness levels gradually diminish such that it is often difficult to hear a person with Parkinson disease when he or she is talking. Case Study 10.2 provides a firsthand account of an individual living with Parkinson disease.

Parkinson Disease

Parkinson disease (PD) is a common degenerative neurological disease that affects 1% to 2% of people over age 50. Average life expectancy after diagnosis is approximately 15 years (Duffy, 2013). Parkinson disease is idiopathic, meaning that there is no known cause; genetic and environmental factors are believed to play a role. More information about Parkinson disease can be found at www.michaeljfox.org

CASE STUDY 10.2

The Story of Carlos, a Man with Parkinson Disease

Carlos is 64 and retired. He had to retire because the effects of Parkinson disease prevented him from continuing to work as a foreign language professor. His wife, 3 years younger, has also retired in order to take care of her husband. About 15 years ago, Carlos noticed tremors in his hands, usually when he was at rest. At first they were intermittent, and he thought they were caused by nervousness, stress, or muscle fatigue. As they became more frequent, Carlos found it harder and harder to ignore the symptoms.

Carlos's disease has progressed to the point where he walks by shuffling his feet, and he can climb stairs only with assistance and support. In danger of falling when he walks, Carlos has found that even getting over the upturned edge of a carpet can offer a genuine challenge. For this reason, he and his wife rarely go out, although they daily walk the lightly traveled road in front of their house, which is flat and easy for him to manage. Carlos calls it his "workout routine."

Carlos finds meals less satisfying than he used to because the consistency of some foods makes them difficult for him to chew. Although Carlos eats independently, his food must be cut beforehand into small pieces. If he uses a knife at all, it is for spreading, not cutting.

Although his speech is affected and is spoken in short quiet bursts, Carlos has maintained his sense of humor and his sarcastic wit. He still loves to tell stories of growing up in New York City.

Along with resting tremors and decreased range of movement, Carlos has experienced other physiological changes related to Parkinson disease. He tires easily, quickly becomes short of breath, and has difficulty concentrating. At other times, he seems to become lost in seemingly repetitive tasks, such as picking up lint. Medication that raises his dopamine level gives him smoother movement, but provides only temporary relief. He is sometimes frustrated by his response to the medication and his inability to time its effect on his movement for special times, such as a visit by his grandchildren.

by clicking on "Understanding Parkinson's." The Mayo Clinic website is also a useful resource (www.mayoclinic.com). Click on the "Health Information" tab, then "Diseases & Conditions A–Z." Click on "P" and scroll down until you see the tab for Parkinson's disease.

Hypokinetic dysarthria may not be apparent in the first several years following the initial signs of PD, but it is eventually present in 90% of cases of PD over the course of the disease (Duffy, 2013). As mentioned previously, voice and speech difficulties associated with hypokinetic dysarthria include reduced loudness, accelerated rate of speech, disfluencies, and imprecise articulation due to reduced range of motion of the articulators. In addition, voice quality may be breathy and harsh or hoarse, and pitch and loudness variability is significantly reduced, resulting in monopitch and monoloudness.

Hyperkinetic Dysarthrias

Hyperkinetic dysarthrias are also due to damage to the basal ganglia control circuitry; however, in this case the indirect pathway and/or structures of basal ganglia that help to inhibit unwanted movements are damaged. As a result, hyperkinesia (i.e., increased movement) occurs. Hyperkinetic dysarthria is essentially the production of motorically normal speech that is interrupted in some fashion by abnormal involuntary movements (Duffy, 2013). A number of hyperkinetic movement disorders can result in hyperkinetic dysarthria.

Tremor, the most common involuntary movement disorder, involves rhythmic movement of a body part, such as the limbs, head, or voice (Duffy, 2013). The best way to determine whether an individual has voice tremor is to ask him or her to sustain the vowel /a/ for as long as possible. Voice tremor may go unnoticed during conversational speech but is quite evident during vowel prolongation.

Tics are rapid, patterned movements that are not completely involuntary and can be suppressed for brief periods with effort. Tics are commonly associated with Tourette's syndrome, which affects more males than females (approximately 3:1 ratio) with onset prior to age 18; they can be motor in nature (e.g., eye blinking, head twitches) or vocal (e.g., throat clearing; snorting; sniffing; compulsive swearing). Vocal tics are the hallmark of hyperkinetic dysarthria in individuals with Tourette's syndrome, with rapid production of these noises, sounds, or words causing significant interruption to the normal flow of speech.

Dystonia is a slow hyperkinesia that may involve the entire body (i.e., generalized dystonia) or may be localized to just one body part (i.e., segmental dystonia). Involuntary movements are characterized by slow, sustained abnormal posturing, with possible twisting of body parts (e.g., arm, leg, head). Hyperkinetic dysarthria in individuals with dystonia may include excessive pitch and loudness variations, irregular breakdowns in articulation, variable rate, and inappropriate silences (Duffy, 2013).

Unlike dystonia, **chorea** is characterized by rapid and unpredictable movements of the limbs, face, and tongue. The term is derived from the Greek word meaning "dance," and patients with chorea appear to move continuously, in an unstable dance-like fashion. Hyperkinetic dysarthria in individuals who exhibit chorea is characterized by variable speech rate, irregular articulatory breakdowns, and significant prosodic abnormalities.

Huntington's Chorea

Huntington's chorea, also known as Huntington's disease, is an inherited progressive disease that results in degeneration of structures in the basal ganglia. Initial symptoms, which appear between the ages of 30 and 50, include involuntary choreatic movements and changes in behavior. As the disease progresses, involuntary movements worsen and become more generalized. Significant changes in mood and personality become evident, with subsequent development of depression and dementia. Average survival rate is about 20 years; however, individuals diagnosed with Huntington's chorea have a higher risk of suicide than do those with other neurodegenerative diseases, although the mechanisms for this are poorly understood.

Mixed Dysarthrias

When two or more types of dysarthria are present in an individual, an SLP diagnoses the individual with mixed dysarthria. Mixed dysarthrias are common in neurodegenerative diseases that cause damage to multiple areas of the central nervous system. This is the case in *amyotrophic lateral sclerosis (ALS)*, also known as Lou Gehrig's disease. In ALS, both upper and lower motor neurons degenerate, thereby causing both spastic and flaccid paralysis. Thus, the individual with ALS will exhibit a mixed spastic-flaccid dysarthria. The speech characteristics of spastic dysarthria are often more pronounced in ALS; therefore, the patient will have a slow rate of speech, hypernasality, imprecise articulation, and a strain-strangled voice quality. The primary features of lower motor neuron damage in patients with ALS will be the presence of fasciculations and atrophy of the tongue. Recall that fasciculations are visible, isolated twitches in resting muscle due to spontaneous firing of nerve impulses in response to nerve degeneration (Duffy, 2013). The severity of mixed dysarthria in individuals with ALS becomes worse as the disease progresses, and 75% of those affected are unable to speak at the time of death. Age of onset is usually in the mid-50s, and males are affected more often than females. Death usually occurs within 5 years after initial diagnosis.

Traumatic brain injury (TBI), discussed in Chapter 7, also causes mixed dysarthria. Typically, a mixed spastic-ataxic dysarthria is seen following TBI, such as a motor vehicle accident or a fall. In these particular cases of trauma, the axons of neurons that enable one neuron to communicate with another are severely damaged. This is called *axonal shearing*, and it results in diffuse damage throughout the brain. Males are at greater risk than females for sustaining traumatic injury, and approximately 70% of injuries resulting in TBI occur in the under-35 age group.

Lifespan Issues

Most acquired dysarthrias occur in adulthood. An individual with even mild dysarthria may be reluctant to speak, perhaps leading others to assume that the person is tense, shy, or unfriendly. For some individuals, even a slight speech abnormality can be cause for embarrassment or depression. In more severe cases of dysarthria, individuals may be frustrated as loved ones and acquaintances attempt to communicate for them by finishing their sentences or ordering for them in restaurants. In turn, these individuals may communicate or socialize less. Difficulty communicating may limit opportunities to participate in social, occupational, and educational activities, leading to feelings of isolation. As an SLP, you can provide a person with dysarthria and his or her communication partners various strategies to promote increased communicative participation and significantly improve the quality of their lives.

In the later stages of progressive degenerative diseases, an individual with dysarthria may be unable to live independently and may need daily living assistance or institutional care. Movement may become difficult, and the person may be unable to care for himself or herself. The person may eventually be unable to speak at all, and you as an SLP can continue to work to improve the quality of life for such individuals with profound dysarthria, with the help of augmentative and alternative communication (AAC) devices.

> Motor speech disorders are not limited to speech production and may have a negative effect on many aspects of an individual's life.

Apraxia of Speech

Apraxia of speech is a clinically distinct neurological speech disorder that impairs the ability to plan or program the sensory and motor commands needed for speech production. Unlike dysarthria, apraxia of speech is not a result of damage to speech muscles, nor does it involve muscle weakness; rather, it is a higher-level deficiency in motor control. The motor speech production process begins with a motor program being retrieved from memory. A motor program is an organized set of motor commands that specify all the necessary parameters of movement for speech production; they are learned and consolidated in memory over time. Apraxia of speech results in an inability to adequately retrieve these speech motor programs, thereby causing disordered articulation of vowels and consonants, slowed rate, and prosodic disturbances (e.g., inappropriate pausing or lengthening of speech segments; incorrect word and sentential stress patterns). It generally occurs following damage to the left cerebral hemisphere, particularly the motor and premotor areas of the left frontal lobe.

The speech of individuals with apraxia is characterized by groping attempts to find the correct articulatory position, with great variability (inconsistency) over repeated attempts. Frequent sound substitutions, omissions, and additions of sounds occur, along with significant difficulties sequencing sounds when producing multisyllabic words. Unlike a person with dysarthria who produces predominately sound distortion errors and/or related sound substitution errors, a person with apraxia often produces unrelated substitutions, repetitions, or additions. A person with apraxia of speech recognizes his or her errors and will make repeated attempts to correct them. As the person tries to produce the correct sound or word, there may be frequent pauses, lengthened sound segments, and re-initiations of words and sentences. As a result, speech production may appear as stuttering-like in nature. Unlike a person with dysarthria who repeats the same error, an individual with apraxia of speech often produces widely varying productions on repeated attempts. Such inconsistencies are specific to apraxia of speech, and thereby help you as an SLP correctly diagnose apraxia of speech from dysarthria. A speech sample from a person with apraxia follows:

> O-o-on . . . on . . . on our cavation, cavation, cacation . . . oh darn . . . vavation, oh, you know, to Ca-ca-caciporenia . . . no, Lacifacnia, vafacnia to Lacifacnion . . . on our vacation to Vacafornia, no darn it . . . to Ca-caliborneo . . . not bornia . . . fornia, Bornifornia . . . no, Balliforneo, Ballifornee, Balifornee, Californee, California. Phew, it was hard to say Cacaforneo. Oh darn.

Consonants and consonant clusters and blends are particularly challenging for those with apraxia, although more frequently used phonemes and words are produced with more accuracy. As you might expect, complex, long, and unfamiliar words are most difficult to produce.

Individuals with apraxia of speech may have no difficulty producing words on one occasion that they struggle to produce on another. In fact, clients may exhibit periods of error-free speech during automatic or emotional utterances. It is not uncommon to have a client struggle with volitional production of a word such as *vacation* only to hear the client easily say later, "Wow, I sure had a lot of trouble with *vacation!*"

A person with apraxia of speech is usually aware of his or her errors, as mentioned previously, and may even anticipate them but be unable to correct them. Monitoring of speech in anticipation of these errors tends to result in a slowed, almost cautious rate of speech, with equal stress and spacing, although prosodic abnormalities such as slow rate and equalized stress patterns are hallmark characteristics of this disorder. Clients frequently report that they know what they want to say but can't initiate the sequence or keep it going. Faced with a naming task, these individuals frequently respond, "I know it, but I can't say it."

Although apraxia and aphasia often co-occur, the two are not the same. Aphasia is a language disorder, while apraxia is a motor speech disorder. An individual with aphasia has difficulty with word recall in all modalities, whereas a person with apraxia of speech may be able to recall a word more easily when writing but be unable to say it correctly. In addition, apraxia of speech can be an individual's only diagnosis, and thus language structure may be perfectly intact. Case Study 10.3 is a story of a woman with apraxia of speech.

CASE STUDY 10.3

Personal Story of a Woman with Apraxia of Speech

Ruth is a 75-year-old woman who suffered a stroke in the frontal lobe of the left cerebral hemisphere. After being discharged from the hospital, Ruth began receiving services twice weekly at a rehabilitation center for her speech and for other motor difficulties related to her stroke.

Six months after the incident, she continues to exhibit severe apraxia of speech, characterized by consonant cluster reduction, inconsistent sound omissions, distorted consonant substitutions, and primary use of single words during conversation. When she is reading, her speech intelligibility decreases with increasingly complex material. She has difficulty initiating speech and difficulty with sound and syllable sequencing. Ruth's speech appears to improve with pre-formulation of the message and when using gestures.

Auditory comprehension during conversation and silent reading comprehension are both intact. Although Ruth reads the newspaper, she seems less interested in the more substantial pleasure reading that occupied much of her time previously. Her memory and attention skills seem unaffected.

A retired schoolteacher and widow, Ruth lives alone. She has six children. Her two oldest daughters are attempting to supplement the home health care she receives in order to help her to progress more quickly with her rehabilitation.

While there appear to be overlapping characteristics between the dysarthrias and apraxia of speech, the two are distinctly different types of motor speech disturbances. Correct diagnosis of a client is essential for speech treatment to be effective. Table 10.2 presents the major differences between the disorders, although there will be many individual variations.

Lifespan Issues

The impact of acquired apraxia of speech on an individual's life depends on the etiology of the disorder, as well as the severity. Most individuals who acquire apraxia of speech do so following a stroke in the left hemisphere, specifically

TABLE 10.2

Differences between dysarthria and apraxia

Dysarthria	Apraxia of Speech
Speech-sound distortions	Speech-sound substitutions
Substitution errors related to target phoneme	Substitution errors often not related to target phoneme
Highly consistent speech-sound errors	Inconsistent speech-sound substitution
Consonant clusters simplified	Schwa (/ə/) often inserted between consonants in a cluster
Little audible or silent groping for a target speech sound	Audible or silent groping for a target speech sound
Rapid or slow rate	Slow rate characterized by repetitions, prolongations, and additions
No periods of unaffected speech	Islands of fluency
Little difference between reactive or automatic speech and volitional speech; both affected	Often very fluent reactive or automatic speech, nonfluent volitional speech

Broca's area in the left frontal lobe. Depending on the severity of the stroke, individuals can make a full recovery and speech may return to normal. In other cases, speech may recover to some extent, but mild prosodic abnormalities such as slow rate and incorrect stress patterns may persist. For an individual who has apraxia of speech secondary to a progressive neurological disease (e.g., corticobasal degeneration), an SLP should get the client to think about AAC early, as such individuals are likely to lose most or even all ability to speak. It is important for an SLP to always encourage clients to continually practice speaking when they can and to utilize their AAC device as often as possible to promote communicative participation. It's also important to promote a positive attitude in clients with apraxia of speech, as well as all other types of motor speech disorders, as helping to maintain a satisfactory quality of life throughout the course of a degenerative disease is an essential role of an SLP.

Etiologies of Motor Speech Disorders in Children

Motor speech disorders can be either acquired (i.e., occurring after the neuromotor system is fully mature) or congenital (i.e., occurring at or before birth). Thus far, we have discussed a number of diseases that typically affect individuals in adulthood and, therefore, represent acquired disorders, including neurodegenerative diseases such as Parkinson disease or speech disturbances caused by stroke or traumatic brain injury. Motor speech disorders, such as dysarthria, can also occur in children due to congenital impairments that were present either at or just before birth.

Thought Question 10.1

How might a motor speech disorder differ for an individual with a congenital impairment versus an acquired impairment?

Cerebral Palsy

Cerebral palsy (CP), a heterogeneous group of non-progressive, permanent disorders of movement and postural development, is a congenital disorder that causes dysarthria in children. CP often results from oxygen deprivation to the brain (i.e., anoxic brain injury) that occurs either during development of the fetus, during the birth process, or shortly after birth. Hemorrhages in the brain can also cause CP. Any interruption in the blood supply, as occurs in a hemorrhage in the vascular system, can cause damage to a developing brain.

Infections and toxins may also disrupt brain development. Bacterial and viral infections, such as HIV, may infiltrate the brain from other bodily organs or may be transported within the blood supply. During the first few months of pregnancy and before the development of the placental barrier, the embryo is especially susceptible to infections of the mother, such as influenza, rubella, and mumps, that can damage the developing brain. Toxic agents such as heavy metals, mercury, and lead may accumulate in brain tissue and disrupt development. Malnutrition and/or the use of alcohol or drugs by pregnant women can also result in children being born with brain dysfunction. Finally, accidents during pregnancy and in the neonatal period can result in fetal brain injury. These may include automobile accidents and, unfortunately, physical abuse of the mother while she is pregnant, or of the infant.

CP is the most common etiology of chronic physical disability in the pediatric population (2 and 3 per 1000 children). It causes abnormal muscle tone (often hypertonia), loss of selective motor control, muscle weakness, and impaired balance (Narayanan, 2012; Rosenbaum et al., 2007).

Individuals with CP vary in age, culture, education, and type and severity. The type of CP varies with the areas of the central nervous system that are damaged. Injury may occur in the motor cortex, the pyramidal or extrapyramidal tracts, and the cerebellum. Most types of CP can be classified in one of three ways: spastic, athetoid, or ataxic. The primary features of each are summarized in Table 10.3.

Spastic Cerebral Palsy

For about 60% of individuals with CP, the prominent characteristics include spasticity and increased muscle tone. Recall that spasticity is increased resistance to passive stretch due to damage to upper motor neurons, meaning that when the muscle of someone with **spastic cerebral palsy** contracts, the opposing muscle may react abnormally to stretch by increasing muscle tone to a greater-than-normal degree. This is referred to as an *exaggerated stretch reflex*.

The damaged upper motor neurons are unable to inhibit signals that increase muscle tone; the result is hypertonicity. With increased muscle tone in the muscles opposing the muscle movement attempted, the desired movement ends up jerky, stiff, labored, and slow. In severe cases, the limbs may be rotated inward, with the arms drawn upward and the head turned to one side. Figure 10.4a shows the posture of an individual with severe spastic CP.

TABLE 10.3

Characteristics of cerebral palsy

Type of Cerebral Palsy	Characteristics	Area of Brain Affected
Spastic	Spasticity, increased muscle tone in opposing muscle groups Exaggerated stretch reflex Jerky, labored, and slow movements Infantile reflex patterns	Motor cortex and/or pyramidal tract
Athetoid	Slow, involuntary writhing Disorganized and uncoordinated volitional movement Movements occur accompanying volitional movement	Extrapyramidal tract, basal ganglia
Ataxic	Uncoordinated movement Poor balance Movements lack direction, force, and control	Cerebellum

Figure 10.4 Characteristic posture of severe spastic and athetoid cerebral palsy.

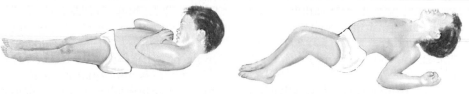

(a) Spastic cerebral palsy   (b) Athetoid cerebral palsy

Athetoid Cerebral Palsy

About 30% of individuals with cerebral palsy have **athetoid cerebral palsy**. *Athetosis* is characterized by slow, involuntary writhing, most pronounced when the individual attempts volitional movement. The resultant movement behavior is disorganized and uncoordinated. Like other involuntary movements, athetosis is due to damage to basal ganglia structures and/or pathways that work to inhibit involuntary movements. Damaged inhibitory mechanisms cannot appropriately monitor the excitation mechanisms of the motor cortex; the result is too much movement. Speech and breathing problems are more severe in individuals with athetoid CP than with any other type.

In its most severe form, athetosis causes an individual's feet to turn inward, the back and neck to arch, and the arms and hands to be overextended above the head. Figure 10.4b shows the posture of a child with severe athetoid CP. The severity of athetoid CP varies, however. For instance, when an individual is quiet or at rest, the athetoid movements might not be evident. Athetosis occurs or is exaggerated when purposeful movement is attempted and/or when the individual is excited or emotionally upset.

Ataxic Cerebral Palsy

Ataxic cerebral palsy, accounting for approximately 10% of the population with CP, is characterized by uncoordinated movement and disturbed balance. Movements are clumsy and awkward, with poor rate and direction control. Walking may be particularly difficult for an individual with ataxic CP, and in extreme cases, it may be characterized by a wide stance, with the head pushed forward and the arms back, in an almost bird-like appearance. Even those who are less affected may have a gait resembling that of someone who is intoxicated.

Recall that ataxia results from damage to the cerebellum. Injury to this part of the brain impairs the monitoring of information about balance from the inner ears, as well as proprioceptive information from the muscles about the rate, force, and direction of movements. Coordination of muscle movement is difficult without accurate feedback. It is easy to see why walking would be especially problematic.

 Thought Question 10.2

What areas of the brain do you believe are damaged in each of the different types of cerebral palsy, and why?

Motor Speech Disorders Associated with Cerebral Palsy

Not everyone with CP has motor speech difficulties. For example, individuals may have spastic CP that involves only their legs (paraplegia). On the other hand, most people with athetoid CP exhibit motor speech abnormalities that affect each of the speech production subsystems: respiratory, phonatory, resonatory, and articulatory. While adults with acquired motor speech disorders once had normal speech, a developing child with CP did not, and consequently may also present with atypical motor patterns of production in the process of learning speech with a faulty motor system. Therefore, you as an SLP must consider both the motor control dysfunction contributing to speech deficits and the overlaid faulty learning.

Speech breathing difficulties are a common problem in children with CP, particularly those with spastic CP. Because vital capacity (i.e., the total amount of air that is expelled after a deep inhalation) may be decreased, there is an insufficient amount of air available to exhale for speech production purposes. Therefore, an individual with CP may produce short phrases or even be limited to single-word utterances.

Inconsistent or inadequate airflow, along with involvement of laryngeal muscles, will affect phonation. Voice quality may vary from a breathy voice with puffs of air to a voice with a strained, harsh quality due to weakness and spasticity. A breathy voice may indicate use of a compensatory strategy to force more air from the lungs.

Resonance may be characterized by hypernasality as a result of velopharyngeal dysfunction. The inability to seal off the nasal cavity from the oral cavity results in loss of the air pressure that is critical for precise production of consonants.

Articulation may be extremely difficult if there is involvement of the tongue, lips, and/or jaw. The tongue of an individual with CP may move as one unit, with limited ability to differentiate its parts. Consequently, speech sounds, particularly those made by moving the tongue tip (e.g., /s/, /z/, /l/, and /r/), will be particularly challenging. Lip movements may be slow and restricted. Articulation deficits will vary, depending on the type of CP. For instance, individuals with athetoid CP may exhibit excessive jaw movements, limited tongue mobility, and velopharyngeal inadequacy.

Prosodic aspects of speech, including pitch, loudness, and duration, may also be affected in individuals with CP. A client may be unable to make the rapid muscular adjustments of the respiratory and phonatory systems to mark lexical stress or convey more subtle meanings of words. Poor muscle control may make it difficult to initiate phonation and sustain it. As a result, speech may be segmented (i.e., choppy), with short phrases or words and frequent interruptions. Speech may be characterized as disfluent, nonrhythmic, and very monotonous.

Other issues may also complicate speech production, including intellectual, attention, auditory processing, and language deficits. While many individuals with CP have average to above-average intelligence, approximately one-third have significant cognitive impairment. Hearing and speech sound discrimination may be problematic, and delayed language development may include immature linguistic structures and use.

Lifespan Issues

Early symptoms of CP may include irritability, weak crying, and sucking, excessive sleeping, minimal interest in surroundings, and persistence of primitive reflexes beyond the newborn stage. Initial parental reactions on learning that their infant has CP vary and may include guilt, grief, anger, and denial. Typically, parents adjust well to their child but may exhibit chronic grief or the continuing desire for their child to be "normal." The parent–child bonding process may be strained as the child fails to respond in predictable ways. In addition, the care of a child with CP may tax the family and introduce stress into the family environment.

It may take up to 2 years to confirm a diagnosis of CP in an infant with mild involvement. The type of CP may change within the first few years, and it is important for the child and family to be in contact with medical and educational professionals. Motor delays associated with CP are often the first sign. As an SLP, you may participate on an early intervention team to address delays in speech, language, and/or feeding and swallowing, as well as help counsel families who struggle with having a child with CP.

Variables such as severity, concomitant disorders, parental involvement, and school system flexibility are important in determining the appropriate educational environment for a child with CP. In general, children with average or higher-than-average intelligence with mild CP are more likely than other children with CP to have a typical educational experience. It is extremely important to assess the cognitive abilities of individuals with severe motor disabilities appropriately, because a physical disability may obscure deficits in intellectual functioning.

Many individuals, especially those with mild physical and cognitive difficulties, obtain higher education and/or go into competitive employment. Often, physical adaptations are made to improve performance in the educational and workplace settings. Other individuals may work and learn in centers run by agencies or the state. Day treatment programs are available to provide training in daily living and vocational skills for individuals with severe motor deficits and/or cognitive impairment. Case Study 10.4 presents the story of a young man with CP.

 Check Your Understanding 10.2

Click here to check your understanding of the concepts in this section.

CASE STUDY 10.4

Personal Story of a Boy with Cerebral Palsy

Jake was born $3\frac{1}{2}$ months prematurely, in a small rural hospital. The delivering obstetrician was concerned about possible oxygen deprivation at the time of his birth, although Jake was put in an incubator shortly after he was born.

Because of their son's prematurity, Jake's parents were counseled to expect developmental delays. They reported that he was irritable and seemed to have difficulty ingesting milk. At 4 months of age, his pediatrician expressed concern because of the continued presence of some reflexive behaviors such as the whole-body response when startled and lack of eye–hand coordination. She referred Jake to a developmental team in a large urban hospital.

The multidisciplinary team consisted of a pediatrician, a neurologist, a physical therapist, an occupational therapist, and a speech-language pathologist. They determined that Jake had cognitive and motor delays, as well as moderate dyskinesia. He was given a diagnosis of athetoid cerebral palsy.

Following the evaluation, it was recommended that Jake participate in home-based early intervention services, provided by the multidisciplinary team's rehabilitation specialists (i.e., physical therapist, occupational therapist, SLP), with periodic follow-up assessments at the hospital. The diagnosis of CP was very disheartening and painful for Jake's parents. Therefore, the team also recommended that the parents receive counseling and participate in a parental support group as part of their son's treatment plan.

By age 3, Jake was able to feed himself finger foods, but he still had some difficulty. Dressing was limited to pulling down a shirt that had been fitted over his arms and head. He could walk but not without significant difficulties, as he needed support to steady himself. His speech consisted of a few words and phrases that were often unintelligible to people other than his family. On the advice of the SLP at the special needs preschool Jake attends, he began training on an AAC device. At first, this involved pointing to pictures on a communication board. Although his pointing response was somewhat imprecise, Jake continued to use the communication board until he entered elementary school.

In first grade, he began using a computer with specialized communication software. Pictures evolved into words and then into individual letters. Now in third grade, Jake is communicating using a combination of his own speech and selection of pictures, words, and simple spelling on his computer. He takes his computer everywhere and can even order his favorite foods at restaurants independently.

EVALUATION OF MOTOR SPEECH DISORDERS

To correctly identify motor speech disorders, you must first obtain a thorough case history from the client or client's caregiver, as motor speech disorders are often accompanied by predictable complaints and symptoms. In addition, it is important to have a client attempt various speech production tasks specifically designed for purposes of differential diagnosis, along with perceptual and objective measures of the speech production subsystems (i.e., respiratory, phonatory, resonatory, articulatory). Such measures will allow you to determine the most effective treatment approach for the client.

As an SLP, you will likely serve on a diagnostic team with medical professionals, particularly when your client is exhibiting generalized neurological impairments. By correctly identifying different speech patterns consistent with a particular type of motor speech disorder, you as an SLP provide valuable information to other members of the team responsible for differential diagnosis of underlying neurological conditions.

When assessing a child or adult client, the purposes of the motor speech evaluation are many and include the following:

- To determine whether a significant long-term problem exists
- To describe the nature of impaired functions, specifically the types of problems, their extent/severity, and the effect of these impairments on everyday functional communication
- To identify functions that are not impaired
- To establish appropriate goals and decide where to begin intervention
- To form a well-reasoned prognosis, based on the nature of the disorder, the client's age, the age or stage of injury or disease, the presence of other accompanying conditions, client motivation, and family support

You as a speech-language pathologist will evaluate the structure and function of a client's oral mechanism, connected speech, and speech in special tasks. Although a few commercial test procedures are available, many SLPs working in hospitals or outpatient clinics have a standard assessment protocol that they use for their motor speech evaluations in pediatric and adult populations. These procedures may or may not rely on the use of instrumental approaches and computerized analysis.

To begin, you examine the oral peripheral mechanism and note the following with particular interest:

- Symmetry, configuration, color, and general appearance of the face, jaw, lips, tongue, teeth, and hard and soft palate at rest
- Movement of the jaw, lips, tongue, and soft palate
- Range, force, speed, and direction of the jaw, lips, and tongue during movement

You also need to either directly (using instrumental and computerized methods) or indirectly (during nonspeech tasks or perceptual speech production tasks) determine the following:

- Lung capacity, respiratory driving pressure, and control during speech production
- Phonatory initiation, maintenance, and cessation

- Pitch and pitch variability
- Loudness and loudness variability
- Volitional pitch–loudness variations
- Velopharyngeal function

For adults who may have acquired apraxia of speech, the following speech production tasks will help in differential diagnosis:

- Imitation of single words of varying lengths
- Sentence imitation
- Reading aloud
- Spontaneous speech
- Rapid repetition of "puh," "tuh," "kuh," and "puh-tuh-kuh" (or "buttercup")

Note that these tasks are repetitive and imitative. Recall that performance in apraxia of speech will likely vary with repeated performance, and thus errors will be inconsistent. Modes of stimulus presentation are also important, because the person with apraxia responds better to auditory-visual stimuli than to either auditory or visual stimuli alone. Additional assessment techniques for children suspected of having childhood apraxia of speech are specifically discussed in Chapter 5.

 Thought Question 10.3

How do the assessment techniques used for dysarthria and apraxia of speech differ, and how are they similar?

 Video Exercise 10.2

Examining Structural Function

Click on the link to a watch a video of a speech-language pathologist examining the structures and function of the articulatory/resonating system in an older adult male client, and complete an exercise.

 Check Your Understanding 10.3

Click here to check your understanding of the concepts in this section.

TREATMENT OF MOTOR SPEECH DISORDERS

Some basic principles underlie treatment of motor speech disorders in children and adults. These include (1) restoring lost function, (2) using compensatory strategies, and (3) making adjustments for lost function (Duffy, 2013). For adults with acquired motor speech disorders such as dysarthria or apraxia, a full recovery is quite possible, particularly in mild cases of stroke, for instance. However, generally speaking, residual motor speech deficits persist for long periods of time in many individuals with acquired disorders, and especially in those with congenital disorders such as cerebral palsy. Therefore, compensation for inadequate functioning of the motor speech system will be necessary. For degenerative diseases such as ALS or Parkinson disease that are progressive, ongoing adaption to lost function will be necessary, and compensatory strategies and the use of prosthetic devices may be effective throughout the course of the disease.

Management of Dysarthria

Because dysarthria affects all aspects of speech production, management must address a client's difficulties with respiration, phonation, resonation, articulation, and prosody. Specific intervention techniques to target increased respiratory drive for purposes of speech breathing might include speech practice production using a pausing/phrasing strategy. In this way, clients (both adults and children, when appropriate) learn to pause more often, using shorter phrases as a means to take in more air and start their speech utterances at a higher lung volume. As a result, speech utterances will be louder (although shorter in length) and, often, more clear. If respiratory muscle weakness impedes the use of such a strategy, as in the case of ALS or in some children with spastic cerebral palsy, the use of an abdominal binder is an effective prosthetic for increasing respiratory drive and, therefore, improving loudness and voice quality. Patients with severe respiratory weakness and significantly reduced loudness levels may also use voice amplifiers.

Specific medical interventions and voice techniques for improving voice and voice quality are described in Chapter 9. An evidence-based behavioral approach to increasing phonatory competence in adults with Parkinson disease and for treating respiratory and phonatory deficits in children with spastic cerebral palsy is the *Lee Silverman Voice Treatment (LSVT)*. LSVT is an intensive 4-week speech treatment program that has been shown to produce marked and long-term improvement in voice and speech function. LSVT trains speakers to use a louder voice and to self-monitor use of this new loud voice.

While voice and voice quality improve as a result of LSVT, indirect benefits of this treatment have also been seen in velopharyngeal function, articulation, and swallowing. Computer software is available that allows an individual to participate in LSVT treatment at home. Visit the LSVT Global website at www.lsvtglobal.com, and click on "Products." Then click on "LSVT Companion System" to see demonstrations of the software and learn more about its application.

Techniques and prosthetic devices to improve velopharyngeal function were described in detail in Chapter 9, including continuous positive airway pressure (CPAP) and use of a palatal lift. These same management techniques may prove useful in individuals with dysarthria secondary to palatal weakness. As mentioned previously, LSVT has also been shown to improve velopharyngeal function in adults and children with dysarthria of varying etiologies.

Intensive, repetitive speech production drill practice with meaningful words and phrases is an effective way to increase articulatory accuracy and thus improve speech intelligibility. Slowing speech rate is also an effective means of increasing articulatory precision in both pediatric and adult populations. Electropalatography (EPG), mentioned in Chapter 8, has utility in increasing articulatory precision in children with dysarthria due to CP and in adults with acquired dysarthria by providing visual feedback of tongue movement placement for articulatory accuracy. Although the device may be awkward at first, wearing an EPG palate for as little as 2 hours in a period of a day results in speech that sounds typical (McLeod & Searl, 2006). Through a combination of EPG computer display, speech monitoring, and biofeedback, some pediatric and adult clients with dysarthria learn better tongue control for improved articulation of speech sounds.

Historically, intervention to improve articulation in individuals with dysarthria has included nonspeech oral-motor treatments (NSOMTs), including exercise, massage, blowing, positioning, icing, cheek puffing, and other nonspeech activities. Data on the value of this methodology are weak. Despite popularity of

NSOMTs, evidence-based practice suggests that there is insufficient evidence to support their use, and NSOMTs are therefore not recommended at this time as a means to improve articulation in adults and children with dysarthria.

Speech supplementation strategies have been shown to increase listener comprehension of speech produced by adults with dysarthria. In particular, using alphabet cues, where the speaker points to the first letter of each word on an alphabet board as he or she says the word, is very effective in improving speech comprehensibility. In addition, combined cues, including using alphabet cues along with topic cues (stating the topic of conversation and indicating topic changes), has also been shown to be effective in increasing speech comprehensibility (Hustad et al., 2003; Yorkston & Beukelman, 2013). Such strategies may also be effective for older children with dysarthria.

For children and adults with markedly severe to profound dysarthria, the use of AAC (see Chapter 13) in conjunction with verbal forms of communication is most beneficial. Individual assessment is needed to determine the optimal system, including the client–device interface or input mode.

Management of Acquired Apraxia of Speech

One of the most effective treatments for acquired apraxia of speech continues to be *integral stimulation*, a speech production approach developed by Rosenbek et al. (1973) that utilizes the basic process "watch me, listen to me, and do what I do." Integral stimulation procedures involve an eight-step continuum comprising a hierarchy of cuing techniques (e.g., tactile, simultaneous production, immediate repetition, delayed repetition) that an SLP uses to help a client with apraxia retrain his or her motor planning/programming abilities necessary for correct speech production. The treatment approach also utilizes a core set of functional vocabulary words or phrases such that stimuli practiced are meaningful and, thus, motivating.

Integral stimulation techniques also incorporate the principles of motor learning (e.g., intensive practice distributed throughout the week), which is important for relearning motor skills that can no longer be accessed following brain injury (e.g., stroke). For a comprehensive discussion of the principles of motor learning, see Maas et al. 2008).

Other useful therapeutic approaches for acquired apraxia of speech include *melodic intonation therapy (MIT)*, an approach that focuses on prosody, emphasizing the melody, rhythm, and stress patterns of spoken utterances. With this approach, an SLP models an utterance for a client by essentially "singing" the phrase and tapping out the rhythm while the client attempts to imitate. As the client is producing the utterance, the SLP works to fade the rhythmic cues until the client is able to imitate speech without such cues (Yorkston et al., 2010). Because acquired apraxia of speech typically involves an infarct in the left hemisphere, melodic intonation therapy is believed to facilitate motor planning/programming for speech production by accessing functions of the right hemisphere (i.e., singing).

Another treatment approach for acquired apraxia of speech that focuses on prosody is contrastive stress. In this approach, the client practices producing sentences by emphasizing stress on particular words in the sentence and thus changing the meaning of that sentence (e.g., *I* didn't say he stole the money"; "I *didn't* say he stole the money"; "I didn't say *he* stole the money"). Contrastive stress practice is most effective for clients with mild to moderate apraxia of speech who continue to exhibit prosodic abnormalities while having otherwise

Thought Question 10.4

How are treatment techniques for childhood apraxia of speech (see Chapter 5) and acquired apraxia of speech in adults similar, and how and why do they differ?

adequate speech articulation skills (Yorkston et al., 2010). Box 10.1 summarizes the evidence-based treatment approaches that may be beneficial for individuals with motor speech impairments.

BOX 10.1 | **Evidence-Based Practice with Motor Speech Impairments**

Repetition/Practice

- Repetition is important for maintaining changes in the brain and their related functional benefits. In general, maintenance of intervention gains requires long-term, consistent use of a skill.

Intensity of Intervention

- Given the need for repetitive motor speech production practice, intensive and individualized treatment is stressed for individuals with acquired apraxia of speech, nonprogressive dysarthria, and in some cases of slowly progressive dysarthria (e.g., Parkinson disease). There are more beneficial results from prolonged practice distributed over time than from intensive massed practice to promote speech motor learning.

Specific Techniques

- Electropalatograph (EPG) technology offers modest gains in speech production.
- Evidence does not support the use of nonspeech oral motor treatments (NSOMTs) as standard treatments. These methods should not be used as speech production interventions.

Apraxia of Speech

- Integral stimulation is beneficial when addressing speech production difficulties in individuals with acquired apraxia of speech.
- Melodic intonation therapy (MIT) is useful during the early stages of acquired apraxia of speech, when speech production may be very difficult.
- Contrastive stress is beneficial for mild to moderate apraxia of speech when prosodic abnormalities persist.

Parkinson Disease

- The Lee Silverman Voice Treatment (LSVT) produces marked and long-term improvement in voice, speech, and swallowing functions in individuals with PD.
- Surgical interventions, such as deep brain stimulation (DBS), may improve limb motor function but may cause further motor speech and/or swallowing deficits.

Dysarthria

- Using a pausing/phrasing strategy, where backslashes are strategically placed in reading passages to remind the client to pause, is an effective way to slow speech rate and increase intelligibility. It is difficult to generalize this strategy to conversational speech, however.
- Over-enunciating and maximizing prosody (i.e., stress and inflection) can improve articulation and overall speech intelligibility in individuals with ataxic dysarthria.
- Supplementation strategies such as specifying the topic of conversation and using an alphabet board (pointing to the first letter of every word produced) have been shown to significantly improve the listener's ability to comprehend speakers with dysarthria, particularly those with severe to profound dysarthria secondary to neurodegenerative disease (e.g., amyotrophic lateral sclerosis).
- Familiarizing listeners with dysarthric speech, even with only brief exposure, is very effective in improving the listener's ability to subsequently understand a speaker with dysarthria.

Source: Based on: Lansford et al. (2016); Ludlow et al. (2008); Tjaden & Liss (1995); Wambaugh et al. (2013); Yorkston et al. (2010), and Yorkston & Beukleman (2013)

☑ Check Your Understanding 10.4

Click here to check your understanding of the concepts in this section.

SUMMARY

The two main types of motor speech disorders are dysarthria and apraxia of speech. Dysarthria is a group of speech impairments that affect the speed, range, direction, strength, and timing of motor movement as a result of paralysis, weakness, or discoordination of the speech muscles. Five distinct types are flaccid, spastic, ataxic, hyperkinetic, and hypokinetic dysarthria. Disorders affecting multiple motor systems may yield a mixed dysarthria.

Dysarthria can be acquired in adulthood as a result of neurological disease, such as Parkinson disease, or it can be congenital, as in the case of children with cerebral palsy (CP). CP is characterized as a group of developmental, non-progressive neurological difficulties resulting from brain injury that occurs very early in fetal or infant development, and affects motor movement, communication, cognition, growth and development, learning, and sensation. The three main types of CP—spastic, athetoid, and ataxic—result in very different motor patterns and speech difficulties.

Apraxia is an acquired disorder in voluntary motor planning and programming of movement gestures for speech that is unrelated to muscle weakness, slowness, or paralysis. Acquired apraxia of speech often results from a lesion in the central programming area for speech in the left frontal lobe that details and plans the coordination of sequenced motor movements for speech.

Motor speech disorders, both congenital and acquired, offer a special challenge to the affected individual, family, friends, and speech-language pathologist. Many clients are in the very frustrating position of being able to formulate a message but unable to produce it intelligibly.

Intervention methods differ greatly. A child with CP may learn to communicate using an augmentative and alternative communication (AAC) device. Meanwhile, an older adult with motor speech deficits may relearn or retrieve previously learned speech patterns. Finally, an individual with a progressive degenerative disease, such as Parkinson disease or amyotrophic lateral sclerosis (ALS), may attempt to maintain the level of effective communication that was previously possible or may explore additional methods of communication. Changing intervention techniques and promising new surgical procedures and medical management continue to offer hope to individuals with motor speech disorders of neurogenic origin.

SUGGESTED READINGS/SOURCES

Duffy, J. (2013). *Motor speech disorders: Substrates, differential diagnosis, and management* (3rd ed.). St. Louis, MO: Elsevier, Mosby.

Yorkston, K., Beukelman, D., Strand, E., & Hakel, M. (2010). *Management of motor speech disorders in children and adults* (3rd ed.). Austin, TX: PRO-ED.

Yorkston, K. M., Miller, R. M., & Strand, E. A. (2004). *Management of speech and swallowing disorders in degenerative disease* (2nd ed.). Austin, TX: PRO-ED.

11

Disorders of Swallowing

LEARNING OUTCOMES

When you have finished this chapter, you should be able to:

- Describe the normal and disordered processes of swallowing

- List and describe the correlates of pediatric and adult dysphagia

- List and describe the important components of the swallowing evaluation

- Describe evidence-based swallowing treatments for children and adults

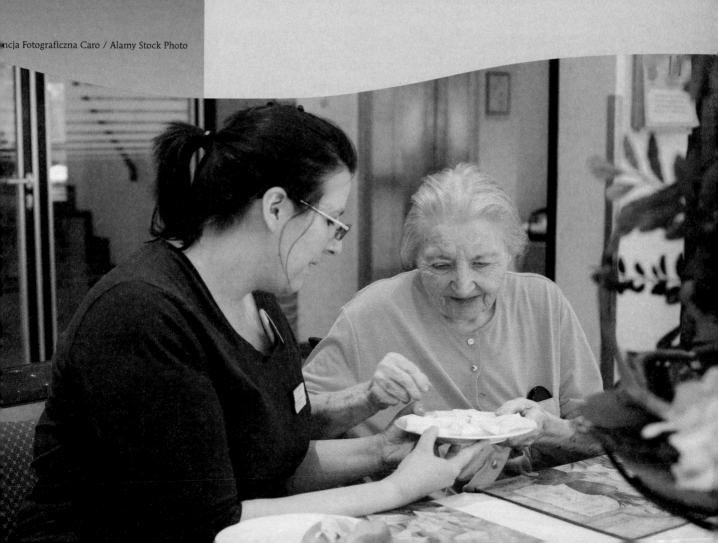

S peech-language pathologists (SLPs) play a major role in the evaluation and management of *dysphagia*, or swallowing disorders. The American Speech-Language-Hearing Association's (ASHA's) 2015 *Health Care Survey in Speech-Language Pathology* found that SLPs who work in adult settings spend the most time (41%) providing treatment in the area of swallowing compared to any other area of intervention (e.g., aphasia, cognitive-communication). In this same survey, 31% of SLPs working in pediatric hospital settings reported that they provide feeding and swallowing services to infants and children (ASHA, 2015). Furthermore, SLPs may be required to manage dysphagia in children in their school-based setting (e.g., Homer & Carbajal, 2015).

An SLP is responsible for identifying, evaluating, and treating individuals with feeding and swallowing disorders. With the continually growing number of adult and pediatric patients identified every year with clinically significant dysphagia, specific knowledge about normal and abnormal swallowing is essential for effective evaluation and management of feeding and swallowing disorders. Case Study 11.1 describes a middle-aged woman with swallowing difficulties following a stroke similar to what you as an SLP will encounter in the acute hospital setting. SLPs do not function alone in much of the work they do. SLPs who treat patients with swallowing problems are generally part of a team consisting of a physician, a nurse, a nutritionist, a radiologist, a gastroenterologist, a dentist, an otolaryngologist, a

CASE STUDY 11.1

Case Study of a Woman with Dysphagia: Adilah

Adilah is a 46-year-old woman who is married with three teenage boys. She works 70 hours per week as a criminal defense attorney. Her medical history is significant for high blood pressure and moderately high cholesterol. While watching her son's fencing tournament last Sunday, Adilah suddenly developed right lower facial weakness, and right arm weakness. Her husband, who was sitting next to her, immediately called 911 and Adilah was rushed to the emergency room; she was having a stroke in the left frontal lobe. Within hours of arriving at the hospital, Adilah's speech and swallowing abilities were screened by the speech-language pathologist. Initially, the SLP recommended "nothing by mouth" for the first couple of days while Adilah's stroke was evolving. After 48 hours, Adilah's swallowing was re-evaluated by the SLP and multidisciplinary dysphagia team.

During the structural-functional examination, the SLP observed Adilah's head and neck control, posture, and the anatomy and general health of Adilah's mouth. The sensory-motor function and strength of the oral and pharyngeal muscles used for swallowing, and her ability to produce a strong cough, were also evaluated. The SLP determined that Adilah had decreased movement and sensation on the right side of her face and tongue. She also had a weak cough. A videofluoroscopic swallow study (modified barium swallow) showed poor tongue control, delayed initiation of laryngeal closure, and penetration of thin liquids into the airway above the vocal folds without aspiration. Difficulty managing regular solid foods in her mouth and pocketing of chewed food on the right side of her mouth were also observed. Upon reviewing the swallow examination results, the multidisciplinary team agreed that Adilah was exhibiting a swallowing disorder, and recommended thickened liquids, pureed foods, and compensatory postural maneuvers to ensure food or liquid did not enter her airway.

As you read this chapter think about:

- Adilah's risk factors for stroke.
- How damage to the left frontal lobe could interfere with swallowing.
- How certain textures of food or consistencies of liquid could be more difficult to swallow.
- How a swallowing disorder might affect a person's daily life.

neurologist, an occupational therapist, a physical therapist, a respiratory therapist, and family members. The role of each of these specialists will become clear when we discuss evaluation and treatment later in this chapter.

Swallowing and the efficient intake of food have both medical and psychosocial implications. Eating is essential to physical health. Without proper nourishment, one cannot grow, develop, or survive. Swallowing disorders increase the risk of choking and may lead to *aspiration* of food into the lungs and respiratory illnesses such as pneumonia. Problems or weakness related to the anatomy of swallowing may result in **gastroesophageal reflux (GER)**, the movement of food or acid from the stomach back into the esophagus. Eating is also one of our major social activities. Feeding difficulties in children may stress the parent–child relationship. Among older people, dysphagia may lead to isolation, depression, frustration, and diminished quality of life.

In this chapter, we describe the normal processes involved in feeding and swallowing, characteristics and correlates of disordered swallowing, evaluation, and treatment.

 Thought Question 11.1

What special skills and knowledge does the SLP bring to swallowing therapy?

The term *dysphagia*, which comes from the Greek, literally means "difficulty with eating."

NORMAL AND DISORDERED SWALLOWING

Most of us don't typically think about how we swallow food. We know very generally that we put something edible in our mouth, chew for a while, and then swallow. Sometimes, however, we experience difficulty that calls attention to the process. For example, we might eat and cough or feel that the food has "gone down the wrong pipe." Occasionally while drinking, we might laugh and find that fluid comes out of our nose. Once in a while, we feel "all choked up" for an emotional reason and feel unable to eat and swallow. Before we can understand disorders of swallowing, we need to examine the basics of normal swallowing.

Normal Swallowing

Normal swallowing can be described in four stages: oral preparation, oral, pharyngeal, and esophageal. The following section describes each of these stages in detail.

Oral Preparation Phase

When you are ready to eat, you put food or liquid into your mouth and close your lips. In the oral preparation stage of drinking, the tongue forms a cupped position and holds the fluid in a liquid **bolus**, the substance that is to be ingested, against the front portion of the hard palate. In preparation for swallowing solid foods, the tongue and cheeks move the food to the teeth for chewing and mixing with saliva to form a solid bolus. The prepared liquid or solid bolus is held in the mouth by the soft palate, which moves forward and down to touch the back of the tongue and close the passage to the pharynx or throat.

Oral Phase

Once the bolus is formed, the oral stage begins. This stage consists of the movement of the bolus from the front to the back of the mouth. When the substance reaches the anterior faucial pillars at the rear of the mouth, the pharyngeal swallow reflex is triggered. Oral transit typically takes about 1 to 1.5 seconds. Figure 11.1 depicts the oral phase of swallowing, which relies heavily on the tongue to propel the bolus back toward the oropharynx.

Figure 11.1 The oral phase of a normal swallow, with food depicted in green. (A) After the food is chewed and mixed with saliva during the oral preparation stage, it forms a bolus that is arranged on the back of the tongue. (B) The tongue tip moves upward and forward to contact the hard palate. (C) The back of the tongue pushes downward and backward toward the soft palate to propel the bolus into the oropharynx.

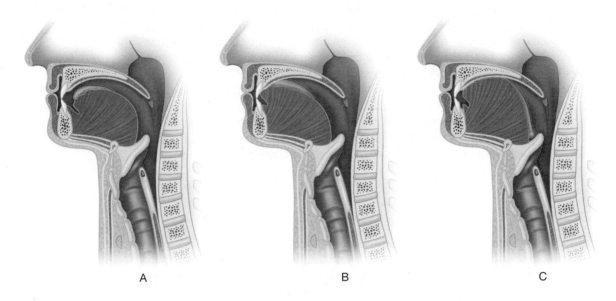

A   B   C

Pharyngeal Phase

The oral and pharyngeal phases of swallowing involve much of the same anatomy that is used in speaking. There is wisdom to the traditional advice "Don't eat and talk at the same time."

During the pharyngeal phase (see Figure 11.2), the velum moves up to meet the rear wall of the pharynx and to prevent the bolus from going into the nasal cavity. The base of the tongue and the pharyngeal wall move toward one another to create the pressure that is needed to project the bolus into the pharynx. The pharynx contracts and squeezes the bolus down. While this is occurring, the hyoid bone rises, bringing the larynx up and forward. The larynx prevents the bolus from entering the trachea by closing the true and false vocal folds and lowering the epiglottis, covering the airway. The pharyngeal phase is complete when the upper esophageal or pharyngeal esophageal segment opens and the food or liquid moves into the esophagus. The pharyngeal phase occurs very quickly and is usually complete in less than 1 second.

Esophageal Phase

The last stage of the swallowing process occurs when the muscles of the esophagus move the bolus in peristaltic, or rhythmic, wavelike contractions from the top of the esophagus into the stomach. This typically takes 8 to 20 seconds in an unimpaired individual.

Disordered Swallowing

Problems in swallowing can occur in any or all phases of the process. A person may have difficulty chewing food, or be unable to form a bolus and move it to the rear of the mouth. In addition, difficulties may arise later if the bolus moves inadequately, or is blocked as it passes through the pharynx and esophagus to the stomach.

Figure 11.2 The pharyngeal phase of a normal swallow, with food depicted in green. (A) As the tongue moves upward, the velopharyngeal port closes, and the larynx begins to elevate. (B) The tongue pushes back into the pharynx, squeezing the bolus downward through the pharynx. The larynx moves upward and forward, which causes the upper esophageal segment (UES) to relax. (C) The tongue continues pushing backward, and the bolus moves through the UES into the esophagus.

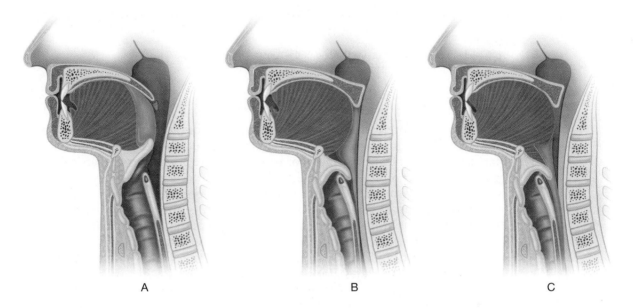

A   B   C

Oral Preparation/Oral Phase

If the lips do not seal properly, drooling can occur. Chewing may be impaired because of poor muscle tone or paralysis involving the mouth or because of missing teeth. Insufficient saliva will impede adequate bolus formation. Food may pocket, or get stuck in the cheek. The muscles of the tongue might not function purposefully or efficiently enough to move the food to the teeth for chewing and to transport the bolus from the front to the rear of the mouth to prepare for the pharyngeal phase.

Pharyngeal Phase

Several serious problems are associated with limitations during the pharyngeal phase. If the swallow is not triggered or is delayed, material may be *aspirated*, or fall into the airway and eventually into the lungs. Failure to close the velopharyngeal port, the passageway to the nose, can lead to substances going into and out of the nose. Poor tongue mobility may result in insufficient pressure in the pharynx, which is needed to drive the bolus into the esophagus.

 Video Example 11.1

As you watch this videofluroscopic video, notice how the liquid bolus spills over into the airway.

Thought Question 11.2

What connections can you think of between swallowing and speech?

Esophageal Phase

If peristalsis is slow or absent, the complete bolus might not be transported from the pharynx to the stomach. Residue might be left on the esophageal walls, resulting in infection and nutritional problems.

 Check Your Understanding 11.1

Click here to check your understanding of the concepts in this section.

CORRELATES OF PEDIATRIC AND ADULT DYSPHAGIA

Infants and children with feeding and swallowing disorders may experience malnutrition, inadequate growth, dehydration, ill health, prolonged feeding times, fatigue, difficulty learning, and poor parent–child relationships. Pediatric dysphagia results from multiple medical problems that develop either before, during, or after birth, with 90% of cases having at least one specific medical diagnosis (Murray, Carrau, & Chan, 2018). Children with central or peripheral nervous system deficits or immaturity, neuromuscular disease, and craniofacial anomalies are particularly vulnerable to feeding and swallowing disorders.

In the adult population, approximately one in 25 individuals (about 4%) living in the United States alone will experience a swallowing disorder each year (Bhattacharyya, 2014). However, because dysphagia is often a symptom secondary to a medical diagnosis (e.g., stroke), it is likely the prevalence of swallowing difficulties in the adult population is underestimated.

Feeding and swallowing difficulties are even more common in older individuals; Roy and colleagues (2007) reported a lifetime dysphagia prevalence rate of 38% in 117 individuals between 65 and 94 years of age who were living independently. Prevalence rates are even higher for elderly people living in long-term care facilities, increasing to 40% to 50% (Easterling & Robbins, 2008).

As a result of the growing numbers of individuals experiencing dysphagia at any given time, there is an increased demand for qualified SLPs who can provide feeding and swallowing services to pediatric and adult clients in various clinical settings. The next sections describe some of the more common correlates of feeding and swallowing disorders in pediatric and adult populations that you will likely encounter as a future SLP.

Lifespan Issues

Feeding and swallowing problems exist in both children and adults. They may occur at any point in the lifespan. Newborns may be unable to suckle and/or ingest nutriment. As they age, infants may refuse food and develop unhealthy food preferences. Neuromotor problems and structural anomalies that are congenital or acquired at any age can interfere with feeding and swallowing, as can a host of psychosocial factors. Dysphagia may be related to many diverse conditions; therefore, we describe only some of the most common ones. The correlates of swallowing disorders are not mutually exclusive; for example, an individual may be impaired in swallowing because of intellectual disability or laryngeal cancer. Whatever the etiology, the outcomes of a swallowing disorder at any age include dehydration, malnutrition, poor health, weight loss, fatigue, frustration, respiratory infection, aspiration, and even death. Table 11.1 lists some of the common correlates of swallowing disorders in children and adults.

Pediatric Dysphagia

Feeding disorders can describe difficulties children may have with accepting varied food textures or an age-appropriate diet; swallowing disorders generally describe difficulty with eating or swallowing that results from physiological or anatomical issues. Feeding disorders in children can develop as a result of a child's history with dysphagia, which may have caused uncomfortable or painful eating experiences, subsequently impacting the child's willingness to try new foods (Olson, 2012). As a result, feeding and swallowing disorders are often described under the umbrella term, "pediatric dysphagia."

However, feeding difficulties may occur in children who have neuromuscular impairments that primarily affect their limbs, making it difficult for them to get the food from their plate into their mouths. In such cases, swallowing may be normal but feeding is clearly impaired. Occupational therapists (OTs), who frequently work on multidisciplinary teams with SLPs with such individuals, specialize in the delivery of treatment aimed at improving activities of daily living, such as eating. The OT may recommend specialized adaptive equipment such as a curved or bent spoon, or a bowl with a suction bottom to assist the child in getting the food into the mouth; or the OT may suggest postural or positional changes that can facilitate feeding.

SLPs may collaborate with OTs when treating children who have feeding difficulties related to fear and avoidance of foods with certain textures, smells, or tastes due to sensory processing disorders. Swallowing difficulties may or may not be present in these children; therefore, where appropriate, we will specifically differentiate "feeding" from "swallowing" disorders. Otherwise, the term "feeding and swallowing disorders" will be used when describing pediatric dysphagia in this chapter. SLPs specialize in the treatment of dysphagia, particularly the oral and pharyngeal phases of dysphagia. The most prevalent correlates of pediatric oral-pharyngeal dysphagia will be discussed in the next.

TABLE 11.1

Correlates of swallowing disorders in children and adults

Congenital Difficulties	Acquired Conditions
Prematurity (infants born before 37 weeks gestation)	Stroke
Cerebral palsy	Head and neck cancer
Intellectual disability and developmental delay	Parkinson disease
Autism	Amyotrophic lateral sclerosis
Cleft lip or palate	Multiple sclerosis
22q11.2 Deletion Syndrome	Traumatic brain injury
Pierre Robin sequence	Medications and drugs
Treacher Collins syndrome	HIV/AIDS
HIV/AIDS	Dementia
	Depression and social isolation

Prematurity

About 1 out of 10 births in the United States are preterm, with a gestation period of less than 37 weeks (World Health Organization, 2016); many of these infants present with a variety of medical and developmental complications including respiratory distress, temperature instability, seizures, feeding/swallowing difficulties, and higher rates of rehospitalization compared to term infants (Raju et al., 2006). Premature infants often have difficulty with feeding and swallowing due to immature sucking, and/or a discoordinated suck, swallow, breathe pattern (e.g., Lau, 2006) which may lead to delays in successful breast- or bottle-feeding, subsequent difficulties with weight gain and dehydration, and risk of aspiration (Arvedson et al., 2010). Some preterm infants may require tube feedings until their sucking and swallowing development is sufficient and safe to transition to total oral feeding (Arvedson et al., 2010).

Cerebral Palsy

As discussed in Chapter 10, cerebral palsy (CP) is a nonprogressive neuromotor disorder that occurs as a result of brain damage prior to or during birth, or soon thereafter. Because the central nervous system is damaged in children with CP, they frequently have feeding and swallowing problems that place them at risk for aspiration with potential respiratory consequences (Arvedson, 2013). An infant with spastic CP exhibits excessive muscle tone, abnormal postures and movements, and possibly a hyperactive gag reflex. The child may be difficult to hold because of his or her increased tone, causing excessive flexion of the arms, an arched posture, and abnormal posturing of the legs. As a result, maintaining a stable posture during feeding is very difficult, and can affect swallowing by altering the position and alignment of the oral and pharyngeal structures (Benfer et al., 2013). The infant may also gag during breastfeeding or may be unable to move the tongue rhythmically to suckle. The unpleasantness of the feeding situation will undoubtedly have adverse effects on the quality of the child–mother interaction.

Gastroesphogeal reflux (GER) is common in infants and children with CP, and ingestion of food may become painful. Reduced lip closure, drooling, poor tongue function, exaggerated bite reflex, delayed swallow initiation, and reduced pharyngeal motility are types of oral and pharyngeal problems exhibited by children with CP (Arvedson, 2013). In severe cases of dysphagia, children with CP require gastrostomy tube feedings.

Intellectual Disability and Developmental Delay

About 2 to 3 of every 100 individuals are considered to have intellectual functioning below average that qualifies as an intellectual disability or developmental delay. Children with intellectual disability (e.g., Down Syndrome) and developmental delay frequently have delayed motor coordination skills; this delay may interfere with feeding and the oral phase of swallowing. Communication disorders are common in this population, and children may be limited in their ability to express food desires and preferences.

Autism Spectrum Disorder

Although children with autism spectrum disorder (ASD) do not usually exhibit swallowing disorders, they may have significant feeding problems. Recall that children with ASD may be socially withdrawn, have impaired communication, and exhibit repetitive or stereotypic behaviors. Social withdrawal and communication deficits may impede the child's ability to indicate hunger or thirst to an adult or caregiver. Repetitive patterns of behavior or sensory issues may restrict the types of food that are consumed, possibly leading to poor nutrition. For instance, children with ASD with sensory processing deficits may be hypersensitive to sound, light, pain, smell, and touch. Avoidance is common when children with sensory disorders are introduced to new foods, and negative responses like spitting, gagging, and/or vomiting may occur when novel foods are presented (Boggs & Ferguson, 2016).

Congenital Structural Abnormalities

Feeding and swallowing are frequently disrupted in children born with craniofacial anomalies such as cleft lip and/or palate; some of these infants and children will experience only mild difficulties. For instance, infants with an isolated cleft lip may have difficulty at first with achieving a lip seal on the nipple, but usually adapt well with minimal feeding alterations (e.g., Bessell et al., 2011). Infants with cleft lip and palate, on the other hand, have more severe feeding and swallowing difficulties, including an inability to create negative intraoral pressure due to the inability to seal the nasal cavity and nasopharynx from the oral cavity and oropharynx, resulting in an impaired ability to express milk from the nipple, and nasopharyngeal regurgitation along with milk remaining in the nose and mouth due to the lack of separation between the oral and nasal cavities (Dailey, 2013).

Certain syndromes are frequently associated with cleft palate and/or velopharyngeal dysfunction, or other congenital structural abnormalities that interfere with normal feeding and swallowing. In **22q11.2 deletion syndrome**, also known as Velocardiofacial syndrome, congenital heart defects are frequent, causing poor feeding endurance and thereby decreasing the total volume of oral intake. Palatal abnormalities may include low tone of the velopharyngeal muscles and/or velopharyngeal insufficiency, leading to nasal regurgitation during feeding (Miller & Madhoun, 2016; Rommel et al., 2008).

Another congenital condition, **Pierre Robin sequence (PRS)**, is characterized by a small, underdeveloped jaw (i.e., micronathia), which subsequently leads to a retracted and elevated tongue, and a cleft of the palate. Airway obstruction due to the tongue's position is the primary medical concern for infants with PRS; feeding and swallowing deficits also result from these anatomical abnormalities (Miller & Madhaun, 2016). Visit http://www.cleftline.org and type "feeding your baby" into the search bar to watch videos of infants with cleft palate using specialized bottles and nipples for feeding.

Pierre Robin sequence can be associated with **Treacher Collins syndrome (TCS)**, an inherited disorder which causes severe anatomical abnormalities of the head and face, including cleft of the lip and/or palate. In addition to feeding and swallowing difficulties, airway compromise due to the small jaw and retracted tongue is the primary concern at birth, and infants with TCS may require a **tracheostomy**, a surgical procedure that involves creating a hole in the trachea and inserting a tube, enabling the infant to breathe (Miller & Madhoun, 2016).

Infants who are born at term (>37 weeks gestation) do not spend much time in a hospital. Rapid diagnosis of and attention to congenital defects are essential for the welfare of the child.

HIV/AIDS

HIV (human immunodeficiency virus) causes the illness known as **AIDS (acquired immunodeficiency syndrome)**. It infects white blood cells, the brain, skin, and other tissues of the body. Children infected with HIV often acquire the disease from their mothers in utero, during the delivery process, and/or through the mother's breast milk. The number of HIV-positive children increases daily in the United States, and feeding difficulties and swallowing abnormalities frequently occur in this population (Nel & Ellis, 2012). One study found that 20.8% of 150 children were determined to have feeding or swallowing problems (Pressman, 1992, 2010). These may be due to reduced immunity to infections such as oral herpes that can cause pain, resulting in difficulty sucking, chewing, and/or swallowing.

In the final stages of the disease, HIV-positive children have difficulty managing oral secretions and exhibit **odynophagia**, or painful swallowing. Because HIV is a progressive disease, HIV-positive children often exhibit developmental delays, language impairments, phonological disorders, and poor attention skills (McNeilly, 2005; Narayanan & Kalappa, 2017).

Adult Dysphagia

Common neurological etiologies of dysphagia include stroke, traumatic brain injury, and progressive neurological disease. Swallowing problems can be seen in patients treated for head and neck cancer who require surgical resection of their tumors. Many other conditions can also cause feeding and swallowing problems in the adult population. These are addressed in the following section.

Stroke

Dysphagia frequently occurs following stroke, and can result in serious health complications including pneumonia, malnutrition, dehydration, and even death (Rogus-Pulia & Robbins, 2013). Prevalence estimates vary because of different assessment methods, timing of assessment, and individual characteristics of stroke patients studied. However, immediately following a stroke, prevalence data indicate that up to 56% of patients have dysphagia (Blackwell & Littlejohns, 2010).

Oral-motor and sensory deficits frequently occur post-stroke, causing swallowing difficulties and increasing the risk for aspiration. For instance, tongue weakness may make it difficult for the patient to adequately control the bolus and/or propel it posteriorly into the oropharynx. Swallow initiation may be delayed, causing the patient to hold the bolus in his/her mouth for an abnormally long time. Patients may have difficulty feeling that a portion of the bolus is still in their mouth; pocketing of food inside the cheek is a common problem in patients with facial weakness following stroke. Patients may also have sensory deficits in the larynx and pharynx, and a decreased cough reflex which can result in **silent aspiration**, or aspiration with no apparent sign or response (Rogus-Pulia & Robbins, 2013).

Patients with dysphagia following stroke are at increased risk of developing **aspiration pneumonia**, a respiratory infection caused when food or liquid enters the lungs (Rogus-Pulia & Robbins, 2013). Aspiration pneumonia affects up to one third of stroke patients, which often leads to death in this population (Sellars et al., 2007). Early detection and management of dysphagia following stroke is critical in preventing aspiration pneumonia.

Head and Neck Cancer

Surgery, radiation, and chemotherapy are used to treat tumors of the mouth, throat, and larynx. Swallowing problems are likely after any type or combination of treatments. Surgery requires removal of the tumor and closing of the wound.

For larger lesions, tissue from another area may be excised and used to help patch the deficit. The degree of swallowing impairment is closely related to the size and location of the original tumor and the surgical procedure used to close or reconstruct the area. For example, if a relatively small area of the tongue has been removed, a short-term swallowing problem is likely, due to the swelling following surgery. In more radical surgical procedures in which the tongue is sewn into the mandible to close the floor of the mouth, swallowing is severely affected (Logemann, 1998).

Radiation therapy may result in decreased salivation and dry mouth, causing the patient to swallow less frequently. Taste changes, swelling, and sometimes mouth sores that cause pain may decrease the patient's motivation to continue an oral diet (Starmer, 2017). These interferences with normal feeding and swallowing may occur during, soon after, or even a year or two after oral radiation therapy. Chemotherapy may cause weakness, nausea, vomiting, and loss of appetite, which also interferes with the eating process (Murray, Carrau, & Chan, 2018; Tierney, 1993).

> The human papillomavirus (HPV), most commonly transmitted sexually, is the leading cause of cervical cancer in women; it is also a significant risk factor for head and neck cancer.

Parkinson Disease

Parkinson disease (PD), also discussed in Chapter 10, is a progressive degenerative disorder, typically of midlife, and is characterized by slowness of movement, muscle rigidity, and tremor resulting from basal ganglia control circuit dysfunction. More than 80% of individuals with Parkinson disease develop swallowing difficulties at some point during the course of the disease (Suttrup & Warnecke, 2016).

Any or all of the oral-preparatory, oral, pharyngeal, and esophageal stages of the swallowing process may be impaired. Reduced range of motion of the jaw causes an increase in the amount of time it takes to chew food and form the bolus. Oral transport may be impaired by a front-to-back rolling pattern until the back of the tongue finally lowers sufficiently to permit the bolus to pass to the pharynx. Pharyngeal swallow may be delayed, and laryngeal closure may be impaired in advanced cases of PD. Aspiration sometimes occurs when the patient inhales after a swallow, and material remaining in the pharynx falls into the airway (Logemann, 1998). Esophageal motor abnormalities that impede swallowing may occur in PD, even in early stages of the disease (Murray, Carrau, & Chan, 2018).

> Tremor and rigidity that are visible in a person's extremities may also occur within the body, resulting in swallowing and other difficulties.

Amyotrophic Lateral Sclerosis

Amyotrophic lateral sclerosis (ALS), discussed in Chapter 10, is a rapidly progressive disease that may begin in middle age, and usually leads to death within two to five years. It is characterized by muscle atrophy due to degeneration of motor neurons. Poor tongue movement is sometimes an early sign. ALS may interfere with swallowing in several ways. Reduced tongue mobility may result in spillage into the airway before the pharyngeal swallow has been triggered. The larynx might not elevate and close adequately during the pharyngeal phase. Pharyngeal peristalsis is frequently reduced, causing material to remain in the pharynx. Any of these difficulties could result in aspiration of food or liquid. Dysphagia also leads to secondary complications such as malnutrition and dehydration, eventually requiring the individual with ALS to receive the majority of his/her nutrition via percutaneous endoscopic gastrostomy (PEG) tube feedings (Yorkston, Miller, & Strand, 2004).

Multiple Sclerosis

Multiple sclerosis (MS), a central nervous system disorder, may affect one or more cranial nerves, the cerebellum, and/or the spinal cord. MS is of unknown cause, and is typically characterized by periods of both relapse and remission. The major general symptoms are poor coordination, muscle weakness, and often speech and visual disturbances. Swallowing difficulties usually occur in the later stages of the disease; delayed swallowing reflex and reduced pharyngeal peristaltic action are the primary forms of dysphagia associated with multiple sclerosis (Logemann, 1998). Feeding difficulties may occur due to hand tremor, making it difficult to get food from the plate into the mouth (Yorkston, Miller, & Strand, 2004).

> Numbness or a "pins-and-needles" sensation in the extremities or on one side of the face may be an early sign of MS.

Traumatic Brain Injury

Traumatic brain injury (TBI) frequently results in diffuse neurological deficits that affect neuromuscular control, cognitive-communication skills, speech and language abilities, and behavior, which contribute to or cause feeding and swallowing difficulties in this population. Dysphagia occurs in over 90% of patients, and can affect the oral preparatory, oral, and/or pharyngeal phases of swallowing (Howle et al., 2014).

Impaired attention skills may cause the post-TBI patient to be unaware of food that is presented to him/her; highly distractible patients may have reduced intake of food or liquid, placing them at risk for malnutrition or dehydration. Some patients are so distracted that they may even forget to swallow, increasing their risk of aspiration (Cherney & Halper, 1996). Motor deficits, including reduced range and control of tongue movements and/or delayed or absent swallowing, are common causes of oral-pharyngeal dysphagia post-TBI, as cranial nerves are often damaged following blows to the head such as those experienced during a car accident (Murray, Carrau, & Chan, 2018).

Medications and Nonfood Substances

Although medications are used to cure and manage disease, they may also have negative side effects. Some medications, including decongestants, cough suppressants, and muscle relaxants, might make a patient feel drowsy and/or confused. This condition can interfere with anticipation and the oral phase of swallowing. A dry mouth, or insufficient saliva, has been reported to be a side effect of more than 300 medications (Murray, Carrau, & Chan, 2018). High doses of steroids may impede pharyngeal swallowing. Antipsychotic drugs may result in **tardive dyskinesia** (involuntary, repetitive facial, tongue, or limb movements) after a year or more of use. At the extreme, tardive dyskinesia may result in the inability to chew and swallow.

Behaviors such as smoking and ingesting excessive amounts of caffeine and alcohol may also interfere with normal swallowing. Appetite may be depressed and sensations dulled, resulting in anticipatory phase impairment. Alcohol abuse has been implicated in pharyngeal phase dysphagia (Feinberg, 1997).

Dementia

Unlike intellectual disability associated with developmental delay, dementia is an acquired disorder. Although found in some older people, decreases in intellectual function are not always a consequence of the aging process. We all know people in their 80s and 90s whose minds are sharp and capable. As we learned in Chapter 7, dementia is associated with Alzheimer's disease, several small strokes, PD, MS, and other ailments that may occur among older people. The cognitive deficits of dementia may impede attention and orientation to food. Those with dementia may forget to eat or may eat the same meal multiple times due to memory deficits. Oral preparatory tongue and jaw movements may be lacking in purpose, resulting in poor bolus formation and drooling. Transport of the bolus may be prolonged. Pharyngeal swallow may be delayed and laryngeal elevation reduced, resulting in possible aspiration (Groher & Crary, 2010).

HIV/AIDS

Individuals with HIV/AIDS indicate swallowing difficulties both in the early and later stages of the disease due to their immune deficiency that makes them susceptible to opportunistic infections, such as bacterial infections, that may affect the oral cavity, oropharynx, and/or esophagus. Bacterial infections can also impair the functioning of the cranial nerves involved in swallowing, causing dysphagia. Esophageal ulcers and esophagitis, or inflammation of the esophagus, is a major cause of death in individuals with HIV infection (Murray, Carrau, & Chan, 2018).

Social Isolation and Depression

Life circumstances among elderly people may interfere with several phases of swallowing. Meals are traditionally social events. We eat with family members and friends. As people enter old age, they may find themselves alone and lonely. Spouses and friends have died. Children have moved away. Some may have no experience preparing food, and so do not have adequate meals. Others are not motivated to cook just for themselves. Communal meals in retirement homes or long-term care facilities may feature unfamiliar foods and may be served in a noisy, hurried environment.

Feelings of depression among elderly people are common. Depression is associated with diminished interest in food, restlessness, and fatigue. The throat may feel tight, making swallowing uncomfortable. Some individuals may feel too tired to eat and then are exhausted after they do eat. This may prompt a cycle of inadequate food intake, weight loss, and malnutrition (Sura et al., 2012).

 Check Your Understanding 11.2

Click here to check your understanding of the concepts in this section.

EVALUATION FOR SWALLOWING

Not everyone with the correlates described in the previous sections has a swallowing disorder. Furthermore, swallowing problems are not always readily apparent. Patients may not report difficulties, and some may experience *silent aspiration* (lack of cough when food or liquid enters the airway). Therefore, the first step in evaluation is to identify individuals who are at risk for dysphagia. Following this screening, an SLP will serve on a team to obtain background information and to use clinical and instrumental techniques to assess swallowing. A determination is made about appropriate intervention, and treatment strategies are developed and implemented in coordination with other professionals. SLPs are advocates for their clients and help provide education and counseling to them, their families, and related others.

The speech-language pathologist is often the leader of the dysphagia team, which also may include a dietitian, pulmonologist, radiologist, occupational therapist, social worker, nurse, and gastroenterologist.

Screening for Dysphagia

In the pediatric population, informal screenings by pediatricians, nurses, parents, and daycare providers for feeding and swallowing difficulties occurs frequently (Delaney, 2015). A primary indication of dysphagia in infants is **failure to thrive**. Infants in a neonatal intensive care unit are carefully monitored for weight gain and development. Full-term infants who are not accepting breast or bottle are signaling feeding problems. Such infants are observed during mealtimes to evaluate breathing and physical coordination (e.g., suck/swallow/respiratory sequence), oral-motor functioning (e.g., tongue elevation), and techniques that enable quantification of nutritive and nonnutritive sucking skill (e.g., responsive to stroking around the mouth) (Groher & Crary, 2010). Caregivers can be counseled and instrumental evaluation recommended when warranted.

For adults, a host of specific checklists to screen for dysphagia are available (Murray, Carrau, & Chan, 2018). The *Burke Dysphagia Screening Test* is a relatively quick way to screen patients who have had a stroke (DePippo et al., 1992). The 3-ounce water swallow test used in the *Burke* has been found to identify between 80% and 98% of patients who were aspirating, as later confirmed by more elaborate tests (DePippo et al., 1992; Suiter & Leder, 2008). Figure 11.3 outlines this procedure. There is evidence to suggest that the *Burke* may not identify patients experiencing silent aspiration; however, given that individuals who aspirate silently do not cough, coughing is the predictive feature of aspiration in this screening protocol (Groher & Crary, 2010).

Another screening instrument is the *Gugging Swallow Screen (GUSS)*, developed by Trapl et al. (2007), which is also for stroke patients. It begins with two parts: an indirect swallow test which requires the patient to swallow his/her saliva, and a direct swallow test that requires the patient to first swallow five $1/2$ teaspoons of distilled water thickened to a pudding consistency. Next, there is a liquid swallowing trial where the patient drinks 50 mL of water as fast as possible, and finally a solid swallowing trial where the patient consumes a small dry piece of bread. This screening test has 100% sensitivity, meaning it identifies patients who actually have a swallowing disorder and aspiration risk with 100% accuracy. However, its specificity is only 50%–69%, meaning it correctly identifies patients without a swallowing disorder only 50–69% of the time. The authors of the test, therefore, recommend daily re-evaluation of patients following stroke using the *GUSS* to identify false-positive patients (Trapl et al., 2007).

Self-assessment checklists can be used to obtain information about feeding and swallowing difficulties from the patient's perspective. One such instrument is the *Eating Assessment Tool (EAT-10)*, which requires the patient to answer 10 questions

Figure 11.3 Three-ounce water swallow test.

Task: Patient drinks three ounces of water from a cup without interruption.

Outcome:

1. No problems.
2. Coughing during swallow.
3. Coughing after swallow.
4. Wet-hoarse voice quality after swallow.

Pass: Outcome 1   *Fail:* Outcome 2, 3, or 4.

Source: Based on DePippo et al. (1992).

on a 5-point scale, such as "swallowing solids takes extra effort" or "I cough when I eat," to provide information about dysphagia symptom severity. Another self-report questionnaire is the *Dysphagia Handicap Index (DHI)*, which has 25 items divided into three scales: physical, functional, and emotional. Each item is rated on a 3-point scale (never, sometimes, always); questions such as "I feel depressed because I can't eat what I want" or "I avoid eating because of my swallowing problem" address not only dysphagia symptoms but also quality of life as it pertains to eating and swallowing. Self-assessments require the individual to have adequate cognitive abilities; therefore, these tools are not appropriate for certain clinical populations.

Dysphagia screening is an important first step in the assessment process; when a feeding or swallowing difficulty is suspected based on the screening, or the patient is at risk for feeding/swallowing difficulties (e.g., poor weight gain in infancy; adult with dementia), additional clinical assessment is needed (Coyle, 2015). Instrumental assessment may be recommended following the clinical assessment to confirm clinical findings, determine the underlying nature of the swallowing disorder, or when pharyngeal dysphagia is suspected (Leder, 2015). Clinical evaluation of swallowing will be discussed in the next section, followed by instrumental assessment.

Clinical Swallow Evaluation

Whether evaluating a child or an adult, the *clinical swallow evaluation (CSE)*, or *bedside swallow evaluation*, is an important part of the comprehensive evaluation of dysphagia, and provides the speech-language pathologist with a significant amount of information about an individual's typical feeding and swallowing function, along with information about the feeding/swallowing environment (Beecher & Alexander, 2004). It also serves to establish rapport with the client and client's caregivers, provides diagnostic information about feeding and swallowing rather quickly, and in some settings is the only diagnostic procedure used to assess swallowing function (Coyle, 2015).

Case History and Background Information

The clinical swallow evaluation begins with a thorough case history to obtain detailed information about the chief complaint regarding the feeding and/or swallowing problem, the individual's current physical and neurological status, any medical conditions that may be present, recent surgeries, or medications the individual may be taking. A parent, caregiver, physician, nurse, or professional from an early intervention program or an adult day treatment center may make a referral to a dysphagia team, typically based on three general areas of concern:

- Difficulties have been observed related to feeding and ingestion of food or liquid.
- The client appears to be at risk for aspirating food or liquid into the lungs.
- The client appears to not be receiving adequate nourishment.

An SLP then seeks answers to questions such as those presented in Figure 11.4. The answers to these questions provide preliminary information about the location of the swallowing problem (oral, pharyngeal, or both), the kinds of food substances that are easiest and hardest to swallow, and the nature and severity of the disorder (Groher & Crary, 2010; Logemann, 1998).

Figure 11.4 Important questions pertaining to swallowing.

Does the infant accept breast or bottle?	When was the problem first observed?
Does the individual refuse certain foods? Which ones?	Did it worsen slowly or rapidly?
Does the individual appear to chew food?	What exactly happens when the individual tries to swallow?
Has drooling been observed?	Are certain foods more problematic for the client?
Does the child or adult eat excessively slowly?	Does food seem to get stuck somewhere? If so, where?
Does the child or adult eat excessively rapidly?	What medical diagnoses or conditions may affect the swallow?
Does coughing or choking occur at mealtimes?	Has the individual had surgery that may relate to swallowing?
Do small amounts of food or liquid ever fall out of the individual's mouth?	Is the client using any medications?
Is food or liquid expelled from the nose?	How is the individual's respiratory health?
Is food or liquid regurgitated?	How attentive is the client?
Is the child gaining weight?	Is the client able to follow directions?
Is the adult maintaining weight?	

Source: Based on Groher & Crary (2010) and Hardy & Robinson (1999).

Caregiver and Environmental Factors

A treating clinician will want to observe feeding as it occurs normally between caregiver and client. The therapist will pay special attention to the following:

- Is the caregiver patient and attentive?
- Does feeding take place in a reasonably quiet environment that is free from distractions?
- What position is the individual in when eating or drinking?
- How does the client express feeding preferences?

The parent or caregiver is an important part of the swallowing team. Careful observation and communication will help an SLP assess how best to improve this person's contributions. This is also an opportunity for an SLP to learn about a client's position in the family and cultural and individual factors that may influence intervention techniques. For example, certain foods and spices may be preferred to others. When possible, personal and cultural desires should be respected and accommodated (Logemann, 1998). Case Study 11.2 describes portions of the assessment of a 51-year-old man who was referred for a swallowing evaluation.

Cognitive and Communicative Functioning

Is the client alert and awake during feeding? Can he or she follow directions? What is the client's general level of functioning? Answers to these questions will influence the type of intervention that is most suitable for a client.

CASE STUDY 11.2

The Personal Story of a Man with Dysphagia

Mr. García was 51 years of age when he was referred as an outpatient by the director of Neurology and Rehabilitative Medicine at Municipal Hospital to the staff SLP in charge of swallowing disorders. The referral note read "myotonic dystrophy, dysarthria, dysphagia for solids." The SLP recognized her role in ensuring the patient's safety. Difficulty in swallowing foods could result in choking and/or aspiration pneumonia. The SLP was also concerned about the dysarthria and wondered to what degree this affected Mr. García's communication.

At their first meeting, the SLP learned that Mr. García, a recent immigrant from Colombia, had limited English proficiency. Once again, the SLP was grateful for her own Spanish language skills; the summer she had spent in Spain after her third year of college had been worthwhile in a multitude of ways. Many of the patients and staff at this inner-city hospital spoke Spanish as their primary language. Although Mr. García was mildly dysarthric, his speech was readily intelligible. His responses during the interview were appropriate in form (Spanish) and content. Mr. García reported that he choked on rice, a staple of his diet. Other foods and liquids did not appear to be problematic. He reported that he smoked "a little, just at the Saturday evening dances." A cursory evaluation of the oral mechanism revealed adequate strength and motion of the lips,

tongue, velum, and mandible. Although coughing, choking, and gurgling were not observed during trial feeding, an apparent delay in the pharyngeal swallow reflex was noted with both liquids and solids. The SLP recommended a modified barium swallow study to confirm and document dysphagia.

Several types of foods were mixed with barium in preparation for the X-ray procedure. Mr. García ate a spoonful of applesauce and then a bite of cookie as the radiologist and the SLP watched the X-ray monitor. No difficulties were noted in the oral phase. However, they observed food lingering in the esophagus and building up with each successive swallow. Although the larynx elevated for swallowing, the bolus did not clear, and residue remained on the right **vallecula** and **aryepiglottic fold**. Mr. García was instructed to produce an abdominal cough, but he was unsuccessful, and the food remained on the fold.

The SLP made the following recommendations: Mr. García should not eat alone. He should avoid clear liquids and take only a small amount of food before swallowing. He should try to cough deeply when he feels food stuck in his throat. At the next appointment, in 2 weeks, Mr. García would be instructed in the supraglottic and hard swallow techniques. Because myotonic dystrophy is a progressive disease, Mr. García requires regular monitoring.

Head and Body Posture

It is important to note whether a patient can hold his or her head erect. Does it lean to one side or the other? Does it tend to tilt forward or back? Can the client position the head when asked to do so? An SLP will also note general body posture and tone. Swallowing and ingestion of food and drink involve more than the head, so a complete picture of an individual is important.

Oral Mechanism

The integrity of the anatomy and health of a patient's mouth needs to be determined. Abnormalities of structure of the lips, teeth, tongue, palate, and velum are noted. An SLP looks for facial symmetry and notes weakness (i.e., drooping) when present. Motor difficulties such as tremor, flaccidity, excessive muscle tone, and poor coordination are observed. Oral reflexes are examined. Certain reflexes such as sucking and rooting (turning to the direction of a cheek that is touched) are expected in infants but should disappear as a child matures. An SLP observes for

Myotonic dystrophy is a rare, slowly progressive hereditary disease; it is the most common form of adult-onset muscular dystrophy. It is characterized by an inability to relax the muscles following contraction, and muscle weakness and wasting (atrophy), especially of the face and neck muscles.

any drooling, which may signal neuromuscular deficits, gum and tooth infections, and upper airway obstruction. An SLP also notes a client's response to sensation. Does the client accept touch such as face washing? If the client is an older child or adult, is she or he aware of food residue or saliva on the face?

Laryngeal Function

An SLP cannot directly observe the larynx in the way that he or she can look at the oral mechanism. An SLP therefore looks for indirect signs of difficulty. In older children and adults, a hoarse, wet-gurgly, or breathy voice quality before, during, or after a swallow may signal laryngeal dysfunction. Other indications of laryngeal problems include the following:

- Inability to rapidly repeat the syllable /ha/ with a clearly voiced vowel sound
- Inability to produce changes in vocal pitch, or inappropriate vocal pitch
- Inability to produce a strong cough
- Inability to feel the larynx elevate when you place your finger on the client's thyroid cartilage when the client is asked to swallow

If an SLP observes any of these difficulties, he or she should refer the client to an otolaryngologist for a thorough laryngeal evaluation.

Swallow Trials

An SLP should observe swallowing on more than one occasion. The nature of the food presented and a client's comfort level and hunger will influence the acceptance of foods.

If a client is alert and is managing his/her saliva without any signs of aspirations or respiratory compromise, swallow trials may be completed by the SLP. Usually food or liquid is used, although some SLPs prefer to conduct this assessment with only a spoonful of crushed ice or small amounts of water; if a small amount of water is aspirated into the lungs it is generally harmless (Groher & Crary, 2010). If adequate laryngeal elevation is present, and a strong, protective cough is present, the examination can proceed to other substances of varying textures. If real food substances are used, the oral preparatory and oral phases of swallowing can be assessed.

An SLP evaluates a client's reaction to the appearance of food or drink and the associated utensils, observing whether the client's activity level changes and whether the person appears eager to receive food. A small amount (1 teaspoon) of thin or thick liquid may be placed in the mouth, and the client is then encouraged to swallow. Oral mechanism function is observed throughout the swallow.

An SLP examines a client's lips to see whether they are together before the intake of food. An SLP is interested in answering questions such as the following:

- Do the lips open and then close around the nipple, cup, or spoon?
- Is there sucking activity on the nipple?
- Is food successfully removed from the spoon?
- Is liquid or food dribbled out of the sides of the mouth?

An SLP also observes tongue movement. Again, answers to certain questions are vital:

- When the mouth opens to take in food, does the tongue cup in anticipation?
- Does the client move the tongue to one side of the mouth if food is presented laterally?

- Does the client move the tongue adequately to form a bolus?
- Is the bolus transported efficiently from the front to the back of the mouth?
- Is the tongue used to remove food substances from the lips?

In addition, an SLP notes movements of the jaw and chewing patterns when solid foods are presented:

- Does the client bite food efficiently?
- Does the client isolate tongue and jaw movement?
- Does chewing continue for an adequate period of time?
- Is the jaw clenched?

Several observations pertaining to the adequacy of pharyngeal swallow are performed. If a client is unable to cough, this may suggest difficulty closing the larynx to protect the airway. Nasal regurgitation points to possibly inadequate velopharyngeal closure. An SLP observes the movement of the hyoid bone and thyroid cartilage in the neck by watching and possibly placing a finger gently on this area. These should move up during pharyngeal swallow. **Cervical auscultation**, which involves placing a stethoscope on the client's neck at the level of the vocal folds, may be used to assess the efficiency of the pharyngeal phase of swallowing. It specifically notes whether or not the swallow was heard, and if so whether or not it was delayed (Groher & Crary, 2010).

The SLP records the number of times the client swallows while ingesting each amount of food or drink. Multiple swallows may suggest inadequate pharyngeal contraction. If vocal quality changes after swallowing, this may indicate residue at the level of the vocal folds.

Of importance to an SLP are which food consistencies appear to cause difficulties and which seem to be swallowed efficiently. Similarly, an SLP notices whether there is a preferential placement in the mouth for food or liquid.

Managing a Tracheostomy Tube

Some clients will have a tracheostomy tube in place to facilitate breathing. A swallowing evaluation can still be conducted in most such cases, with a physician's approval. An SLP or nurse deflates the cuff of the tube before assessment and suctions secretions from the mouth and within and below the tracheostomy tube. The swallowing evaluation is similar to the one just outlined; however, the patient is instructed to cover the tube with a gauze pad or gloved finger before each swallow to normalize tracheal pressure (Logemann, 1998).

Instrumental Swallow Examination

Although the clinical swallow evaluation is useful in identifying the presence or absence of a swallowing problem, it cannot adequately determine the nature or severity of dysphagia of the pharyngeal phase (Leder, 2015). Complete, accurate assessment of swallowing function requires the use of instrumentation. An SLP collaborates with other team members, such as a physician, a radiologist, and an X-ray technician, in the use of diagnostic technology. Some of the most commonly used instrumental procedures are described in the following section.

Accurate interpretation of videofluoroscopic swallowing studies requires a strong knowledge base in anatomy and physiology.

Videofluoroscopic Swallowing Study

Videofluoroscopy, also referred to as a **modified barium swallow study**, is an X-ray procedure that is considered the "gold standard" in dysphagia diagnosis in children or adults. This procedure is used when clinical evaluation or screening suggests dysphagia and/or aspiration. Barium, a substance that can be seen on X-rays, is coated onto or mixed into the food or beverage to be ingested. An SLP typically determines the size, texture, and consistency of the food or liquid to be presented and the head and body position of the patient during the study. A radiologist and an X-ray technician use fluoroscopic (X-ray) equipment to observe the movement of the barium throughout the swallow. These views are digitally recorded for further analysis by the physician and SLP. The study provides real-time visualization of the swallowing process and is highly useful in determining whether the client should be fed orally or nonorally, what food textures are safest, and what types of treatment are appropriate.

The FEES procedure is increasingly being used because of its convenience, portability, and absence of radiation exposure.

Fiberoptic Endoscopic Evaluation of Swallowing

Fiberoptic endoscopic evaluation of swallowing (FEES) may be used with pediatric and adult patients who are too ill to be brought to a radiology department for the videofluoroscopic swallow study. FEES is not an X-ray procedure. Instead, following topical or localized anesthesia, an otolaryngologist inserts a flexible fiber-optic laryngoscope through the patient's nose and down into the pharynx. A specially trained SLP can also perform this procedure in consultation with a physician. When the scope is in place, the patient may be asked to cough, hold his or her breath, and swallow foods of different textures and thickness that have been dyed for better visualization. FEES may reveal bolus spilling into the pharynx before swallowing, and residue may be seen after the swallow. The actual swallow cannot be viewed with FEES due to a "white-out" period when the epiglottis obscures the view. Oral and esophageal phases of swallowing are also not visible with FEES. Nevertheless, observations with FEES can be performed at the bedside and provides valuable information about desirable body and head posture during feeding, preferred food types, and aspiration.

FEES may be a more effective instrumental technique than videofluoroscopy, particularly for patients with head and neck cancer who may require repeated swallow studies (e.g., Starmer et al., 2011). Additionally, because of its superiority in the inspection of pharyngeal anatomy and the ability to observe how a patient manages his/her own secretions, FEES is beneficial for patients with anatomical changes following surgery or trauma, or for those with paralysis following cranial nerve damage (Groher & Crary, 2010). It is also useful for biofeedback during treatment. To see video examples of FEES go to ASHA's website www.asha.org and type in "Endoscopic Evaluation of Swallowing Videos" in the search bar, click on "Endoscopic Evaluation of Swallowing" and then scroll down to the bottom of the page and click on "Video Examples of Endoscopy from YouTube."

Scintigraphy

Scintigraphy is a computerized technique sometimes used with adults to track the movement of the bolus and measure the amount of residue in the oropharynx, pharynx, larynx, and/or trachea (Murray, Carrau, & Chan, 2018). It is also used to identify and quantify aspiration during or after a swallow. A specialized physician such as a radiologist, a gastroenterologist, or an otolaryngologist performs scintigraphy; however, an SLP plays a role in positioning the patient, suggesting swallowing procedures, and interpreting test results. A radioactive tracer is mixed with the food or liquid to be ingested. Radioactive markers may be placed externally on the chin, lip, thyroid notch, and other anatomical landmarks to facilitate measurement. A specialized gamma scintillation camera is used. When scintigraphy is used, it is generally to supplement information obtained from other tests. Scintigraphy provides insight regarding esophageal function and may help in the determination of the safety of oral feedings (Szacka et al., 2016).

Ultrasound

Ultrasound, or **ultrasonography**, is an imaging technique that uses sound waves at a frequency that is inaudible to human ears, over 20,000 Hz. It is a non-invasive procedure that is safe to use with infants and children as well as adults. A transducer that generates and receives sound waves is placed below the chin for views of the oral cavity and on the thyroid notch for visualizing the laryngeal area. The acoustic images are videotaped. Ultrasonographic real-time measures are particularly helpful in assessing the duration of the oral phases of swallowing as well as the structure and movement of the tongue and hyoid bone. One drawback is that ultrasound does not permit visualization of the pharyngeal stage of swallowing (Murray, Carrau, & Chan, 2018).

 Video Exercise 11.1

Assessing a Swallow

Click on the link to watch a video of a normal swallow, and complete an exercise.

 Check Your Understanding 11.3

Click here to check your understanding of the concepts in this section.

TREATMENT OF SWALLOWING DISORDERS

Disorders of feeding and swallowing present medical, nutritional, psychological, social, and communicative problems, so many individuals are involved in working toward their resolution. As previously mentioned, the SLP is usually the dysphagia team leader, and thus the coordinator of services and the professional who is most likely to implement dysphagia treatment. Nevertheless, input from other team members is essential to a satisfactory outcome.

The dysphagia team will work together to determine the most effective rehabilitation options for individuals with feeding/swallowing disorders. Generally, treatment can be divided into three categories: compensatory strategies, indirect rehabilitation strategies, and direct rehabilitation strategies. Compensatory strategies or techniques are often used as temporary measures to maintain client safety with oral intake of food or liquids until recovery or improvement of swallowing function occurs with direct or indirect rehabilitation treatments. Compensatory strategies do not involve changes to swallowing physiology (Rogus-Pulia & Robbins, 2013). Indirect and direct rehabilitation treatments, on the other hand, are aimed at changing swallowing physiology by accelerating recovery of swallowing function after a stroke or other acquired, non-progressive disorder; maintaining swallowing function in progressive diseases for as long as possible; or, in the case of pediatric disorders like prematurity, helping to develop the skills needed for feeding and swallowing effectiveness and efficiency.

Feeding Environment

Whether a patient is an infant, a young child, or an adult, the environment for feeding sets the stage for a satisfactory experience. It is especially important for clients with swallowing problems to have their meals in an environment that is conducive to success. Visual and auditory distractions should be minimized. This means that the eating area should not contain nonrelevant objects. Lighting should be comfortable—neither too bright nor too dark—and noise should be reduced.

The caregiver should have a relaxed, unhurried manner. He or she must be tuned in to the client's signals regarding feeding speed, food choices, and quantity. When necessary, these communication strategies may be developed and trained. The caregiver should indicate an interest in the person being fed and reinforce his or her healthy, effective eating behaviors. When possible, the goal is the development of self-feeding skills.

Utensils for feeding need to be appropriate to a patient's functioning. For infants, a slow-flow nipple may be helpful in controlling the amount of liquid taken at a time. A Teflon or latex-covered spoon may be used for children with infantile tonic bite reflex, who will bite hard on any object that is placed on the teeth or gums. Children and adults with motor coordination difficulties may benefit from the use of a shallow-bowled spoon. Special cutout cups may help to improve tongue positioning in drinking.

Whereas children who have excess muscle tone (hypertonia) benefit from low lighting, soft music, and minimal stimulation, children with insufficient muscle tone (hypotonia) often respond better to bright lights, upbeat music, and physical stimulation.

Body and Head Positioning

Body posture and stability have a strong influence on oral-pharyngeal movements; altering body and head positions represent compensatory treatment strategies for swallowing. The basic premise is that controlled mobility stems from a solid base (Woods, 1995). An upright, symmetrical position with a 90-degree hip angle and sufficient postural support to provide stability is generally needed. The individual's head and neck must be positioned and prevented from making extraneous movement.

Occasionally, a child or an adult may benefit from a body posture that is not upright with a hip angle of 90 degrees. For example, some infants with severe respiratory and swallowing difficulties may feed better when placed on their sides. For some adults with pharyngeal weakness on one side, lying on their side with the stronger pharyngeal side in the down position allows gravity to assist in bolus transit toward the stronger side of the pharynx (Groher & Crary, 2010).

An SLP works closely with a physical therapist and an occupational therapist in obtaining optimum positioning for swallowing. Additional compensatory techniques include the **chin tuck** posture, which is often recommended for patients with delayed pharyngeal swallow. This position helps prevent food and liquid from entering the airway. The **head-back position** is useful for patients with poor tongue mobility if they have excellent airway closure. **Head tilt** and **head rotation** postures are used when an individual has impairment on one side. In these positions, the head may be moved in the direction of (rotation) or away from (tilt) the impairment. Compensatory positioning strategies require patient compliance, adequate cognition, and the physical capability to complete such maneuvers to effectively manage swallowing disorders in the short term (Groher & Crary, 2010).

Modification of Foods and Liquids

During an assessment, liquids and foods of varying consistencies, amounts, and possibly temperatures will have been presented to a patient. On the basis of the findings of these tests, appropriate recommendations will be made. Diet modification is a commonly used compensatory management strategy for swallowing disorders; for certain individuals it will be a short-term solution, but for others it will represent their new "normal" to enable them to safely participate in oral-intake of food and liquids (Rogus-Pulia & Robbins, 2013).

Certain foods that are hard to chew, are small or slick when wet, or are thick and sticky may need to be eliminated from the diets of some individuals, like those with neuromotor difficulties. The elimination of certain unsafe or difficult to swallow diet items may be sufficient to eliminate the risk or aspiration. For others, however, a range of food consistency requirements may be recommended. For instance, they might not tolerate any food by mouth, may accept only thin or thick liquids, or they may require a pureed consistency.

The National Dysphagia Diet (NDD), published in 2002, was developed to establish standard terminology and best-practice procedures for the modification of dietary textures for the treatment of dysphagia (McCullough et al., 2003). It specifies the classification of foods based on four food texture levels:

- *NDD Level 1:* Dysphagia–pureed (i.e., cohesive, pudding-like; minimal chewing required)
- *NDD Level 2:* Dysphagia–mechanical altered (semisolid, cohesive, moist foods; some chewing required)
- *NDD Level 3:* Dysphagia–advanced (soft foods requiring more chewing)
- *NDD Level 4:* Regular (all foods permissible)

The NDD also specifies four levels of liquid: thin, nectar-like, honey-like, and spoon-thick (McCullough et al., 2003). The texture level of food, liquid level, and amount of food and liquid that clients can manage in their mouths is determined by the videofluoroscopic swallow study. With regard to amount of food and liquid, the goal is typically to reduce the amount that is presented. Drinking through a straw typically causes too much fluid to enter the mouth, so straws are usually not advised. Spoons with a shallow bowl are helpful in limiting food amounts. Caregivers and patients must avoid placing food in the mouth until the previous bolus has been swallowed. Finally, patients may be encouraged to swallow twice per bite or sip.

Providing foods of varying temperatures may increase a client's sensory awareness of the food and improve swallowing. Cold food or drink sometimes improves tongue movement during the oral transport phase and helps to stimulate pharyngeal swallow, although some patients with respiratory problems prefer all substances to be ingested at room temperature. Some consider bolus temperature alterations as an indirect rehabilitation technique, whereas others characterize it is a compensatory strategy (cf., Rogus-Pulia & Robbins, 2013; Murray, Carrau, & Chan, 2018).

Placement

Food or drink should be placed in the mouth where the patient has intact sensation and adequate muscle strength. For example, an individual who has had oral cancer has diminished sensation in the region where surgery occurred. Similarly, the ability to feel may be reduced after radiation therapy. Neurological disease and damage may also impair a person's full awareness of foods that are placed in the mouth. Surgery and neurological problems may also compromise muscle tone and make the person less able to move parts of the tongue, lips, or cheeks.

Appropriate placement along with adjustments in texture, quantity, and temperature may serve as beneficial compensatory strategies for some pediatric and adult clients with swallowing disorders. Box 11.1 provides more specific information regarding the treatment efficacy of some of these techniques with specific populations.

BOX 11.1 | **Evidence-Based Practices for Individuals with Dysphagia**

General Intervention

- Clinical and instrumental methods of assessment are both necessary to accurately evaluate dysphagia and guide selection of intervention goals.
- Patient status changes over time; therefore, ongoing assessment of feeding and swallowing function during therapy is necessary to continually update treatment goals.
- Involving patients and/or caregivers in treatment planning increases motivation and compliance with treatment recommendations and strategies.
- Ensuring that eating occurs in a familiar environment and keeping the environment free from distractions is beneficial for individuals with feeding or swallowing difficulties.

Specific Behavioral Treatment Techniques for Adults

- Postural adjustments to the body and head can facilitate safe swallowing in many patient groups; research has shown that the chin tuck posture prevented aspiration in 55% of adult patients with dysphagia secondary to stroke or trauma.
- Adults with severe reflux, including those that are tube-fed, benefit from maintaining an upright posture during and after eating to prevent aspiration of stomach acids.
- The chin tuck technique eliminated signs and symptoms of aspiration in 15 adult patients with dysphagia that resulted from neurological damage.

- The head rotation technique has been shown to be effective in eliminating aspiration of liquids for some patients with dysphagia of neurological origin, as well as those with head and neck cancer post-surgery.
- Diet modification, particularly modification of thin liquids, is highly effective, at least in the short term, in patients with dysphagia associated with dementia and/or PD. Honey-thickened liquids were most effective for both patient populations, followed by nectar-thickened liquids plus use of the chin tuck technique. Patient endurance must be taken into consideration when interrupting results, however, because the benefit of thickened liquids is not maintained as patients become fatigued.
- Maintaining oral intake during radiation treatment has been shown to help prevent radiation-associated dysphagia in patients with head and neck cancer.
- Respiratory muscle strength training targeting increased force generation of expiratory muscles improved swallowing safety and function for patients with Parkinson disease with mild dysphagia.
- Systematic lingual resistance exercise training programs increased lingual strength and swallowing ability in patients with dysphagia following stroke.
- Patients with pharyngeal dysphagia who participated in a 6-week exercise program involving head-raising exercises (referred to as the *Shaker technique*) three times per day

showed significant increases in swallowing functioning and reduced post-swallow aspiration.

- The supraglottic technique is difficult for many patients, but is effective for some patients with dysphagia associated with neurological disease.
- The super-supraglottic swallow technique has shown positive changes in swallowing in patients with head and neck cancer.
- Studies examining the effects of neuromuscular electrical stimulation (NMES) applied to the neck via surface electrodes on functional swallowing outcomes in adults with dysphagia are promising. Well-controlled experimental trials are needed to establish the treatment efficacy of NMES procedures, however.

Specific Behavioral Treatment Techniques for Children

- Specialized feeding equipment such as bottles that reduce air intake during feeding, nipples with slower or faster flow rates, or assisted bottle-feeding delivery systems are beneficial for infants with craniofacial anomalies such as cleft lip and palate.
- Oral-motor interventions, such as non-nutritive sucking to allow sucking practice and oral stimulation to reduce hypersensitivity and improve function of the oral structures, have shown positive preliminary evidence for preterm infants, including reduced hospital stays, increased alertness for feeding, and earlier transition to full oral feeding. Evidence is limited, however, and more research with larger sample sizes is needed.
- Case study research has shown that individualized swallowing programs that use principles which promote motor learning (e.g., maximized practice trials, random practice, and systematic feedback) are effective for young children with dysphagia.

Source: Based on Arvedson (2009); Ashford et al. (2009a, 2009b); Boggs & Ferguson (2016); Clark et al. (2009); Gosa & Dodrill (2017); Groher & Crary (2010); Logemann et al. (1989), Logemann et al. (1997), Logemann et al. (2008); Nagaya et al. (2004); Rogus-Pulia & Robbins (2013); Shaker et al. (2002); Starmer (2017); Troche & Mishra (2017)

Direct and Indirect Rehabilitative Swallowing Treatments

Each of the procedures described here is used only after clinical and instrumental assessment has demonstrated its safety and appropriateness. Clients also need to be able to follow instructions. All the techniques may be practiced without food; however, the swallowing techniques are specific to improving the actual swallowing process. Direct rehabilitative techniques are those that are accomplished during swallowing, while indirect rehabilitative techniques are exercises that theoretically serve to improve swallowing (e.g., tongue strength training) without the patient actually having to swallow. The evidence bases for these treatments are presented at the end of the chapter.

Strengthening Exercises

Swallowing physiology may be indirectly improved through exercise. Clients with impaired swallowing may have restricted mouth opening, tongue or lip movement, and laryngeal elevation. **Range of motion** may be improved by practicing specific exercises. Bite blocks of differing sizes may be used to encourage lowering the mandible. Flavored gauze or a toothette may be placed in various places around the mouth to stimulate tongue and lip movement. A licorice stick or a Life Saver candy on a string may also be used to improve tongue movement. The client may be instructed in moving her or his lips from pucker to smile and back again. Exercises to facilitate awareness of laryngeal movement may involve placement of the hand on the neck at the level of the hyoid bone. A mirror is often used to provide visual feedback to the patient.

Lip strength and seal may be improved by having a client attempt to hold a tongue depressor with the lips. Pushing the tongue against a tongue depressor is a technique for strengthening that muscle. Improved coordination is taught by asking the client to follow instructions such as moving the tongue to explore the outside and then inside the upper and lower front teeth. Pharyngeal muscle strengthening exercises involve head-lift exercises, where the patient lies flat on his or her back and then raises the head and holds this position for 1 minute. After three sustained head raisings, the patient rests for 1 minute. The patient then performs 30 additional head raisings (Shaker et al., 2002). Clark (2004) provides an excellent tutorial regarding neuromuscular treatment of swallowing disorders.

Effortful Swallow

A hard or effortful swallow may be helpful for patients whose tongues do not retract enough to trigger pharyngeal swallow. In such a case, the client is instructed to swallow forcefully and try to feel the tongue moving backward. This technique is helpful as swallowing practice with or without food or drink, and is aimed at reducing abnormalities within the swallow response itself (Groher & Crary, 2010; Rogus-Pulia & Robbins, 2013).

Supraglottic and Super-Supraglottic Swallow

In a normal swallow, the vocal folds are closed to prevent food from entering the airway. A supraglottic swallow may be used for individuals who do not fully close the glottis during swallowing or who close the glottis late. This technique teaches voluntary closure of the glottal area and reduces the depth of misdirected swallows (Bulow et al., 2001). The client is instructed to do the following:

1. Breathe in and hold your breath.
2. Put a small amount of food or liquid in your mouth.
3. Swallow.
4. Cough or clear your throat while exhaling.
5. Swallow again.

Results of physiological studies reveal that the supraglottic swallow technique does in fact close the vocal folds earlier in the swallow, and it keeps them together longer (Wheeler-Hegland et al., 2009). The super-supraglottic swallow technique is like the supraglottic swallow, except that it requires an *effortful* breath hold. This is to ensure complete glottal closure during the swallow (Groher & Crary, 2010). In patients who have had a stroke with or without heart disease, however, breath holding may be dangerous. Abnormalities in cardiac function have been observed while patients performed these techniques; therefore, the supraglottic and super-supraglottic swallow techniques are not recommended for individuals with a history of stroke (Rogus-Pulia & Robbins, 2013).

Mendelsohn Maneuver

The Mendelsohn maneuver is useful for clients who do not have adequate laryngeal elevation during swallowing. A patient is taught to hold the larynx manually at its highest point during the swallow. The instructions are as follows (Groher & Crary, 2010):

In the Mendelsohn maneuver, the client manually holds the larynx at its highest position to facilitate swallowing.

1. Place a small amount of food or liquid in your mouth.
2. Chew if necessary.
3. Swallow while placing your thumb and forefinger on either side of your larynx.
4. Manually hold the larynx for 3 to 5 seconds during and after swallowing in the highest position it reached during swallowing.
5. Let go of your larynx and let it drop.

The iSwallow app by Infonet, Inc. provides comprehensive instructions and video tutorials for patients and SLPs on how to perform each of these swallowing techniques.

During the assessment process, an SLP determines which of these exercises and techniques are appropriate for a particular client. Modifications in treatment approaches are often made as treatment proceeds.

Medical and Pharmacological Approaches

Patients with progressive neurological diseases (e.g., PD) who are taking medications to improve their condition benefit from taking their drugs before eating. For those with GERD, over-the-counter prescription may help manage oral-pharyngeal dysphagia caused by reflux of stomach acid. Some medical conditions (e.g., stroke) and medical treatments (e.g., radiation) can reduce the amount of saliva, causing dry mouth and interfering with normal swallowing function. Some medications are available that may increase the amount of watery secretions in the mouth, and some over-the-counter remedies may be externally applied to the mouth, providing increased lubrication (Groher & Crary, 2010). As discussed earlier in this chapter, some medications actually cause or contribute to swallowing disorders. In these cases, an SLP needs to work with a physician to determine whether alternatives can be used.

A current reference app describing prescription drugs is helpful for the practicing SLP in the medical setting.

Prostheses and Surgical Procedures

Patients who lack an intact swallowing mechanism because of malformation, surgery, or another cause may benefit from using a prosthetic device. For example, individuals who had oral cancer and have had a significant portion of the soft palate excised may have a palatal obturator, a permanent or removable plate, that helps close this area during speaking or eating. Patients requiring a partial or complete glossectomy (removal of the tongue) due to oral cancer may be fitted with a tongue prosthesis. Additional treatment strategies provided by the SLP are needed to optimize the use of a tongue prosthetic device, however (Murray, Carrau, & Chan, 2018).

If less invasive approaches have been unsuccessful, surgery to improve swallowing and prevent aspiration is sometimes needed. Some techniques attempt to correct organic defects. For example, if a patient has bony growths on the cervical vertebrae that displace the rear pharyngeal wall, these may be reduced surgically. Other surgical procedures are used to increase the dimensions of the vocal folds or elevate the larynx. In severe cases of aspiration, the true or false vocal folds may be sutured closed, and breathing will have to occur through a tracheostomy (Logemann, 1998).

Nonoral Feeding

Clients who require more than 10 seconds to swallow a liquid or food bolus or who aspirate more than 10% of either will likely require at least some nonoral feeding (Logemann, 1998). Several approaches are used.

With **nasogastric tube (NG tube)** feeding, a tube is placed from the nose to the pharynx, the esophagus, and finally the stomach. Liquefied food and water are inserted through this opening. Unlike the more long-term procedures described later, NG tubes are typically not used for periods of more than 5 or 6 months.

In **pharyngostomy**, a feeding tube is inserted into a **stoma**, or hole in the external neck region skin, which extends into the pharynx. **Esophagostomy** is a similar procedure; however, a hole is made into the esophagus from the upper chest/neck area and a food tube is inserted through it.

In percutaneous endoscopic gastrostomy (PEG, or G-tube), a hole is surgically made from the abdomen to the stomach. A soft tube is placed through this hole, and blended regular food can be inserted into the tube. This procedure is used in cases of severe dysphagia and may be a permanent means for nutrition and hydration.

Treatment Effectiveness and Outcomes for Swallowing Disorders

The overriding objectives of swallowing treatment are improved intake of food and liquid and prevention of aspiration of these materials into the lungs. The potential for treatment success is determined largely by the cause of the disorder, the severity of aspiration, and the onset of treatment. Early identification and successful intervention for swallowing disorders reduces the risk of aspiration and death, shortens the length of time patients need to stay in the hospital, and improves quality of life. Box 11.1 provides a brief overview of the research evidence supporting the use of various treatment approaches and techniques for pediatric and adult clients with dysphagia.

SLPs are successful in preventing dysphagia in some cases. Caregivers of youngsters who are at risk are instructed in feeding techniques soon after the child's birth, including positioning that is most optimal for breastfeeding, attending to the infant's cues regarding readiness to eat, and paced bottle-feedings to facilitate slower intake and reduce over- or under-feeding. Information for the older population is also valuable. Among elderly people, swallowing disorders are sometimes related to poor dentition, which might be corrected by appropriate dental care. Speech-language pathologists can also provide education and training to caregivers who assist elderly individuals with feeding to prevent malnutrition and dehydration. In particular, overly restrictive diets can lead to poor oral intake and reduced quality of life; therefore, more liberal diets that are still safe are recommended for elderly individuals (Dorner, 2010).

 Check Your Understanding 11.4
Click here to check your understanding of the concepts in this section.

SUMMARY

Speech-language pathologists who want to focus their careers in the area of dysphagia become specially trained to assess and treat swallowing disorders in pediatric and adult populations. They work with infants who are unable to nurse adequately, children with feeding problems, and adults with oral-pharyngeal dysphagia secondary to progressive and nonprogressive medical conditions. The oral preparation, oral, pharyngeal, and/or esophageal phases of swallowing may be impaired. Causes include congenital or acquired neurological problems, stroke, cancer, developmental disability, dementia, and trauma. Swallowing affects not only nutrition and health but also social and personal aspects of life. A team approach is used for both assessment and intervention. Evaluation includes a careful history and direct observation of a client while he or she is feeding. The videofluoroscopic swallow study uses X-ray equipment and is considered the gold standard in dysphagia evaluation. Compensatory and rehabilitative treatment procedures address the feeding environment, the client's body and head posture, food textures and liquid consistencies, oral-motor function, and specific swallowing techniques. Medical, prosthetic, and surgical approaches are used when necessary. Nonoral feeding may be required in severe cases.

SUGGESTED READINGS/SOURCES

Clark, H. M. (2004). Neuromuscular treatment for speech and swallowing: A tutorial. *American Journal of Speech-Language Pathology, 12,* 400–415.

Hall, K. (2001). *Pediatric dysphagia resource guide.* San Diego, CA: Singular.

Logemann, J. A. (1998). *Evaluation and treatment of swallowing disorders* (2nd ed.). Austin, TX: PRO-ED.

Mabry-Price, L. (2015, Feb. 1). Treating dysphagia in schools: Making it easy to swallow: If a child with dysphagia enters your caseload, will you know how to help that student? Enhance your knowledge with the basics. *The ASHA Leader, 20,* 36–37.

The 2009 issue of the *Journal of Rehabilitation Research and Development, 46*(2), 175–222, provides a systematic review of evidence-based practice in dysphagia treatment.

12

Audiology and Hearing Loss

David A. DeBonis, Ph.D.

LEARNING OUTCOMES

When you have finished this chapter, you should be able to:

- Describe statistics regarding the incidence and prevalence of hearing loss as well as the psychosocial consequences of hearing loss

- Describe the role of the audiologist, common employment settings, and educational requirements

- Describe the mechanics of sound production, including frequency and intensity.

- Identify key anatomic structures of the auditory system

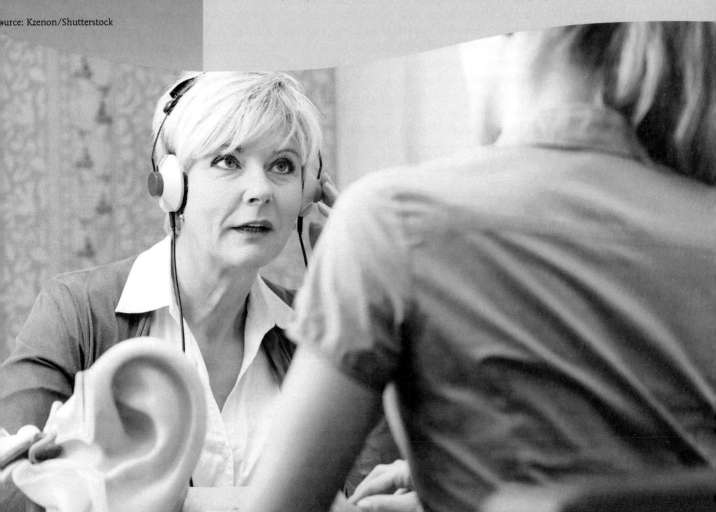

- Associate various auditory disorders with the general types of hearing loss

- Identify the components of the audiological test battery, including air conduction, bone conduction, speech audiometry, and pediatric testing.

- Describe common techniques that are used to reduce the effects of hearing loss on communication, including hearing aids, use of sign language, and communication strategies

T hose of you who are unfamiliar with the topic of hearing loss may have the misconception that it is a disorder that primarily affects the elderly population and is caused by age. In reality, hearing loss is common in people of all ages—from newborns to school-aged children, from teenagers and young adults to seniors—and it can be caused by a number of factors. You might also think that hearing loss is a disorder that simply affects your ability to hear. In fact, hearing loss can affect the overall quality of your life. It can have a very negative impact on speech and language development, reading skills, educational achievement, job performance, social interactions, and psychological well-being. It can also have a significant negative impact on your family members and close friends. In this chapter, we provide an introductory overview of how hearing loss occurs, the many ways it impacts people's lives, how it is diagnosed, and how it is treated.

INCIDENCE, PREVALENCE, AND CLASSIFICATION OF HEARING LOSS

One of the first questions that comes to mind when introducing students to the topic of hearing loss is "How many people are we talking about?" Although this question is difficult to answer precisely, a general estimate is that approximately 20 percent of Americans, 48 million, report some degree of hearing loss. (http://hearingloss.org/content/basic-facts-about-hearing-loss). This number has doubled since the mid-1980s and is expected to reach 40 million by 2025. Approximately 3 in every 1000 births results in a child with hearing loss, making it the most frequently occurring birth defect (Centers for Disease Control and Prevention, 2009). Also, approximately 1 in every 1000 births results in a child with a severe to profound degree of hearing loss. Approximately 83 in every 1000 children in the United States exhibit what is termed an "educationally significant" hearing loss that can have lifelong consequences (National Dissemination Center for Children with Disabilities, 2003). The World Health Organization (WHO) provides important and alarming statistics regarding hearing loss worldwide (World Health Organization, 2017: http://www.who.int/mediacentre/factsheets/fs300/en/) in 2017. It reports that 360 million people worldwide have disabling hearing loss, including 32 million children. Approximately one third of individuals who are older than 65 years of age have disabling hearing loss, and the majority of hearing loss that impacts children could be prevented. The WHO urges the following to prevent hearing loss: immunizing children to prevent disease and screening to identify disease early, greater access to medications to treat infections, improved hygiene practices, avoidance of medications that damage inner ear structures, early hearing testing, and providing better information to young people regarding noise-induced hearing loss. The WHO predicts that 1.1 billion individuals between the ages of 12 and 35 years are at risk of developing hearing loss from their recreational activities.

Classification of Impairment, Disability, and Handicap

When it comes to describing the effects of hearing loss, terminology can be confusing, especially for those who are new to the subject. Terms such as *impaired*, *disabled*, and *handicapped* can seem to overlap in meaning. The International Classification of Functioning (ICF; http://www.who.int/classifications/icf/en/) provides a system that defines and distinguishes these terms. **Impairment** is defined as a loss of structure or function. As related to audiology, examples of impairments could include trauma to the eardrum, damage to the bones of the middle ear, or damage to the sensory cells in the inner ear. Do all impairments lead to a disability? The answer is "no." Activity limitation is the term used to refer to the functional consequences associated with a particular impairment, and **disability** is a broad term that includes the impairment as well as the environmental factors that interfere with functioning. For those with hearing loss, examples of disability could include an inability to understand speech in the presence of background noise, difficulty understanding conversations on the phone, or difficulty hearing low-intensity speech sounds. When audiologists guide their clients with treatment recommendations, they are often addressing the person's hearing disability. Finally, impairment and disability may lead to *participation restriction*, which is defined as restriction of the ability of a person to participate in life situations. Examples here could include hearing loss that makes employment impossible or that interferes with the ability to maintain positive social relationships. It is important to remember that many individuals who have hearing loss do not have a hearing handicap, because their loss does not interfere with their ability to participate in life situations. For example, despite problems hearing on the phone or understanding conversations in noisy settings, many people who have hearing loss are well-adjusted, independent, fully participating members of society.

Effects of Hearing Loss

Knowing that hearing loss can negatively impact access to speech and language and knowing how critical speech and language are to all aspects of development, we now examine the broader effects of hearing loss on individuals.

Children

It is relatively easy to understand that a profound hearing loss (i.e., thresholds of 90 dB or greater) would have a very negative impact on speech and language development. An individual demonstrating such a loss would have no access to the speech sounds in our language without amplification. What is perhaps less broadly understood is that all degrees of hearing loss, including mild losses, can interfere with speech and language. In addition, all degrees of hearing loss in children can interfere with their ability to succeed in school. This includes not only their academic abilities but also the development of their social interaction skills.

A review of the literature on this topic reveals a number of broad principles that may serve as the foundation for understanding the important relationships that exist between hearing loss, speech and language development, and school success. Some of the themes noted are:

- Children with mild hearing loss typically perform well on basic auditory tasks presented in favorable acoustic environments. However, when the task becomes more challenging and/or the environment becomes less favorable (e.g., due to noise), the negative effects of the hearing loss become more obvious. In addition, because of the added burden of the hearing loss, children must rely more on their memory and attention abilities than their hearing peers. Over time, this additional effort can be difficult for the child to maintain, resulting in reduced academic performance.

- Because grammatical morphemes are perceptually subtle compared to other language structures, children with hearing loss are at great risk for delays in their morphological development. Use of hearing aids to increase the child's access to these subtle grammatical markers can promote the age-appropriate development of morphemes.

- Even though children with unilateral hearing loss have normal hearing in one ear, they are still at risk for academic difficulties due to their loss. This includes difficulty in both localizing sound and hearing in noise. In addition, because of the impact of their hearing loss, these children must work harder in school to receive and understand incoming information; therefore, they become more fatigued than their peers throughout the day. The use of assistive devices, such as an FM system, may be helpful.

- Hoffman et al. (2015) compared the social interaction skills of two groups of children, all between the ages of 2.5 and 5.3 years. One group all had profound hearing loss, and the other all had normal hearing. As expected, the children without hearing loss performed better than those who were deaf. The researchers also found that the social competence of the children could be predicted (using statistics) by the child's hearing status and the child's degree of language development. Other factors related to social competence in the group of children who were deaf included the age at which the hearing loss was diagnosed and the age at which they started using amplification. In both cases, the earlier these things occurred, the better for the development of social interaction abilities.

Adults

Although adults do not have the same kinds of challenges as children who are receiving new information on a daily basis, they still rely on their hearing to meet their own unique challenges at home and at work and to foster their physical and emotional health. The Better Hearing Institute (www.betterhearinginstitute.org) summarizes themes related to the effects of untreated hearing loss among adults, including:

- increased irritability and fatigue due to the extra cognitive effort required to receive needed information
- increased stress

- greater likelihood of becoming isolated due to difficulty participating successfully in conversations
- increased risk of injury related to being less auditorily aware of surroundings
- reduced earning power and less confidence in ability to perform job duties
- reduced self-esteem
- overall reduced psychological health.

Think for a moment about the following surprising statistic: Approximately 95% of children who have hearing loss are born to parents with normal hearing (Mitchell & Karchmer, 2004). Now think about the implications of this for the parents of these children. Most of them have little knowledge or experience related to hearing loss and the challenges it presents when raising a child. The understandable joy, hopefulness, and optimism that parents feel at the birth of a child can quickly turn to feelings of fear and helplessness when their newborn baby is identified as having significant hearing loss. Parents may feel as if their lives are suddenly spiraling out of control as they face the reality of raising a child who has a disorder. The stages of grief that are usually associated with the dying process are also applicable to those dealing with hearing loss. Parents of children with hearing loss often experience shock, denial, anger, and depression before they are finally able to accept the reality of the situation.

Adults who have acquired hearing loss over the course of their lifetime, whether suddenly or gradually, are certainly also at risk for psychosocial problems. Many go through the same stages of grief as parents of children with hearing loss. An adult with hearing loss who is no longer able to enjoy social activities to the same degree as in the past or understand conversations on the phone, at meetings, or during family gatherings may experience a variety of emotions, including anger and frustration that may eventually lead to depression (Mullins, 2004). Having to rely on others can lead to feelings of inadequacy, guilt, decreased self-sufficiency, and reduced self-worth; in addition, family relationships may become strained. It is very important that professionals pay attention to these psychosocial issues to determine the full impact of a hearing problem on an individual client and his or her family members.

Deafness, the Deaf Community, and Deaf Culture

Our discussion of impairment and disability leads us to a brief discussion about individuals who are deaf. As you will learn in more detail later in this chapter, when a person's hearing loss reaches 90 dB or greater the loss is categorized as profound; that is, we say the person is **deaf**. It might seem logical to think that if you had such significant hearing loss, you would be most interested in wearing hearing aids or getting a cochlear implant and receiving speech and language services. The truth, however, is that if your parents were deaf and you grew up around other people who were deaf, you might view your deafness not as a disability that needed to be fixed but rather as a cultural trait. Individuals who have this perspective make up what is referred to as the **Deaf community**, a group who views deafness with a sense of pride that serves to unite its members and positively shape their sense of self-identity.

You might be wondering at this point how deafness could be considered a culture. Consider that a culture is created when a group of people share a common background of language, traditions, and values. Those who identify with Deaf culture in the United States share a common language, **American Sign Language (ASL)**, which is considered the natural language of the Deaf that serves to foster group cohesion. **Deaf culture** is further characterized by its rich history, traditions, folklore, and various contributions to the arts, including poetry, dance, and theater. At this point, an important distinction needs to be made between the labels *deaf* with a lowercase *d* and *Deaf* with an uppercase *D*. Individuals who are "deaf" share a common physiological condition: severe to profound hearing loss. In contrast, "Deaf" refers to individuals who are members of the Deaf community.

Think for a moment about recent technological advances that have occurred that allow individuals who are deaf to receive cochlear implants via a surgical procedure discussed in detail later. This surgery has allowed many individuals to receive speech and language information and to develop oral language skills. Although this is a positive development for these individuals, there has been some very heated discussion in the literature about the effect it might have on Deaf culture. As fewer and fewer individuals attend schools for the deaf and greater numbers choose to get cochlear implants, learn oral English, and integrate more fully with hearing individuals, some people fear that the future of the Deaf community and culture is threatened. Possibly for this reason, leaders in the Deaf community were originally quite forceful in their opposition to the use of cochlear implants. But as Hossain (2012) notes, as the benefits of cochlear implants have become clearer the Deaf community has become more accepting of the device and more open to the fact that this is a personal choice that should be respected.

Living and working in today's culturally diverse society, it is important for professionals in the fields of speech-language pathology and audiology to develop an awareness and understanding of Deaf culture and to think carefully about the complex and hard-to-answer questions surrounding deafness. Even though many academic training programs have traditionally seen all hearing impairments from a pathological perspective that assumes they need to be treated, those who are considering a career in speech-language pathology or audiology should be aware that this is not the only perspective. Also, in order to use evidence-based practice, we must value and respect the beliefs and preferences of our clients. Our role is not to tell our clients what to do, but rather to listen to their goals and priorities and coach them in ways that are consistent with those beliefs and with their culture. We certainly can expose clients to new information and perhaps new ways of thinking, but they must make the final decisions about their communication goals and how to achieve them.

 Thought Question 12.1

Do you believe that deafness is a cultural difference, or do you view it as a disability?

 Check Your Understanding 12.1
Click here to check your understanding of the concepts in this section.

WHAT IS AUDIOLOGY?

The American Speech-Language-Hearing Association (ASHA) defines **audiology** as the discipline involved in "the prevention of and assessment of auditory, vestibular, and related impairments as well as the habilitation/rehabilitation and maintenance of persons with these impairments." (ASHA, 2004, p. 2). Note that audiology consists of work related to both assessment *and* habilitation/rehabilitation. Often, people perceive audiology as a discipline that deals strictly with the diagnosis of hearing loss. Although assessment is a critical part of audiology, treatment and management of a client diagnosed with a hearing problem are equally important. Audiologists must be skilled at providing habilitative/rehabilitative services including counseling, prescribing and fitting **amplification**, and various therapeutic services designed to support communication and improve one's overall quality of life.

Educational Requirements and Employment for Audiologists

According to the American Academy of Audiology website (www.audiology.org), from the 1960s until 2007 the degree that audiologists needed for clinical practice was a master's degree in audiology. In 2007, a clinical doctorate degree, designated the Au.D., became the entry-level degree for clinical audiology practice. This change in degree requirements was made so that those of you who choose to enter audiology programs would be better prepared to meet the broad range of skill requirements that are needed in many employment settings. Most Au.D. training programs require 4 years of study beyond the bachelor's degree. Although the Au.D. degree prepares you to understand research and perform clinical research, if you are primarily interested in performing audiology research and/or working at the college level you should pursue a Ph.D. in audiology.

Once you had completed your Au.D program, you would be able to seek employment in a wide range of settings. A survey of ASHA-certified audiologists revealed that more than half work in nonresidential health care settings (e.g., private practices, community speech and hearing centers, physician's offices), and 27% are employed in hospital settings, 11% in schools, 9% in universities, and a smaller percentage in industry (ASHA, 2010).

 Check Your Understanding 12.2

Click here to check your understanding of the concepts in this section.

FUNDAMENTALS OF SOUND

Several conditions must exist in order for sound to occur and be perceived. For the purpose of this discussion, let's focus specifically on the speech signal. The following must be available: (a) an energy source, such as exhalation of air from the lungs; (b) an object capable of vibrating, such as the vocal folds of the larynx, for the energy source to act on; (c) a medium, such as air, that is capable of conducting the resulting vibrations; and (d) a receptor to receive and interpret the resulting sound.

How is it that sound is able to travel great distances through the air to reach our ears? Let's take a step back and first consider how an object, such as a simple guitar string, vibrates. Vibration can be thought of as a series of rhythmic back-and-forth movements. As the guitar string is plucked, it vibrates to and fro. As it moves in one direction, an increase in pressure occurs as air molecules that are close to each other are displaced and become compressed or packed together tightly. As the guitar string reverses and moves in the opposite direction, the air molecules that were initially compressed begin to rebound or spread apart, creating a decrease in pressure referred to as a rarefaction. Sound, then, is a series of **compressions** and **rarefactions** that move outward from a vibrating source. It is important to realize that the individual air molecules themselves do not travel from their original position to the listener's ear, but their movement creates the sound wave that travels to the ear.

A vibrating object that moves back and forth from its normal resting position has special qualities. First, the vibrating object travels a measurable distance in either direction. This is referred to as the *amplitude* of the vibration. The amplitude of a sound determines its **intensity**, which is measured in decibels (dB). Second, this back-and-forth movement regularly repeats itself, resulting in a certain number of complete cycles during a specified period of time. This is referred to as the **frequency** of the vibration and is expressed in cycles per second, or hertz (Hz). Every sound, therefore, can be described in terms of its unique intensity and frequency characteristics. This information is decoded or interpreted by the auditory system, allowing the listener to differentiate the infinitesimal number of sounds he or she is exposed to throughout the course of a day.

 Check Your Understanding 12.3

Click here to check your understanding of the concepts in this section.

ANATOMY AND PHYSIOLOGY OF THE AUDITORY SYSTEM

Before we can begin our discussion of the various types and causes of hearing loss, a general understanding of the anatomy and physiology of the auditory system is essential. Anatomically, the auditory system can be divided into several general areas. They include the outer ear, the middle ear, the inner ear, the vestibulocochlear nerve, the auditory brain stem, and the auditory cortex of the brain. The first four areas (Figure 12.1) are commonly referred to as the **peripheral auditory system**; the latter two are part of the **central auditory system**. Typically, when we say that someone has a hearing loss, we are referring to a peripheral problem. When someone has a deficit in the central auditory system, we usually say that this person has a processing or an auditory processing problem.

Figure 12.1 The peripheral auditory system.

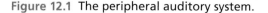
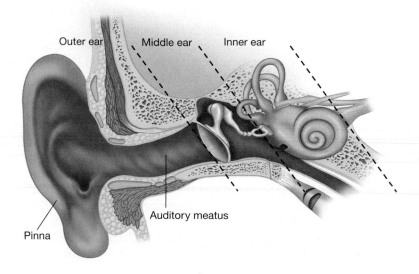

The Outer Ear

Your **outer ear** is comprised of the **pinna**, or auricle, and the **external auditory meatus**, or external auditory canal. The pinna is the most visible structure of the auditory system and is made of cartilage covered with skin. If you take a look at someone's pinna, you will note various ridges and depressions; these are important because they provide a natural boost to certain sounds as they enter the ear. The pinna also collects and funnels sound into the ear canal and helps the listener to identify where sound originates in space, a process called **localization**.

Your external auditory meatus, which is also called the ear canal, is a tube lined with skin that extends from the bowl-like depression of the pinna, known as the **concha**, to the **tympanic membrane**, or **eardrum**. The ear canal is approximately 1 inch in length in adults and has a slight "S-shaped" curve as it progresses toward the eardrum. The outer region of the canal contains hair follicles and glands that produce **cerumen**, more commonly known as earwax. Similar to the pinna, the ear canal also enhances certain high frequency sounds as they travel to the eardrum.

The Middle Ear

Your external auditory canal leads to the tympanic membrane, which marks the boundary between your outer ear and the **middle ear**. Your tympanic membrane is a thin concave-shaped structure that vibrates in response to sound waves that travel down your ear canal. Most of the surface area of your tympanic membrane is composed of three distinct layers of tissue. The middle layer is made of fibrous tissue that provides both the strength and elasticity of the eardrum. A healthy eardrum is often described as appearing "pearl gray" in color. Because your eardrum is semitransparent, it is possible to view some of the structures of the middle ear when conducting a visual examination of the eardrum.

Located behind your tympanic membrane is the **middle ear space**. This air-filled cavity is lined with a mucous membrane, and includes the opening to your **Eustachian tube**. This important tube connects your middle ear with the **nasopharynx**, the space located behind the nose and above the roof of the mouth. Your Eustachian tube is normally closed but opens periodically, providing a passageway for air to ventilate the middle ear space and equalize air pressure on each side of the eardrum.

Also located in your middle ear space is a chain formed by three small bones. These bones, called the **malleus**, **incus**, and **stapes**, are collectively referred to as the **ossicles**, or **ossicular chain** (see Figure 12.2). The first bone in the chain, the malleus, is the largest of the three and is embedded in the fibrous layer of the eardrum. The upper portion of the malleus makes contact with the incus, which makes contact with the stapes, the smallest bone in the human body. The footplate of the stapes rests against the **oval window**, a thin membrane that marks the entrance to the inner ear.

The Inner Ear

At this point, you should be able to begin to think about how you hear. We now know that sound waves travel through the air, down the ear canal, and cause the eardrum to vibrate. These vibrations are then carried across the ossicular chain to the footplate of the stapes, which makes contact with the oval window, which is

Figure 12.2 Structures of the middle ear.

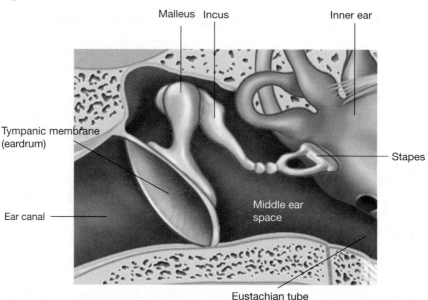

Malleus Incus

Inner ear

Tympanic membrane
(eardrum)

Stapes

Ear canal

Middle ear
space

Eustachian tube

the entry point to the inner ear. The **inner ear** is a complex structure that serves two important roles. One major component, the **cochlea**, is responsible for providing auditory input to the central auditory system. The other major component, the **vestibular system**, is responsible for supplying information regarding balance.

Let's turn our attention first to your cochlea, a structure the size of a pea that resembles a snail's shell. Your cochlea is the portion of the inner ear that contains special nerve cells designed to respond to auditory stimuli; these are referred to as *auditory sensory receptor cells*. Your cochlea is composed of two complicated networks of passages, referred to as *labyrinths*. The outer labyrinth is composed of bone and filled with a fluid called **perilymph**; the inner labyrinth is composed of membranous material and contains a fluid called **endolymph**.

Running along the center of the membranous labyrinth is a structure called the **organ of Corti** (see Figure 12.3). The floor of the organ of Corti is formed by the basilar membrane. The **basilar membrane** is narrower, thinner, and stiffer at the base and wider, thicker, and more flaccid at the apex. Think for a moment about a guitar string; the thinner, stiffer strings produce high frequency sounds and the thicker, looser strings produce low frequency sounds. Although the process is not completely understood, we know that these anatomical differences of your basilar membrane enable it to respond differently to sounds of different frequencies. That is, the portion of the basilar membrane closest to the stapes responds best to high frequency sounds, and the portion nearest the tip or apex of the cochlea responds best to low frequency sounds.

It is very important to note here that located on your basilar membrane are thousands of tiny **hair cells**, which are considered to be your sensory receptor cells of the auditory system. Located on the top of each cell are small hairlike projections called **stereocilia**. Also, forming the roof of the organ of Corti is a structure called the **tectorial membrane**. The tectorial membrane is fixed at one end, while

Figure 12.3 The organ of Corti.

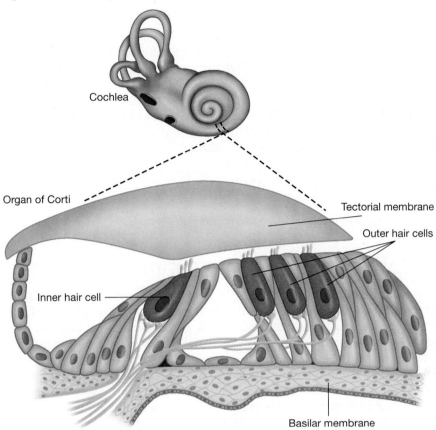

the opposite end is free to move up and down in response to displacement of the surrounding fluid.

At this point, take a look back at the pathway of sound from the sound wave in the air to movement of the stapes in the oval window, described above. Now add to that understanding the following: As your stapes rocks in and out of the oval window, fluid is displaced in the membranous labyrinth. As the stereocilia are bent through the movement of the tectorial and basilar membranes, chemical transmitters are released at the base of the cochlear hair cells, and neuroelectric energy is generated and transmitted to auditory nerve fibers that form the acoustic branch of the **vestibulocochlear**, or **VIIIth cranial nerve**. This information is then directed to your brain stem and eventually the brain.

Before we end our discussion of the inner ear, a brief mention of your vestibular system should be made. Your vestibular system is also made up of bony and membranous sections and contains sensory receptor cells that sense head movement. Nerve fibers innervating the sensory cells of the vestibular system form the vestibular branch of the VIIIth nerve. The anatomical connections that exist between the balance and hearing mechanisms help explain why both balance testing and nonmedical intervention of balance disorders are included in the audiologist's scope of practice (ASHA, 2004).

The Central Auditory System

Your central auditory system, which consists of nuclei, nerve fibers, and nerve tracts, includes pathways that carry auditory information to your brain (ascending pathway) and pathways that receive information from your brain (descending pathways) Although it may appear that the anatomical structures leading to your brain simply send neural impulses, they actually play a key role in ensuring that information about the frequency, intensity, and duration of the auditory stimuli remains intact until it reaches the auditory cortex for interpretation. Further exploration of the central auditory system is typically presented to students in anatomy and physiology and audiology courses.

 Check Your Understanding 12.4

Click here to check your understanding of the concepts in this section.

TYPES OF HEARING LOSS AND AUDITORY DISORDERS

The previous section described the ear from an anatomical and physiological standpoint. The outer and the middle ear serve to collect, amplify, and conduct sound to the cochlea. The outer and middle ear, therefore, are referred to as the **conductive system**. The cochlea is the actual sensory organ of hearing, and the auditory branch of the VIIIth nerve is responsible for transmitting the resulting neural signal to the brain stem and eventually to the auditory cortex for processing. The cochlea and auditory nerve, therefore, make up the **sensorineural system**. When audiologists describe peripheral hearing loss, they typically use terms like *conductive* and *sensorineural*. When deficits are noted in the central auditory system, these are typically described in terms of how they impact a person's auditory processing abilities.

Conductive Hearing Loss

If you had a conductive hearing loss, the cause would most likely be the result of a deformation, a malfunction, or an obstruction of the outer or middle ear. Not all disorders of the outer and middle ear result in a loss of hearing. In many cases, however, problems in these areas reduce or eliminate the ear's natural conduction of sound as it travels to the cochlea. As a result, the intensity of sound arriving at the inner ear is reduced. This usually prevents low- to moderate-intensity sounds from being heard at all, and higher-intensity sounds are perceived as much softer than normal. It is important to remember that the primary consequence of conductive hearing loss is a loss of loudness or audibility. As long as the sensorineural system remains intact, sound can be heard without difficulty if it is made loud enough for the individual, such as by turning up the volume of a radio or TV, or by raising the level of one's voice.

There are a few other key things you should remember about conductive hearing loss. First, it does not result in a total loss of hearing. In other words, a person who is considered deaf would not have lost hearing solely as a result of a conductive deficit. Second, most conductive losses are not permanent. Some resolve without any treatment, and most others are medically treatable. In rare cases when medical treatment cannot be given or when the client prefers not to pursue it, a hearing aid or hearing aids may be possible if medical clearance is given by the physician.

Disorders of the Outer Ear

Several conditions of the outer ear can occur due to the malformation of structures during embryonic development. If you had anotia, your pinna would be absent on one or both sides; if you had **microtia**, you would have a small malformed pinna. These conditions alone do not result in a loss of hearing, but with microtia there is an increased likelihood that you would also have some other congenital condition, such as *atresia*. **Atresia** is a disorder in which there is complete closure of the external auditory meatus; because sound cannot travel through the ear canal in the usual manner, hearing loss results. Stenosis, a severe narrowing of the external canal, may occur in some individuals. Unlike atresia, however, stenosis does not result in significant hearing loss unless debris or earwax becomes trapped in the narrow opening. These conditions most frequently occur in conjunction with other craniofacial disorders (see Chapter 11).

A much more common cause of conductive hearing loss in the outer ear and one that you may have experienced is impacted wax (cerumen) or a foreign object. Although many people view cerumen as a problem, it actually protects the ear, at least to some degree, from insects and other foreign bodies entering the canal. It also traps dirt and debris, naturally cleansing the external canal as it migrates outward. Cerumen acts as a lubricant to prevent the skin that lines the canal from drying out and serves as a chemical barrier to bacterial and fungal infection. In view of these positive attributes of wax, you should not use cotton swabs or other tools to remove cerumen. In fact, aggressive use of cotton swabs often pushes more wax further into your ear canal, which can create a wax blockage that needs to be removed by a physician. In many states cerumen management (removal) is within the audiologist's scope of practice, although it should be conducted with caution and only after proper training.

Overuse of cotton swabs can cause two additional disorders of the outer ear. The first, and one that you or someone you know may have experienced, is external otitis, more commonly known as swimmer's ear. This can occur when too much wax has been removed from the ear canal, making the canal more vulnerable to infection by bacteria or fungus. This condition is typically painful as the ear canal begins to swell. In some cases, drainage from the ear is noted. External otitis is typically treated by an **Ear, Nose, and Throat physician (ENT),** also referred to as an otolaryngologist. This physician will examine the ear canal carefully, clean it, and apply medication. Often, the physician will provide you with medicated eardrops to use at home.

Aggressive use of cotton swabs can also result in a perforation, or hole in the tympanic membrane, if the swab is pushed too deeply into the canal. Another possible cause of this condition is a blow to the head, or a rupture caused by excessive fluid pressing against the eardrum. Symptoms of a perforated eardrum can be subtle or extreme, ranging from slight discomfort to significant pain and bleeding. The degree of conductive hearing loss resulting from this condition can also be subtle or significant, depending on size and location. Perforations can be identified by the ENT physician through examination of the eardrum using an otoscope, and in some cases also a high-powered microscope. Perforations may heal spontaneously without any treatment, but often need to be repaired by the ENT. The physician typically uses tissue from the outer ear to patch the perforated area. Case Study 12.1 presents the story of one child with several disorders of the outer ear.

CASE STUDY 12.1

Anotia and Atresia

Joshua was born with bilateral anotia and canal atresia, which means that his pinnae are not developed and his ear canals are absent. Because sound is unable to travel to the eardrum through the ear canal, Joshua is experiencing the maximum conductive hearing loss of 60 dB in each ear. Although audiological testing indicates that Joshua's cochleas are functioning normally, results of the CT scan suggest that Joshua is not a good candidate for surgery to open up his ear canals. Joshua's parents bring their son to the audiologist to be fit with a bone anchored hearing aid (BAHA) attached to a soft headband. This device delivers sound to Joshua's normally functioning inner ear by bypassing the outer and middle ears. Once Joshua reaches the age of 5 years, he will have surgery to secure the BAHA to the back of his head either by an implanted abutment or a magnet placed underneath the skin. This is done so that he will no longer have to wear the head band.

Disorders of the Middle Ear

Several conditions can occur due to problems in the middle ear. For example, **otosclerosis** is a disorder that affects primarily young adults, particularly females, and in the majority of cases is linked to genetic factors. If you had this condition, healthy bone would be replaced with spongy bone in the area of the stapes footplate, most likely causing reduced mobility of the stapes and hearing loss. If your hearing loss was interfering with your ability to understand speech at school, at work, or in social situations, you could pursue surgery to remove all or part of the stapes footplate followed by insertion of a prosthetic device that acts as an artificial stapes.

Another middle ear condition involving the ossicles is ossicular discontinuity, which refers to a break somewhere in the ossicular chain. This condition can be caused by head trauma and typically creates a large conductive hearing loss in the affected ear. Surgical repair for this condition is done by the ENT, who examines the condition of the ossicles, identifies where the break has occurred, and either repairs the ossicle or replaces it with a prosthetic one.

One of the most common causes of conductive hearing loss, particularly in children, is **otitis media**, an inflammation of the mucous membrane lining the middle ear cavity. Otitis media generally results from **Eustachian tube dysfunction**, which prevents proper ventilation of the middle ear cavity. A normally functioning Eustachian tube opens and closes regularly as you chew, yawn, or swallow, allowing for the equalization of air pressure between your middle ear and the external environment. In children the Eustachian tube is less efficient than it is in adults, and therefore is less effective in ventilating the middle ear. Another factor that can interfere with Eustachian tube function and middle ear ventilation is enlarged adenoids.

When the middle ear is not consistently ventilated, oxygen within the cavity is absorbed into the mucous membrane lining, forming a partial vacuum. This, in turn, results in a condition known as *negative middle ear pressure*, which causes your eardrum to retract into the middle ear cavity, reducing its ability to vibrate freely. If this situation goes untreated or does not respond to treatment, the secretion of fluid may occur in the middle ear; this is a condition referred to as **otitis media with effusion (OME)**. As fluid fills the cavity, sound must be conducted through fluid, instead of the usual air-filled environment. If the fluid is sterile, the condition is classified as **serous otitis media**. However, when bacteria are present pus may form within the middle ear cavity, causing a condition referred to as **purulent (or suppurative) otitis media**. In these cases, in addition to conductive hearing loss you may also experience restlessness, irritability, ear pain, fever, and vomiting. During this process your tympanic membrane may appear reddish in color or bulging. In some cases, the eardrum may rupture due to the pressure created by the fluid behind it.

Otitis media is not rare. In fact, it is the most frequently diagnosed disorder in the United States in children younger than 15 years. More than 90% of children experience at least one episode by the age of 7 years, with peak incidence generally occurring during the period from 6 months to 2 years of age (Jung & Hanson, 1999).

Treating otitis media is a complex process because no one treatment works best for everyone. In some cases, your physician may recommend that you wait and monitor the condition because a number of these cases resolve without treatment. In other cases, use of a decongestant or an antihistamine helps resolve the underlying problem of inadequate Eustachian tube function. If you had acute otitis media with infected fluid, antibiotics such as amoxicillin would likely be used, but this must be done carefully because some people have difficulty tolerating antibiotics, and there is concern among medical professionals about the overuse of antibiotics.

Some treatment options cannot be pursued by a child's pediatrician and require a referral to an ENT. When nonsurgical treatments have been ineffective, ENTs often perform a surgical treatment that research and clinical observation have shown to restore hearing and reduce the likelihood of further middle ear pathology. The procedure, called a **myringotomy**, involves making an incision into the tympanic membrane in order to drain fluid from the middle ear cavity. This is frequently followed by insertion of a **pressure equalization (PE) (or tympanostomy) tube** into the tympanic membrane. These tubes serve the same purpose as the Eustachian tube, allowing air to pass into the middle ear space. However, instead of passing from the nasopharynx in the usual manner, air enters the middle ear from the external auditory canal via the open PE tube situated in the eardrum. Images of various outer and middle ear disorders are available on Roy Sullivan's video otoscopy website at http://www.rcsullivan.com/www/ears.htm#2.0

The treatment of otitis media in children can be stressful for both parents and professionals because resolving the problem is often not an efficient process. From a physician's point of view, it certainly makes sense to choose treatment options that are more conservative first and to gradually move to more aggressive options. But in cases where the treatment is not working, the hearing loss that accompanies the otitis media can remain unresolved for many months in a child who is in a very critical period for speech and language development. This can be of great concern to parents, speech-language pathologists (SLPs), and audiologists. In addition, the fact that some treatment options are only available through an ENT can add more waiting time to this process.

At this time, there is disagreement in the literature regarding whether early otitis media with hearing loss has negative effects on a child later in life. For example, Zumach et al. (2010) found that the early negative effects on receptive and expressive language from otitis media that were measured in children who were 27 months of age disappeared by the time the same children were 7 years old. In contrast, Shapiro et al. (2009) found that children who had a history of otitis media prior to the age of 2 years performed more poorly at 9 years of age on measures of reading and phonological awareness than did those who did not have this history and those who had otitis media after the age of 2 years. This question of the possible long-term impact of early hearing loss is an important one. If long-term effects do exist, greater efforts to quickly resolve early hearing loss in children who have otitis media will have to become part of our treatment protocols. The story of an 18-month-old with otitis media is presented in Case Study 12.2.

Sensorineural Hearing Loss

A second general type of hearing loss is sensorineural hearing loss. If you had this type of loss, it would most often be due to the absence or malformation of, or damage to the structures of, the inner ear, including the hair cells within the cochlea. Sensorineural hearing loss may be present at birth or may develop over the course of one's life. It may be sudden in onset, occurring over a matter of hours, or gradual, occurring over a period of years. Some forms of sensorineural hearing loss have a genetic basis; other forms are acquired. Some cases of sensorineural hearing losses may remain stable; some become worse; and some fluctuate. Unlike conductive hearing losses, which are most commonly temporary, sensorineural losses are usually permanent.

CASE STUDY 12.2

Otitis Media

Brittany is an 18 month-old female. Her parents note that their daughter has recently been tugging at her ears and at times does not seem to be hearing normally. She also has not been sleeping well. In addition, Brittany uses only about 10 one-word labels to communicate expressively. A visit to the pediatrician reveals the presence of fluid in each of Brittany's middle ears, and a visit to the audiologist reveals abnormal responses to speech and tones and flat tympanograms, suggesting that her eardrums are not vibrating well. These findings are also consistent with middle ear pathology. Based on these findings, the audiologist refers Brittany back to the pediatrician and also recommends that she be seen by a speech-language pathologist. The pediatrician prescribes a combination of allergy medication and an antibiotic, which Brittany uses for several weeks in an attempt to clear up the middle ear fluid. When it is determined that this is unsuccessful, the pediatrician refers Brittany to an ENT, who confirms the presence of fluid and prescribes a different combination of medications. Three weeks later the condition is still unresolved, and the ENT recommends that Brittany have a procedure to remove the middle ear fluid and have pressure equalization (p.e.) tubes inserted. These tubes will take over the function of the Eustachian tubes. In addition, an examination of Brittany's adenoids reveals that they are quite large and possibly interfering with the normal functioning of her Eustachian tubes. The ENT decides that they should be removed during the same surgical procedure. Brittany's parents are back at the ENT office two months later to report that the repeat hearing evaluation conducted one month ago revealed responses to speech and tones that were within normal limits and that speech-language therapy is going very well. Brittany's parents report that their daughter is responding positively to speech and environmental sounds and her vocabulary is beginning to increase.

Although sensorineural hearing loss may affect hearing sensitivity for any range of frequencies, in most cases the higher frequencies are affected. Unlike conductive hearing loss, where the problem stems from sound not being loud enough, sensorineural hearing loss can involve both a lack of loudness and a lack of clarity. Not only are certain sounds inaudible or difficult to hear, but sounds that are audible are often perceived as being distorted. To illustrate this point, consider the following example. Talking on your cell phone at a low volume level simulates a conductive hearing loss. That is, sound is softer than normal, making it difficult to perceive. If, however, the volume is increased (i.e., the conductive disorder is resolved), the signal not only becomes easier to hear but the signal also becomes clear. If we now take the same phone but add distortion or static, the signal remains audible but is harder to understand. Increasing the volume sometimes makes the distorted signal louder, but it is still not clear.

As you might expect, sensorineural hearing loss can have a negative impact on speech, language, and cognitive development. Factors that influence the effects of the loss on these aspects of development include (a) the degree of the loss, (b) the age of the person when the loss occurred, referred to as *age of onset*, (c) the age of the person when the loss was identified, and (d) the age of the person when appropriate intervention was begun.

Age of onset is usually described as **congenital** (present at birth) or acquired (occurring sometime after birth). Another way of looking at this is to consider whether the hearing loss occurred **prelingually** (i.e., before speech and language skills have developed) or **postlingually** (i.e., after the person has acquired spoken language skills). There is no precise age that defines these two terms, but traditionally hearing loss that occurs prior to the age of 2 years is considered prelingual in onset, and hearing loss that occurs after the age of 5 years is considered postlingual. Think about a child who is born with a moderate hearing loss that is not detected until he or she is 4 or 5 years of age, compared to a child whose loss is identified when the child is a newborn. The negative effects on speech and language will be much greater for the first child. For the second child, early intervention services can be provided during a critical time of development to reduce these negative effects.

Disorders of the Inner Ear

Now that we have a general understanding of sensorineural hearing loss, let's take a look at some of the causes, starting with those that are congenital and hereditary. When a hearing loss is due to the absence or malformation of inner ear structures during embryonic development, it is referred to as **aplasia**, or **dysplasia**. There are several types of aplasia, depending on which part of the inner ear is affected. Very often, congenital hereditary sensorineural hearing loss is one component of a group of disorders associated with a syndrome. For example, **Usher's syndrome** is a genetic disorder characterized by significant sensorineural hearing loss as well as degenerative visual changes that result in night blindness and reduced peripheral vision. **Waardenburg's syndrome** is another genetic disorder characterized by mild to severe sensorineural hearing loss, as well as changes in the coloring of the hair, skin and eyes. Children with **Alport's syndrome** often have sensorineural hearing loss and kidney disease.

Although sensorineural hearing loss may be present at birth, it is not always a result of genetic factors. Instead, an illness or toxic agent experienced by the mother during pregnancy may be the cause. One of the most well-known examples is hearing loss resulting from **maternal rubella** (German measles), which occurred in approximately 10,000 to 20,000 children born in the early to mid-1960s. Although a rubella vaccine is now available, other viruses, such as the human immunodeficiency virus (HIV) and cytomegalovirus (CMV), continue to be major causes of congenital sensorineural hearing loss when contracted by the mother during pregnancy. Sexually transmitted bacterial diseases such as syphilis can seriously damage the central nervous system of a developing fetus, leading to intellectual and developmental disabilities, as well as hearing loss. Sensorineural hearing loss can occur as a result of circumstances encountered at any point during one's lifetime. Acquired hearing loss may be due to viral infections such as mumps or due to bacterial infection such as **meningitis**, an inflammation of the tissue covering the brain that can lead to a severe or profound hearing loss in young children and adults. The structures of the inner ear are vulnerable to damage either from the bacteria that caused the disease or from the high fever that often accompanies the illness. In addition, in some cases bacterial meningitis requires treatment with high doses of strong antibiotics that can be **ototoxic** (i.e., poison to the ear). Hearing loss resulting from ototoxicity may be permanent or reversible. Frequent monitoring of hearing is often recommended for individuals being treated with ototoxic medications so that drug type and dosage can be adjusted if changes in hearing are noted.

Meniere's disease is a disorder which can produce hearing loss that is rather sudden in onset. First described by Prosper Meniere in 1861, Meniere's disease is believed to be caused by pressure resulting from the buildup of endolymph fluid within the membranous labyrinth of the inner ear. Both the cochlear (hearing) and vestibular (balance) portions of the inner ear may be involved, or the disorder may be specific to only one region. The classic symptoms associated with Meniere's disease are fluctuating and progressive sensorineural hearing loss, tinnitus, vertigo, and a feeling of fullness in the ear. In addition, symptoms typically come and go unpredictably, and may be so severe that the person must lie still until he or she feels better. There is no known cure for Meniere's disease, but drug therapy, surgical intervention, and changes in diet to reduce symptoms have all been used with varying amounts of success.

Another type of inner ear disorder, referred to as **auditory neuropathy spectrum disorder (ANSD)**, has received considerable attention in recent years. In general, ANSD is characterized by normal outer hair cell function (as seen in normal otoacoustic emissions) and abnormal responses from the inner hair cells or auditory nerve fibers (as seen in an abnormal auditory brain stem response). A lack of synchrony in the firing of auditory nerve fibers in response to sound appears to be the underlying problem in these cases. Individuals who have ANSD may exhibit pure tone hearing that is anywhere from within normal limits to profoundly impaired, and this pure tone hearing does not typically correlate well with their real-world difficulties or their potential to develop language. These individuals also usually have considerable difficulty understanding speech, even when their pure tone loss is not significant. According to Berlin et al. (2010), hearing aids are helpful to only a small number of these individuals; cochlear implants have been shown to be helpful to greater numbers of these clients. Some of the challenges in working with individuals who have ANSD is that the diagnosis is often not made in a timely manner (if at all), which means the resulting treatment plan does not provide the needed supports. Also, once the diagnosis is made, there is some disagreement regarding the best treatment approach to use. When working with children who have this disorder, many audiologists start by fitting the child with hearing aids and then monitoring closely the development of the child's auditory behaviors and skills. Lack of progress may lead to a discussion with parents about possible use of a cochlear implant.

Another cause of sensorineural hearing loss is the presence of a vestibular schwannoma, more commonly referred to as an acoustic neuroma. These terms refer to a non-malignant growth that develops on the cells near the VIII nerve. Because of the location of this tumor, symptoms that you might experience include decreased hearing, tinnitus, some type of balance difficulty, and a plugged feeling on the affected side. The particular combination of symptoms and the severity of those symptoms depend on the size of the tumor. Audiologists are trained to attempt to rule out acoustic neuroma as a diagnosis in all cases where a client demonstrates an unexplained unilateral hearing loss and to inform the client's physician when unilateral losses are seen. Diagnosis of this condition is typically made by an ENT or neurologist based on identification of the tumor using MRI. For the majority of individuals who have an acoustic neuroma, surgery is recommended. In addition to removing the tumor, the surgeon's goal is to preserve the patient's hearing and avoid trauma to important surrounding structures, including the facial nerve. In a small number of cases the tumor grows very slowly; for these clients, a wait-and-watch approach may be taken rather than intervening right away.

Let's now turn our attention to a cause of sensorineural hearing loss that in most cases is avoidable: hearing loss resulting from excessive exposure to high levels of sound (noise). We live in an age where we are surrounded by ever-increasing amounts of noise. From machines at factories and construction sites to common everyday items such as power tools, motorcycles, and musical instruments, it is almost impossible to escape noise. It should come as no surprise, then, that **noise-induced hearing loss** is one of the leading causes of acquired sensorineural hearing loss in young and middle-aged adults. Now even children are at risk for noise exposure because many of today's popular toys, electronic games, and ear-level personal stereos emit sound levels that are potentially hazardous. Research now reveals some disturbing facts about personal music devices. Overwhelming majorities of both high school and college students own one, nearly 75% of the college students who own one use it every day, and young people, in general, are not well-informed about listening levels that are unsafe (Danahauer et al., 2012; Punch et al., 2011; Vogel et al., 2010). Exposure to high-intensity sound exposes the delicate structures of your cochlea to considerable stress that may lead to irreversible damage.

Hearing loss that occurs from exposure to high levels of noise can be temporary or permanent. If you experience short-term exposure to a loud sound that causes a hearing loss which recovers spontaneously, you have experienced a **temporary threshold shift (TTS)**. To understand TTS better, think about the last time you went to a loud concert and later noticed a slight reduction in hearing accompanied by tinnitus (ear or head noises). After several hours of rest the ringing noise stopped, and hearing returned to normal. You experienced a TTS. Although we have long believed that TTS is not a problem as long as hearing thresholds return back to normal, research by Truong and Cunningham (2011) suggests that even when hearing ability has returned to normal after TTS, permanent damage to both the cochlea and auditory nerve can be measured.

Now consider the factory worker who is exposed to loud sounds every day? Frequent exposure to high levels of noise over time may eventually lead to **permanent**

threshold shift (PTS). A PTS is typically characterized by a loss of hearing sensitivity in the high frequency range (between 3000 and 6000 Hz). As damage resulting from long-term exposure increases, more hearing is lost, and the ability to understand speech decreases, particularly in the presence of background noise.

The Occupational Safety and Health Administration (OSHA) has attempted to reduce the number of individuals who are at risk for getting PTS; it has established guidelines limiting the amount of time a worker can remain in a high-noise area. In addition, OSHA has policies for the use of hearing protection for workers and the annual monitoring of hearing with hearing testing. Unfortunately, these guidelines are not practical in all cases. For example, military personnel who are exposed to sudden, unpredictable blasts of sound remain at great risk for noise-induced hearing loss.

Finally, most of us will eventually experience some degree of sensorineural hearing loss in our lifetimes through the aging process. This hearing loss is referred to as **presbycusis**, and can be due to loss of cochlear hair cells, reduced responsiveness of the hair cells, or loss of auditory nerve fibers. Because changes that occur with age can affect not just the ear but also the central auditory system, presbycusis may involve not only reduced hearing sensitivity but also deficits in auditory perception. Cruickshanks et al. (1998) estimate that approximately 45% of adults between the ages of 48 and 92 years have some degree of hearing loss, with men demonstrating a higher prevalence than women. Knowing that the elderly population continues to be one of the fastest-growing segments within the United States, it is important that SLPs and audiologists have a good understanding of presbycusis and how it can impact people's lives.

 Thought Question 12.2

What kinds of information might you provide to a teenager who is exposing him/herself to very loud levels of music on a regular basis?

It is very exciting to conclude this discussion of sensorineural hearing loss with information about research conducted by Mizutari et al. (2013). Using mice that were deaf, these researchers demonstrated that they could stimulate certain existing cells so that they would function like cochlear hair cells. This resulted in a partial recovery of hearing. Certainly, our hope is that this type of research will one day lead to a cure for hearing loss due to hair cell damage. Case Study 12.3 presents the narrative of a man with adult sensorineural hearing loss.

CASE STUDY 12.3

Adult Sensorineural Hearing Loss

Michael is a 45-year-old male who has worked in a factory for the past 20 years. Although ear protection is available to him at work free of charge, Michael has decided not to use it because he feels that it prevents him from hearing his coworkers when they speak to him. Michael recently noticed a high-pitched ringing sound in both of his ears and his wife and children have been complaining that he does not hear them, particularly when they're in a noisy environment. During the audiological assessment, Michael is asked about sources of noise exposure other than at his work. In answering these questions, Michael realizes that he has a long history of noise exposure from listening to loud music when younger, use of power tools for home projects, and shooting guns at a shooting range. The audiological exam reveals that the source of Michael's tinnitus is a high frequency sensorineural hearing loss in each ear. Michael is fit with two hearing aids to support his understanding of speech, and he now regularly uses ear protection in all situations involving loud noise. Michael is also provided with a list of communication strategies to further support his understanding of speech in various environments.

Mixed Hearing Loss

If you had a mixed hearing loss, the third general type of hearing loss, you would have the simultaneous presence of conductive and sensorineural hearing loss. For example, if the hair cells of your cochlea have been damaged by listening to loud music through a personal music device, and you have congestion in your middle ear due to a head cold, you have a mixed hearing loss. An older individual with an age-related sensorineural hearing loss who also has impacted cerumen, which temporarily decreases their hearing sensitivity even further, also has a mixed hearing loss. In most cases, the conductive component can be medically treated, leading to some improvement in overall hearing sensitivity. However, because the sensorineural component remains, the person's hearing cannot be restored to normal levels.

(Central) Auditory Processing Disorders

The three types of hearing loss described in the preceding section refer to impairment of the peripheral auditory system or the structures of the ear spanning from the pinna to the auditory nerve. The function of the peripheral auditory system is routinely assessed during a comprehensive audiological evaluation. Because what we hear needs to be processed in order to be useful, audiologists must consider the *entire* auditory system, including problems that affect the central auditory system. This can generally be thought of as the auditory structures, pathways, and neural synapses that span from the level of the brain stem to the cortex of the brain (see Figure 12.4). Problems associated with the central auditory system may or may not cause hearing loss. Often, they interfere with the ability to efficiently and effectively use and interpret acoustic information. This is often reflected in problems such as difficulty hearing subtle differences between similar sounding words and misunderstanding of speech when presented in a background of noise. These types of difficulties in an individual who has normal peripheral hearing are commonly referred to as central auditory processing deficits (CAPD) or auditory processing deficits (APD). Additional information regarding auditory processing is found on pages 366–367 and 380–381 of this chapter.

Hearing Loss Through the Lifespan

With the information covered at this point about the various types of hearing loss, it should now be clear that our hearing is something that should be attended to at all ages and stages of life, beginning immediately after birth. As discussed, newborns may be at risk for hearing loss due to a number of factors, including difficulties that occur during the birth process, genetic disorders, and syndromes. Over the past two decades, we have seen the development of numerous **early hearing detection and intervention (EHDI) programs** across the United States. Some of these programs are state-mandated and some are voluntary. All these programs are designed to identify significant hearing loss in newborn babies and follow up with prompt audiological intervention services. As of 2010, in the United States nearly 98% of babies were being screened for hearing loss within the first month after birth (Centers for Disease Control and Prevention, 2009). The goal is that babies who fail their newborn hearing screening and any follow-up rescreening should have a comprehensive audiological and medical evaluation

Figure 12.4 Schematic representation of the central auditory nervous system.

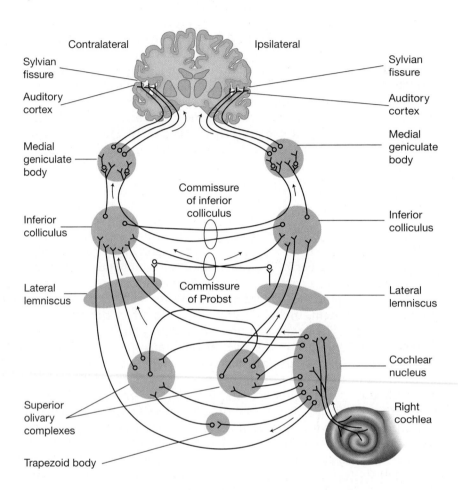

before the age of 3 months to confirm or rule out the presence of hearing loss. Although the diagnosis of hearing losses that are present at birth is occurring at an earlier age in recent years due to these universal newborn hearing screening programs, this is only the first step in the audiological intervention process. It is equally important that appropriate early intervention services be planned and delivered as soon as possible after a hearing loss has been identified, preferably by 6 months. In fact, research strongly suggests that children who are diagnosed with hearing loss and receive hearing aids and early intervention by 6 months of age develop significantly better language skills than do similar children who are identified after 6 months of age as having hearing loss (Meinzen-Derr et al., 2011; Yoshinaga-Itano et al., 1998). For up-to-date information on the status of early hearing detection and intervention programs in the United States, visit the National Center for Hearing Assessment and Management website at http://www.infanthearing.org/

Both newborns and preschoolers are particularly susceptible to hearing loss due to Eustachian tube dysfunction and otitis media, which can create a temporary, but often difficult to resolve, hearing loss that may negatively affect speech and language development. During the school-age years, students with listening difficulties often find themselves struggling to process the more complicated language structures that are part of academic learning, particularly when they are in the poor acoustic setting of the classroom. School-age, adolescent, and college-age students are all now at risk for noise-induced hearing loss due to the widespread use of ear-level music devices that can deliver very intense levels of sound directly to the ear.

By middle age, some adults with a history of early noise exposure begin to experience hearing loss as the effects of noise and aging impact their ability to understand speech. In addition, disorders such as Meniere's disease and otosclerosis are more common in middle-aged individuals. Also, some research suggests that by middle age, listeners may experience changes in their processing abilities, despite having normal hearing.

Finally, in older individuals age-related changes can affect both the cochlear hair cells and auditory nerve fibers, resulting in reduced speech understanding, sometimes even with good amplification. When these auditory changes combine with changes in memory or cognitive function, the effects on communication can be even greater.

 Check your Understanding 12.5

Click here to check your understanding of the concepts in this section.

AUDIOLOGICAL ASSESSMENT PROCEDURES

Now that we have discussed the basic principles of sound, the anatomy and physiology of the auditory system, the various types and causes of hearing loss, and their effect on one's life, we are ready to take a look at how this knowledge is applied in the assessment of hearing. It is important to stress that no single test can accurately capture the full extent of a person's hearing loss or how that loss may be affecting the person in terms of his or her communication or psychological health. Instead, an audiologist must rely on a battery of tests and other measures, combined with careful questioning of and listening to the client, in order to obtain an accurate picture of an individual's hearing problem.

Before continuing, now is a good time to differentiate assessment, as we discuss in this section, from screening, referred to earlier in this chapter. Screening is the process used to determine which individuals, whether children or adults, are *likely* to have a hearing loss. If you ever had your hearing tested in school, it is likely that you participated in a screening. As previously mentioned, newborn hearing screening programs have been set up across the country in an effort to identify infants who are suspected of having a significant hearing impairment and who therefore should be referred for further testing. The screening equipment and procedures used vary with different screening programs. For example, a newborn screening performed in a hospital with automated equipment is quite different from a screening program using a traditional audiometer performed at a senior center. In general, individuals who pass a screening are not referred for further testing, and those who fail a screening are. It is important to note that even if someone does not pass a screening, we cannot conclude that he or she has a hearing loss. Screenings are frequently performed in environments where background noise or distractions can interfere with the person's ability to respond accurately. It is not uncommon for students to fail their school hearing screening but have a comprehensive hearing test done in a sound-treated booth and find normal hearing. Finally, it is important to be aware that performing hearing screenings is part of the scope of practice of both an audiologist and an SLP.

The remainder of this section focuses on the types of tests that may be included in a comprehensive audiological assessment battery, as performed by an audiologist. For students who one day hope to work as SLPs, it is important to remember that as professionals you will need to have an understanding of the hearing assessments that have been performed on your clients and how to use this information to better meet their speech and language needs.

Referral and Case History

Before conducting any tests, an audiologist spends time interviewing a client and collecting case history information. This process provides an opportunity to obtain background information from the client's perspective and helps the audiologist gain a better understanding of the client's communication challenges and goals. During this interview, the audiologist may ask questions about why the client has come in for the evaluation, whether he or she has been exposed to noise, whether there is a history of ear infections or ear surgery, and what communication situations are difficult for the client.

Another way to gain valuable information about a client's communication challenges and feelings about his or her hearing loss is by use of published self-assessment questionnaires. For example, a particular item on a questionnaire might ask the client to rate the degree of difficulty he or she experiences when listening in a noisy restaurant. Another item might ask whether the client feels left out of social activities because of his or her hearing loss. Several of these questionnaires contain a companion version that can be completed by the client's significant other or a family member. Obtaining input from someone the client is close to can be very important, particularly if the client is not fully aware of how much he or she is missing and how much others in the family have to change their speaking pattern to accommodate the hearing loss. Finally, when these self-assessment tools are given before and after a hearing aid fitting, they can provide information about improvements that have occurred due to hearing aid use.

Otoscopic Examination

One of the first procedures performed if you were being seen for an audiological evaluation is a visual ear exam, or **otoscopic examination**. You are most likely familiar with the small handheld device that is used by an audiologist because it is the same device that physicians use to examine the ear canal and ear drum. The device is called an **otoscope**, and the otoscopic exam is an important early step in the assessment process because it alerts the audiologist to any conditions that may interfere with sound conduction during testing, such as excessive cerumen or any conditions that require immediate medical referral, such as drainage from the ear. Another version of this device, called a video otoscope, projects the image of the ear being viewed onto a television or computer monitor, allowing the client and family members to observe simultaneously. This technology allows the audiologist to print and store images that can then be shared with other medical personnel, such as the client's physician.

Electroacoustic and Electrophysiological Testing

Electroacoustic measures record acoustic signals from within the client's external auditory canal; **electrophysiological tests** record neuroelectric responses (nerve impulses) that are generated by the auditory system in response to sound. Both of these categories of tests evaluate the integrity of the peripheral and central auditory systems without requiring the client to provide any observable behavioral responses, such as repeating words or responding to tones. Because these tests do not assess a client's ability to recognize and use sound, they are not considered true hearing tests. Nevertheless, these tests do provide data that an audiologist can use to make some inferences about the functioning of the client's auditory system and his or her hearing.

The two types of electroacoustic measures that are commonly performed on children and adults are tests of acoustic immittance and otoacoustic emissions.

Acoustic immittance measures are useful in the diagnosis of conductive pathology. Because they can be completed in a short period of time and do not require any behavioral responses, they are frequently used with both children, including infants, and adults. Acoustic immittance testing is performed using an electronic device that assesses the admittance of the middle ear as a function of changes in air pressure within the ear canal. This process results in a graph called a **tympanogram** (see Figure 12.5). Data obtained as part of this process can assist in identifying the presence of conductive pathology and distinguishing between a break in the ossicular chain, otitis media with effusion, or a perforation of the eardrum, for example.

Otoacoustic emissions (OAEs) are a second type of electroacoustic measure that has received considerable attention during the past two decades. Discovered by David Kemp (1978), otoacoustic emissions are low-intensity sounds, commonly referred to as "echoes," that are generated within the cochlea as a result of movement of the outer hair cells. These tiny emissions move outward from the cochlea through the middle ear to the external auditory canal, where they can be recorded by a microphone placed in the ear canal. For clinical uses, otoacoustic emissions are produced by presenting a moderate-intensity acoustic stimulus to the ear canal and then determining if the emissions were present or not. Generally, when OAEs

Figure 12.5 Schematic of three common tympanogram patterns: (a) normal middle ear function, (b) somewhat reduced admittance due to otosclerosis, (c) minimal admittance due to otitis media with effusion.

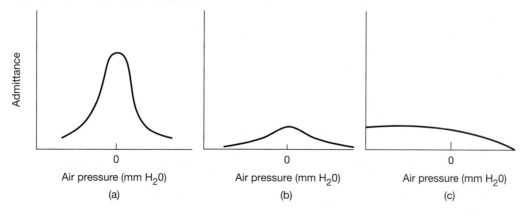

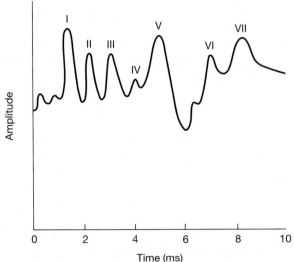

Figure 12.6 Schematic drawing of a typical auditory brain stem response (ABR) waveform for a normal ear.

are present hearing sensitivity is presumed to be normal or no worse than a mild loss (Glattke & Robinette, 2007). Perhaps the most important use of OAE testing is in newborn hearing screening programs. This noninvasive and quick test has provided an inexpensive and efficient way to test millions of newborns each year.

In addition to electroacoustic tests, several electrophysiological tests are available to audiologists. Recall that electrophysiological tests record neuroelectric responses (nerve impulses) generated by the auditory system in response to sound. These responses are collectively referred to as **auditory evoked potentials (AEPs)**. To measure these neuroelectric responses, small electrodes would be placed on your head and sound would be delivered to your ear. These tiny responses are captured and recorded using specialized computer equipment, and the pattern that is generated would be compared to normative data. **Auditory brain stem response (ABR)** test is commonly used to assess the neuroelectric activity of the auditory nerve and structures in the lower brain stem in individuals suspected of having neurological issues, such as a tumor on the eighth cranial nerve or auditory neuropathy/dyssynchrony disorder. In addition, it can be used to estimate the auditory thresholds in individuals who are unable or unwilling to be evaluated using conventional behavioral techniques, such as infants, young children, and individuals who have developmental delays. Because this testing can often be conducted while a child sleeps, it is often used as part of newborn hearing screening programs.

Behavioral Testing

One major limitation of electroacoustic and electrophysiological measures is that although they provide information about the integrity of the auditory system, they do not provide information on how the individual perceives or responds to sound. For this reason, testing a person with behavioral measures is necessary to fully understand a person's ability to hear and process sound.

Most behavioral tests are administered using a specialized piece of electronic equipment called an **audiometer**, which contains controls that allow an audiologist to select, manipulate, and present various stimuli, such as tone and speech, to assess hearing. Testing is usually carried out in a specially treated sound booth that limits the amount of external and internal noise that can interfere with hearing; this supports the reliability of the test results.

Behavioral Observation (BO)

The most basic form of behavioral assessment used with infants is a process referred to as **behavioral observation (BO)**. As the term implies, an audiologist presents a stimulus such as speech or tones through a loudspeaker and observes the child's reaction. Basic responses to sound that the audiologist looks for are gross body movements such as startling, widening of the eyes, and facial grimacing. Although fairly simple to administer, BOA has been criticized for its poor reliability and validity (Hicks et al., 2000). Audiologists often have difficulty making judgments about whether a child's bodily movement was in response to a stimulus or was just a random movement. In addition, a child may quickly habituate to the task, losing interest in it after only a few presentations of the stimulus. For these reasons, electroacoustic and electrophysiological measures are preferred over BOA when assessing children younger than 5 months of age.

Visual Reinforcement Audiometry (VRA)

Once a child reaches the age of 5 to 6 months, the natural ability to localize, or turn toward a sound, has developed, and this means an audiologist can use a technique called **visual reinforcement audiometry (VRA)** to test behavioral responses to speech and frequency-specific tones. With VRA, the child is rewarded for turning toward the stimulus. As soon as the child responds, the audiologist activates an animated or lighted toy. This reinforcement helps maintain the child's interest in the task, giving the audiologist more time to collect hearing data. VRA is more reliable than BOA, and has been shown to be an effective tool for accurately assessing hearing sensitivity in young children (Diefendorf, 1988). Despite the value of VRA, most audiologists would combine VRA test results with an electrophysiological measure prior to fitting a child with hearing aids.

Pure Tone Audiometry

By $2^1/_2$ years of age, a child should be able to perform many of the same procedures that are used with adults, but often with some modifications. For example, when testing a child's responses to pure tones, rather than ask a child to raise his or her hand or press a response button, **conditioned play audiometry (CPA)** is often used. This procedure involves the use of toys such as blocks, puzzle pieces, or stacking rings to engage the child in a listening game. The child is conditioned to put a block in a bucket or a ring on a post each time the test signal is heard. Conditioned play audiometry can be used until a child is able to be tested using conventional pure tone audiometry, which usually occurs somewhere around the age of 5 to 8 years.

A great deal of information can be obtained about a person's hearing through **pure tone audiometry**. In fact, the pure tone test is considered to be one of, if not *the* most fundamental behavioral tests in the standard audiometric assessment battery. **Pure tones** are sounds that contain energy only at a single frequency. Standard practice is to test a range of frequencies from 250 Hz to 8000 Hz so that information is collected about the person's ability to perceive the speech sounds of the language. The purpose of pure tone testing is to determine a person's threshold at each test frequency for the right and left ears. **Threshold** is defined as the lowest (quietest) intensity level, measured in decibels, at which a person can just barely detect a given stimulus approximately 50% of the time.

An example of a blank audiogram is shown in Figure 12.7. To help orient the reader to the audiogram, let's discuss briefly some of the frequency and intensity characteristics of sound in the environment and in speech. Chirping birds, for example, tend to be low in intensity but quite high in frequency. In contrast, an air conditioner has much greater intensity and is low in frequency. Both a lawn mower and large truck create high-intensity and low frequency sounds. Regarding speech sounds, vowels have their primary energy in the lower frequencies, whereas stops and fricatives are high frequency sounds.

Degree of Hearing Loss

At this point, it will be helpful to discuss briefly the degree of hearing loss. As noted previously in this chapter, when describing a person's hearing loss audiologists use terminology such as *conductive*, *sensorineural*, and *mixed* to specify the region of the auditory system affected. These terms describe the type of hearing loss a person has. Although this is a critical part of the diagnostic process, it is also important to quantify the degree of hearing loss, and this is typically expressed in units called decibels (dB). A decibel is a mathematical unit based on the pressure exerted by a particular sound. The lowest decibel level at which a given sound

Figure 12.7 Blank audiogram used to record patient thresholds in pure tone audiometry. Note frequency in hertz on the *x* axis and intensity in decibels on the *y* axis.

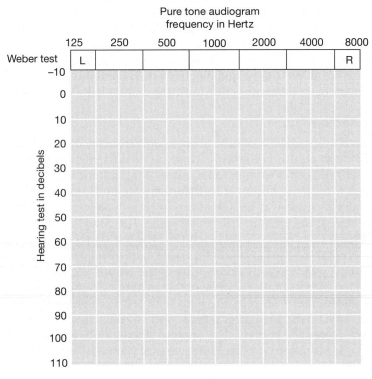

is barely audible represents a person's auditory threshold. The greater the decibel value required to reach a person's threshold (compared to what is considered "normal"), the greater the degree of hearing loss.

Many audiologists use the terms presented in Table 12.1 to label the degree of hearing loss (HL). Notice that the range considered "normal" is different for children than for adults. Specifically, although adult thresholds up to 25 dB HL are considered within normal limits, the cutoff for children is set at 15 dB HL. Think for a moment about why this makes sense. What is different about the process of hearing for children than for adults? According to Bess et al. (1998), children who are in the process of developing speech and language may miss some of the subtle information found in the acoustic speech signal when auditory thresholds are in the 16 to 25 dB range. Adults, in contrast, typically experience no difficulty with these thresholds because their language is more developed, and they have a better ability to "fill in" missing pieces of information that they did not hear. They do this using their prior knowledge and experience. This process is referred to as *auditory closure*.

In general terms, individuals whose degree of hearing loss falls within the slight/mild-to-severe range are classified as *hard of hearing* or *hearing impaired*. These individuals depend on their remaining hearing (also referred to as *residual hearing*) for receptive communication and for the learning of new concepts. For people whose auditory thresholds fall in the profound range, however, the auditory system provides limited or no access to speech without the use of amplification. As previously mentioned, these individuals are often referred to as *deaf*.

It is important to note that the descriptors used in Table 12.1 should be interpreted with caution. For example, both research and clinical observation reveal that children with mild hearing losses are more likely to have delays in receptive and expressive vocabulary, phonological awareness, and syntax (grammar). In addition,

TABLE 12.1

Degrees of hearing loss

Threshold	Degree of Hearing Loss		Description
	Children	Adults	
−10 to 15 dB HL	Normal	Normal	
16–25 dB HL	Slight	Normal	Children who are in the process of developing speech and language may miss some of the subtle nuances of speech.
26–40 dB HL	Mild	Mild	Difficulty with faint or distant speech.
41–55 dB HL	Moderate	Moderate	Difficulty following conversational-level speech.
56–70 dB HL	Moderately severe	Moderately severe	Can hear only loud speech.
71–90 dB HL	Severe	Severe	Difficulty understanding even loud speech without amplification.
>90 dB HL	Profound	Profound	Usually considered deaf; without amplification, cannot depend on auditory system alone to obtain information.

Audio simulations of different degrees of hearing loss are available at http://www.starkey.com/hearing-loss-simulator.

they are more likely to have reduced speech understanding in noise and are at risk for emotional health difficulties.

Air Conduction and Bone Conduction Testing

It is very important for students to understand that during hearing testing, pure tone thresholds are established by delivering pure tones in two different ways: through **air conduction** and **bone conduction**. Air conduction testing is administered while a client wears earphones delivering the sound to the cochlea via the outer and middle ear. This is the typical way that we hear. Hearing loss resulting from disorders in any of the three major sections of the peripheral auditory system (the outer, middle, or inner ear) will be identified with air conduction testing. Once air conduction testing is completed, the process is repeated using a bone oscillator, a small vibrating device that is positioned against the skull, behind the pinna. When a stimulus is presented through the oscillator, the bones of the skull are set into vibration, and this vibration directly stimulates the cochlea. So, with bone conduction the person is able to hear the stimulus even though it has bypassed the outer and middle ears.

By comparing the results of air conduction testing to those obtained from bone conduction testing, it is possible to identify the type of hearing loss. Take a look at the audiograms in Figures 12.8 and 12.9. In Figure 12.8, the right ear air

Figure 12.8 Audiogram representing a moderate conductive hearing loss in the right ear. (Note: The symbol used to denote bone conduction thresholds depends on the method used to assess it.)

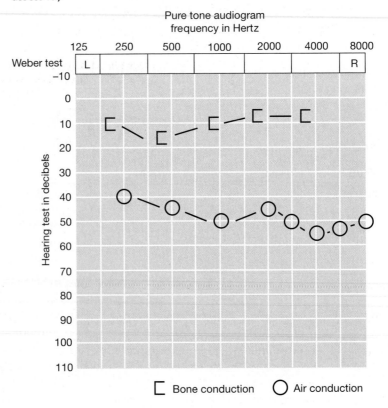

Figure 12.9 Audiogram representing a moderate sensorineural hearing loss in the right ear.

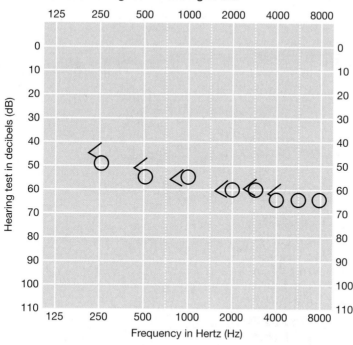

conduction thresholds (represented by the circles) fall within the mild to moderate hearing loss range. However, the bone conduction thresholds (represented by the brackets) fall within the normal range of hearing. From this, the audiologist can infer that the client has difficulty hearing sound when it is introduced in the conventional manner—that is, through the external auditory meatus. Notice, however, that the client has no difficulty hearing sound if the outer and middle ear are bypassed and the cochlea is stimulated directly. Therefore, this client has a conductive hearing loss occurring in the outer or middle ear. In Figure 12.9, both the air and bone conduction thresholds fall outside the normal limits and within the moderate to severe range of hearing loss. Because the results are the same when the inner ear is stimulated by air conduction or by bone conduction, the audiologist can conclude that the inner ear itself must be affected. Therefore, this client has a sensorineural hearing loss.

In Figure 12.10, again both the air and bone conduction thresholds fall outside the normal range. However, the degree of hearing loss represented by the air conduction thresholds is greater than the degree of hearing loss represented by the bone conduction thresholds. In this case, although there is obvious damage to the inner ear, as evidenced by the bone conduction results, the person has the potential to hear better if the outer and middle ear are bypassed. Therefore, there is evidence that both a sensorineural and a conductive hearing loss exist simultaneously. In other words, the client has a mixed hearing loss. You can find the latest information about hearing disorders and hearing loss at the National Institute on Deafness and Other Communication Disorders (www.nidcd.nih.gov) website. Use the search box provided and type in your topic of interest or choose from several featured topics in the middle of the home page.

Figure 12.10 Audiogram representing a moderate to severe mixed hearing loss in the right ear.

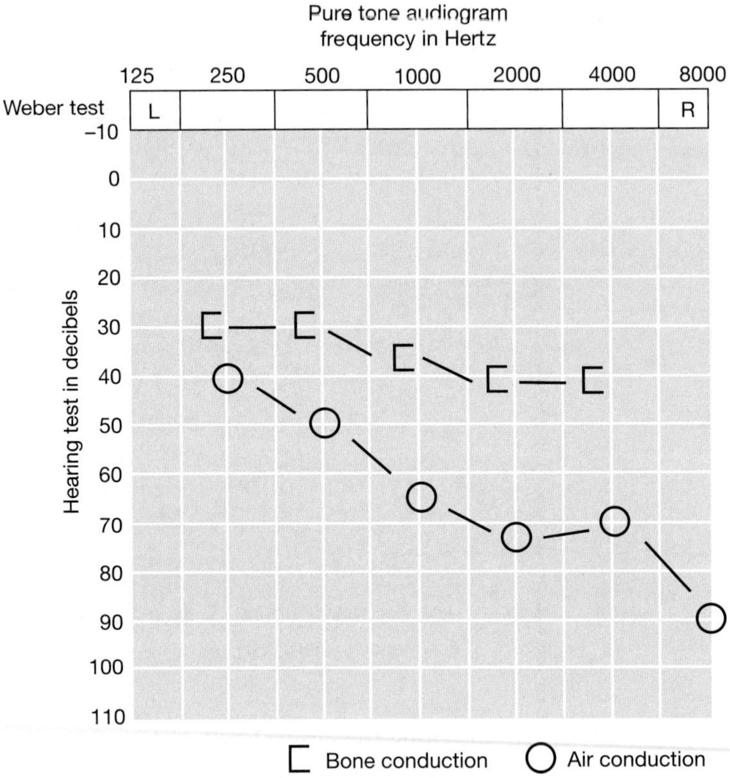

Pure tone audiogram
frequency in Hertz

Weber test	L						R

Bone conduction   Air conduction

Speech Audiometry

Although pure tone audiometry is often considered to be the most fundamental component of an audiological evaluation, we must keep in mind that people typically seek the services of an audiologist because they are having difficulty understanding speech, not pure tones. It is only natural, then, that we evaluate a client's ability to hear and understand speech as part of the assessment battery.

A variety of tools are available to assess a client's auditory skills for speech. Two speech audiometry measures that are typically included in routine hearing tests are the Speech Recognition Threshold and the Word Recognition Test. The **Speech Recognition Threshold (SRT)** is a measure of the lowest (softest) intensity where a person can recognize two-syllable words, and the **Word Recognition Test (WRT)** assesses how well a client is able to identify one-syllable words presented at some level above the threshold.

Auditory Processing Assessment

According to ASHA (2005) and the American Academy of Audiology (2010), tests of auditory processing can be used on school-age children to determine if they have a fundamental impairment of their central auditory processing system. The tests used are different from those used during the conventional hearing test, and often involve testing the client's understanding of speech in challenging conditions, including in a background of noise, as well as when more than one piece of information is presented simultaneously. Sometimes non-speech tests are also used in an effort to reduce the impact of language on the client's performance. The ASHA document states that tests of auditory processing should not be done on individuals younger than seven years old or on those who have language or cognitive deficits that could interfere with the test results.

To understand some of the important issues related to this topic, it may be helpful to review briefly the earlier use of tests of auditory processing. Years ago, before advanced imaging techniques such as CT scans and MRIs were readily available, tests of auditory processing were used with patients to identify what brain regions might be impaired and to provide some information about the kinds of tasks that were challenging to them. A person, for example, with a tumor on the right side of the brain would demonstrate a different pattern of responses on these tests than would someone with a tumor on the left side. Similarly, a person with a temporal lobe problem would perform differently than would someone with a frontal lobe impairment.

Today, tests of auditory processing are used most often by audiologists not on patients with medical issues such as tumors or strokes but rather with school-age children who are experiencing difficulties functioning in the classroom. These children may be demonstrating some of the following: distractibility, difficulty comprehending rapid speech or speech in poor acoustic environments, difficulty following complex auditory directions, or difficulty paying attention.

Despite the great interest and increased awareness among professionals and the public about CAPD, the disorder remains controversial for a number of reasons. First, individuals who have deficits of the central auditory system often demonstrate a variety of different symptoms, and often those symptoms are the same as or similar to those associated with other disorders, such as learning disabilities, language impairment, and attention disorders. This raises the question as to whether the auditory processing diagnosis is truly a unique disorder.

Second, if the language and cognitive testing that are done prior to performing tests of auditory processing are not thorough, a child with language, learning, or cognitive deficits may perform poorly on the auditory processing tests and that child may be misdiagnosed as having an auditory processing disorder. Such a child would then not receive the appropriate diagnosis and resulting intervention to address their difficulties.

Third, the current literature includes greater awareness that processing of auditory stimuli involves many systems (e.g., auditory, language, cognitive) and it is difficult if not impossible to create tests that assess only auditory abilities. It is also more widely understood that although there are children who demonstrate normal peripheral hearing with reduced listening abilities, tests of auditory processing may not be the most effective tools to identify such children.

Fourth, there is a tendency for the public to believe (incorrectly) that an auditory processing deficit may be the underlying cause of other disorders, such as autism or attention deficits. The important point to note here is that even though individuals with autism and attention deficits frequently display problems in their ability to understand/process auditory information, the fundamental, underlying cause of their processing difficulty is neurological, not auditory.

Finally, this testing is controversial because there is still a lack of evidence from research regarding how to improve the way the auditory processing system works. It is understandable that this would be frustrating to parents who are seeking to help their children.

For information regarding support for children who have been diagnosed with auditory processing disorders or who are suspected of having listening difficulties, see pages 380–381 of this chapter.

 Check Your Understanding 12.6
Click here to check your understanding of the concepts in this section.

HELPING PEOPLE WHO HAVE HEARING LOSS

Before beginning the next section of this chapter which addresses ways to help individuals who have hearing loss, it may be helpful to preview the information that follows by briefly describing four broad ways that audiologists can help their clients.

One of the first and most important things that audiologists can do when meeting a new client is to listen to the client. This may seem like an obvious and simple thing, but too many professionals are very good at telling clients what to do, yet not very good at listening to what clients have to say. When we listen to our clients we not only learn a great deal of information about their perspective of the challenges that they face, but we also communicate respect to them and start to build a rapport with them that will enhance the effectiveness of any other recommendations we make.

As experts in matters related to hearing, audiologists are in a unique position to provide valuable information to clients about their hearing and ways to decrease their communication difficulties. Sometimes this information not only serves to inform the client but also to ease some of the client's fears. For example, clients who are concerned that because they have a hearing loss they will one day lose all of their hearing will likely be comforted in knowing that their hearing loss has been stable for the past several years and that sudden changes in hearing are not likely. In addition to providing information to clients, audiologists can, with client permission, also provide information to family members, friends, parents, teachers, caretakers, etc. The more broadly the audiologist can provide information to people with whom the client comes in contact, the more knowledgeable these communication partners will be and the greater the support the client will have.

It is very important for audiologists to put in writing specific recommendations that they have for the client. This does not mean that the client will agree to pursue all of the recommendations, but it is important for audiologists to document a management plan that they believe will be beneficial for the client. The types of things that audiologists regularly recommend, and which are discussed in this chapter, include hearing aids or cochlear implants, the use of assistive devices such as an amplified telephone, and the use of communication strategies.

It is the ethical obligation of any clinician to make a referral to another professional when the client needs something that the clinician cannot provide. For example, for people with conductive hearing losses, the audiologist would most likely refer the client to a medical professional. If the client reports difficulty coming up with the funds to pay for new hearing aids, the audiologist might refer the client to a local agency that does charitable work. If the audiologist notes that a client would benefit from therapy by a trained counselor, the audiologist could make such a referral.

Aural (Audiological) Habilitation/Rehabilitation

After an audiological assessment has been completed and various tests analyzed, it is time to work with the client in creating an appropriate course of treatment. In some cases, this requires a referral to a physician for a medical evaluation. It may also involve various therapy services referred to as **aural (or audiological) habilitation/rehabilitation**, which can be defined as "intervention aimed at minimizing and alleviating the communication difficulties associated with hearing loss" (Tye-Murray, 2009, p. 2).

Before discussing the specific intervention options available, it is important to differentiate the terms *aural habilitation* and *aural rehabilitation*. **Aural habilitation** refers to intervention conducted with individuals whose hearing loss occurred at an early age and therefore prevented normal development of auditory and spoken language skills. In general, this refers to services and therapies used primarily with children who are prelingually hearing impaired and also their families. In contrast, **aural rehabilitation** refers to services and therapies provided to individuals who have lost their hearing later in life, after spoken language skills have fully developed. In this case, the focus is on preserving and restoring communication skills that have been negatively impacted by a loss of hearing. Frequently, the term *aural rehabilitation* is used to refer to both habilitative and rehabilitative aspects of intervention, as is done in the remainder of this chapter.

An important early step in the aural rehabilitation process is to work with a client to gain detailed information about his or her communication problems resulting from the hearing loss. This can usually be accomplished by synthesizing information obtained from the case history interview, self-assessment questionnaires, and results of the audiometric test battery. In some cases, collaboration with medical personnel, SLPs, special education teachers, teachers of those who are deaf and hard of hearing, psychologists, and vocational rehabilitation counselors may also be needed in order for the rehabilitation plan to be strong. By identifying the specific needs of the individual and selecting treatment methods using principles of evidence-based practice, both the client and the clinician can feel confident that the rehabilitation process will be based on the best available information.

Counseling

At this point, it is important to discuss briefly the critical role of counseling. Although counseling can be used from the very first minute that you meet a new client, it is introduced here because our efforts to help an individual with communication challenges related to a hearing loss (or any communication disorder) can be enhanced considerably if we use effective counseling techniques. Counseling is an essential component of all the audiological services we provide.

Counseling is usually thought of as the process of giving a client information, sometimes referred to as **informational counseling**. Some examples of this include explaining the results of individual tests, providing technical information on the anatomy of the ear, or explaining how hearing loss occurs so the client can better understand the nature of his or her problem. The audiologist might also present possible courses of treatment, including hearing aids and rehabilitation options, to support spoken communication. This type of counseling is critical and requires great skill on the part of the clinician so that information is communicated in a way that is easily understood and remembered. It has been reported that only 50% of the information conveyed by health care providers is actually remembered by clients, and that approximately half of this information is remembered inaccurately (Kessels, 2003; Margolis, 2004). For this reason, it is a good policy to provide a written summary of information discussed so that the client can refer back to it. Some clinical providers are now providing clients access to a website where they can find information that specifically relates to their condition.

Although important, informational counseling is only one part of the counseling process. A second broad category of counseling is **personal adjustment counseling**, which involves providing assistance to the client and family in dealing with the emotional consequences of hearing loss. As noted earlier in this chapter, hearing loss can have a profound impact on a person's psychological, social, and emotional well-being. Clients may struggle as they try to come to terms with feelings of anger, anxiety, fear, frustration, and despair that are a direct result of their hearing loss. These feelings are often seen not only in the client but also in others who are in close contact with the individual, such as parents or a spouse. Often, unless these individuals receive support from an empathetic clinician, they cannot move forward to address their communication problems.

Most audiologists and SLPs are comfortable providing informational counseling because they feel confident that they can provide accurate information about the factual aspects of hearing loss. Personal adjustment counseling is more intimidating to many clinicians because it involves skills that many of us believe are less well developed. It is important to note that the literature on personal adjustment counseling clearly indicates that one of the most important skills we can use as clinicians is to be good listeners. An audiologist, then, must pay close attention to what a client reports and what questions the client asks in an effort to uncover any underlying personal adjustment issues. The audiologist must try to distinguish between the client's request for factual information and the client's need for the audiologist to acknowledge some personal feelings the client is having about the hearing problem (English, 2007).

Personal adjustment counseling involves encouraging clients to "tell their stories" of what it's like to live with a hearing loss. Eventually, as a rapport develops between a client and an audiologist, the client can be helped to accept and assume ownership of the hearing loss and move forward to solving his or her communication challenges. Simply telling a client what he or she should do will not lead to progress if the client does not first acknowledge and accept the fact that a problem exists.

Some final points regarding counseling should be made. First, clinicians must attend to the client's/family's cultural background and linguistic needs so that appropriate and effective communication is used (Scott, 2000). Second, audiologists should provide counseling whenever the opportunity presents itself, not only at the conclusion of a clinical session. Finally, clinicians should always be aware of their professional boundaries. When you suspect that a client is dealing with potential psychological or mental health issues that are beyond those related to the hearing loss, a referral to a qualified professional counselor should be made.

Amplification

Amplification is considered the core of most aural rehabilitation plans. For this reason, one of the first steps in the aural rehabilitation process is the selection, fitting, and evaluation of amplification. In most cases, amplification consists of **personal hearing aids**, although other amplification options, described later, are also available.

Hearing Aids. Hearing aids come in a variety of styles and sizes, ranging from tiny custom-made models that fit entirely in the ear canal to custom in-the-ear models that fit into the concha region of the pinna to slightly larger instruments that are worn behind the ear (see Figure 12.11). Regardless of the style, every hearing aid contains certain basic components: a microphone, an amplifier, a receiver, and some type of computer processor. The microphone picks up acoustic energy from the environment, converts it to an electrical signal, and sends it to the amplifier. The amplifier increases the voltage of the electrical signal and sends it to the receiver, which in turn converts it back into acoustic energy and routes it to the user's ear canal.

There have been numerous advances in hearing aid technology in recent years. Nearly all hearing aids dispensed today incorporate sophisticated digital signal processing. Sound entering the hearing aid is converted into a digital code that can be processed and manipulated in various ways to improve audibility while also reducing unwanted background noise and eliminating acoustic feedback (the annoying "whistle" that hearing aids sometimes create). Most modern hearing aids are programmed by an audiologist using a computer and special software. The primary goal in most hearing aid fittings is to make speech audible to the user to improve intelligibility. This is not a simple task because, unlike with eyeglasses which, in many cases, can restore a person's sight to 20/20, a hearing aid will not return hearing to normal.

Let's consider for a moment a person whose hearing loss prevents him from hearing some sounds at all and for whom other sounds are softer than usual. Obviously, this will interfere greatly with his ability to understand speech. But if audibility is the main problem, the use of hearing aids should be quite helpful because they amplify the specific sounds that he is missing. Once this person has access to those sounds, he will hopefully understand speech much more easily.

Unfortunately, however, in some cases clients report that their hearing aids have made things louder but not clearer, and they still cannot understand speech. These individuals may be experiencing distortion due to the type of damage they have to their auditory system. The intelligibility issue that results from this is more difficult to resolve, and the audiologist may need to provide strategies and supports to be used in conjunction with the hearing aids to increase speech understanding. In some cases, an SLP can be very helpful in providing communication strategies to address these clients' needs. When a person is considering whether to purchase amplification, he or she must be counseled so that his or her expectations for improvement remain realistic.

 Video Exercise 12.1

Checking the Functionality of Hearing Aids

Click on the link to watch a video about styles of hearing aids, and complete an exercise.

Figure 12.11 Styles of hearing aids.

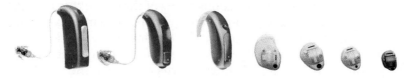

(Photographs courtesy of Oticon Hearing Instruments)

We mentioned previously in the chapter that most conductive hearing losses can be treated with either medication or surgery. In cases where conductive hearing loss is not medically treatable, such as a chronically draining ear, use of a bone conduction hearing aid may be useful. This device consists of a headband and bone vibrator attached to a conventional hearing aid. With the bone vibrator placed against the skull, sound is converted to mechanical vibration that stimulates the inner ear, bypassing the impaired outer or middle ear. A newer version of this device, called a **bone-anchored hearing aid**, functions in the same manner, but rather than having to wear the device on the head, a small external device containing a microphone and other electronic components attaches to a screw that has been surgically implanted into the skull, directly behind the pinna.

A new and disturbing trend related to hearing aids is the emergence of companies that sell hearing aids on the Internet. In some cases, hearing aids are sent directly to the consumer, along with fitting software, and the client is expected to program his or her own hearing aid! This is certainly not in the client's best interest, and audiologists must continue to educate the public about the role of audiologists in successful hearing aid fittings (Bramble, 2013).

Cochlear Implants. Some people with severe to profound hearing losses receive little or no benefit from traditional hearing aids because these devices fail to provide enough amplification to make sound audible. For this group of individuals, a cochlear implant (Figure 12.12) may be an option. A cochlear implant is a prosthesis designed to bypass the damaged hair cells of the cochlea and directly stimulate the surviving auditory nerve fibers with electrical energy.

A cochlear implant consists of externally worn and internally implanted components. The external components are the microphone and speech processor, which are typically housed in the same unit (and worn either behind the ear or off the ear), and the external transmitter. The internal components include the receiver–stimulator that is surgically attached to the skull and a group of electrodes that are inserted into the cochlea. The microphone of the cochlear implant picks up sound, converts it to electrical energy, and transmits it to the speech processor. The speech processor is a sophisticated microcomputer that is programmed for each client so that the information sent to the impaired ear includes those features of the speech signal that are critical to understanding speech. The signal is sent through a cable to the external transmitting coil that is magnetically secured to the head. Using FM radio waves, the signal is transmitted across the skin to the internal receiver–stimulator and finally to the individual electrodes implanted in the cochlea. Modern cochlear implants contain multiple electrodes that provide electrical stimulation to many sites along the basilar membrane, allowing the client to receive information of different frequencies. The resulting neural impulses are transmitted to the brain in the usual manner, by way of the ascending auditory pathways.

In the past, when the procedure was more invasive, only one ear was selected for implantation, even when there was significant hearing loss in both ears. Today, due to improvements in the internal components of the device that has made it less traumatic to the cochlea, bilateral implantation has become more common in children and adults in an effort to improve overall hearing ability, particularly in noise. Also, in some cases a client may choose to wear a cochlear implant on one ear and a hearing aid on the other ear. This might be the case when the cochlear implant is not successfully delivering certain frequency information. This is referred to

Figure 12.12 Components of an ear-level cochlear implant. (a) Internal and external components of a cochlear implant. (b) External components of a cochlear implant positioned on the head and ear: Microphone and speech processor (located behind the ear) and external transmitter. (c) Internal components of a cochlear implant: Receiver stimulator (surgically attached to skull) and electrode array inserted into the cochlea.

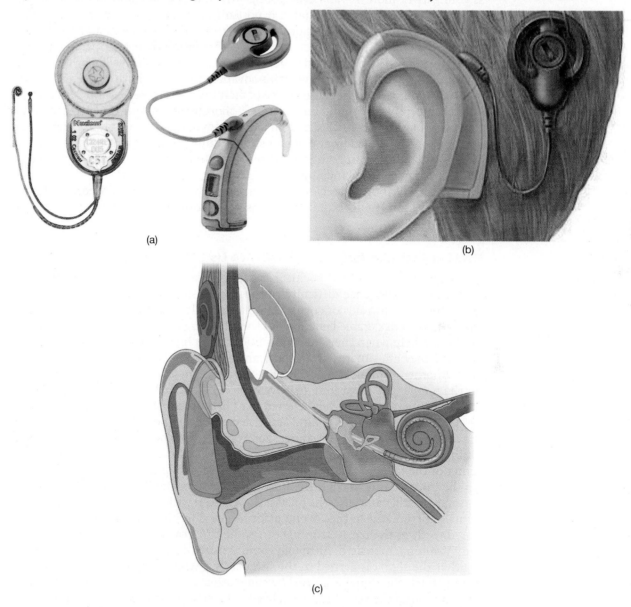

(a)

(b)

(c)

as bimodal hearing because both acoustic "hearing aid" and electrical "cochlear implant" stimulation is used. Another option that now exists is a hybrid device that makes use of both hearing aid and cochlear implant technology within the same unit. Such a device can now also be used on individuals who have severe high frequency hearing loss that cannot be addressed with hearing aids. The cochlear implant component of the device is used to address the high frequency hearing loss, and the hearing aid component provides amplification to those frequencies where hearing is less impaired.

When cochlear implants were originally introduced, only adults who were post-lingually deafened were candidates for them. Today, cochlear implant surgery is routinely conducted on children with severe to profound hearing loss who are as young as 12 months—and even younger in certain cases—and adults of all ages, including those with prelingual and postlingual onset. The success of cochlear implants with adults who became deaf postlingually may be related to the fact that they acquired spoken language skills before losing their hearing and are able to use this knowledge when interpreting the auditory cues provided by the device. Children are who deaf do not have this advantage, but they have a different advantage; they do not have the same degree of auditory nerve degeneration because they have been deprived of sound for a relatively short period of time compared to adults (Won & Rubinstein, 2012). Children who are implanted at an early age and receive intensive auditory therapy also demonstrate significant gains in speech perception, language acquisition, speech production, and literacy development (Papsin et al., 2000; Waltzman & Roland, 2005).

Communication strategies often serve as a very effective addition to the use of amplification. Table 12.2 summarizes some common strategies with rationale for their use.

Hearing Assistive Technology/Assistive Listening Devices

Although hearing aids and cochlear implants provide benefit in many situations, clients often experience difficulty in specific environments or specific situations where their hearing aids or cochlear implants are less helpful. For example, people who receive considerable benefit from their hearing aids regularly report that they need more help when they are communicating in high levels of background noise or when they are situated at a significant distance from the person they want to hear. Another example is a client who hears speech very well except when talking on the phone. Use of various assistive devices can be helpful in overcoming these problems, and are collectively referred to as hearing assistive technology (HAT).

One of the principles behind assistive devices is to position the microphone of the device close to the sound source. For example, an older person sitting in a noisy dining room at the nursing home where she lives can place a microphone at the center of the table so that the intensity of the speech of her conversation partners will be increased more than the unwanted noise in the background. Similarly, a person who still can't hear the television well even with his hearing aids can attach a small microphone to the TV and place receivers in his ears. The TV signal is then sent directly to the receivers in his ears so he can hear it without the need to have the TV volume increased. Although some assistive devices are still "wired," meaning that the signal is carried to the listener by a wire, many use wireless technology in which the signal is carried by some other means, such as a radio signal. In addition, often the signal can be delivered directly to the listener's hearing aids or cochlear implant.

One type of assistive device that is very popular, particularly in educational settings, is a personal **FM system**. Such a device operates on the same principle as conventional FM radio. The talker speaks into a lapel or headset microphone attached to a small body-worn transmitter that "broadcasts" on a frequency or channel. The listener receives the FM signal through a receiver tuned to the same FM radio frequency as the transmitter. In cases in which the person uses a hearing aid or cochlear implant, this receiver can be plugged directly into the hearing instrument.

TABLE 12.2

Rationale for common communication strategies for individuals who have hearing loss

Communication Strategy	Rationale
Reduce the distance between yourself and the person with whom you are speaking.	As sound travels it decreases in intensity, so it makes good sense to be sure that the distance between the speaker and the listener is reduced. In addition, high frequency sounds cannot travel as far as low frequency sounds, and many people with hearing loss have greater hearing loss in the high frequencies. Finally, most hearing aids become less effective when sound is coming from more than 4 to 6 feet away.
Use the visual modality.	Most communicators gain with least some information by watching the face and body gestures of the person with whom they are speaking. For listeners, this means that they should be attending to these nonverbal cues, and for speakers, it means that they should not be speaking with their hand in front of their face or while chewing food. Other examples of the great value of the visual modality include the use of texting and email by people with hearing loss.
Reduce background noise.	One of the most common concerns expressed by individuals who have hearing loss is that they have difficulty following conversations when in a noisy or crowded environment. This most likely occurs because noise tends to cover over or "mask" important speech sounds that the listener is relying upon to understand the message. In addition, hearing in background noise requires greater attention and memory skills. Many people with hearing loss choose their social activities and the location of these activities based on the noise levels in the particular environment. For example, it would be particularly difficult for a person with a significant hearing loss to follow conversation with friends at a bowling alley, even if wearing effective hearing aids.
Use context clues.	If you are speaking with a person who has hearing loss and you begin your conversation by saying "I'd like to talk to you about our vacation plans," you have provided that person with context. The value of this for the listener is that he or she now knows that the vocabulary that you will be using will be related to the topic of vacation. This increases the listener's ability to predict some of what you might say and fill in some information that may be missed based on their knowledge of the topic. Another example of using context is the employee who reviews the agenda before the meeting begins. By familiarizing herself with the focus of the meeting, she can better follow the conversation even if she does not hear all of it.
Use assistive devices.	As discussed in this chapter, there are a variety of assistive listening devices that can allow individuals with hearing loss to have access to information that may be difficult to deliver using hearing aids alone. One of the problems that arises when audiologists recommend assistive devices is that some individuals with hearing loss believe that hearing aids alone (which typically are costly and not covered by insurance) should meet all of their hearing needs. Despite the additional expense involved in purchasing assistive devices, research is clear that such devices can sometimes reduce the challenges imposed by hearing loss in ways that hearing aids cannot.
Communicate your needs to your communication partners.	It is important that individuals who have hearing loss be proactive in providing to their communication partners specific suggestions that will facilitate their understanding of the spoken message. The suggestions could be related to the manner in which the partner is speaking (e.g., "Please slow down," "Please don't speak when chewing") or related to the environment ("Can we move to a quieter location,?" "Please do not speak to me from another room").

Sound field amplification is similar to a personal FM, except that instead of broadcasting the signal to individual receivers, the signal is sent to loudspeakers placed around the room. With sound field systems, all students in a room can benefit from the device, including those with fluctuating hearing loss due to otitis media, those who have attending issues, and those with language impairments.

A number of other assistive devices are available for use with telephone listening. Many clients purchase amplified telephones so that they can adjust the volume of the incoming voice to meet their hearing needs. In recent years, the availability of email, text messaging, synchronous chat, and videoconferencing have been very helpful for those who have difficulty using the phone. Captioning has recently become available for phone use. The telephone of the listener includes a small screen where the talker's message is displayed in written form. Shaw (2012) reports that engineers at the University of Washington have developed a new cellphone program called MobilASL that is able to broadcast communication between ASL signers. When available, the program will be able to be used "on any 3G phone and can be integrated into any mobile device that has a camera on the screen side" (p. 22).

Assistive devices are also helpful for individuals who want to be alerted to sounds occurring from a distance. For example, a new mother who is concerned that even with her hearing aids on she might not hear her crying infant from another room can use a system that will alert her when the baby is crying by activating a flashing light. Such devices are available to visually alert a person of a ringing phone, an alarm clock, and a smoke detector.

Before leaving this topic of assistive technology and devices, brief mention should be made of the term *connectivity*. On a basic level, this term can refer to allowing a person who wears hearing aids to wirelessly access auditory information from a device such as a television, telephone, or computer directly into the aids. More broadly, this term refers to being connected not only with other devices but also with other people in ways that were not possible in the past due to hearing loss. As Beck and Fabry (2011) note, advances in consumer electronics have led to the development of new opportunities for individuals who have hearing loss and hearing aids to successfully access new information and new interactions with others. As an extension of this, the term *tele-audiology* refers to the use of electronic and telecommunications technology to provide distance audiology services. This is particularly important for clients who have difficulty getting to an audiologist for services, such as those who have poor health, lack transportation, or live in remote areas.

Auditory Training and Auditory Communication Modality

Once a client has been fitted with an appropriate amplification device, he or she may need to learn (or relearn) how to make sense of what is being heard through some type of guided listening practice. This process is referred to as auditory training. The goal of auditory training is to maximize a person's use of his or her **residual hearing** to enhance their perception of speech and non-speech cues (Schow & Nerbonne, 2007). Particularly in young children, improvements in these skills should lead to progress in other areas, including speech and language development, cognition, reading, and learning.

The principle of **neural plasticity** is very important to our understanding of the process of auditory training. Neural plasticity, as it relates to the auditory system, refers to physiological and functional changes within the central nervous system in response to auditory stimulation (Greenough, 1975). By providing certain types of auditory input on a regular basis, we hope to change the way the central auditory system works and thereby improve the individual's ability to make effective use of speech and language information that is delivered by the peripheral auditory system. Because there is a greater likelihood that we can change a younger central auditory system than an older one, early identification and early intervention must remain high priorities in our profession.

Before discussing three cases to illustrate how auditory training might differ with various clients, it is important to note that each of the following clients (or their parents, in the case of children) has decided to pursue a communication modality that is auditory-based. In other words, regardless of the degree of hearing loss, these clients (or their parents) have decided that they want their main method of communication (or their child's) to emphasize speaking and listening. Choosing to make use of auditory information is rarely in question for individuals who have mild or moderate hearing losses, because hearing aids are usually very successful in giving such clients access to the important speech sounds in our language. But in cases where the hearing loss is severe to profound, some individuals may choose to use a visual communication system, such as sign language, as their primary communication mode. In recent years, as hearing aids and cochlear implants have become more effective and identification of hearing loss has occurred earlier in life, greater numbers of individuals with very significant hearing losses and parents of such children are choosing to develop auditory skills and use oral English. Those who support this choice believe that this will help these individuals integrate more easily into the hearing world and will enhance their social, educational, and employment opportunities. With these concepts in mind, we now discuss three cases—Case Studies 12.4, 12.5, and 12.6—to illustrate the application of auditory training programs. As you review these cases, note the importance of the following factors: the age of the client, the degree of hearing loss, and the age at which the hearing loss occurred. Case Study 12.4 and Case Study 12.5 present the stories of two different children with hearing losses, while Case Study 12.6 focuses on an elderly man's hearing loss.

CASE STUDY 12.4

Child with Congenital Sensorineural Hearing Loss

The first case is a child who was born with a severe sensorineural hearing loss in each ear. He was identified by an audiologist at 5 months of age and was fitted with hearing aids by 6 months. He also started receiving speech and language services by 6 months of age. Because of the child's degree of hearing loss and in order to make use of the neural plasticity of the child's system (discussed previously), the aural rehabilitation program will be developmentally-based and intense. It will most likely start with basic awareness of environmental sounds and then move to discriminating different sounds.

Of course, work will be done on speech sounds, moving from consonants and vowels to syllables, words, phrases, sentences, and eventually connected discourse. Labeling what is heard will also be part of this training, along with work on comprehension of spoken messages. In some philosophies, this work is done without allowing the child to use any visual cues, like watching the speaker's face; in other approaches, both auditory and visual cues are used together. Parents would most likely be given tasks that they could work on at home in the normal course of communicating with their child.

CASE STUDY 12.5

Five-Year-Old with High Frequency Hearing Loss

The second case involves a 5-year-old girl who was born with a mild high frequency sensorineural hearing loss in each ear. Because of the mild nature of the loss, it was not identified until the child was $4\frac{1}{2}$ years old, as part of a pre-K hearing screening. The child also had a speech-language evaluation and exhibited some speech sound errors of the /s/, /t/, and /k/ sounds; some vocabulary deficits; and some delays in the use of certain morphological markers. For this child, two hearing aids would be critical in order to provide her with access to the high frequency sounds she is missing. Also, an FM device would be beneficial in the classroom to help her understand the teacher's voice in noisy conditions and when she is listening from a distance. In addition, speech and language therapy would be necessary to build her vocabulary, work on morphological markers, and provide articulation therapy. Parents would be most likely encouraged to read to their daughter regularly to support vocabulary development. You can see that this program of aural rehabilitation is less intense than that described in the previous case, but note that even this mild loss has negatively affected the child in several ways.

CASE STUDY 12.6

Elderly Man with Moderate Sensorineural Hearing Loss

Finally, consider a case involving an adult who was born with normal hearing in each ear but now, at age 74, finds himself with a moderate sensorineural hearing loss, due to his age and a history of noise exposure. Although retired, he is very active, doing volunteer work each week and enjoying a robust social life with friends and family members. This client has become somewhat discouraged at the effect that his hearing loss is having on his life, and he is now ready to use hearing aids. In addition to use of the aids, his aural rehabilitation program would most likely also include teaching him about barriers in the environment that could interfere with his speech understanding. These include background noise, poor lighting, and distance. He also will need to learn to politely let others know what they can do to improve his ability to understand. For example, he can request that a communication partner speak more slowly or move to a quieter part of a room. He can also ask the speaker to look at him when speaking. Finally, the audiologist will most likely talk to this client about the value of using context to support his understanding of speech. By using prior knowledge about the topic of the conversation, he can fill in missing information. With this in mind, the audiologist may suggest that this client ask his communication partners to start conversations by telling him the general topic.

One popular program that has been used with adults who have hearing loss and are wearing hearing aids is the Listening and Communication Enhancement program by Sweetow and Sabes (2006). This program can be used at home on the client's computer and includes practice listening in noise, with rapid speech and when more than one speaker is talking. Research suggests that many individuals who use this program improve their ability to understand speech in various conditions.

Visual Communication Modality

The three cases just discussed were about clients whose focus was to use oral English as their primary means of communication. There are, of course, clients who choose to use a visual system of communication. As noted previously, these clients typically have hearing loss that is in the severe to profound range. This choice could be based on cultural factors related to an allegiance to the Deaf community. For example, some parents who are deaf believe that the use of ASL with their deaf child will help that child gain acceptance into the Deaf community, which will be beneficial to the child's social and emotional development. In other cases, this choice may be made because the client's hearing loss is so great that he or she is not able to learn oral English sufficiently for it to be a functional and efficient communication system. As noted earlier in the chapter, audiologists and SLPs must respect the choices that their clients make.

A helpful tool for understanding the options and differences among the visual approaches is the continuum found in Figure 12.13. Note that manually coded English signing systems are at one end and ASL is at the other. ASL is a language unto itself, with its own unique set of grammatical rules; it is not a visual form of English. ASL is often described as a conceptual language because a single sign can convey an entire thought. Unlike ASL, which is a natural language, forms of **manually coded English (MCE)** were developed for use in educational settings with children who are deaf to expose them to certain grammatical markers such as *-ed* and *-ing*. Some believe that this exposure to English language structures, which are not explicitly used in ASL, support the development of English literacy skills and overall academic achievement. In MCE much of the vocabulary comes from ASL, but the word order is the same as it is in oral English. Because of this, English can be modeled using both visual and auditory modalities at the same time.

Pidgin Signed English (PSE) is usually the type of manual communication taught in basic sign curricula for hearing people interested in learning to sign. New users of PSE tend to communicate using a structure that is more English-like, whereas experienced users tend to incorporate more features of ASL. One final popular form of manual communication to be mentioned is **fingerspelling**, which consists of hand shapes used to visually represent each of the 26 letters of the English alphabet. Although this would not be a very efficient way to communicate,

Figure 12.13 Sign language continuum.

Manually Coded English Signing Systems	⟶	*American Sign Language (ASL)*
Signed Exact English (SEE)	Pidgin Signed English (PSE)	
Word meaning is NOT considered (e.g., the word "right" will have the same sign regardless of context)	Signs used are more conceptual. One word may have many signs depending upon meaning.	Has its own vocabulary, grammar, and sentence structure. One sign may represent an entire thought.
All grammatical markers (articles, auxiliary verbs, plurals, etc.) are signed.	Grammatical markers may or may not be signed.	Does not have specific signs for grammatical markers.
	Facial expression and gestures are incorporated.	Facial expression, body position, space, and repetition are used extensively.

fingerspelling is very helpful when used in conjunction with ASL, PSE, or MCE systems to communicate proper names, technical vocabulary, and other English words that have no known signs.

To view samples of ASL in action, visit the Signing Online website: www.sign-ingonline.com. Click on the dictionary tab to the left and enter a word of your choice. Then, on the right side of the page, view a video of that word being signed.

Treatment and Management of (Central) Auditory Processing Disorders

Regardless of whether an audiologist accepts the view of central auditory processing described by ASHA and the American Academy of Audiology, we do know that there are individuals who have normal peripheral hearing and difficulty understanding speech under certain difficult conditions. These conditions could involve hearing in noisy or reverberant environments as well as understanding rapid speech or speech that is presented with an accent, for example. It is the responsibility of the audiologist and speech pathologist to attempt to help such people.

ASHA and AAA recommend that three broad areas of intervention be used in attempting to support these individuals. These areas include modifying the environment, teaching compensatory strategies, and providing direct auditory therapy.

Environmental accommodations refer to changes we can make to the listening environment that will improve a listener's ability to receive auditory/verbal information clearly. Some examples of environmental accommodations include adding carpeting or drapes to a classroom in an effort to reduce noise and reverberation, seating the individual closer to the sound source, fitting the individual with a personal FM or sound field system, or providing written notes to supplement verbal information. Accommodations may also include instructional techniques such as speaking clearly at a moderate rate, providing clear and concise directions, using familiar vocabulary and age-appropriate sentence structure, breaking multistep directions into smaller segments, and use of hands-on activities that include visual supports.

Work on compensatory strategies is designed to strengthen other broader cognitive areas, such as attention and language. This could include work on using memory and organizational techniques, using linguistic and contextual cues, and developing problem-solving strategies.

Finally, direct therapy consists of intensive auditory training, designed to attempt to strengthen the specific auditory deficits identified during the assessment. Although some authorities believe that this formal training of specific deficit areas has great potential, currently there is a lack of evidence that such training alone can result in changes in the functional communication abilities of students who have CAPD. For this reason, many of the recommendations made by audiologists focus on improving the listening environment and building other cognitive areas.

One final point should be made about CAPD. The role of an SLP in working with children who have or are suspected of having a listening or processing disorder is critical because students' challenges frequently show up at school where complex messages need to be understood and listening environments tend to be poor. In addition, even if the auditory processing diagnosis is valid and does apply to a student, one of the primary methods of supporting this student's listening and learning will be by increasing his language competence. For example, increasing his vocabulary and understanding of sentence structure will decrease the likelihood that he will experience communication breakdowns. In his 2011 article addressing students diagnosed with CAPD disorders, Kamhi states that our approach to helping these students should be the same as that used with students who have language and learning disabilities. In addition, thorough testing of these students' speech, language, and literacy skills is urged, including higher-level language abilities such as problem-solving and inferencing. In addition, Kamhi states that testing should be completed by the psychologist in order to assess areas of working memory and attention and to identify undiagnosed learning issues.

Box 12.1 summarizes some of the evidence-based research that validates the exciting progress being made in audiology for the benefit of children and adults with hearing and balance difficulties.

 Thought Question 12.3

How might the recommendations that we might make for a person with a hearing loss be similar to those that we might make for a person with unexplained listening deficits?

BOX 12.1 | Evidence-Based Practice in Audiology

Auditory Neuropathy Synchrony Disorder

A comparison of males and females diagnosed with ANSD revealed that females tended to demonstrate poorer hearing, poorer speech understanding, and less significant help from hearing aids compared to males. (Narne et al., 2016)

Tele practice

Efforts to reach more individuals who have hearing loss and live in remote and rural communities include the use of Tele practice. Williams-Sanchez et al. (2014) and Margolis et al. (2016) have studied a hearing screening and hearing threshold test that can be done at home. The screening test, called the US National Hearing Test (NHT), is performed over the phone, with the client responding to a series of tones. The test results were found to yield data that were consistent with conventional auditory measures. The threshold test, called the Home Hearing Test (HHT), requires the patient to respond to tones presented through the personal computer, and these results were found to be consistent with hearing thresholds measured in a clinic.

Cochlear implants

- Although in the past cochlear implant surgery had resulted in destroying the remaining hearing in the implanted ear, new surgical techniques available today allow some hearing to be preserved. Sheffield et al. (2015) found that using amplification in the implanted ear can result in improved hearing compared to the use of a cochlear implant alone.
- Saxena et al. (2015) investigated the availability of online social media sources related to cochlear implants, and found more than 350 sources. Facebook and Twitter were the most active sites, but other sources included YouTube, forums, and

blogs. Researchers also report that these online tools can be the source of important information for users as well as personal support.

Hearing aids

- The hearing aid effect was identified in the literature in 1977, and refers to the negative perceptions attached to individuals who wear hearing aids. Using a very similar research design as that of the original study, Rauterkus and Palmer (2014) investigated whether the hearing aid effect still existed to the same degree as in the past. The researchers found that individuals wearing hearing aids were not seen as more negative than individuals wearing non-hearing aid devices, such as earbuds or Bluetooth. This suggests that the hearing aid effect is lessening.
- Many individuals who are told that their hearing loss is mild are hesitant to purchase hearing aids. Johnson et al. (2016) reviewed the literature regarding the effects of hearing aids on adults who exhibited mild sensorineural hearing loss. The data supported the effectiveness of such devices.

Assistive technology

Individuals who wear hearing aids or cochlear implants regularly report that they receive considerably more benefit in quiet environments and that speech understanding in noise remains particularly difficult. Recent research demonstrates that the use of a remote microphone placed on the body of the conversational partner, typically below the mouth, significantly improves hearing in noise by directing speech to the hearing aids without significantly increasing the background noise (Rodermerk & Galster, 2015; Wolfe et al., 2015).

Check Your Understanding 12.7

Click here to check your understanding of the concepts in this section.

SUMMARY

The profession of audiology is a diverse field that offers opportunities to work with many populations in a wide variety of settings. An audiologist has the responsibility to assess auditory and vestibular function and to provide aural (audiological) habilitation/rehabilitation services. A hearing loss is caused by an interruption at one or more points along the auditory pathway from the outer ear to the brain. The three types of hearing loss that affect the peripheral auditory system are conductive, sensorineural, and mixed. Audiologists are also concerned with problems affecting the central auditory system, including the auditory areas of the brain stem and brain. Problems along these pathways generally result in an inability to use and interpret auditory information efficiently and effectively, referred to as auditory processing disorder.

When describing hearing loss, audiologists use terminology such as conductive, sensorineural, mixed, and central to identify the portion of the auditory system that is affected. Another important set of terms describes the degree of hearing loss measured in decibels. Each degree of hearing loss corresponds to a specific decibel range. Individuals with hearing loss in the slight/mild to moderately severe range are often referred to as hard of hearing or hearing impaired, and depend as much as possible on the use of residual hearing for communication. For people with profound hearing loss, often referred to as deafness, the auditory system provides little or no access to sound without proper amplification.

When evaluating the auditory system, audiologists rely on electroacoustic, electrophysiological, and behavioral measures. They administer a battery of tests to identify the presence of a hearing loss, determine its type, quantify its degree, and assess its impact on communication. Informational and personal adjustment counseling are critical to the process.

Aural (audiological) habilitation/rehabilitation refers to the services and procedures that are designed to minimize and resolve communication difficulties presented by a hearing loss. Aural habilitation refers to therapies that are used primarily with children to teach missing communication skills, and aural rehabilitation refers to services provided to those who have lost their hearing later in life, after spoken communication skills have been established. The focus of aural rehabilitation is to help the person recover lost skills and to use compensatory strategies effectively. Areas typically considered in creating an individual aural rehabilitation program are the evaluation and fitting of amplification and hearing assistive technology, auditory training, communication strategy training, and determination of an appropriate mode of communication.

SUGGESTED READINGS/SOURCES

Bellis, T. J. (2003). *Assessment and management of central auditory processing disorders in the educational setting: From science to practice.* San Diego, CA: Singular.

Clark, J. G., & English, K. (2004). *Audiologic counseling in clinical practice: Helping clients and families adjust to hearing loss.* Boston: Allyn & Bacon.

DeBonis, D., & Donohue, C. (2008). *Survey of audiology: Fundamentals for audiologists and health professionals.* Boston: Allyn & Bacon.

Kamhi, A. (2011). What speech-language pathologists need to know about auditory processing disorder. *Language Speech Hearing Services in Schools, 42,* 265–272.

Tye-Murray, N. (2009). *Foundations of aural rehabilitation: Children, adults, and their family members* (3rd ed.). Clifton Park, NY: Delmar Cengage Learning.

Welling, D. & Ukstins, C. (2015). *Fundamentals of audiology for the speech-language pathologist.* Burlington, MA: Jones & Bartlett.

13 Augmentative and Alternative Communication

James Feeney, Ph.D.

LEARNING OUTCOMES

When you have finished this chapter, you should be able to:

- Define augmentative and alternative communication (AAC)
- Describe various types of aided and unaided AAC systems, access methods, and AAC output
- Identify a number of considerations in AAC assessment

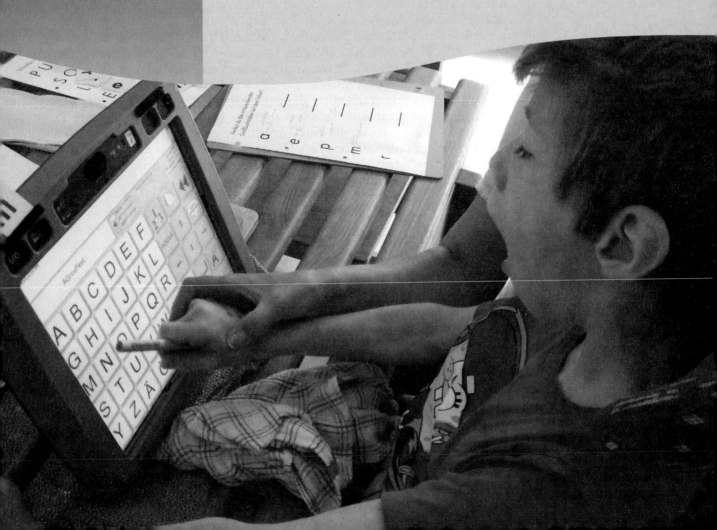

- Describe methods for AAC system selection and the concept of feature matching

- Explain how interactive competence and communicative competence are critical in AAC assessment and intervention practices across the lifespan

DEFINING AUGMENTATIVE AND ALTERNATIVE COMMUNICATION (AAC)

At times, all of us use some form of augmentative and alternative communication (AAC) to communicate, although most of us still rely on speech as a primary means of communication. When you text a friend, in essence you are using a form of AAC. Let's focus for a few paragraphs on what AAC use means to individuals who have difficulty using the speech channel.

As much as it is important to understand what AAC is, it is also important to understand what it is not. A common misconception about AAC is that this area of practice in speech-language pathology focuses solely on the things people use to communicate. To be sure, AAC includes how people use things such as *speech-generating devices (SGDs)* to make known their wants and needs. But limiting the scope of AAC to the objects, electronic gadgets, handheld devices such as tablets and smart phones, or any of the other things a person might use to communicate is like watching your favorite music video with the volume off. Without sound, a viewer can only make use of the visual experience offered in the video, but in doing so, the person only *sees* the artist. Without the benefit of the sounds that make the music, the viewer loses the very essence of what makes the artist's song a song—the music. In a similar way, when viewing or defining AAC, it is necessary to consider not just the things a person uses to get a message across but the interplay between the *communication technologies* used to support individuals with *complex communication needs (CCNs)* and the interactive competence of everyday communication partners.

One of the most useful and broad-based conceptualizations of AAC is found in the American Speech-Language-Hearing Association's (ASHA's) definition of AAC from Special Interest Division 12: Augmentative and Alternative Communication. Based on the work of many professionals (Beukelman & Mirenda, 2013; Glennen & DeCoste, 1997; Lloyd et al., 1997), this definition states:

> Augmentative and alternative communication (AAC) refers to an area of research, clinical, and educational practice. AAC involves attempts to study and when necessary compensate for temporary or permanent impairments, activity limitations, and participation restrictions of individuals with severe disorders of speech-language production and/or compensation, including spoken and written modes of communication. (ASHA, 2005a)

In the definition, the terms *activity limitations* and *participation restrictions* relate directly to concepts found in the World Health Organization's (WHO's)

International Classification of Functioning, Disability, and Health (ICF) framework (WHO, 2001). This framework is used to inform clinical decision making in assessment and intervention planning. In other words, it helps professionals examine a person's ability to use AAC in relation to functional abilities, contextual factors that influence functioning, and other variables that play a part in clinical decision making. While a full review of the WHO/ICF framework is beyond the scope of this chapter, there are several excellent online resources that provide comprehensive reviews of the WHO/ICF framework for interested parties; for example, see www.asha.org and www.who.int.

As noted in other assessments of communication impairment, assessment for AAC use is a team effort.

Although ASHA situates its definition of AAC within the WHO/ICF framework, it also states the following on its website (www.asha.org) in response to the question, "What is AAC?":

> Augmentative and alternative communication (AAC) includes all forms of communication (other than oral speech) that are used to express thoughts, needs, wants, and ideas. We all use AAC when we make facial expressions or gestures, use symbols or pictures, or write.

The statement "We all use AAC . . ." provides a clear connection between AAC and the reader's own experiences in communicating with others. This is an important aspect of the definition of AAC, in that it emphasizes how it is not something that only people with communication challenges use to make their wants and needs known. It is a part of any communication culture, community, group, or setting in which people interact. Put simply, *AAC includes anything that supplements an existing communication system.* Think of your own life and consider the many ways you use AAC each day—the possibilities are endless!

Who Uses AAC?

It is estimated that approximately 4 million people in the United States are not able to use natural speech to express their wants and needs (Beukelman & Mirenda, 2013). While this number does not provide an exact count of people who use AAC, it suggests that there is a large group of people in the United States alone who have the *potential* to use AAC. Other estimates of the prevalence of AAC use in the United States range from 0.8% to 1.3% of the total population (Beukelman & Ansel, 1995). Expressed differently, of the 324 million people who are estimated to live in the United States (www.census.gov), somewhere between 2.5 and 3.8 million of them are not able to communicate with others using natural speech. With such a large number of individuals in mind, it is clearly important for speech-language pathologists (SLPs) and other helping professionals—possibly you in the future—to remain diligent in efforts to collaboratively serve and advocate for individuals who use, or have the potential to use, AAC systems.

All typical communicators augment speech with other means of communication, such as gestures and facial expressions.

Although it is true that we all use AAC in our everyday communication routines in the form of gestures and body movements, texting, and emails, it is also important to accept the premise that "there is no typical person who relies on AAC" (see Beukelman & Mirenda, 2013, p. 4). In fact, there are many groups of people who, for some reason, use AAC and also share a common diagnosis or condition. For example, individuals with developmental disabilities such as cerebral palsy (CP), autism spectrum disorder (ASD), or intellectual disability (ID), may have difficulty communicating using natural speech as a result of the physical, cognitive, and communicative limitations associated with their specific disability. Other

Thought Question 13.1

What is Augmentative and Alternative Communication (AAC)?

individuals who might benefit from AAC include, but are not limited to, people with aphasia, people who have experienced a traumatic brain injury (TBI), people who have undergone a glossectomy or a laryngectomy, and people who have motor speech problems (e.g., dysarthria and/or apraxia of speech).

Throughout human history, people with disabilities have managed to overcome huge social, cultural, and civil barriers to living independent, productive, and satisfying lives. As technology grows with incredible speed, it is necessary to help professionals across disciplines so they can collaboratively support individuals with CCN in their pursuit of *efficient* and *effective* communication with others.

 Check Your Understanding 13.1

Click here to check your understanding of the concepts in this section.

TYPES OF AAC

AAC has long been separated into two well-conceived and broad categories: *aided* and *unaided systems* (Lloyd et al., 1997; http://www.asha.org/NJC/AAC/; http://www.asha.org/public/speech/disorders/AAC/). In general, unaided systems have not been considered to involve any external equipment but to rely only on the individual's body. Aided systems have been considered to include the use of some type of equipment or device, and range from very simple to extremely sophisticated options. In more recent AAC taxonomies used to group AAC systems (e.g., Beukelman & Mirenda, 2013; Schlosser, 2003), however, two major distinctions are noted. First, an additional category for *combinations of aided and unaided systems* is offered. Second, *symbols*, or "anything that stands for or represents something else" (Vanderheiden & Yoder, 1986, p. 15), are viewed as central to the process of classifying AAC systems.

Unaided AAC: Gestures and Vocalizations

Any time a person uses a gesture, a body movement, or an observable signal with a communication partner, he or she is using unaided AAC. For example, imagine talking with a friend about a movie. With each gesture, change in tone of voice, or change in body posture, you are using unaided symbols to send messages to your conversational partner. This does not mean, however, that the *intent* of your message(s) is perceived accurately by your partner! That is another area of exploration altogether.

Manual Sign Systems

Manual sign language is a highly developed form of communication, as is speech. American Sign Language (ASL), for example, is a language that has its own vocabulary and syntax. Other sign systems in use in the United States are translations of English into sign and include Signed English, Signing Exact English (SEE), and Tactile Signing.

Also in this category is Amer-Ind, a gestural or hand communication system that some nonspeaking individuals use. It is a relatively grammar-free, nonsign system involving 250 concept signals. Almost all gestures in Amer-Ind can be made with one hand, making it easier than ASL and other signing systems for those with hemiplegia (i.e., paralysis on one side of the body) or hemiparesis (i.e., weakness on one side).

Some signs are easy to comprehend because they look like what they represent. These signs are called *iconic*. For example, the sign for *drink* in most systems is made by miming drinking from a cup. Unfortunately, few signs are of this type. Signs that are easily guessable, explainable, and memorable are called *transparent*. Amer-Ind has a high proportion of transparent signs. Signs, such as the one for *apple*, which are difficult to interpret, are called *opaque*. Examples of iconic, transparent, and opaque signs are presented in Figure 13.1.

Figure 13.1 Examples of iconic, transparent, and opaque signed English signs.

ICONIC

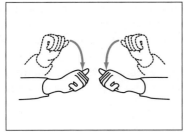

coat

Make an "A" shape with both hands. With thumbs, trace shape of jacket lapels.

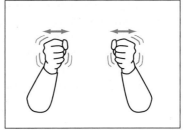

cold *(adj.)*

Make an "S" shape with both hands. Draw hands close to body and shiver.

TRANSPARENT

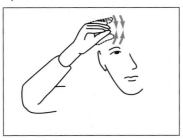

boy

With hand by forehead, snap a flat "O" shape twice, indicating the brim of a baseball cap.

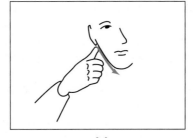

girl

Make an "A" shape with right hand. Place thumb by right earlobe and move down jaw line.

OPAQUE

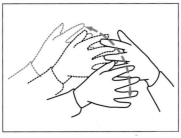

gray

Make a "5" shape with both hands, thumbs up, palms facing body. Move hands back and forth with Ⓡ fingers passing between Ⓛ ones.

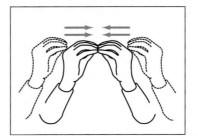

more

Make a flat "O" shape with both hands, fingertips facing each other. Tap fingertips together twice.

Gestural communication systems can be differentiated based on their grammatical structure. As we have discussed, sign languages, including ASL, have their own syntax or grammar, whereas sign systems such as Signed English are based on, and follow, the rules of American English grammar; thus, these systems are not separate languages.

For most deaf signers, fingerspelling is mixed with signs and used for new words or names. Fingerspelling, or the manual alphabet, may be a promising alternative for older clients with both good cognitive and fine motor abilities. The client has ultimate flexibility because any word in the language can be spelled for transmission.

Unaided systems are not appropriate for every individual who needs either to enhance or replace his or her current method of communicating. For example, an individual with severe motor involvement in the limbs, as in some forms of CP, may be unable to make the fine motor adjustments necessary for many signs. Another problem with gestural communication systems has to do with the number of communication partners who understand the system. Unfortunately, many individuals in the community (e.g., outside a signer's home or school environments) are not familiar with signing and may not be able to understand what a signer is trying to communicate.

Aided AAC

Aided systems, in general, range in terms of the representations used within a system, the input and output modes of a system, and the degree to which the symbols in a system are transparent to others. AAC systems also vary according to the amount of technology in a particular system, and while there is some variation in how AAC systems are specifically categorized, in general they are typically grouped within categories described as no-tech, low-tech, mid-tech, or high-tech and can be represented by a continuum of technology (see Figure 13.2). No-tech systems are those that do not involve the use of any technology and use readily available materials or symbols sets (e.g., paper and pencil, gesture systems, Picture Exchange Communication System (PECS; www.pecsusa.com), writing the letters of the alphabet on a piece of paper so the user can spell out a message) or a home-made communication book or wallet with familiar pictures and/or symbols. Low-tech systems are those that are fairly simple to use, often require little or no power source, or electrical components, and contain few moving parts (Mann & Lane, 1991; http://www.ussaac.org/aac-devices). Examples of low-tech AAC

Figure 13.2 Continuum of aided AAC technology, with examples of each.

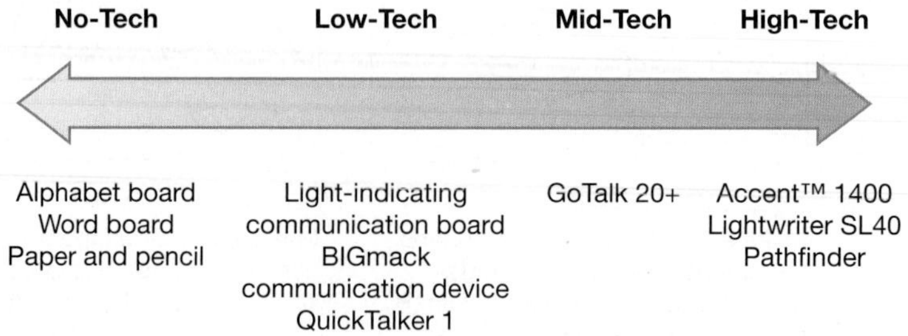

No-Tech	Low-Tech	Mid-Tech	High-Tech
Alphabet board Word board Paper and pencil	Light-indicating communication board BIGmack communication device QuickTalker 1	GoTalk 20+	Accent™ 1400 Lightwriter SL40 Pathfinder

systems include such devices as The BIGmack, the QuickTalker 1, or the iTalk2 with Levels (https://www.ablenetinc.com/technology/speech-generating-devices), to name a few. Mid-tech systems typically use some amount of electrical power, have speech-generation ability, and have limited programming options and capacity to hold stored messages. Examples of mid-tech systems are the GoTalk 20+ or the QuickTalker 23 (http://www.mayer-johnson.com/gotalk-20). High-tech AAC systems are electronic devices that are considerably more sophisticated, require some amount of training related to programming, and make use of computer technology (e.g., software used for speech production). Examples include such devices as Accent™ 1400, the PRiO (https://store.prentrom.com/communication-devices), or the Lightwriter SL40 Connect (https://www.tobiidynavox.com/en-us/products/devices/). Also included in this category are tablet devices, such as the iPad (https://www.apple.com/ipad/) (www.apple.com), or Microsoft products, such as the Surface (https://www.microsoft.com/en-us/surface). For a review of AAC apps for the iPad, see Andrew Leibs' 2016 review at https://www.thoughtco.com/top-alternative-and-augmentative-communication-198828. From the home page, click on the "Learning Centre" tab and then click on "AAC Feature Comparison Grid."

Aided Symbols: Tangible Symbols

Tangible symbols include real objects, miniature objects, partial objects, and artificially associated and textured symbols. Much of what we know about using tangible symbols can be captured under the heading *visual schedules*, originally described by Stillman and Battle (1984) in their work with individuals with visual and hearing impairments. Visual schedules that include tangible symbols, such as real objects, are often organized according to the daily activities that occur in an individual's life. Figure 13.3 shows an example of a visual schedule made up of objects and Picture Communication Symbols for an adult with severe intellectual disability. Similarly, with very young children SLPs may choose to use actual objects, as these are very concrete and may not represent anything beyond the referent displayed. A system called Tangible Symbols (Rowland & Schweigert, 2000) attempts to bridge the gap between actual objects and graphic representations by using objects or pictures that have a clear relationship to the referent. For example, a key might represent *car* or a shoelace might represent *shoe*.

Aided Symbols: Pictorial Symbols

Whether on a communication board or an electronic device, graphic symbols are just as important to aided AAC as words are to speech or signs to signing. Symbols may include pictures, various representational systems, and/or line drawings. Some symbol systems have been specifically designed for AAC use. Graphic symbol systems include iconic representations, such as Picture Communication Symbols (PCS) and some Rebus Symbols; less iconic representations, such as Pictogram Ideogram Communication (PIC); and opaque symbol systems, such as Blissymbolics or spelling. These are presented in Figure 13.3. Symbolic systems are relatively rule-governed and generative, allowing for symbol combination and the creation of new symbols.

Graphic symbol systems may use a variety of means to express different concepts. Rebus symbols are line drawings of both concrete and abstract concepts and

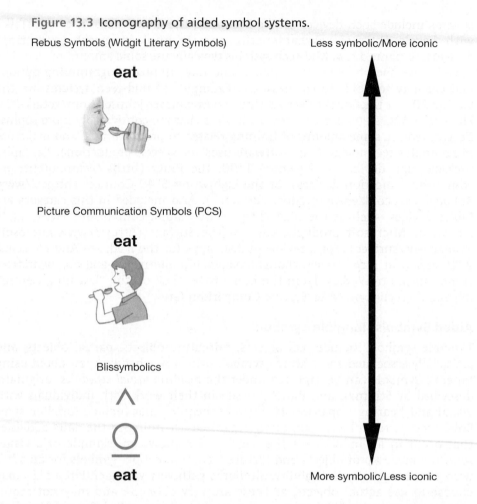

Figure 13.3 Iconography of aided symbol systems.

Rebus Symbols (Widgit Literary Symbols)

eat

Less symbolic/More iconic

Picture Communication Symbols (PCS)

eat

Blissymbolics

eat

More symbolic/Less iconic

Graphic symbols may be selected directly by an AAC user or scanned, with each symbol highlighted in turn until the desired one is reached.

of sound sequences, originally developed as an aid for teaching reading. PIC contains ideograms used to represent an idea rather than the way a referent or concept appears in the real world. Ideograms and symbols, such as those used in Blissymbolics, can be used for abstract concepts just as words can. Blissymbols consist of 100 pictographic representations and arbitrary symbols that can be combined to create words.

Aided Symbols: Orthography and Orthographic Symbols

This category of AAC includes such systems as Braille, fingerspelling, writing, and other ways a person uses symbols for language. English orthography, for example, includes the use of the letters of the alphabet to transcribe thoughts and ideas into words in print. Any process like this, regardless of the language being transcribed, is considered a type of AAC that involves orthography.

Combinations of Aided and Unaided Systems

If there is a common theme among all definitions and classifications of AAC, it is that it is multimodal. That is, people invariably use multiple methods or modes of communication when interacting with others, and AAC is no exception. For example, a woman with severe physical limitations due to CP may use a high-tech AAC system with synthesized speech to express herself in a business meeting. She may also use a letter board and a partner's assistance to spell a quick message while having coffee with a friend. In both scenarios, AAC is appropriately used to address communication goals.

Access

A person's use of an AAC system invariably involves a selection technique or method to *access* the system. Access might include touching buttons, pointing to symbols, or holding an object. The means of access is especially important, and great care must be exercised in choosing the appropriate interface between a client and a device.

Two primary means of access are *direct selection* and *indirect selection*. With direct selection, individuals may select an item in a selection set directly by pointing with a finger, hand, head pointer, optical head pointer, or by operating a joystick. In cases of severe neuromuscular involvement, eye gaze, sometimes referred to as eye pointing, may be used to select symbols. Most people who use communication boards indicate their message by direct selection.

Pointing may be aided by the use of either hand splints or pointing sticks that strengthen or enable the person's response. Optical head pointers may be used with both electronic and non-electronic systems. For example, something as simple as a small flashlight, laser pointer, or penlight attached by a headband to an individual's head can be used to access a communication board (e.g., a letter board). An electronic communication device may have sensors built into the device itself. The optical head pointers used with these devices typically utilize infrared (IR) technology. As the optical head pointer moves across the symbol display, the device's sensors light up, indicating to the user what symbol it is on. When the individual gets to the desired symbol, he or she stops for a predetermined period of time (called *dwell time*). Once the user has rested on that location for that period of time, the device "knows" that the user is selecting that symbol. The dwell time on most devices can be set depending on the needs and abilities of the user.

Individuals using eye gaze may look at symbols on a clear acrylic board located between the user and the communication partner. The user gazes at desired symbols, which appear on both sides of the board.

Direct selection methods can be difficult, especially for those with severe motor problems. The main challenge in using direct selection relates to the person's efficiency and effectiveness. *Efficiency* in this context refers to the speed with which a person is able to use an AAC system to send a message to a partner. *Effectiveness* refers to the degree to which a person is able to use an AAC system to achieve his or her communication goal. Difficulty with access will almost certainly slow the communication process (i.e., decrease efficiency) and, in turn, negatively impact a person's ability to say what he or she wants to say (i.e., negatively impact effectiveness). Although word prediction programs, including context-specific prediction, have been proposed to increase efficient use, there do not seem to be statistically significant process and performance differences in actual performance using keystroke-based measures (Higginbotham et al., 2009).

Indirect selection methods or techniques, such as scanning and partner-assisted selection/scanning, may also be used to access AAC systems. *Scanning* is often an available option in mid- to high-tech AAC systems, and it is suitable for

Thought Question 13.2

Why is it important to consider various forms of aided and unaided AAC systems for people with complex communication needs?

individuals with limited motor abilities. With electronic AAC systems, scanning typically involves a process in which an individual assembles a message through a series of switch activations, during which choices are presented sequentially to the user, who then signals when the desired item in a selection set has been presented. In partner-assisted scanning, the options in a selection set are presented by another person, who might be pointing to symbols on a communication board, while the user signals when the symbol/message he or she wants to communicate has been presented. People with motor limitations can use many different types of input—simple pressure switches, devices with touch screens, pneumatic "sip and puff" switches, and eye blink switches. The type of switch an individual uses depends on his or her particular needs and abilities. Often, an SLP, maybe you, along with an occupational therapist (OT), is involved in selecting the most appropriate type of switch for an individual to use to access his or her AAC system.

Auditory scanning works in a similar way, but in addition to the symbols being presented visually, there is also an auditory cue present. For example, imagine a lunch page on which the device has the symbols hamburger, hot dog, and pizza present. For visual scanning, when those symbols are presented, an illuminated frame appears first around the hamburger. If no selection is made, the frame moves to the hot dog, and then if this selection is not made the frame moves to pizza. To select pizza, when the pizza symbol is highlighted the individual activates his or her switch, and the device speaks the message, "I'd like pizza for lunch today." If the individual is using auditory scanning, the device works as just described here, but with the addition of an auditory cue. So when the hamburger symbol is highlighted, the device says "hamburger." If no selection is made, the illuminated frame moves to the hot dog, and the device says "hot dog." If no selection is made again, the illuminated frame moves to pizza, and the device says "pizza." If the individual activates his or her switch to select pizza, the device speaks the message programmed into that location: "I'd like pizza for lunch today."

 Video Example 13.1

Watch this brief video showing a student with CCN interacting with a teacher in a classroom. Think about how many other ways a person might access an AAC system or an activity with others in order to participate in a learning activity. Which types of aided and unaided communication did you observe the student and the teacher using in this video? Would you characterize the student's AAC system(s) as high-tech, mid-tech, low-tech, or no-tech, and why? https://www.youtube.com/watch?v=mxkzBB4SJ6A]

As mentioned, scanning is a very effective option for individuals with significant motor limitations. However, it can be an extremely slow and laborious process. The majority of an individual's time is spent waiting while extraneous things are presented. Scanning requires extended concentration and has the potential to be very frustrating, especially when symbols are missed and the process must be repeated.

In many cases, *efficiency*, or the speed with which a person is able to assemble a message using an AAC system, can be enhanced by placing symbols so that those that are most frequently used are scanned most frequently. For example, if the cursor or indicator begins at the top of the display and returns there after each symbol selection, then the most frequently used symbols are placed at the top. Obviously, such an arrangement requires that communication partners understand the person's AAC system in order to ensure peak efficiency. Various scanning methods can also increase efficiency (Venkatagiri, 1999), but there are many variables that might impact a person's overall competence in using a scanning system, such as the individual's literacy skills (Roark, Fried-Oken, & Gibbons, 2015), the cognitive profile of the individual, and the display or organizational characteristics of the AAC system (Thistle & Wilkinson, 2017). For example, a person might use a dynamic display that allows for linear scanning, and each possible selection is presented in sequence. This process requires that the individual have the cognitive, visual, and motoric capacity to use the system successfully. In both row/column and group/zone scanning, the user must scan areas and then refine the scan once the desired area has been highlighted. For example, the user might press the switch to begin the scanning process. Rows are lighted in sequence until the desired one is found. The user presses the switch again, and individual symbols within that row are highlighted, one at a time. Once the system highlights the target word or symbol in the person's message, the user triggers a switch to make a selection. In group/zone scanning, the person scans groups of related symbols (group/zone display), such as food items, from which the AAC user then selects the desired symbol.

> In order for AAC training to generalize to everyday use, important people in a user's life should be included in the intervention.

Obviously, the type of access method is as important as the symbol system used. In general, an SLP and a client determine the most efficient and accurate access method given the individual's cognitive and physical abilities, along with the environmental, social, and educational demands of the person's life.

Output

Electronic AAC devices almost invariably have a wide range of outputs that are available to the user. Electronic output or transmission may be as simple as a light over or behind a symbol or as elaborate as a voice and printed message. SLPs help clients to find the most appropriate output for their needs. Several types of output options exist. In some situations, an individual may need written or printed output. For example, at school a device user may need to submit a hard copy of a speech he or she delivered in class, necessitating written output. In many other situations, spoken output or voice output would be most natural and appropriate.

Voice output communication (VOC) can be either recorded or digitized, synthesized, or a combination of both. Because digitized output is actually prerecorded by a person, it is much more natural sounding, and it is relatively easy to age- and gender-match the voice on the device with the individual using it. However, a disadvantage of digitized VOC is that the only output an individual can produce on his or her device is messages that have already been anticipated and programmed, or stored, in the system's memory. In contrast, synthesized speech has more flexibility but often sounds mechanical or robotic. Instead of recording actual words or phrases, the speech synthesizer contains sounds and rules for combining them. Generally, messages are programmed into a device with synthesized speech by simply typing in the words and phrases/messages. The speech synthesizer then converts that text string into spoken output, using the sounds and rules for combining them contained in its program.

In general, AAC systems with voice output capability are designed to facilitate communication by supplementing or replacing the speech of the individual using the system. In some cases, the voice produced by the AAC system is more efficient in facilitating communication compared to speaking. Figure 13.4 lists reasons why AAC may facilitate communication better than speech.

> AAC use can change the communication process in ways that are not always predictable.

Figure 13.4 Why AAC may facilitate communication better than speech.

Simplification of input
  Irrelevant and parenthetical comments eliminated.
  Slower rate permits more processing time.

Response production advantages
  Pressure to speak removed.
  Physical demands decreased compared to speech.
  Physical manipulation of client's hands or other parts of body by trainer is possible.
  Client observation of physical manipulation facilitated.

Advantages for individuals with severe cognitive impairment
  Limited and functional vocabulary.
  Individual's attention easier to maintain.

Receptive language/auditory processing advantages
  Structure of language is simplified.
  Auditory short-term memory and/or auditory processing problems minimized.

Simultaneous processing/stimulus association advantages
  Visual nature of the symbol makes it more obvious.
  Visual symbols have more consistency.
  Duration of symbol is greater than spoken word.
  Visual symbols more easily associated with visual referents.

Symbolic representation advantages
  Supplement speech symbols.
  Symbols visually represent referents.

Source: Based on information from "Augmentative and Alternative Communication," by L. L. Lloyd and K. A. Kangas (1994). In G. H. Shames, E. H. Wiig, and W. A. Secord (Eds.), *Human Communication Disorders* (4th ed.). Boston: Allyn & Bacon.

Compared to natural speech, comprehension of synthesized speech, found on devices such as the Lightwriter SL40, requires increased focused attention by the partner. When attention is divided, partners comprehend significantly less synthesized speech (Drager & Reichle, 2001). In addition, partners tend to respond more slowly to synthesized speech (Reynolds & Jefferson, 1999). Although more research is needed on intelligibility, listeners to synthesized speech can improve their speech-sound perceptions through word recognition training (Francis et al., 2007). Even individuals with severe intellectual disabilities can become more proficient at recognizing synthetic speech as a result of repeated exposure to it (Koul & Hester, 2006). For preschool children, intelligibility of synthesized speech is increased if single words are placed within longer language units, such as sentences (Drager, Clarke, Serpentine et al., 2006).

Decisions on the appropriate type of AAC are made only after careful evaluation. As part of this evaluation, it is important for an SLP, in collaboration with an individual using systems, his or her everyday communication partners, and other members of the assessment team, to identify an AAC system that will change as the communicative needs of the individual change.

 Check Your Understanding 13.2
Click here to check your understanding of the concepts in this section.

ASSESSMENT CONSIDERATIONS

Up to this point in this chapter, a great deal of attention has been paid to terms, concepts, and ideas related to AAC, without specific case illustrations to link these concepts to real people. There is perhaps no more useful way to show this link than in the area of AAC assessment. It will be your responsibility, as an SLP, to pull together all that you know about AAC and the abilities and needs of each individual client. In AAC assessment, it is paramount that an SLP, along with members of the assessment team, understand an individual's cognitive-communicative strengths, the everyday communication routines of the individual, and the barriers and/or facilitators to the individual's successful communication.

In the interaction described in Case Study 13.1, Jackie, an individual using AAC to communicate, employs a range of AAC systems. While reading, try to keep track of Jackie's cognitive-communicative strengths, as this is a useful step in the process of selecting an AAC system.

All members of an intervention team should use an AAC system to provide multiple partners and multiple situations.

CASE STUDY 13.1

An Encounter with Jackie

Jackie is a 26-year-old woman with profound physical impairments secondary to CP, a diagnosis of intellectual disability, and profound speech challenges requiring the use of an electronic AAC system to communicate. My first encounter with Jackie occurred when I was walking down a hallway in a vocational day program for adults with developmental disabilities. Jackie was moving toward me in her electric wheelchair, which she controlled by touching any of four small round switches attached to the lap tray on her wheelchair. As she approached, I noticed some pictures taped to her lap tray. They depicted family and friends engaging in a range of social activities. Jackie's arms were straight and rigid, with her hands in fist-like positions. She stopped her wheelchair in front of me, and I noticed that her entire body was flexing and relaxing, causing her facial expressions to change severely as her body tension changed. Hanging off the side of her wheelchair was a metal apparatus which I assumed to be a device that allowed Jackie to use her head to point to objects or to control her electronic communication device. The device was made of lightweight flat metal bars covered with padding, shaped like a hat designed to fit Jackie's head. It also had a large piece of Velcro hanging from it, which looked like a strap for the pointer to be secured to Jackie's head. The apparatus had a large (approximately 24-inch) protruding piece of metal (about the width of a pencil) stemming from its front. As I would learn, when this device was attached to Jackie's head,

it allowed her to touch buttons on her electronic communication device. Jackie made eye contact with me and vocalized. Her electronic communication device, a Liberator made by Prentke-Romich, was situated about 2 feet from her face, directly in front of her. It was attached via a metal arm bracket connected to the frame of her wheelchair.

It was obvious that Jackie wanted to tell me something. I asked her if I should place the pointing device on her head, and she responded with a loud vocalization and head movement to indicate "no"—or, at least, that was my interpretation of her behavior. I looked at her communication device and noticed that it was not turned on. After a series of fruitless interactions with me in which I attempted to guess what she wanted to say and pointed to pictures of people on her lap tray, I noticed that Jackie was moving her eyes in a well-controlled up-and-down, side-to-side, and sometimes circular motion. As I observed this behavior pattern, a staff member named Stan, who knew Jackie very well, approached. He said, "She's spelling with her eyes." Jackie smiled and vocalized, apparently confirming Stan's statement. I looked closely at her eye movements and noticed that she was, in fact, moving her eyes to "write" letters in space. After about a minute of "eye spelling" to Stan, he said to Jackie, "You missed the bus?" to which Jackie responded with a smile and a vocalization. Jackie had spelled the word *bus* with her eyes to indicate that she had missed the bus to

(continued)

go home. Interestingly, when Jackie used her eyes to spell words, she did so from her perspective, causing a communication partner to observe eye movements from the opposite perspective of Jackie's. In other words, from a communication partner's perspective, the shapes of letters were reversed as Jackie produced them. Imagine two people standing on either side of a window. One person uses a marker to write messages on the window. The person reading the message from the other side would see letters and words backward, making it extremely difficult to decipher messages.

Stan placed the head pointer on Jackie's head, secured the Velcro strip, and asked her what happened. Jackie assembled a message using her Liberator by touching several icons with her head pointer. Jackie's communication device produced the following message: "Eleanor [a staff person working with Jackie] says I'm sick." Stan responded saying, "Eleanor told the bus driver you were sick, so he left without you?" Jackie smiled and vocalized loudly to confirm Stan's interpretation of her comment.

Clearly, Stan's understanding of Jackie's idiosyncratic communication style (i.e., her use of eye spelling) facilitated their interaction. Stan and Jackie seemed to have a shared communication code as they interacted. That is, they both knew that Jackie's

use of eye spelling, an undeniably literate behavior, was the conduit through which communication occurred.

After observing Jackie interact with Stan, I could not help but wonder about the way she learned this unique method of communication. I thought, if Jackie is considered to be a person with intellectual disability, how is it that she learned that she could use her eyes to spell words? I also wondered how Stan learned to interact so competently with Jackie and what I could do to interact competently with her.

Considering all the layers in the interaction described, it is easy to create a list of Jackie's cognitive-communicative strengths. For example, she (a) initiated interaction with an unfamiliar communication partner to solve a problem; (b) demonstrated the ability to solve communication breakdowns with a familiar communication partner and an unfamiliar communication partner; (c) made use of multiple modes of communication in her interaction (e.g., eye gaze, body movements, vocalizations, high-tech AAC system); (d) used her understanding of English orthography to spell single words with her eyes; and (e) used her AAC systems to accurately to convey messages across contexts to communication partners. There are easily 50 more of Jackie's strengths in this interaction.

Jackie's story not only provides an appropriately human element to the topic of AAC assessment, but it allows us to consider how the interactive competence of her partners varied so drastically and directly impacted her communicative success. The emphasis placed on understanding the *competency* of the person using AAC is well described in the work of Light (Light & McNaughton, 2014). Light's framework for AAC assessment includes four competencies that relate to a person with CCN: *linguistic competence, operational competence, social competence,* and *strategic competence.* As Jackie's story suggests, each of these competencies can also be connected to the communication partner and can be used in making intervention-planning decisions.

Linguistic competence is a broad term used to describe an individual's language ability across all dimensions of language. This includes, but is not limited to, a person's receptive and expressive language ability, understanding and use of symbolic representations, and use of linguistic codes across contexts. A person's strengths in the area of meta-linguistic awareness and metacognition would also fall in this area, as they directly relate to how an individual uses an AAC system. Understanding linguistic competence also requires that helping professionals understand the interrelationship between AAC and an individual's culture and background. In other words, exploring a person's linguistic competence should invariably include an understanding of the person's culture and background, because language and culture are inextricably intertwined.

Operational competence has to do with how a person uses an AAC system. For example, a person might need to turn on an electronic AAC system by pressing a button or flipping a switch. Also in this area are procedures such as programming new vocabulary, changing a recorded message, changing a voice setting on the system, and managing software issues.

Social competence relates to how well a person is able to manage the social aspects of communication, such as turn taking, topic maintenance, and using balanced and reciprocal interaction with a partner. Without doubt, a person's use of AAC invariably impacts the social-interactive dynamic between partners in an interaction. Think about how many times you have quickly and effortlessly used a glance, a wave, and one or two words to respond to a friend saying, "How are you?" or "What's up?" or "Yo!" For individuals using AAC, however, "quick" and "effortless" communication can be very difficult to achieve. In many cases, a person using AAC must use the very same communicative resources a person not using AAC uses to respond immediately (e.g., eye contact, hand movements, vocalizations) to access and use an AAC system to create a message. In other words, many of the natural social interactive routines that we all use for efficient and effective interaction with others are simply not available to many individuals with CCN who use AAC.

Strategic competence relates to a person's ability to solve problems. An individual who uses AAC may experience a range of communication breakdowns that require the use of a strategy to manage the breakdown. A strategy in this context is essentially a way to solve a communication problem. For example, a person who uses a mid- or high-tech AAC system might prepare an audible message to be played for unfamiliar communication partners to describe what they can do to help in moments of communication breakdown. Such a message might say, "Please be patient. I use an electronic device to talk, and it takes me a few minutes to say what I want to say. Thank you."

Since the competencies described above were published over two decades ago, advances in AAC have caused Light and other contributors to return to the literature to re-examine and re-emphasize the more general idea of *communicative competence*, which takes into account each competency discussed above in addition to issues such as quality of life, a person's autonomy in using communication that supports the pursuit of meaningful goals, and how communication is a human right (Light & McNaughton, 2014; Light & McNaughton, 2012). A logical extension of this orientation is to include communication partners in the assessment process, given their important role in either facilitating or creating barriers to communication success (Light & Drager, 2007; Blackstone & Hunt-Berg, 2012).

Specific Assessment Considerations

With the emphasis placed on understanding the interactive competencies a person and his or her partners possess, AAC assessments ideally include multi-contextual observations of an individual with CCN. Such observations, along with structured and/or appropriately chosen standardized assessments, are used to provide a

Vocabulary should reflect a person's culture, current needs, and communication potential.

 Thought Question 13.3

How do interactive competence and communicative competence relate to AAC assessment and intervention planning for people with CCN?

comprehensive evaluation. As mentioned, a client's current communication skills are very important. The desire to communicate or to improve communication is often thought to be the basis for AAC intervention and the motivation for learning. Although individuals with severe disabilities have great difficulty making clear and intentional signals, they often create their own individualistic gestures (Chan & Iacono, 2001). The multimodal nature of AAC necessitates a systematic exploration of the roles these gestures and other forms play in communication (Johnston et al., 2004).

As you recall from Jackie's story, one of the roles of an SLP is to determine the communication method (or methods) currently used by a client. This is often more difficult than it sounds, because sometimes the manner in which an individual is communicating is not recognized as communication. For example, a young girl with severe disabilities was frequently observed tapping her cheek after coming in from the playground. It was not until an SLP began to look at this behavior more closely that people realized she was using this cheek tapping to indicate that she wanted a drink. Communication is often demonstrated when an individual engages in a consistent behavior (e.g., cheek tapping) in the same situations over time (e.g., after coming in from the playground). As an SLP, you should attempt to determine the current and future communication needs of a client.

An occupational and/or physical therapist can aid in motor assessment. Of interest are ambulation, or the ability to move about; fine-motor dexterity for signing or pointing; range of movement, especially of the upper limbs; motor imitation skills; and the consistency and accuracy of motor responses. Data in these areas are extremely important in determining the appropriate aided or unaided system and the placement and size of graphic symbols.

> For children with good manual motor control, signing may offer a good means of communication.

Visual and auditory acuity and perception are important for system selection and intervention. Vision and motor skills are used to decide the size of graphic symbols. A vision specialist is an invaluable member of the team in assessing these abilities.

Occasionally, the environment will not support the use of AAC. Caregivers may be uncomfortable, feel inadequate, or just not want to be involved. An SLP may need to educate caregivers about the benefits of AAC to the client and to the home or school. Explaining the likely course of intervention may increase caregiver comfort levels.

> Caregivers are part of an AAC intervention team.

Finally, an SLP is interested in collecting a list of client preferences and possible symbols to train. Likes and desires of the client are important for intervention. This information can be gathered from client responses or choices, from caregiver suggestions, or through observation of the client. This portion of the assessment can be very positive, with the focus on communication potential rather than on impairment. It is especially important for those with acquired communication disabilities, such as dysarthria, in which the focus tends to be on loss rather than potential (Insalaco et al., 2007). A positive shift is welcome.

The actual assessment is only a first step. An SLP, in coordination with a client's family members and other professionals, such as the occupational and physical therapists, audiologist, vision specialist, psychologist, rehabilitation engineer, and/or classroom teacher, uses the data from the assessment to make decisions on the appropriate AAC method, AAC symbol system, and potential vocabulary. These decisions will be adjusted and modified as the client progresses. A good fit increases the likelihood of success.

Check Your Understanding 13.3
Click here to check your understanding of the concepts in this section.

AAC SYSTEM SELECTION OR FEATURE MATCHING

In deciding on an appropriate AAC system or method, an SLP considers a client's motor and cognitive abilities, the potential size of the client's vocabulary, the ease of learning and using the system, the acceptability of the system to the user and potential communication partners, and the flexibility and intelligibility of the system. For example, unaided systems are very portable and can be expanded easily without concern for limited storage or display space, but allow for no permanent record, thus necessitating use of some graphic system for purposes such as doing homework. Many graphic symbols appear with the printed word, making them easy for communication partners to use, but these same symbols require the partner to concentrate on the graphic message to the exclusion of the user's face.

AAC system selection is much more than merely matching a client and a system.

The potential user's motor abilities are very important in determining the best system to use. Individuals with severe motor impairments in their upper extremities may be poor candidates for unaided systems. However, poor pointing skills need not deter an individual from using a communication board or a device and accessing it via head pointing or eye gaze, or with an assistive device like a T-stick that allows the individual to hold the pointer in both hands while the bottom leg of the "T" serves to point to the desired symbol or location. In addition, poor motor abilities may dictate the use of certain selection methods (e.g., scanning) to access an electronic communication device.

Everyday communication partners must also be able to provide input into the assessment process. In some cases, this is to express a concern about the lack of portability in an AAC system or to report their embarrassment about using the AAC system with someone in a social setting. No matter what the challenge, communication partners play a critical role in assessment and intervention planning.

The selection of an AAC system includes the consideration of several features that might be suitable to a particular person. These include, but are not limited to, aesthetics of the system, overall size of the system, arrangement and size of the symbols, placement and organization of the symbols, and the output of the system.

AAC Symbol Selection

Decisions related to choosing an appropriate symbol system flow naturally from the method of communication chosen. If signing is deemed to be the appropriate method, an SLP must make decisions about the best gestural or sign system to use. In addition to the cognitive and motor abilities of the potential user, the SLP might consider the gestural or signing system used most frequently in the client's school or workplace and in the local community, the availability of teaching materials, and the ease in using these materials.

Selection of aided symbol systems may be guided by the potential user's cognitive abilities, the ease of learning different graphic AAC systems, and the willingness of potential communication partners. Aided symbols form a continuum from actual objects, which may represent only themselves, to letters that can be used to spell words. As we move from concrete objects to abstract symbols and letters, the client gains increased communication flexibility. Although not all clients can spell or use an encryption code, potential partners may be uneasy with interpretation of pictures, photographs, or other symbols. If we expect a client to use a system at home or in school, then these partner concerns must be considered when planning intervention.

AAC Vocabulary Selection

The vocabulary chosen for an AAC system will likely have a significant impact on future communication, language, and/or literacy development (Clendon & Erickson, 2008; Barker, Akaba, Brady, & Thiemann-Bourque, 2013). Decisions about potential vocabulary will continue to be made as long as the client uses AAC. The best guideline is to select vocabulary that reflects the user's needs, desires, likes, and preferences and is functional or useful, based on observation of the client and the communication environment. The resultant vocabulary should be highly individualized.

Several lists of potential vocabulary are available and may serve as a guide when matched with a client's communication needs (see Dark & Balandin, 2007). These lists may also suggest various communication intentions and semantic categories of language that are important for early language development with presymbolic clients. Individuals with acquired speech and language impairments may have very different needs and rarely must relearn language.

 Thought Question 13.4

What are some major considerations in AAC assessment?

The order of teaching signs or symbols must also be guided by a client's immediate needs. In addition, the iconicity and transparency of different signs/symbols must be considered. Selecting appropriate and useful vocabulary can make or break the success of an AAC system for an individual (Yorkston et al., 1990). The impact of vocabulary selection on AAC use cannot be underestimated.

> ✔ Check Your Understanding 13.4
>
> Click here to check your understanding of the concepts in this section.

INTERVENTION CONSIDERATIONS

Although intervention is a team effort, it is important for services not to become fragmented (Beukelman & Mirenda, 2013). Rather, a coherent, holistic approach is needed—one that includes the user's natural environment and communication partners. Family members, whether parents of a child with a developmental communication impairment or spouses and children of an adult with an acquired communication impairment, must be integral members of the intervention team.

As discussed previously, an SLP must be concerned with linguistic, operational, social, and strategic competence in an individual using AAC and his or her partner. It is not enough, however, for an individual with CCN to have assistive technology and the skills to operate it. A child needs to be able to communicate spontaneously in family interactions and in everyday settings (Granlund et al., 2008; Singleton & Shulman, 2014)

AAC users may have other needs that call for the use of additional assistive technologies.

Some important considerations for you as an SLP are as seemingly simple as the location of symbols on a communication board, whereas others involve the teaching of complex syntactic constructions. For example, both typically developing children and those with Down syndrome like drawings that share a color and are clustered together to create a subgroup, such as clothing or food, to facilitate both the speed and accuracy of locating the target symbol (Wilkinson et al., 2008).

Children with ID do not seem to induce English word order rules from the language spoken around them and apply these rules to their sign output (Grove & Dockrell, 2000; Morford et al., 2008). Occasionally, they change the form of the signs creatively, such as performing the sign for *hit* in the location where a blow occurred, to indicate changes in meaning. In this way, signs are used more as gestures (Grove & Dockrell, 2000; Woll & Morgan, 2012).

Production of longer grammatical utterances is slow if users are forming them from single symbols. One option for increasing the rate of production is to pre-store potential utterances in a device. The disadvantage of this approach is that the utterance may not exactly fit a communication situation. However, partners seem to prefer these less-than-precise but more quickly produced messages (McCoy et al., 2007).

Modeling is one method for teaching production of multisymbol messages (Binger & Light, 2007). With modeling, an SLP points to two symbols on a child's AAC device, such as *mommy* and *eat*, while providing a grammatically complete spoken model, such as "Mommy is eating." This teaching can be enhanced by the use of matrix strategies in which all actions needed are combinable with all objects and by milieu language teaching strategies (Nigam et al., 2006). In milieu teaching, an SLP might perform an action while asking, "What am I doing?" If a child fails to respond or responds incorrectly, the SLP models the correct response and then asks again. A sample matrix is presented in Figure 13.5.

Intervention must include both the short-range and long-range needs of a client (Beukelman & Mirenda, 2013). As users move beyond the school years, there is a need for easily accessible vocabulary that reflects socially valued adult roles, such as being a college student or engaging in intimate relationships (Nelson Bryen, 2008).

Figure 13.5 Possible matrix format.

	Pencil	Book	Wagon	Car	Cocoa	Tea
Drop	Drop pencil	Drop book				
Pick up	Pick up pencil	Pick up book				
Push			Push wagon	Push car		
Pull			Pull wagon	Pull car		
Drink					Drink cocoa	Drink tea
Make					Make cocoa	Make tea

Although many of the good intervention practices described in Chapter 2 are equally important when working with individuals using AAC, there are other intervention considerations you will need to keep in mind which apply more specifically to AAC (Cunningham et al., 2005; Erickson, 2003; Granlund et al., 2008; Koppenhaver, 2000; Schlosser, 2003). These include, but are not limited to, the following:

- Establishing a positive AAC culture
- Understanding AAC as being critical in literacy development, especially for children
- Using everyday experiences as a teaching context
- Individualizing the content, as discussed earlier
- Teaching partners to modify their interaction style
- Considering positioning for those with severe motor impairments
- Making communication based on meaningful interaction

Although individual client factors are important, a number of external factors contribute to positive outcomes in AAC intervention (Lund & Light, 2007a; Rackensperger, 2012). Such environmental support is very important. Abandonment of AAC technology usually is related to loss of facilitator/partner support rather than to rejection of the technology (Angelo, 2000; Louise-Bender et al., 2002).

Creating a positive AAC culture is very important and highlights the need to have others, such as caregivers and teachers, involved. An AAC system should be used by others, and aided systems should always be available for a user. We are reminded of one teacher who constructed a huge communication board on a wall of her classroom so that she could use it when addressing the entire class. Naturally, integration into the classroom requires a collaborative strategy involving both the classroom teacher and maybe you as an SLP. AAC training for the entire educational team—teachers, instructional aides, SLPs, and parents—is a key element in success with children (Soto et al., 2001).

 Video Example 13.2

Watch this brief video showing students with CCN interacting with a teacher in a classroom. Think about how many ways the teacher has created a culture in the classroom that promotes the use of multiple modes of communication, modeling for all students involved in the teaching lesson, and individualized supports for each student with CCN. https://youtu.be/n0no1Pmg-14?list=PLocplddh5SS RBGRsR0tOFXIJd5wh6i89k

Intervention will be maximally effective if caregivers also use AAC, along with speech. Caregivers can be taught a few simple signs, or they can learn to use an individual's communication board and point to a symbol while speaking their message. For individuals using an electronic device, caregivers can and should learn to use the device, and, again, pair what they are saying with using the voice output of the device. This is referred to as *augmented input,* and it serves as a model for use of the communication device (Romski & Sevcik, 1996).

Caregivers are sometimes fearful that they will be expected to sign as if they are interpreting for a deaf audience. Nothing could be further from reality with most clients. Signs or graphic symbols can be used as gestures for important words in an utterance as the caregiver continues to speak.

One unintended consequence of AAC use by nonsymbolic children with profound multiple disabilities is that over time, a child becomes more and more dependent on one or two skilled interaction partners within the family. As a result, the child is less likely to interact with a range of partners within the family (Stadskleiv, 2017; Wilder & Granlund, 2006). This is especially true if a child learns to use an AAC mode, but family members do not develop sufficient skills in that mode (Thunstam, 2004). As much as possible, we want to plan intervention so that a client has multiple competent partners in multiple situations to increase social integration, especially among peers. In one classroom, we trained partners to interact with AAC users and reinforced them when they did. Educators can also organize clubs and experiences, such as an integrated dramatic arts program, to promote AAC use (McCarthy & Light, 2001; Clarke et al, 2012).

In short, as an SLP you must identify opportunities for communication, create a need for communication, and maximize the instructional benefit of these opportunities (Sigafoos, 2000). Partners will need instructional support if they are to function as effective communication partners for AAC users.

One method that holds some promise for children with ASD is *aided language modeling* (*ALM*), which consists of engaging children in interactive play activities and providing models of AAC symbol use during play (Drager, Postal et al., 2006). ALM is implemented in a natural play context in which the child is provided models of use of the AAC symbols on a communication board.

Clients with acquired communication impairments may elect, if possible, to continue to work. Self-reports indicate that access to appropriate AAC systems is an important factor in facilitating continued employment (McNaughton et al., 2001). In addition, job-related social networks can be maintained by email and the Internet (Nelson Bryen, 2006).

Everyday events and routines provide *scripts,* or personalized event sequences, that enable each of us to participate. When circumstances are modified, as in the use of AAC, we rely heavily on a script to help us. Use of a script frees "cognitive energy" to be applied to other aspects of the situation. In addition, the use of everyday events teaches a client to use AAC as the need arises. An SLP must use instructional strategies that integrate AAC into the different communication environments of a user (Ball et al., 2000; Rainforth et al., 1992). Even children using low-tech communication boards can have ample opportunities to use their AAC systems to communicate during the school day in greetings, academics, snack, sharing, and recess (Downey et al., 2004).

Acceptance of AAC is the degree to which a system is integrated into the life of a user (Lasker & Bedrosian, 2000). Optimal use occurs when AAC is used willingly and at every opportunity. Community-based training approaches in which the client becomes more comfortable and efficient using AAC in public may lead to optimal use (Lasker & Bedrosian, 2001). In these approaches, venues such as the post office, grocery store, and fast-food outlets are identified. Training begins with scripted interactions that are modified gradually to more spontaneous communication.

In some situations, well-meaning communication partners may assume too active a role in their interaction with an AAC user. In such cases, it is particularly important to include the partner in the assessment process, with the intent of identifying specific interactive competencies, choice-making routines, and environmental supports that can be used to facilitate the person's communicative success. Communication partners may learn or teach others how to interact with the individual using AAC in order to offer real choices, to acknowledge the user's communication attempts, and to allow time for the user to express his or her message.

Often because of the size, location, and other aspects of an AAC system, communication takes place at a very close distance, with the partner near or in the AAC user's personal space. Fortunately, there are a number of ways AAC intervention plans can address such issues. For example, a person could be involved in creating orientation materials for unfamiliar communication partners that describe what helps and what does not help facilitate meaningful communication. A person might engage in other self-advocacy efforts, such as making an orientation video, a book, or a presentation to share with others. The use of self-advocacy projects to help the person understand their strengths and weaknesses and to help others know how to interact successfully was originally described by Ylvisaker and Feeney (1998), in their work with individuals with traumatic brain injury (see also Feeney & Capo, 2002).

Because communication partners may be unfamiliar with AAC, it is important that systems and their purpose be explained carefully and demonstrated (Cress, 2001; Kent-Walsh & McNaughton, 2009). Partners should also be taught to use AAC expressively—not because they need AAC to be understood but because they can help the user acclimate to this method of communication (Kent-Walsh et al., 2015). Communication partners should be consulted for their observations, suggestions, and ideas for intervention. As members of the intervention team, they become invested in the outcomes for the client.

For clients with severe motor impairments such as CP, positioning is very important and can often be the determining factor in successful motor movement. Control of the head, shoulders, spine, and hips and alignment along the midline are essential.

Finally, a user of AAC must be involved in real communication that is versatile and has meaningful outcomes. Otherwise, for individuals with progressive disorders such as ALS and Parkinson's disease, communication becomes solely a means of regulating the behavior of others for basic needs and wants (Fried-Oken et al., 2006). It is all too easy for intervention to evolve into drill in which the client touches objects or pictures with no real outcome except a reinforcing word by an SLP or another partner. Ideally, person-centered and context-sensitive interventions are employed to promote real communication choices, not just performance of a sign or locating a symbol. With meaningful communication, the grief and sense of loss that accompany acquired communication impairments and laryngectomy and glossectomy can be replaced by a sense of empowerment (Fox & Rau, 2001).

For more information related to AAC assessment, intervention, policies, and laws, please take a look at the resources in Table 13.1.

Evidence-Based Practice (EBP) in AAC

Schlosser and Raghavendra (2004) describe EBP as:

> the integration of best and current research evidence with clinical/educational expertise and relevant stakeholder perspectives to facilitate decisions for assessment and intervention that are deemed effective and efficient for a given stakeholder. (p. 3)

Each client seen by an SLP is unique, and those with AAC needs are especially so. This, plus the relatively small number of users seen by any one SLP, makes conducting clinical research especially difficult. As a result, many studies include

TABLE 13.1

Online resources related to AAC

Name of Resource and Website	Description
Closing the Gap (www.closingthegap.com)	Closing the Gap has an online, searchable version of its resource directory for computer-related products for people with special needs, including software and hardware. It also has an online archive of articles from *Closing the Gap Newsletter*.
Center for Literacy and Disability Studies (www.med.unc.edu)	The Center for Literacy and Disability Studies is a unit within the Department of Allied Health Sciences, School of Medicine, at the University of North Carolina at Chapel Hill. There are a vast number of resources on this website related to helping people with complex communication needs address communication, language, and literacy issues.
The International Society for Augmentative and Alternative Communication (ISAAC) (www.isaac-online.org)	ISAAC provides excellent information about AAC, conferences, educational resources, evidence-based practice, and many other connections to people and groups involved in AAC around the world.
Rehabilitation Engineering Research Center (https://rerc-aac.psu.edu/)	The AAC-RERC functions as a collaborative research group dedicated to the development of effective AAC technology. AAC refers to methods (other than speech) that are used to send a message from one person to another.
Quality Educators for Assistive Technology (QIAT) (www.qiat.org)	QIAT is "a nationwide collegial endeavor dedicated to the Development and Implementation of Quality Indicators for Assistive Technology Services in School Settings," managed by Joy Zabala. Check this site for excellent resources on quality indicators for assistive technology. Sign up for the QIAT listserv for quality information and discussion regarding assistive technology.
Iowa State Dept. of Education (2016) https://www.youtube.com/playlist?list=PLocplddh5SSRBGRsR0tOFXIJd5wh6i89k	This is an excellent video playlist assembled by Iowa State Dept. of Education, and includes a range of high quality illustrations of students with CCN using AAC in the classroom and across settings.
Resource on laws related to AAC/AT SpeciaLaw from EDLAW, Inc. (www.edlaw.net)	Full texts of statutes, regulations, and administrative interpretations.
AACIntervention.com (http://aacintervention.com)	This site is full of useful tips and strategies for using AAC with children. Make sure to check out the Tips, Tricks, and Cheat Sheets as well as the Tip of the Month. Software setups and other products from Caroline Musselwhite and Julie Maro are available from this site.

only a single subject or a very small number of subjects, resulting in conclusions that cannot be generalized to most users. Table 13.2 provides a list of some current topics in AAC intervention in which integrated reviews are available.

While an exhaustive list of the outcomes stemming from evidence available in the field of AAC is beyond the scope of this chapter, consider the following:

- Little long-term research in AAC exists. Longitudinal studies are needed that focus on everyday communicative routines of children and adults who use AAC.
- Improved speech intelligibility coming from high-tech systems doesn't necessarily lead to a person's participation in social interactions. Therefore,

TABLE 13.2

Evidence reviews in AAC

Focus of Review	Author(s)
AAC, people with developmental disabilities, peer interactions	Schlosser, Walker & Sigafoos, 2006; Sigafoos et al., 2004; Therrien, Light, & Pope, 2016
Individuals with severe cognitive disabilities	Snell et al., 2006; Snell et al., 2010
AAC and supportive communication partners	Shire & Jones, 2015
Literacy, AAC, and individuals with physical and developmental disabilities	Machalicek et al., 2010
AAC and infants and toddlers with disabilities, early intervention	Branson & Demchak, 2009; Romski, Sevcik et al., 2015
AAC and individuals with chronic severe aphasia	Corwin & Koul, 2003; Russo et al., 2017
Use of AAC with individuals on the autism spectrum	Osser et al., 2013; Schlosser & Koul, 2015; Kagohara et al., 2013.
Review of iPad Applications for AAC and mobile technologies	Alliano, Herriger, Koutsoftas & Bartolotta, 2016; Wendt & Miller, 2013; Alzrayer, Banda & Koul, 2014

in-context intervention designed to promote generalization and transfer must be considered.

- Scanning as an access option is especially difficult for young children. Direct selection is often easier to teach.

- For children with ASD or intellectual disabilities, AAC intervention does not impede speech production. Most studies report an increase in speech production, albeit rather modest in most cases. These results indicate that SLPs must help families and clients to have realistic expectations about speech gains.

- For children with ASD, the gains in overall communication from the use of sign are modest.

- Although many individuals who use AAC can comprehend and express a wide range of grammatical structures, they tend to produce shorter utterances when they use graphic symbol-based AAC systems.

- Few studies have investigated the effectiveness of AAC-specific aspects of intervention in a family context, making it difficult to draw any empirically based conclusions about the effectiveness of these interventions in family environments.

Source: Based on Beukelman & Mirenda (2013); Therrien, Light, & Pope, (2016); Binger & Light (2007); Granlund et al. (2008); Lund & Light (2006, 2007a); Millar et al. (2006); Schlosser & Wendt (2008); Schlosser & Koul (2015); Schwartz & Nye (2006); Snell et al. (2006).

 Check Your Understanding 13.5

Click here to check your understanding of the concepts in this section.

SUMMARY

Put simply, augmentative and alternative communication (AAC) includes anything that supplements an existing communication system. It takes many forms, is based on the interactive competence of a person and a partner, and includes the strategies and methods individuals use to meet their communication needs. AAC may enhance or augment an individual's speech, or it may become a person's primary means of communication.

Although the specific goals of AAC intervention vary with each individual user, treatment aims include the following:

- Assist individuals with their everyday communication needs.
- Help facilitate the development of speech, language, and literacy.
- Help facilitate the return of speech and language in cases where there is a temporary loss of speech.

Decisions related to the appropriate type of AAC for a specific person typically include a feature-matching process (Beukelman & Mirenda, 2013) that may need to be revised as the user's abilities or needs change. People using AAC may also employ multiple types of systems for successful communication that require others in their environment to learn about ways to facilitate maximum efficacy. Involvement of everyday communication partners in the assessment and intervention planning process cannot be overstated. An SLP, in coordination with a client's family members and other professionals, uses the data from an assessment to make decisions about the appropriate AAC method, AAC symbol system, and potential vocabulary.

In planning interventions to address both the short-range and long-range communication needs of a client, an SLP must be concerned with the linguistic, operational, social, and strategic competencies of a person using AAC and his or her partners.

SUGGESTED READINGS/SOURCES

Beukelman, D. R., & Mirenda, P. (2013). *Augmentative and alternative communication: Supporting children and adults with complex communication needs* (4th ed.). Baltimore: Paul H. Brookes.

Lloyd, L. L., Fuller, D. R., & Arvidson, H. H. (1997). *Augmentative and alternative communication: A handbook of principles and practices*. Boston: Allyn & Bacon.

Reichle, J., Halle, J. W., & Drasgow, E. (1998). Implementing augmentative communication systems. In A. Wetherby, S. Warren, & J. Reichle (Eds.), *Transitions in prelinguistic communication* (pp. 417–436). Baltimore: Brookes.

Professional Organizations

AMERICAN SPEECH-LANGUAGE-HEARING ASSOCIATION (ASHA)

ASHA is a nonprofit organization of speech-language pathologists, audiologists, and speech and hearing scientists that was founded in 1925. As of 2012, ASHA represents 155,000 speech-language pathologists, audiologists, and speech scientists from throughout the United States and the world. It is the largest association for those concerned with communication disorders. ASHA's mission is to empower and support speech-language pathologists, audiologists, and speech, language, and hearing scientists by:

- Advocating on behalf of persons with communication and related disorders
- Advancing communication science
- Promoting effective human communication (ASHA, 2009c)

Scientific Study of the Processes and Disorders of Human Communication

ASHA encourages study of typical and disordered communication by mandating a curriculum of study for prospective speech-language pathologists and audiologists. In addition, ASHA provides financial grants to individuals who are engaged in research that furthers our knowledge of communication and assessment, treatment, and prevention of pathologies. ASHA works closely with governmental agencies that sponsor relevant scientific investigation.

To dispense knowledge among professionals, ASHA publishes several scholarly periodicals: *Journal of Speech, Language, and Hearing Research*; *Language, Speech, and Hearing Services in Schools*; *American Journal of Speech-Language Pathology: A Journal of Clinical Practice*; and *American Journal of Audiology: A Journal of Clinical Practice*. ASHA also holds an annual convention at which members and others share information and learn through scientific sessions, exhibits, seminars, and short courses. Additional institutes, workshops, conferences, and teleseminars are held throughout the year. ASHA fosters continuing education for professionals through these activities.

Clinical Service in Speech-Language Pathology and Audiology

Programs that provide clinical services to people with communicative disorders may be accredited by ASHA. This means that representatives of ASHA will review the procedures that are used in diagnosis and treatment. A site visit will ensure that equipment, materials, and record keeping adhere to the highest professional standards. Clinical service will be the responsibility of individuals who meet ASHA standards for the Certificates of Clinical Competence-Speech Language Pathologist (CCC-SLP) or Certificates of Clinical Competence-Audiologist (CCP-A).

Maintenance of Ethical Standards

To ensure that the highest moral and ethical principles are followed in the professions of speech-language pathology and audiology, ASHA provides a code of ethics, which is found on the ASHA website. The basic principles are as follows:

1. The welfare of the persons served by communication disorders specialists is paramount.
2. Each professional must achieve and maintain the highest level of professional competence. The ASHA Certificates of Clinical Competence (CCC) are considered the minimal achievement for independent professional practice. Clinicians should provide service only within their own areas of competence. Professional development and continuing education should be ongoing. New technology requires that speech-language pathologists and audiologists continually update their skills in order to safely and accurately address patient needs.
3. Professionals must promote understanding and provide accurate information in statements to the public.
4. Professionals are responsible for ensuring that ethical standards are maintained by themselves, colleagues, students, and members of allied professions. All members of ASHA are responsible for the monitoring and maintenance of ethical standards throughout the profession (ASHA, 2010).

Advocacy for Individuals with Communicative Disabilities

ASHA is active in encouraging members of Congress and state legislatures to pass legislation that provides for appropriate services for communication-impaired individuals. Bills such as the Individuals with Disabilities Education Act and the Americans with Disabilities Act became law in part because of the extensive promotional activities of ASHA and other organizations.

The needs and characteristics of people with speech, language, and hearing disabilities are clarified and publicized by ASHA on radio, on television, and through print media. In May, which is "Better Speech and Hearing Month," you are especially likely to hear public service announcements that advocate for understanding, prevention, and treatment of communication disorders.

RELATED PROFESSIONAL ASSOCIATIONS

Although ASHA is the largest organization for communication disorder professionals, other groups are also active and worthwhile. Some speech-language pathologists and audiologists belong to several associations. Table A.1 lists some of the ones that are most closely affiliated. Prospective speech-language pathologists and audiologists are advised to take courses in biology, psychology, and sociology to better understand their clients and to work more effectively with professionals from other disciplines.

TABLE A.1

Selected professional associations relevant to communication disorders

Academy of Dispensing Audiologists	American Auditory Society	National Hearing Conservation Association
Academy of Rehabilitative Audiology	American Speech-Language-Hearing Association	National Student Speech-Language-Hearing Association
American Academy of Audiology	Audiology Foundation of America	Orton Dyslexia Society
American Academy of Otolaryngology–Head and Neck Surgery	Canadian Association of Speech-Language Pathologists	Stuttering Foundation of America
	Council on Education of the Deaf	

22q11.2 deletion syndrome A genetic condition caused by deletion of a small segment of the long arm of chromosome 22 on the 22q11.2 band. It is the second most common multiple anomaly syndrome in humans, and is frequently associated with heart abnormalities, cleft palate, velopharyngeal dysfunction, developmental delay, and speech, language, resonance, voice, feeding, and/or hearing impairments; also known as Velocardiofacial syndrome or DiGeorge sequence.

Abduction When the vocal folds open or spread apart during vibration.

Acoustic immittance The term used to refer to either the flow or opposition to the flow of energy through the middle.

Acquired Occurring after birth.

Acquired immunodeficiency syndrome (AIDS) A viral disease in which a person becomes susceptible to an assortment of other illnesses.

Acute laryngitis Temporary swelling of the vocal folds, resulting in a hoarse voice quality.

Addition In articulation, the insertion of a phoneme that is not part of the word.

Adduction When the vocal folds close or come together during vibration.

Affricate A combination of a stop and fricative phoneme.

AIDS See *Acquired immunodeficiency syndrome.*

Air conduction A method of evaluating hearing by transmitting sound to the inner ear via the outer ear and middle ear.

Allophone A phonemic variation.

Alport's syndrome A hereditary disorder characterized by kidney disease and bilateral progressive sensorineural hearing loss.

Alveolar Related to the alveolar, or gum, ridge of the mouth. In speech, alveolar consonants are those produced with the tongue on the alveolar ridge.

Alveolar pressure Pressure inside the lungs.

Alzheimer's disease (AD) A cortical pathology that affects primarily memory, language, or visuospatial skills as a result of diffuse brain atrophy; presenile dementia.

American Sign Language (ASL) A complex nonvocal language that contains elaborate syntax and semantics. Proficiency in its use is one of the primary methods by which a deaf individual becomes part of the Deaf community.

Amplification Technology such as hearing aids, cochlear implants, and assistive listening devices that improve access to sounds by electronically increasing their intensity.

Amyotrophic lateral sclerosis (ALS) Commonly called Lou Gehrig's disease, a rapidly progressive degenerative disease in which an individual gradually loses control of his or her musculature. It is characterized by fatigue, muscle atrophy or loss of bulk, involuntary contractions, and reduced muscle tone. Speech in the later stages is labored and slow, with short phrasing, long pauses, hypernasality, and severely impaired articulation.

Anatomy The study of the structures of the body and the relationship of these structures to one another.

Aneurysm A type of hemorrhagic stroke that results from the rupture of a sac-like bulge in a weakened artery wall.

Anomic aphasia A fluent aphasia characterized by naming difficulties and mild to moderate auditory comprehension problems.

Aphasia An impairment due to localized brain injury that affects understanding, retrieving, and formulating meaningful and sequential elements of language.

Aphonia A complete loss of voice.

Aplasia (or dysplasia) Hearing loss due to the absence of the inner ear structures during embryonic development.

Apraxia of Speech A disorder in the planning or programming of movements for speech production

Arteriovenous malformation A poorly formed tangle of arteries and veins that may result in a rare type of stroke in which arterial walls are weak and give way under pressure.

Articulation Rapid and coordinated movement of the tongue, teeth, lips, and palate to produce speech sounds.

Articulatory/resonating system Structures used during sound production, including the oral cavity, nasal cavity, tongue, and soft palate.

Aryepiglottic folds The membrane and muscle that connect the sides of the epiglottis to the arytenoid cartilages in the larynx.

Aspiration Inhalation, especially the inhalation of fluid or food into the lungs; in phonology, a puff of air that is released in the production of various allophones.

Aspiration pneumonia A respiratory infection that occurs when foreign material (e.g., food, saliva, liquids) enters the lungs.

Assessment of communication disorders The systematic process of obtaining information from many sources, through various means, and in different settings to verify and specify communication strengths and weaknesses, identify possible causes, and make plans to address them.

Assistive listening devices (ALD) The general term applied to electronic devices designed to enhance the reception of sound by those whose hearing is impaired.

Ataxic cerebral palsy A congenital disorder characterized by uncoordinated movement and disturbed balance. Movements lack direction, and hypotonic muscles lack adequate force and rate and have poor directional control.

Ataxic dysarthria A motor speech disorder involving problems with muscle coordination; the problem involves the accuracy, timing, and direction of movement. Speech is characterized by irregular articulatory breakdowns, slowness, excessive and equal stress, and imprecise articulation.

Athetoid Cerebral Palsy A congenital disorder that is characterized by slow, involuntary writhing movements, particularly during attempts at voluntary movement. It is caused by damage to basal ganglia structures and/or pathways that work to inhibit involuntary movements

Atresia A congenital disorder resulting in complete closure of the external auditory meatus.

Atrophy Wasting away or loss of cells.

Attention-deficit/hyperactivity disorder (ADHD) Hyperactivity and attentional difficulties in children who do not manifest other characteristics of learning disabilities.

Audible nasal emission Perception of nasal air flow during speech. Commonly occurs in individuals with cleft palate.

Audiologist A professional whose distinguishing role is to identify, assess, manage, and prevent disorders of hearing and balance.

Audiology Professional discipline involving the assessment, remediation, and prevention of disorders of hearing and balance.

Audiometer A device used to regulate and deliver pure tone and speech stimuli during audiometric testing.

Auditory brain stem response (ABR) A type of electrophysiological test that records neural responses along the ascending auditory pathways occurring within the first 5 to 6 milliseconds following stimulus presentation.

Auditory evoked potentials (AEPs) Small neuroelectric responses to auditory stimulation by the ascending auditory pathways leading from the cochlea to the cortex of the brain.

Auditory neuropathy spectrum disorder (ANSD) Condition characterized by normal outer hair cell function with abnormal cranial nerve VIII function.

Auditory-oral A training method for hearing impaired persons that emphasizes the use of residual hearing and speech reading (lipreading).

Auditory training Listening activities designed to maximize a hearing-impaired person's ability to detect, discriminate, identify, and comprehend auditory information.

Augmentative and alternative communication (AAC) Gestures, signing, picture systems, print, computerized communication, and voice production used to complement or supplement speech for persons with severe communication impairments.

Aural (audiological) habilitation/rehabilitation Services and procedures designed to improve communication deficits that result from hearing loss.

Authentic data Information about an individual that is based on real life.

Autism spectrum disorder (ASD) Term used to characterize individuals at the severe end of the pervasive developmental disorder (PDD) continuum. ASD is an impairment in reciprocal social interaction with a severely limited behavior, interest, and activity repertoire that has its onset before 30 months of age.

Automaticity The ease with which a person uses a particular skill without apparent thought.

Babbling Single-syllable nonpurposeful consonant–vowel (CV) or vowel–consonant (VC) vocalizations that begin at about 4 months of age.

Basal ganglia Large subcortical nuclei that regulate motor functioning and maintain posture and muscle tone.

Baseline data Information about client performance before intervention begins.

Basilar membrane The membrane that forms the floor of the organ of Corti. It is nonuniform in width, thickness, and stiffness, and it responds differently to different frequencies of sound (tonotopically). The basilar membrane contains thousands of hair cells, the receptor cells for the auditory system.

Behavior modification A systematic method of changing behavior through careful target selection, stimulation, client response, and reinforcement.

Behavioral observation audiometry (BOA) A method of assessing infant hearing by presentation of different stimuli and watching for any changes in activity that signal a response.

Bilabial Pertaining to two lips, such as phonemes produced with both lips.

Blend Create a word from individual sounds and syllables.

Bolus A chewed lump of food ready for swallowing. Or, the substance to be ingested when eating or drinking.

Bone-anchored hearing aid A type of amplification in which some of the components are surgically implanted into the temporal bone of the skull, stimulating the cochlea via bone conduction.

Bone conduction A method of evaluating hearing by transmitting sound to the inner ear by mechanically vibrating the bones of the skull.

Booster treatment Additional therapy, based on retesting, offered after treatment has been terminated.

Bound morpheme A morpheme that must be attached to a free morpheme to communicate meaning; grammatical morpheme.

Breathiness Perception of audible air escaping through the glottis during phonation.

Broca's aphasia A nonfluent aphasia that is characterized by short sentences with agrammatism; anomia; problems with imitation of speech because of overall speech problems; slow, labored speech and writing; and articulation and phonological errors.

Broca's area Located in the left frontal area of the brain and responsible for working memory and enabling the motor cortex for speech.

(Central) Auditory processing disorder (C)APD A disorder resulting from impairment to the auditory structures leading from the brain stem to the cortex of the brain.

Central auditory system Part of the auditory system that includes structures beyond the auditory nerve and extending to the auditory cortex.

Central nervous system (CNS) The brain and spinal cord.

Cerebellum A lower brain structure consisting of two hemispheres that smoothly regulates and coordinates the control of purposeful movement, including very complex and fine-motor activities. The cerebellum revises the transmission from the cortex's motor strip to produce accurate, precise movements. It is also important for motor skill learning.

Cerebral arteriosclerosis A type of ischemic stroke resulting from a thickening of the walls of cerebral arteries in which elasticity is lost or reduced, the walls become weakened, and blood flow is restricted.

Cerebral palsy (CP) A heterogeneous group of neurogenic disorders that result in difficulty with motor movement; were acquired before, during, or shortly after birth; and affect one or more limbs.

Cerebrovascular accident (CVA) Stroke, the most common cause of aphasia, results when the blood supply to the brain is blocked or when the brain is flooded with blood.

Cerumen (or earwax) A substance produced by glands in the ear canal that provides lubrication and protects the ear from the invasion of insects and other foreign objects.

Cervical Auscultation A technique that involves placing a stethoscope on the neck at the level of the vocal folds to amplify breathing sounds in relation to the pharyngeal swallow to determine the efficiency of the pharyngeal phase of swallowing.

Chin tuck A posture with the chin down that is helpful with some patients who have a swallowing disability.

Chorea A form of hyperkinetic dysarthria characterized by rapid or continual, random, irregular, and or abrupt hyperkinesia. Speech, when affected, may be characterized by inappropriate silences caused by voice stoppage; intermittent breathiness, strained harsh voice, and hypernasality; imprecise articulation with prolonged pauses; and forced inspiration and expiration resulting in excessive loudness variations.

Chronemics The study of the effect of time on communication.

Chronic laryngitis Vocal abuse during acute laryngitis that leads to vocal fold tissue damage.

Closed syllable A syllable, or basic acoustic unit of speech, that ends in one or more consonants.

Cochlea The portion of the inner ear that contains the sensory cells of the auditory system. It is composed of two concentric labyrinths. The outer one is composed of bone and the inner one of membrane.

Cochlear implant An electronic amplification device that is surgically placed in the cochlea and provides electrical stimulation to the surviving auditory nerve fibers.

Code switching The process in which bilingual speakers transfer between two languages, based on the listener, context, or topic.

Cognitive impairment An umbrella term for pathological conditions and syndromes that result in declining of memory and at least one other cognitive ability that interferes with daily life activities.

Cognitive rehabilitation A treatment regimen for individuals with traumatic brain injury that is designed to increase functional abilities for everyday life by improving the capacity to process incoming information.

Communication An exchange of ideas between sender(s) and receivers(s).

Communication disorder An impairment in the ability to receive, send, process, or comprehend concepts of verbal, nonverbal, or graphic symbol systems.

Compression Part of the sound wave where the displaced molecules are in close proximity to each other.

Concha The deep bowl-like depression on the pinna.

Conditioned play audiometry (CPA) A method of assessing the hearing of children ages $2\frac{1}{2}$ to 3 years and older by instructing them to put a block in a bucket, place a ring on a peg, or carry out another action whenever they hear the test signal.

Conduction aphasia A fluent aphasia in which the individual's conversation is abundant and quick. Characterized by anomia, auditory comprehension that is impaired mildly if at all, extremely poor repetitive or imitative speech, and paraphasia.

Conductive hearing loss A loss of auditory sensitivity due to malformation or obstruction of the outer ear and/or middle ear.

Conductive system Part of the auditory system made up of the outer and middle ears.

Congenital Present at birth.

Consonant A phoneme that is produced with some vocal tract constriction or occlusion.

Contact ulcer A benign lesion that may develop on the posterior surface of the vocal folds.

Conversion aphonia Psychologically based loss of voice.

Conversion disorder A condition in which emotion is suppressed and transformed into a sensory or motor disability.

Correlate Something that tends to exist in the presence of something else or be associated with it, but without a demonstrated causal relationship.

Cranial nerves The 12 pairs of nerves in the peripheral nervous system that innervate the muscles of speech production, as well as mediate the sensations of vision, hearing, balance, smell, and touch from the face.

Craniofacial anomalies Congenital malformations involving the head (*cranio* = above the upper eyelid) and face (*facial* = below the upper eyelid).

Critical literacy A reader's ability to actively interpret between the lines, analyze, and synthesize information and to be able to explain content.

Criterion-referenced An evaluation of an individual's strengths and weaknesses with regard to specific skills.

Deaf Term used to describe a person whose hearing loss is in the severe to profound range.

Deaf community A group of persons who share a common means of communication (American Sign Language) that facilitates group cohesion and identity.

Deaf culture A view of life manifested by the mores, beliefs, artistic expression, understandings, and language (ASL) that is particular to members of the Deaf community.

Decibel (dB) A mathematically derived unit based on the pressure exerted by a particular sound vibration.

Decoding Breaking or segmenting a written word into its component sounds and then blending them together to form a recognizable word.

Decontextualized Outside a conversational context. When we write, we construct the context with our writing rather than having it constructed by our conversational partner(s).

Diagnosis A statement distinguishing an individual's difficulties from the broad range of possibilities.

Diagnostic therapy Ongoing assessment and evaluation as intervention takes place.

Dialect A linguistic variation that is attributable primarily to geographic region or foreign language background. It includes features of form, content, and use.

Dialogic reading Picture book interactive sharing between a caregiver and a young child, in which parents try to get children involved in the reading process by asking them questions about the story or allowing a child to tell the story.

Dichotic The simultaneous presentation of different stimuli to each ear.

Diphthong Two vowels said in such close proximity that they are treated as a single phoneme.

Diplophonia The perception of two vocal frequencies.

Disability The functional consequence of an impairment.

Distortion In articulation, a deviant production of a phoneme.

Dynamic Characterized by energy or effective energy, changing over time.

Dynamic assessment A nonstandardized assessment approach that can take the form of test–teach–test to determine a child's ability to learn.

Dynamic literacy A reader's ability to interrelate content to other knowledge through both deductive and inductive reasoning.

Dysarthria One of several motor speech disorders that involve impaired articulation, respiration, phonation, or prosody as a result of paralysis, muscle weakness, or poor coordination. Motor function may be excessively slow or rapid, decreased in range or strength, and have poor directionality and timing.

Dysphagia A disorder of swallowing.

Dysplasia See *aplasia*.

Dystonia A form of hyperkinetic dysarthria that is characterized by a slow, sustained increase and decrease of hyperkinesia involving either the entire body or localized sets of muscles. As a result, there are excessive pitch and loudness variations, irregular articulation breakdowns, and vowel distortions.

Dysphonia An impairment in normal voice production.

Ear, nose, and throat physician (ENT) Medical doctor specializing in diagnosis and treatment of diseases of the ear, nose, and throat.

Early hearing detection and intervention (EHDI) programs Public health initiative designed to facilitate early detection of hearing loss through universal hearing screening, followed by appropriate referral for diagnostic testing and early intervention as necessary.

Eardrum See *Tympanic membrane*.

Edema Swelling due to an accumulation of fluid.

Effectiveness The probability of benefit to individuals in a defined population from a specific intervention applied to a given communication problem under *average everyday* clinical conditions.

Efficacy The probability of benefit to individuals in a defined population from a specific intervention applied for a given communication problem under *ideal* conditions.

Efficiency Application of the quickest intervention method involving the least effort and the greatest positive benefit, including unintended effects.

Electroacoustic measures Tools that record acoustic signals from within the client's external auditory canal.

Electrolarynx A battery-powered device that sets air in the vocal tract into vibration.

Electropalatography (EPG) A technique used to teach correct placement of the articulators for speech production. It uses an artificial palatal plate fitted in the client's mouth that contains electrodes. The electrodes are connected to a computer. When the tongue contacts the electrodes during speech production, the articulatory patterns can be viewed on a computer screen.

Electrophysiological tests Tools that record neuroelectric responses (nerve impulses) that are generated by the auditory system in response to sound.

Embolism A blood clot, fatty materials, or an air bubble that may travel through the circulatory system until it blocks the flow of blood in a small artery. If it travels to the brain, it may cause a stroke.

Endolymph The fluid that fills the membranous labyrinth of the cochlea and vestibular system.

Endoscope A lens coupled with a light source that is used for viewing internal bodily structures, including the vocal folds.

Esophageal speech Speech that is produced by using burping as a substitute for the laryngeal voice.

Esophagostomy A surgical procedure that involves creating a hole in the esophagus in the upper chest/neck region, and inserting a feeding tube so that food can be delivered to the stomach, bypassing the oral and pharyngeal cavities.

Etiology The cause or origin of a problem; also the study of cause.

Eustachian tube The tube that connects the middle ear cavity with the nasopharynx.

Eustachian tube dysfunction Condition in which the Eustachian tube does not adequately equalize middle ear pressure; commonly results in pathology of the middle ear.

Examination of the peripheral speech mechanism Sometimes called oral peripheral exam; assessment of the structure and function of the visible speech system.

Executive function An aspect of metacognition used in self-regulation and including the ability to attend; to set reasonable goals; to plan and organize to achieve each goal; to initiate, monitor, and evaluate your performance in relation to that goal; and to revise plans and strategies based on feedback.

External auditory meatus (or canal) The tubular structure that extends from the concha of the pinna to the tympanic membrane.

External error sound discrimination Perception of differences in the production of the target phoneme in another person's speech. Also known as interpersonal error sound discrimination.

Extrapyramidal tract Motor tract fibers involved in unconscious modulation of motor movements, and the regulation of reflexes, posture, and tone; also known as the indirect activation pathway or indirect motor system.

Failure to thrive The absence of healthy growth and development.

Fasciculations Involuntary localized twitches due to spontaneous motor unit discharges seen in denervated muscle.

Fast mapping A process in which a child infers the meaning of a word form context and uses it in a similar context at a later time. A fuller definition evolves over time. Fast mapping enables preschool children to expand their vocabularies quickly by being able to use a word without fully understanding the meaning.

Figurative language Nonliteral phrases consisting of idioms, metaphors, similes, and proverbs.

Filler Utterances such as "er," "um," and "you know" that are used in productions. Sometimes characteristic of disfluent speech and/or stuttering.

Fingerspelling A form of manual communication consisting of 26 distinct handshapes that visually represent the letters of the English alphabet.

Flaccid dysarthria A speech disorder caused by weak, soft, flabby muscle tone, called hypotonia. May result in hypernasality, breathiness, and imprecise articulation.

Fluency Smoothness of rhythm and rate.

Fluent aphasia Speech characterized by word substitutions, neologisms, and often verbose verbal output. Also called Wernicke's aphasia.

FM system A type of hearing assistive technology that transmits sound to a hearing impaired person via FM radio waves. The system consists of a microphone, a transmitter, and a wireless receiver.

Free morpheme The portion of a word that can stand alone and designate meaning; root morpheme.

Frequency An acoustical term that refers to the number of sound wave cycles that are completed within a specific time period. Subjectively, it is perceived as the pitch of a sound.

Fricative A consonant phoneme that is produced by exhaling air through a narrow passageway.

Fundamental frequency The lowest frequency component of a complex vibration.

Gastroesophageal reflux (GER) Movement of food or acid from the stomach back into the esophagus.

Generative Capable of being freshly created; refers to the infinite number of sentences that can be created through the application of grammatical rules.

Glide A phoneme in which the articulatory posture changes from consonant to vowel.

Global, or mixed, aphasia A profound language impairment in all modalities as a result of brain damage.

Glottal Relating to or produced in or by the glottis, the space between the vocal folds.

Glottis The space between the vocal folds.

Grammar The rules of a language.

Granuloma A nodular lesion due to injury or infection. May occur on the vocal folds and may be caused by a breathing tube being placed through the glottis.

Habitual pitch The basic frequency level that an individual uses most of the time.

Hair cells Auditory receptor cells located in the organ of Corti that are responsible for encoding auditory information.

Harmonics Frequencies in a complex sound that are integer multiples of the fundamental frequency.

Head-back position A posture with the head held back that is useful for some clients with a swallowing disability.

Head rotation A posture with the head turned toward the impairment, used for some clients with a swallowing disability.

Head tilt A posture with the head away from the impairment, used for some individuals with a swallowing disability.

Hearing disorder Impaired sensitivity of the auditory or hearing system.

Hematoma Blood trapped in an organ or skin tissue due to injury or surgery.

Hemianopsia Blindness in the left or right visual field of both eyes caused by lesions on the temporal or lower parietal lobe.

Hemiparesis Muscle weakness on one side of the body, resulting in reduced strength and control.

Hemiplegia Paralysis on one side of the body.

Hemisensory impairment Loss of the ability to perceive sensory information on one side of the body.

Hemorrhagic stroke A type of stroke resulting from the weakening of arterial walls that burst under pressure.

Hertz (Hz) The number of complete vibrations or cycles per second.

Hesitation A pause before or between parts of utterances. If used excessively, it may be considered a sign of disfluency or stuttering.

HIV/AIDS See *Human immunodeficiency virus* and *Acquired Immunodeficiency Syndrome*.

Hoarseness A voice quality that is characterized by a rough, usually low-pitched quality.

Holistic Pertaining to the whole; multidimensional.

Human immunodeficiency virus (HIV) The organism responsible for AIDS.

Huntington's chorea An inherited progressive disease also known as Huntington's disease, that results from a genetic defect on chromosome 4.

Hyoid Bone horseshoe-shaped structure that serves as the point of attachment for laryngeal and tongue muscles.

Hyperadduction Excessive movement toward the midline, often resulting in a tense voice quality.

Hyperfluent speech Very rapid speech found in people with fluent aphasia and characterized by few pauses, incoherence, inefficiency, and pragmatic inappropriateness.

Hyperkinetic dysarthria A speech disorder characterized by increased movement, such as tremors and tics, and by inaccurate articulation.

Hyperlexia A mild form of pervasive developmental disorder (PDD) characterized by an inordinate interest in letters and words and by early ability to read but with little comprehension.

Hypernasality Excessive nasal resonance.

Hypokinesia Abnormally decreased motor function or activity.

Hypokinetic dysarthria A speech disorder that is characterized by a decrease in or lack of appropriate movement as muscles become rigid and stiff, resulting in monopitch and monoloudness and imprecise articulation.

Hyponasality An abnormal resonance characterized by lack of nasal air flow during production of the phonemes /m/, /n/, and / ŋ / resulting from a blockage in the nasopharynx or nasal cavity.

Impairment A loss of structure or function.

Incidental teaching Use of a natural activity to train targets.

Incus The middle bone of the ossicular chain in the middle ear. It articulates with the malleus at the top and has a projection that is joined to the stapes at the bottom.

Infarction Death of bodily tissue due to deprivation of the blood supply.

Informational counseling The process of imparting information to clients and their families.

Inner ear The interior section of the ear, which contains the cochlea and vestibular system. It supplies information to the brain regarding balance, spatial orientation, and hearing.

Intellectual disability (ID) Substantial limitations in intellectual functioning; significant limitations in adaptive behavior consisting of conceptual, social, and practical skills; and originating before age 18.

Intelligibility The ability to understand what has been detected aurally.

Intensity A measure of the magnitude of a sound, generally expressed in decibels.

Intentionality Goal directedness in interactions, which is first demonstrated at about 8 months of age, primarily through gestures.

Interdental Between the teeth; see *Linguadental*.

Internal error sound discrimination Ability to judge the accuracy of one's own phoneme production. Also known as *intrapersonal error sound discrimination*.

Interpersonal error sound discrimination See *External error sound discrimination*.

Intonation Pitch movement within an utterance.

Intrapersonal error sound discrimination See *Internal error sound discrimination*.

Ischemic stroke A cerebrovascular accident resulting from a complete or partial blockage or occlusion of the arteries transporting blood to the brain.

Jargon Strings of unintelligible speech sounds with the intonational pattern of adult speech.

Kinesics The study of bodily movement and gesture. Also known as body language.

Labiodental Pertaining to lips and teeth; phonemes produced with lip and tooth contact.

Language A socially shared code for representing concepts through the use of arbitrary symbols and rule-governed combinations of those symbols.

Language impairment (LI) A heterogeneous group of deficits and/or immaturities in the comprehension and/or production of spoken or written language.

Language sample A systematic collection and analysis of a person's speech or writing. Sometimes called a corpus; used as a part of language assessment.

Laryngeal cancer Carcinoma of supraglottal, glottal, or subglottal structures.

Laryngeal papilloma A wartlike growth on the vocal folds.

Laryngeal system Structures of the larynx used for sound production.

Laryngeal webs Results from extraneous connective tissue growing between the vocal folds.

Larynx The superior termination of the trachea that protects the lower airways and is the primary sound source for speech production.

Language disorder Impairment in comprehension and/or use of spoken, written, and/or other symbol systems

Lexicon An individual's personal dictionary of words and meanings.

Linguadental Pertaining to tongue and teeth; phonemes produced with tongue and tooth contact.

Linguistic intuition A language user's underlying knowledge about the system of rules pertaining to his or her native language; linguistic competence.

Liquid Refers to the oral resonant consonants /r/ and /l/.

Literacy Use of visual modes of communication, specifically reading and writing.

Localization The process of determining where sound originates in space.

Lungs A pair of air-filled elastic sacs that change in size and shape and allow us to breathe.

Maintaining cause The perpetuating cause that keeps a problem from self-correcting; for example, parents of an 8-year-old considering a lisp "cute."

Malleus The largest of the ossicles. It is fastened to the eardrum and articulates with the incus, the next bone in the chain.

Manually coded English (MCE) Sign communication systems designed to manually duplicate spoken English for teaching children who are deaf.

Maternal rubella German measles contracted during pregnancy that may result in various disorders in the developing fetus.

Maximal contrast A minimal pair in which the differing phonemes often differ across place, manner, and voicing (e.g., "mop and "chop").

Mean length of utterance (MLU) The average length of utterances, measured in morphemes. In English, this is an important measure of preschool development because language increases in complexity as it becomes longer.

Meniere's disease A condition resulting from excessive endolymph in the inner ear, involving vertigo, tinnitus, aural fullness, and sensorineural hearing loss.

Meningitis An inflammation of the meninges, or layers of tissue covering the brain and spinal cord.

Metacognition Knowledge about knowledge and cognitive processes, including self-appraisal.

Metalinguistic skills Abilities that enable a child to consider language in the abstract, to make judgments about the correctness of language, and to create verbal contexts, such as in writing.

Metaphon approach An approach to phonological therapy that is based on the premise that phonological disorders in children are developmental language learning disorders.

Metaphonological skills The ability to analyze, think about, and manipulate speech sounds.

Microtia A congenital disorder that results in a small malformed pinna or ear canal.

Middle ear The section of the ear containing the ossicles. It is bounded laterally by the tympanic membrane and medially by the cochlea.

Middle ear space (or tympanic cavity) The cube-shaped area between the outer and middle ear that contains the ossicles.

Minimal pair contrasts Two words that differ in a single phoneme, such as *sip* (/se/) and *ship* (/be/).

Mixed hearing loss The simultaneous presence of conductive and sensorineural hearing loss.

Modified barium swallow study An X-ray procedure that is used to visualize the swallowing process. Also known as videofluoroscopy.

Monoloudness A voice lacking normal variations of intensity that occur during speech.

Monopitch A voice that lacks variation in fundamental frequency and inflection during speech production.

Morpheme The smallest meaningful unit of language.

Morphology An aspect of language concerned with rules governing change in meaning at the intraword level.

Morphophonemic contrast Change in pronunciation as a result of morphological changes.

Motor cortex Located in the posterior portion of the frontal lobe of the brain and responsible for signaling the muscles of motor movement.

Multiple oppositions approach A phonologically based therapy approach that targets multiple sound errors at one time, using phoneme word pairs that are maximally contrasted (i.e., differ according to place, manner, and voicing).

Multiple sclerosis (MS) A progressive disease characterized by demyelinization of nerve fibers of the brain and spinal cord.

Multiview videofluoroscopy Motion picture X-rays recorded from various angles.

Muscular Dystrophy A group of inherited muscle diseases that causes progressive weakness and atrophy of skeletal muscles.

Muscle Tension Dysphonia A functional voice disturbance caused by abnormal tightening of laryngeal muscles in the absence of structural or neurological abnormalities.

Mutational Falsetto A psychogenic voice disorder characterized by inappropriate use of a high-pitched voice by postpubescent males, although it can also occur in postpubescent females. Also known as puberphonia, juvenile voice, or falsetto.

Myelination Development of a protective myelin sheath or sleeve around the cranial nerves.

Myringotomy A small surgical incision made in the surface of the tympanic membrane.

Nasal A phoneme that is produced with nasal resonance.

Nasalance score A numerical score that reflects the magnitude of hypernasality measured by a nasometer.

Nasogastric tube (NG tube) A tube placed into the nose and then through the pharynx and esophagus by which liquefied food may be fed.

Nasometer A commercially available device that is used to measure nasality.

Nasopharynx The space within the skull that is behind the nose and above the roof of the mouth.

Neural plasticity Physiological and functional changes within the central nervous system in response to auditory stimulation.

Neurogenic stuttering A disorder of fluency associated with some form of brain damage.

Neuron The basic unit of the central nervous system, consisting of the cell body, axon, and dendrites.

Noise-induced hearing loss Hearing impairment that results from exposure to high levels of occupational or recreational noise.

Nonfluent aphasia Characterized by slow, labored speech and struggle to retrieve words and form sentences

Nonvocal Without voice.

Norm-referenced A comparison that is usually based on others of the same gender and similar age.

Odynophagia Pain associated with any phase of swallowing; it can occur with or without swallowing difficulties.

Omission In articulation, the absence of a phoneme that has not been produced or replaced.

Open syllable A syllable, or basic acoustic unit of speech, that ends in a vowel.

Organ of Corti The intricate structure that runs along the center of the membranous labyrinth of the cochlea and contains the auditory sensory receptor cells.

Ossicles (or ossicular chain) The small bones—the malleus, the incus, and the stapes—housed within the middle ear.

Otitis media Inflammation of the middle ear.

Otitis media with effusion (OME) Inflammation of the middle ear with fluid.

Otoacoustic emissions (OAEs) Measurable low-level sounds or echoes that occur either spontaneously or in response to acoustic stimulation, due to outer hair cell motility within the cochlea.

Otosclerosis A disorder characterized by the formation of spongy bone in the region of the stapes footplate, resulting in a progressive conductive hearing loss.

Otoscope A small handheld device used to visually inspect the external auditory canal and tympanic membrane.

Otoscopic examinations Visual examination of the ear canal and eardrum using an otoscope.

Ototoxic Refers to drugs and chemical agents that are potentially damaging to the inner ear.

Outer ear The section of the ear comprised of the pinna and the external auditory meatus, or ear canal.

Oval window A small oval membrane located on the lateral wall of the cochlea, behind the stapes footplate.

Palatal Refers to the front area of the roof of the mouth. In speech, palatal consonants are produced with the tongue touching or approximating the hard palate.

Palatal lift A prosthetic device for a weak or immobile soft palate.

Palatal obturator A plate that covers a portion of the soft palate. It is useful for individuals who have had palatal surgery.

Parkinson disease A progressive neurogenic disorder that is characterized by resting tremors, slowness of movement, and difficulty initiating voluntary movements. Speech may be rapid, breathy, and reduced in loudness, pitch range, and stress.

Pedunculated polyp A polyp that appears to be attached to the vocal fold by a stalk.

Perilymph The fluid that fills the bony labyrinth of the cochlea and vestibular system.

Peripheral auditory system Part of the auditory system that includes the outer, middle, and inner ears as well as cranial nerve VIII (the auditory nerve).

Peripheral nervous system (PNS) The cranial and spinal nerves that receive and transmit information from the brain to the body.

Perpetuating cause See *Maintaining cause.*

Permanent threshold shift (PTS) A permanent change in hearing acuity associated with exposure to high-intensity noise.

Personal adjustment counseling The process of assisting clients and their families in dealing with the emotional consequences of hearing loss.

Personal hearing aid A personal amplification device ranging from tiny completely-in-the-canal models to those worn behind the ear.

Pharyngostomy A surgical hole in the pharynx, through which a feeding tube may be placed.

Phonation Production of sound by vocal fold vibration.

Phonemic awareness Ability to manipulate sounds, such as blending sounds to create new words or segmenting words into sounds.

Phonetically consistent forms (PCFs) Consistent vocal patterns that function as meaningful "words" for an infant. PCFs are a transition to words.

Phonics Sound–letter or phoneme–grapheme correspondence.

Phonological awareness (PA) Knowledge of sounds and syllables and of the sound structure of words.

Phonology The study of the sound systems of language.

Phonotactic The study of the way in which phonemes are combined and arranged into syllables and words of a particular language or dialect.

Physiology The branch of biology that is concerned with the process and function of parts of the body.

Pidgin Signed English (PSE) A sign system that incorporates ASL signs while maintaining English word order.

Pierre Robin syndrome A congenital condition resulting in a small mandible, cleft lip, cleft palate, and other facial abnormalities.

Pinna The funnel-shaped outermost part of the ear that collects sound waves and channels them into the ear canal.

Pitch The perceptual counterpart to fundamental frequency associated with the speed of vocal fold vibration.

Pitch breaks Sudden, uncontrolled upward or downward changes in pitch.

Postlingually After the development of speech and language.

Post-therapy testing Assessment following intervention.

Pragmatics The use, function, or purpose of communication; the study of communicative acts and contexts.

Precipitating cause Factors that trigger a disorder (e.g., a stroke).

Predisposing cause Underlying factors that contribute to a problem (e.g., a genetic basis).

Prelingually Prior to the development of speech and language.

Presbycusis Hearing loss incurred as a result of the aging process.

Presbyphonia Voice disorder due to aging of the larynx.

Pressure equalization (PE) tube (or tympanostomy tube) A small-diameter tube that is surgically placed in the eardrum to provide ventilation of the middle ear space via the external auditory meatus.

Prevalence The total number of cases of a disorder at a particular point in time in a designated population.

Primary motor cortex A 2-centimeter-wide gyrus immediately in front of the central sulcus of the brain that controls voluntary motor movements.

Primary progressive aphasia A degenerative disorder of language in which other mental functions and activities of daily living are preserved. There is no marked dementia or loss of cognitive functioning.

Print awareness Knowledge of the meaning and function of print, including recognition of words and letters, and terminology, such as letter, word, or sentence.

Prognosis An informed prediction of the outcome of a disorder.

Prolongation In fluency analysis, the process of holding a phoneme longer than is typical; for example, "sssssso."

Prolonged speech A group of speech rate reduction techniques (e.g., prolonged, continuous phonation; gentle voicing onsets; light articulatory contacts) used to treat stuttering and establish stutter-free speech.

Prosody The flow of speech measured as rate and rhythm.

Proxemics The study of physical distance between people.

Psychogenic Caused by psychological factors.

Pure tone audiometry A procedure that is used to assess hearing sensitivity at discrete frequencies.

Pure tones Sounds that contain energy at only a single frequency, such as 250 Hz, 500 Hz, 1000 Hz, 2000 Hz, 4000 Hz, and 8000 Hz, and are used in pure tone audiometry.

Purulent (or suppurative) otitis media Pus formation and discharge by the tissue of the middle ear cavity.

Pyramidal tract Descending motor fibers that arise from the motor cortex and mediate rapid, discrete, skilled volitional movement; also known as the direct activation pathway or direct motor system.

Range of motion The extent of movement of a joint from maximum extension to maximum flexion.

Rarefaction Part of the sound wave where the displaced molecules are far from each other.

Rate The speed at which something occurs. In speech this may be the number of words or syllables in a given period of time.

Recurrent Laryngeal Nerve A branch of the vagus nerve (cranial nerve X) that supplies the majority of laryngeal muscles used for voice production.

Reduplicated babbling Long strings of consonant–vowel syllable repetitions, such as "ma-ma-ma-ma-ma."

Reformulation An adult response to a child's utterance in which the adult adds to the child's utterance to provide a more complex example of what the child has said.

Reinforcement A procedure that follows a response with the intent of perpetuating or extinguishing it; used in conditioning.

Repetition In fluency analysis, the process of repeating a word or a part of a word, as in "the-the-the" or "b-b-ball."

Representation The process of having one thing stand for another, such as a piece of paper used as a blanket for a doll.

Residual hearing Any hearing that remains following the onset of hearing loss.

Respiratory system Structures, including the lungs, bronchi, trachea, larynx, mouth, and nose, that are used in breathing for life and for speech.

Resting tidal breathing Breathing to sustain life.

Right hemisphere brain damage (RHBD) A group of neuromuscular, perceptual, and/or linguistic deficits that result from damage to the right hemisphere of the brain and may include epilepsy, hemisensory impairment, and hemiparesis or hemiplegia.

Scintigraphy A computerized technique for measuring aspiration during or after a swallow.

Self-monitoring The ability to recognize one's own errors and correct them.

Semantic features Pieces of meaning that come together to define a particular word.

Semantics The study of word and language meaning.

Sensorineural hearing loss Permanent hearing loss that results from absence, malformation, or damage to the structures of the inner ear.

Sensorineural system Part of the auditory system made up of the inner ear and cranial nerve VIII.

Sensory-motor approach Articulatory training that emphasizes tactile and proprioceptive sensations and sound, syllable, and word production.

Serous otitis media Inflammation of the middle ear with sterile fluid.

Sessile polyp A polyp with a broad-based attachment to the vocal fold.

Silent aspiration The entrance of food or liquid into the airway that is not accompanied by coughing.

SLP See *Speech-language pathologist*.

Sociolinguistics The study of influences such as cultural identity, setting, and participants on communicative variables.

Sound field amplification A type of assistive listening device that transmits sound from a microphone to loudspeakers that are strategically placed within a room.

Spasmodic dysphonia (SD) A voice disorder characterized by hyperadduction of the vocal folds, resulting in strained/strangled voice production with intermittent stoppages.

Spastic cerebral palsy A congenital disorder that is characterized by increased muscle tone such that when a muscle contracts, the opposing muscle may react abnormally to stretch by increasing muscle tone too much. Muscle movements are described as jerky, labored, and slow.

Spastic dysarthria Speech that is characterized as slow, with jerky, imprecise articulation and reduction of the rapidly alternating movements of speech because of stiff and rigid muscles.

Specific language impairment (SLI) A language impairment in the absence of hearing, oral structural or functioning, cognitive, or perceptual deficits.

Speech bulb obturator An obturator that fills the velopharyngeal space, closing the velopharyngeal portal.

Speech-language pathologist (SLP) A professional whose distinguishing role is to identify, assess, treat, and prevent speech, language, communication, and swallowing disorders.

Speech Recognition Threshold (SRT) A test procedure used in speech audiometry that measures the lowest (quietest) level at which a person can recognize approximately 50% of the spondees presented for a given number of trials.

Speech sample A systematic collection and analysis of a person's speech, a corpus; used in language assessment.

Speech disorder Atypical production of speech sounds, interruption in the flow of speaking, or abnormal production and/or absences of voice quality, including pitch, loudness, resonance, and/or duration.

Spinal nerves Any of the 31 pairs of nerves in the peripheral nervous system, containing sensory and motor fibers that arise from each side of the spinal cord to innervate the body.

Spondees Two-syllable compound words that are spoken with equal emphasis on both syllables and used in Speech Recognition Threshold testing.

Spontaneous recovery A natural recovery process that proceeds without professional intervention.

Stapes The third and smallest of the ossicles in the middle ear.

Stereocilia Small hairlike projections situated on the top of the hair cells in the organ of Corti.

Stimulability The ability to imitate a target phoneme when given focused auditory and visual cues.

Stimulus Anything that is capable of eliciting a response.

Stoma A small opening, such as a surgical hole in the external neck region that extends into the pharynx to permit breathing following laryngectomy.

Stop consonants A consonant phoneme produced by building air pressure behind the point of constriction.

Story grammar Common elements and event sequences in narratives.

Stridor Noisy breathing or involuntary sound that accompanies inspiration and expiration.

Stroke A cerebrovascular accident (CVA), the most common cause of aphasia, which results when the blood supply to the brain is blocked or when the brain is flooded with blood.

Stuttering A disorder of speech fluency characterized by hesitations, repetitions, prolongations, tension, and avoidance behaviors.

Substitution In articulation, the production of one phoneme in place of another.

Support group Individuals with similar problems who meet together to share feelings, information, and ideas.

Suppurative otitis media See *Purulent otitis media.*

Synapse The minuscule space between the axon of one neuron and the dendrites of the next, where "communication" between neurons occurs.

Syntax How words are arranged in sentences.

Symbolization Use of an arbitrary symbol, such as a word or sign, to stand for something.

Tactiles Touch behaviors, such as a hand on the shoulder, that signal communication.

Tardive dyskinesia Involuntary, repetitive facial, tongue, or limb movements that sometimes occur as a side effect of certain medications.

TBI See *Traumatic brain injury.*

Tectorial membrane The gelatinous tongue-shaped structure that forms the roof of the organ of Corti.

Teletypewriter (TTY) A portable keyboard used for remote text conversations over regular phone lines by those who are deaf.

Temporary threshold shift (TTS) A temporary change in hearing acuity followed by spontaneous recovery that is associated with short-term exposure to high-intensity noise.

Threshold The lowest (quietest) presentation level (measured in decibels) at which a person can barely detect a stimulus 50% of the time it is presented.

Thrombosis The formation or presence of a blood clot within a blood vessel of the body. It may result in an ischemic stroke.

Thyroid cartilage Largest of the laryngeal cartilages that forms most of the front and sides of the laryngeal skeleton and protects the inner components of the larynx.

Thyroid prominence anterior outward projection of the thyroid cartilage that is more prominent in males than females; also called the Adam's apple.

Tics Involuntary, rapid and repetitive, stereotypic movements.

Trachea A cartilaginous membranous tube by which air moves to and from the lungs.

Tracheoesophageal puncture (TEP) or tracheoesophageal shunt A device that directs air from the trachea to the esophagus for esophageal speech.

Tracheostomy Surgical procedure that involves creating a stoma (hole) in the trachea and inserting a tube to relieve a breathing obstruction.

Traditional motor approach An articulation treatment approach that emphasizes discrete skill learning, beginning first with auditory discrimination of the error sound, followed by production training of the sound in isolation, in nonsense syllables, and then in words, phrases, sentences, and conversations.

Transcortical motor aphasia A nonfluent aphasia that is characterized by impaired conversational speech, good verbal imitative abilities, and mildly impaired auditory comprehension.

Transcortical sensory aphasia A rare fluent aphasia that is characterized by word substitutions, lack of nouns and severe anomia, and poor auditory comprehension, but featuring the ability to repeat or imitate words, phrases, and sentences.

Transient ischemic attack (TIA) Sometimes called a mini-stroke, it is a condition that occurs when blood flow to some portion of the brain is blocked or reduced temporarily.

Traumatic brain injury (TBI) Damage to the brain that results from bruising and laceration caused by forceful contact with the relatively rough inner surfaces of the skull or from secondary edema or swelling, infarction or death of tissue, and hematoma or focal bleeding.

Treacher Collins syndrome An inherited disorder that is characterized by excessive muscle tone in the face and jaw.

Tremor Involuntary, rhythmic movement of a body part.

Tympanic membrane (or eardrum) The thin cone-shaped structure composed of three layers of tissue located at the end of the external auditory meatus. It is set into vibration as acoustic energy strikes its surface.

Tympanogram A graph generated during acoustic immittance testing that depicts compliance of the eardrum relative to changes in air pressure.

Tympanostomy tube See *Pressure equalization (PE) tube.*

Ultrasonography See *Ultrasound.*

Ultrasound (or ultrasonography) A technique that uses high-frequency sound waves to visualize internal bodily organs.

Unilateral hearing loss Loss of hearing on one side.

Usher's syndrome A hereditary disorder characterized by sensorineural hearing impairment and progressive blindness.

Uvula A small, pendulous structure suspended from the soft palate.

Vallecula Wedge-shaped space or "pocket" between the epiglottis and the base of the tongue on each side of the mouth.

Variegated babbling Long strings of consonant–vowel syllables, in which adjacent and successive syllables in the string are not identical.

Velar Refers to the posterior area of the roof of the mouth. In speech, velar consonants are produced with the tongue touching or approximating the velum or soft palate.

Velopharyngeal closure Contact of the velum with the lateral and posterior pharyngeal walls, thus separating the oral and nasal cavities.

Velopharyngeal dysfunction (VPD) Inability of the velopharyngeal mechanism to separate the oral and nasal cavities during swallowing and speech.

Vestibular system Structures of the inner ear that are responsible for supplying information to the brain regarding balance and spatial orientation.

Vestibulocochlear nerve (or VIIIth cranial nerve) The cranial nerve that runs from the base of the cochlea to the cochlear nucleus of the brain stem. It is composed of the vestibular and cochlear branches.

Videofluoroscopy See *Modified barium swallow study.*

Videonasendoscopy An invasive instrumental procedure involving a flexible fiberoptic nasopharyngoscope that allows direct observation of velopharyngeal function during speech production.

Visual reinforcement audiometry (VRA) A method of hearing assessment in which a child is rewarded for localizing to a test signal through the use of moving toys and/or flashing lights.

Vocal abuse Any of several behaviors, including smoking and yelling, that can result in damage to the laryngeal mechanism.

Vocal fold paralysis Immobilization of the vocal fold, usually due to nerve damage.

Vocal hygiene Proper care of the voice.

Vocal nodules Localized growths on the vocal folds that are associated with vocal abuse.

Vocal polyp A fluid-filled lesion of the vocal fold that results from mechanical stress.

Voice tremor Variations in the pitch and loudness of the voice that are involuntary.

Voice Vocal tone and resonance.

Vowel Any of several voiced phonemes that are produced with a relatively open vocal tract.

Waardenburg's syndrome A hereditary disorder characterized by pigmentary discoloration, particularly in the irises and hair; craniofacial malformation of the nasal area; and severe to profound hearing impairment.

Wernicke's area Located in the left temporal lobe of the brain and responsible for processing of language.

Wernicke's aphasia A fluent aphasia that is characterized by rapid-fire strings of sentences with little pause for acknowledgment or turn taking. Content may seem to be a jumble and may be incoherent or incomprehensible, although fluent and well-articulated.

Word Recognition Test (WRT) A test procedure used in speech audiometry to measure an individual's ability to recognize single-syllable words presented at a predetermined level above their auditory threshold.

Adams, C. (2005). Social communication intervention for school-age children: Rationale and description. *Seminars in Speech and Language, 26*(3), 181–188.

Aikens, N. L., & Barbarin, O. (2008). Socioeconomic differences in reading trajectories: The contribution of family, neighborhood, and school contexts. *Journal of Educational Psychology, 100*(2), 235–251.

Alliano, A., Herriger, K., Koutsoftas, A., & Bartolotta, T. (2016). A review of 21 iPad applications for augmentative and alternative communication purposes. *Perspectives on Augmentative and Alternative Communication, 21*(2), 60–71. doi: 10.1044/aac21.2.60

Altmann, L., Lombardino, L. J., & Puranik, C. (2008). Sentence production in students with dyslexia. *International Journal of Language & Communication Disorders 43*(1), 55–76.

Alzheimer's Association. (2017). Alzheimer's disease facts and figure. Accessed on October 10, 2017 at http://www.alz.org/facts/overview.asp

Alzrayer, N., Banda, D. R., & Koul, R. K. (2014). Use of iPad/iPods with individuals with autism and other developmental disabilities: A meta-analysis of communication interventions. *Review Journal of Autism and Developmental Disorders.* doi: 10.1007/s40489-014-0018-5

Ambrose, N., Cox, N., & Yairi, E. (1997). The genetic basis of persistence and recovery in stuttering. *Journal of Speech, Language, and Hearing Research, 40,* 567–580.

Ambrose, N., & Yairi, E. (2002). The Tudor study: Data and ethics. *American Journal of Speech-Language Pathology, 11,* 190–203.

American Academy of Audiology. (2010). Clinical practice guidelines: Diagnosis, treatment, and management of children and adults with central auditory processing disorder. Reston, VA: Author.

American Association on Intellectual and Developmental Disabilities. (2009). *Definition of intellectual disability.* Retrieved June 2, 2009, from www.aaidd.org/content_100.cfm?navID=21.

American Cancer Society (2016, February 17). *What are the risk factors for laryngeal and hypopharyngeal cancers?* Retrieved from http://www.cancer.org/.

American Psychiatric Association. (1994). *Diagnostic and statistical manual of mental disorders* (4th ed.). Washington, DC: Author.

American Psychiatric Association. (2000). *Diagnostic and statistical manual of mental disorders* (4th ed.). Washington, DC: American Psychiatric Association.

American Psychiatric Association. (2013). *Diagnostic and Statistical Manual of mental disorders.* (5th ed.) Washington, DC: American Psychiatric Association.

American Speech-Language-Hearing Association. (1994). Functional assessment of communicative skills for adults (FACS). Washington, DC: Author.

American Speech-Language-Hearing Association. (2015). *ASHA SLP Health Care Survey 2015: Caseload characteristics.* Available from www.asha.org.

American Speech-Language-Hearing Association (ASHA). (2000a). Council on Professional Standards. *Back-ground information for the standards and implementation for the certificate of clinical competence in speech-language pathology.* (Effective date: January 1, 2005). Retrieved May 13, 2013, from http://professional.asha.org/library/slp_standards.htm.

American Speech-Language-Hearing Association (ASHA). (2000b). Council on Professional Standards. *Back-ground information for the standards and implementation for the certificate of clinical competence in audiology.* (Effective date: January 1, 2007). Retrieved May 13, 2013, from http://professional.asha.org/library/audiology_standards.htm.

American Speech-Language-Hearing Association (ASHA). (2000c). *Fact sheet: Speech-language pathology.* Retrieved May 13, 2013, from http://professional.asha.org/students/careers/slp.htm.

American Speech-Language-Hearing Association (ASHA). (2001a, December 26). Code of ethics (revised). *ASHA Leader, 6*(23), 2.

American Speech-Language-Hearing Association (ASHA). (2001b). Council on Academic Accreditation. *Stan-dards for accreditation of graduate education programs in audiology and speech-language pathology.* Retrieved May 13, 2013, from http://professional.asha.org/students/caa_programs/standards.htm.

American Speech-Language-Hearing Association (ASHA). (2001c). *Fact sheet: Audiology.* Retrieved May 13, 2013, from http://professional.asha.org/students/careers/audiology.htm.

American Speech-Language-Hearing Association (ASHA). (2001d). *Roles and responsibilities of speech-language pathologists with respect to reading and writing in children and adolescents* [Position paper, technical report, and guidelines]. Rockville, MD: Author.

American Speech-Language-Hearing Association (ASHA). (2004). Scope of practice in audiology. *ASHA Supplement, 24.*

American Speech-Language-Hearing Association (ASHA). (2007). *Childhood apraxia of speech* [Position statement]. Retrieved May 13, 2013, from www.asha.org/policy.

American Speech-Language-Hearing Association (ASHA). (2008). *Treatment efficacy summary: Cognitive-communication disorders resulting from right hemisphere brain damage.* Retrieved on May 5, 2013, from www.asha.org/uploadedFiles/public/TESCognitiveCommunicationDisordersfromRightHemisphereBrainDamage.pdf.

American Speech-Language-Hearing Association (ASHA). (2009) *About the American Speech-Language-Hearing Association (ASHA).* Retrieved May 30, 2009, from www.asha.org/about_asha.htm.

American Speech-Language-Hearing Association (ASHA). (2010). 2010 *Audiology survey summary report: Number and type of responses.* Rockville, MD: Author.

American Speech-Language-Hearing Association. (2005a). *Augmentative and alternative communication: knowledge and skills for service delivery* [Knowledge and skills]. Retrieved May 13, 2013, from www.asha.org/policy.

American Speech-Language-Hearing Association (2005b). *(Central) auditory processing disorders.* [Knowledge and skills]. Retrieved on October 14, 2017 from https://www.asha.org/policy/TR2005-00043/.

American Speech-Language-Hearing Association (2005). (Central) auditory processing disorders. [Technical report]. Available from http://www.asha.org/policy

Andreu, L., Sanz-Torrent, M., & Guardia-Olmos, J. (2012). Auditory word recognition of nouns and verbs in children with specific language impairment (SLI). *Journal of Communication Disorders, 45,* 20–34. doi:10.1016/j.jcomdis.2011.09.003

Andrews, G., Craig, A., Feyer, A. M., Hoddinott, S., Howie, P., & Neilson, M. (1983). Stuttering: A review of research findings and theories circa 1982. *Journal of Speech and Hearing Disorders, 48,* 226–246.

Angelo, D. (2000). Impact of augmentative and alternative communication devices on families. *Augmentative and Alternative Communication, 16*(1), 37–47.

Apel, K., & Masterson, J. (2001). Theory-guided spelling assessment and intervention: A case study. *Language, Speech, and Hearing Services in Schools, 32,* 182–194.

Apel, K., & Self, T. (2003). Evidence-based practice: The marriage of research and clinical practice. *The ASHA Leader, 8*(16), 6–7.

Apel, K., & Werfel, K. (2014). Using morphological awareness instruction to improve written language skills. *Language, Speech, and Hearing Services in Schools, 45,* 251–260. doi:10.1044/2014_LSHSS-14-0039

Archibald, L. M., & Joanisse, M. (2009). On the sensitivity and specificity of nonword repetition and sentence recall to language and memory impairments in children. *Journal of Speech, Language, and Hearing Research, 52,* 899–914.

Aronson, A. E. (1990b). *Clinical voice disorders.* New York: Thieme.

Aronson, A. (1990a). Importance of the psychosocial interview in the diagnosis and treatment of "functional" voice disorders. *Journal of Voice, 4,* 287–289.

Arvedson, J. (2009, June 19). *Pediatric feeding and swallowing disorders. Treatment efficacy summary.* Retrieved June 24, 2009, at www.asha.org/NR/rdonlyres/EEE3706F-215C-428B-A461-3ABFA8C0787A/0/TESPediatricFeedingandSwallowing.pdf.

Arvedson, J. (2013). Feeding children with cerebral palsy and swallowing difficulties. *European Journal of Clinical Nutrition, 67,* S9–S12.

Arvedson, J., Clark, H., Lazarus, C., Schooling, T., & Frymark, T. (2010). Evidence-based systematic review: Effects of oral motor interventions on feeding and swallowing in preterm infants. *American Journal of Speech-Language Pathology, 19,* 321–340.

Ashford, J. R., Logemann, J. A., & McCullough, G. (2009a, June 19). *Swallowing disorders (dysphagia) in adults. Treatment efficacy summary.* Retrieved June 23, 2009, at www.asha.org/NR/rdonlyres/1EC1FFDC-CDD2-4569-AB57-319987BFB858/0/TESDysphagiainAdults.pdf.

Ashford, J. R., McCabe, D., Wheeler-Hegland, K., Frymark, T., et al. (2009b). Evidence-based systematic review: Oropharyngeal dysphagia behavioral treatments: Part III. Impact of dysphagia treatments on populations with neurological disorders. *Journal of Rehabilitation Research & Development, 46,* 195–204.

Associated Press. (2013, April 4). Study: Dementia leader in cost. (Albany, NY) *Times Union,* p. A6.

Baken, R., & Orlikoff, R. (2000). *Clinical management of speech and voice* (2nd ed.). San Diego, CA: Singular Press.

Ball, L. J., Marvin, C. A., Beukelman, D. R., Lasker, J., & Rupp, D. (2000). Generic talk use by preschool children. *Augmentative and Alternative Communication, 16,* 145–155.

Balsamo, L., Xu, B., Grandin, C., Petrella, J., et al. (2002). A functional magnetic resonance imaging study of left hemisphere language dominance in children. *Archives of Neurology, 59,* 1168–1174.

Bankson, N., & Bernthal, J. (1990). *Bankson–Bernthal test of phonology.* Austin, TX: PRO-ED.

Barker, R. M., Akaba, S., Brady, N. C., & Thiemann-Bourque, K. (2013). Support for AAC use in preschool, and growth in language skills, for young children with developmental disabilities. *Augmentative and Alternative Communication, 29*(4), 334–346. doi: 10.3109/07434618.2013.848933

Barkmeier-Kramer, J. (2016, November). *How do principles of speech science inform clinical practice for voice disorders?* Oral presentation presented at the annual convention of the American Speech-Language-Hearing Association, Philadelphia, PA.

Barth, A. E., & Elleman, A. (2017). Evaluating the impact of a multistrategy inference intervention for middle-grade struggling readers. *Language, Speech, and Hearing Services in Schools, 48*, 31–41. doi:10.1044/2016_LSHSS-16-0041

Baum, S., & Dwivedi, V. (2003). Sensitivity to prosodic structure in left- and right-hemisphere-damaged individuals. *Brain and Language, 87*, 278–289.

Bear, D. R., Invernizzi, M., Templeton, S., & Johnston, F. (2000). *Words their way: Word study for phonics, vocabulary, and spelling instruction* (2nd ed.). Upper Saddle River, NJ: Prentice Hall.

Bear, D. R., Invernizzi, M., Templeton, S., & Johnston, F. (2004). *Words their way: Word study with phonics, vocabulary, and spelling instruction* (3rd ed.). Upper Saddle River, NJ: Merrill/Prentice Hall.

Beck, D., & and Fabry, D. (2011, January/February). Access America: It's about connectivity. *Audiology Today*, pp. 24–29.

Bedore, L. M. (2010). Choosing the language of intervention for Spanish–English bilingual preschoolers with language impairment. *EBP Briefs, 5*(1), 1–13.

Bedore, L. M., & Leonard, L. B. (2001). Grammatical morphological deficits in Spanish-speaking children with specific language impairment. *Journal of Speech, Language, and Hearing Research, 44*, 905–924.

Beecher, R., & Alexander, R. (2004). Pediatric feeding and swallowing: Clinical examination and evaluation. *Perspectives on Swallowing and Swallowing Disorders (Dysphagia), 13*, 21–27.

Behrman, A. (2007). *Speech and voice science*. San Diego, CA: Plural Publishing.

Behrman, A., Rutledge, J., Hembree, A., & Sheridan, S. (2008). Voice hygiene education, voice production therapy, and the role of patient adherence: a treatment effectiveness study in women with phonotrauma. *Journal of Speech, Language, and Hearing Research, 51*, 350–366.

Belin, P., Zatorre, R. J., Lafaille, P., Ahad, P., & Pike, B. (2000) Voice-selective areas in human auditory cortex. *Nature, 403*, 309–312.

Behrman, A. (2007). *Speech and voice science*. San Diego, CA: Plural Publishing.

Benelli, B., Belacchi, C., Gini, G., & Lucanggeli, D. (2006). "To define means to say what you know about things": The development of definitional skills as metalinguistic acquisition. *Journal of Child Language, 33*, 71–97.

Benfer, K., Weir, K., Bell, K., Ware, R., Davies, P., & Boyd, R. (2013). Oropharyngeal dysphagia and gross motor skills in children with cerebral palsy. *Pediatrics, 131*, 1553–1562.

Bergman, R. L., Piacentini, J., & McCracken, J. (2002). Prevalence and description of selective mutism in a school-based sample. *Journal of the American Academy of Child and Adolescent Psychiatry, 41*, 938–946.

Bernhardt, B. H., & Holdgrafer, G. (2001). Beyond the basics I: The need for strategic sampling from in-depth phonological analysis. *Language, Speech, and Hearing Services in Schools, 32*, 18–27.

Berninger, V. W. (2000). Development of language by hand and its connections with language by ear, mouth, and eye. *Topics in Language Disorders, 20*(4), 65–84.

Berninger, V. W., Abbott, R. D., Billingsley, F., & Nagy, W. (2001). Processes underlying timing and fluency of reading: Efficiency, automaticity, coordination, and morphological awareness. In M. Worf (Ed.), *Dyslexia, fluency, and the brain* (pp. 383–413). Timonium, MD: York.

Bernstein Ratner, N. (2006). Evidence-based practice: An examination of its ramifications for the practice of speech-language pathology. *Language, Speech, and Hearing Services in Schools, 37*, 257–267.

Bernthal, J., Bankson, N., & Flipsen, P. (2017). *Articulation and phonological disorders: Speech sound disorders in children* (8th ed.). Boston: Pearson Education.

Bess, F. H., Dodd-Murphy, J., & Parker, R. A. (1998). Children with minimal sensorineural hearing loss: Prevalence, educational performance, and functional status. *Ear and Hearing, 19*, 339–354.

Bessell, A., Hooper, L., Shaw, W., Reilly, S., Reid, J., & Glenny, A. (2011). Feeding interventions for growth and development in infants with cleft lip, cleft palate or cleft lip and palate. *Cochrane Database of Systematic Reviews (2)*, CD003315. doi: 10.1002/14651858. CD003315.pub3.

Beukelman, D. R., & Ansel, B. (1995). Research priorities in augmentative and alternative communication. *Augmentative and Alternative Communication, 11*, 131–134.

Beukelman, D. R., & Mirenda, P. (2013). *Augmentative and Alternative communication: supporting children and adults with complex communication needs* (4th ed.). Baltimore: Paul H. Brookes.

Bhattacharyya, N. (2014). The prevalence of dysphagia among adults in the United States. *Otolaryngology-Head and Neck Surgery, 151*, 765–769.

Binger, C., & Light, J. (2007). The effect of aided AAC modeling on the expression of multisymbol messages by preschoolers who use AAC. *Augmentative and Alternative Communication, 23*, 30–43.

Bishop, D. V. M., & McDonald, D. (2009). Identifying language impairment in children: Combining language test scores with parental report. International Journal of Language & Communication Disorders, 44(5), 600–615.

Bishop, D. V. (2014). Ten questions about terminology for children with unexplained language problems. *International Journal of Language & Communication Disorders, 49*, 381–415. doi:10.1111/1460-6984.12101

Blachman, B., Ball, E., Black, R., & Tangel, D. (2000). *Road to the code: A phonological awareness program for young children*. Baltimore: Paul H. Brookes.

Black, L., Vahratian, A., & Hoffman, H. (2015). *Communication disorders and use of intervention services among children aged 3–17 years: United States, 2012* (NCHS Data Brief, No. 205). Hyattsville, MD: National Center for Health Statistics.

Blackstone, S., & Hunt-Berg, M. (2012) Social networks: A communication inventory for individuals with complex communication needs and their communication partners. Verona, WI: Attainment Company.

Blackwell, Z., & Littlejohns, P. (2010). A review of the management of dysphagia: A South African perspective. *Journal of Neuroscience Nursing, 42,* 61–70.

Blake, M. L. (2006). Clinical relevance of discourse characteristics after right hemisphere brain damage. *American Journal of Speech-Language Pathology, 15,* 255–267.

Blake, M. L. (2007). Perspectives on treatment for communication deficits associated with right hemisphere brain damage. *American Journal of Speech-Language Pathology, 16,* 331–342.

Blake, M. L. (2009). Inferencing processes after right hemisphere brain damage: Maintenance of inferences. *Journal of Speech, Language, and Hearing Research, 52,* 359–372.

Blake, M. L., Duffy, J. R., Myers, P. S., & Tompkins, C. A. (2002). Prevalence and patterns of right hemisphere cognitive/communicative deficits: Retrospective data from an inpatient rehabilitation unit. *Aphasiology, 16,* 537–548.

Blake, M. L., & Lesniewicz, K. (2005). Contextual bias and predictive inferencing in adults with and without right hemisphere brain damage. *Aphasiology, 19,* 423–434.

Bloodstein, O. (1995). *A handbook on stuttering.* San Diego, CA: Singular.

Bloodstein, O., & Ratner, N. (2008). *A handbook on stuttering* (6th ed.). Clifton Park, NY: Thomson Delmar Learning.

Blumgart, E., Tran, Y., & Craig, A. (2014). Social support and its association with negative affect in adults who stutter. *Journal of Fluency Disorders, 40,* 83–92.

Boburg, E., & Kully, D. (1995). The comprehensive stuttering program. In C. W. Starkweather & H. F. M. Peters (Eds.), *Stuttering: Proceedings of the First World Congress on Fluency Disorder* (pp. 305–308). Munich: International Fluency Association.

Boey, R., Van de Heyning, P., Wuyts, F., Heylen, L., Stoop, R., & De Bodt, M. (2009). Awareness and reactions of young stuttering children aged 2–7 years old towards their speech disfluency. *Journal of Communication Disorders, 42,* 334–346.

Boggs, T., & Ferguson, N. (2016). A little PEP goes a long way in the treatment of pediatric feeding disorders. *Perspectives of the ASHA Special Interest Groups (SIG 13), 1,* 26–37.

Boone, D. R., & McFarlane, S. C. (2000). *The voice and voice therapy* (4th ed.). Boston: Allyn & Bacon.

Boone, D. R., McFarlane, S. C., Von Berg, S. L., & Zraick, R. I. (2010). *The voice and voice therapy.* Boston: Allyn & Bacon.

Boswell, S. (2004). International agreement brings mutual recognition of certification. *The ASHA Leader, 9*(19), 1, 22.

Bothe, A., Davidow, J., Bramlett, R., & Ingham, R. (2006). Stuttering treatment research 1970–2005: I. Systematic review incorporating trial quality assessment of behavioral, cognitive, and related approaches. *American Journal of Speech-Language Pathology, 15,* 321–341.

Boudreau, D. (2005). Use of a parent questionnaire in emergent and early literacy assessment of preschool children. *Language, Speech, and Hearing Services in Schools, 36,* 33–47.

Boudreau, D. M., & Chapman, R. (2000). The relationship between event representation and linguistic skills in narratives of children and adolescents with Down syndrome. *Journal of Speech, Language, and Hearing Research, 43,* 1146–1159.

Boudreau, D. M., & Larson, J. (2004). *Strategies for teaching narrative abilities to school-aged children.* Paper presented at the annual convention of the American Speech-Language-Hearing Association, Philadelphia.

Bourgeois, M. S., & Hickey, E. M. (2009). *Dementia: From diagnosis to management: A functional approach.* New York: Psychology Press.

Boyle, M. (2015). Relationships between psychosocial factors and quality of life for adults who stutter. *American Journal of Speech-Language Pathology, 24,* 1–12.

Brackenbury, T., Burroughs, E., & Hewitt, L. E. (2008). A qualitative examination of current guidelines for evidence-based practice in child language intervention. *Language, Speech, and Hearing Services in Schools, 39,* 78–88.

Brackenbury, T., & Pye, C. (2005). Semantic deficits in children with language impairments: Issues for clinical assessment. *Language, Speech, and Hearing Services in Schools, 36,* 5–16.

Bramble, K. (2013, March/April). Internet hearing aid sales: Our new reality. *Audiology Today,* pp. 16–18.

Branson, D., & Demchak, M. (2009). *AAC: Augmentative & Alternative Communication,* Dec 2009, Vol. 25 Issue 4, 274–286, 13p, 2 Charts; DOI: 10.3109/07434610903384529, Database: Communication & Mass Media Complete

Brault, M. W. (2005). Americans with Disabilities, 2005. *Current Population Reports,* pp. 70–117. Washington, DC: U.S. Census Bureau.

Brea-Spahn, M. R., & Dunn Davison, M. (2012). Writing intervention for Spanish-speaking English language learners: A review of research. *EBP Briefs, 7*(2), 1–11.

Brinton, B., Spackman, M. P., Fujiki, M., & Ricks, J. (2007). What should Chris say? The ability of children with specific language impairment to recognize the need to dissemble emotions in social situations. *Journal of Speech, Language, and Hearing Research, 50,* 798–811.

Brinton, B., & Fujiki, M. (2004). Social and affective factors in children with language impairment: Implications for literacy learning. In C. A. Stone, E. R. Silliman, B. J. Ehren, & K. Apel (Eds.), *Handbook of language and literacy: Development and disorders* (pp. 130–153). New York: Guilford.

Brooks, G., Torgerson, C. J., & Hall, J. (2008). The use of phonics in the teaching of reading and spelling. *EBP Briefs, 3*(2), 1–12.

Brown, S., Ingham, R., Ingham, J., Laird, A., & Fox, P. (2005). Stuttered and fluent speech production: An Ale meta-analysis of normal neuroimaging studies. *Human Brain Mapping, 25,* 105–117.

Bulow, M., Olsson, R., & Ekberg, O. (2001). Video-manometric analysis of supraglottic swallow, effortful swallow, and chin tuck in patients with pharyngeal dysfunction. *Dysphagia, 16,* 190–195.

Bunton, K., & Leddy, M. (2011). An evaluation of articulatory working space area in vowel production of adults with Down syndrome. *Clinical Linguistics & Phonetics, 25,* 321–334.

Burgess, S., & Turkstra, L. S. (2006). Social skills intervention for adolescents with autism spectrum disorders: A review of the experimental evidence. *EBP Briefs, 1*(4).

Byrd, C., Gkalitsiou, Z., McGill, M., Reed, O., & Kelly, E. (2016). The influence of self-disclosure on school-age children's perceptions of children who stutter. *Journal of Child and Adolescent Behavior, 4,* 1–9.

Byrd, C., McGill, M., Gkalitsiou, Z., & Cappellini, C. (2017). The effects of self-disclosure on male and female perceptions of individuals who stutter. *American Journal of Speech-Language Pathology, 26,* 69–80.

Cabré, M., Serra-Prat, M., Force, L., Almirall, J., Palomera, E., & Clavé, P. (2014). Oropharyngeal dysphagia is a risk factor for readmission for pneumonia in the very elderly persons: Observational prospective study. *The Journals of Gerontoly. Series A Biological Sciences and Medical Sciences, 69*(3), 330–337. doi:10.1093/gerona/glt099. Epub 2013 Jul 5.

Caccamise, D., & Snyder, L. (2005). Theory and pedagogical practices of text comprehension. *Topics in Language Disorders, 25*(1), 1–20.

Cain, K. Patson, N., & Andrews, L. (2005). Age- and ability-related differences in young readers' use of conjunctions. *Journal of Child Language, 32,* 877–892.

Calvert, D. (1982) Articulation and hearing impairments. In Lass, L., Northern, J., Yoder, D., & McReynolds, L. (Eds.), *Speech, language, and hearing* (Vol. 2). Philadelphia: Saunders.

Campbell, T., Dollaghan, H., Rockette, H., Paradise, J., Feldman, H., & Shriberg, L., et al. (2003). Risk factors for speech delay of unknown origin in 3-year old children. *Child Development, 74,* 346–357.

Carding, P., Roulstone, S., Northstone, K., & the ALSPAC Study Team (2006). The prevalence of childhood dysphonia: A cross-sectional study. *Journal of Voice, 20,* 623–629.

Catten, M., Gray, S., Hammond, T., Zhou, R., & Hammond, E. (1998). Analysis of cellular location and concentration in vocal fold lamina propria. *Archives of Otolaryngology—Head & Neck Surgery, 118,* 663–666.

Catts, H. W. (1997). The Early Identification of Language-Based Reading Disabilities. *Language, Speech, and Hearing Services in Schools, 28,* 86–89.

Catts, H. W., Adlof, S. M., & Ellis Weismer, S. (2006). Language deficits in poor comprehenders: A case for the simple view of reading. *Journal of Speech, Language, and Hearing Research, 49,* 278–293.

Catts, H. W., Fey, M. E., Zhang, X., & Tomblin, J. B. (2001). Estimating the risk of future reading difficulties in kindergarten children: A research-based model and its clinical implementation. *Language, Speech, and Hearing Services in Schools, 32,* 38–50.

Catts, H. W., & Kamhi, A. (2005). Causes of reading disabilities. In H. W. Catts & A. G. Kamhi (Eds.), *Language and reading disabilities* (2nd ed., pp. 94–126). Boston: Allyn & Bacon.

Centers for Disease Control and Prevention. (2009). *Summary of 2009 CDC EHDI data.* Retrieved March 1, 2013, from www.cdc.gov/ncbddd/hearingoss/ehdi-data.html.

Centers for Disease Control and Prevention. (2014, March 27). CDC estimates 1 in 68 children has been identified with autism spectrum disorder. Accessed on December 22, 2017 at https://www.cdc.gov/media/releases/2014/p0327-autism-spectrum-disorder.htmlhttps://www.cdc.gov/media/releases/2014/p0327-autism-spectrum-disorder.html

Cha, Y. J., & Kim, H. (2013). Effect of computer-based cognitive rehabilitation (cbcr) for people with stroke: A systematic review and meta-analysis. *NeuroRehabilitation, 32,* 359–368.

Chakrabarti, S., & Fombonne, E. (2001) Pervasive developmental disorders in preschool children. *Journal of the American Medical Association, 27,* 3093–3099.

Chang, S., Angstadt, M., Chow, H., Etchell, A., Garnett, E., Choo, A., Kessler, D., Welsh, R., & Sripada, C. Anomalous network architecture of the resting brain in children who stutter. *Journal of Fluency Disorders* (2017), http://dx.doi.org/10.1016/j.jfludis.2017.01.002

Cherney L., & Halper, A. (1996). Swallowing problems in adults with traumatic brain injury. *Seminars in Neurology, 16,* 349–353.

Civier, O., Tasko, S., & Guenther, F. (2010). Overreliance on auditory feedback may lead to sound/syllable repetitions: Simulations of stuttering and fluency-inducing conditions with a neural model of speech production. *Journal of Fluency Disorders, 35,* 246–279.

Chan, J. B., & Iacano, T. (2001). Gesture and word production in children with Down Syndrome. *Augmentative and Alternative Communication, 17*(2), 73–87.

Chang S., Angstadt M., Chow H., Etchell A., Garnett E., Choo A., Kessler D., Welsh R., & Sripada C. Anomalous network architecture of the resting brain in children who stutter. Journal of Fluency Disorders (2017), http://dx.doi.org/10.1016/j.jfludis.2017.01.002

Charity, A., Scarborough, H., & Griffin, D. (2004). Familiarity with school English in African American children and its relation to early reading achievement. *Child Development, 75,* 1340–1356.

Charman, T., Drew, A., Baird, C., & Baird, G. (2003). Measuring early language development in preschool children with autism spectrum disorder using the MacArthur Communicative Development Inventory (Infant Form). *Journal of Child Language, 30,* 213–236.

Choudhury, N., & Benasich, A. A. (2003). A family aggregation study: The influence of family history and other risk factors on language development. *Journal of Speech, Language, and Hearing Research, 46,* 261–272.

Chouinard, M. M., & Clark, E. V. (2003). Adult reformulations of child errors as negative evidence. *Journal of Child Language, 30,* 637–669.

Church, C., Alisanski, S., & Amanullah, S. (2000). The social, behavioral, and academic experiences of children with Asperger syndrome. *Focus on Autism and Other Developmental Disabilities, 15*(1), 12–20.

Cirrin, F. M., & Gillam, R. B. (2008). Language intervention practices for school-age children with spoken language disorders: A systematic review. *Language, Speech, and Hearing Services in Schools, 39,* 110–137.

Clare, L., & Jones, R. (2008). Errorless learning in the rehabilitation of memory: A critical review. *Neuropsychological Review, 18,* 1–23.

Clark, H., Lazarus, C., Arvedson, J., Schooling, T., & Frymark, T. (2009). Evidence-based systematic review: Effects of neuromuscular electrical stimulation on swallowing and neural activation. *American Journal of Speech-Language Pathology, 18,* 361–375.

Clark, H. M. (2004). Neuromuscular treatment for speech and swallowing: A tutorial. *American Journal of Speech-Language Pathology, 12,* 400–415.

Clarke, M., Newton, C., Petrides, K., Griffiths, T., Lysley, A., & Price, K. (2012). An examination of relations between participation, communication and age in children with complex communication needs. *Augmentative and Alternative Communication, 28*(1), 44–51. doi: 10.3109/07434618.2011.653605

Clendon, S., & Erickson, K. A. (2008). The vocabulary of beginning writers: Implications for children with complex communication needs. *Augmentative and Alternative Communication, 24*(4), 281–293.

Cleave, P. L., Becker, S. D., Curran, M. K., Owen Van Horne, A. J., & Fey, M. E. (2015). The efficacy of recasts in language intervention: A systematic review and meta-analysis. *American Journal of Speech-Language Pathology, 24,* 237–255. doi:10.1044/2015_AJSLP-14-0105

Coelho, C. A., DeRuyter, F., Kennedy, M. R. T., & Stein, M. (2008). Cognitive-communication disorders resulting from traumatic brain injury. *Treatment Efficacy Summary.* Retrieved June 28, 2009, from www.asha.org/NR/rdonlyres/4BAF3969-9ADC-4C01-B5ED-1334CC20DD3D/0/TreatmentEfficacySummaries2008.pdf.

Cohen, S., & Garrett, G. (2007). Utility in voice therapy management of vocal fold polyps and cysts. *Otolaryngology Head and Neck Surgery, 136,* 742–746.

Colton, R., Casper, J., & Leonard, R. (2011). *Understanding voice problems: A physiological perspective for diagnosis and treatment* (4th ed.). Baltimore, MD: Lippincott, Williams & Wilkins.

Colton, R. H., & Casper, J. K. (1990). *Understanding voice problems: A physiological perspective for diagnosis and treatment.* Baltimore: Williams & Wilkins.

Condouris, K., Meyer, E., & Tager-Flusberg, H. (2003). The relationship between standardized measures of language and measures of spontaneous speech in children with autism. *American Journal of Speech-Language Pathology, 12,* 349–358.

Conti-Ramsden, G., & Botting, N. (2004). Social difficulties and victimization in children with SLI at 11 years of age. *Journal of Speech, Language, and Hearing Research, 47,* 145–161.

Conti-Ramsden, G., & Durkin, K. (2008). Language and independence in adolescents with and without a history of specific language impairment (SLI). *Journal of Speech, Language, and Hearing Research, 51,* 70–83.

Conti-Ramsden, G., Durkin, K., & Simkin, Z. (2010). Language and social factors in the use of cell phone technology by adolescents with and without Specific Language Impairment (SLI). *Journal of Speech, Language, and Hearing Research, 53,* 196–208.

Conture, E. G. (1996). Treatment efficacy: Stuttering. *Journal of Speech and Hearing Research, 39,* S18–S26.

Conture, E. G., & Guitar, B. (1993). Evaluating efficacy of treatment of stuttering: School-age children. *Journal of Fluency Disorders, 18,* 253–287.

Conture, E. G., & Yaruss, J. S. (2009, June 19). Stuttering. *Treatment Efficacy Summary.* Retrieved June 23, 2009, from www.asha.org/NR/rdonlyres/85BCEC0C-FBF5-43C7-880D-EF2D3219F807/0/TESStuttering.pdf.

Cooper, E. B. (1984). Personalized fluency control therapy: A status report. In M. Peins (Ed.), *Contemporary approaches to stuttering therapy* (pp. 1–38). Boston: Little, Brown.

Corriveau, K., Posquine, E., & Goswami, U. (2007). Basic auditory processing skills and specific language impairment: A new look at an old hypothesis. *Journal of Speech, Language, and Hearing Research, 50*, 647–666.

Corwin, M., Koul, R. (2003) Augmentative and Alternative Communication Intervention for Individuals with Chronic Severe Aphasia: An Evidence-Based Practice Process Illustration. *Perspectives on Augmentative and Alternative Communication*, Vol. 12 Issue: 4 p11–15, 5p.

Cowan, N., Nugent, L., Elliott, E., Ponomarev, I., & Saults, S. (2005). The role of attention in the development of short-term memory: Age differences in the verbal span of apprehension. *Child Development, 70*, 1082–1097.

Coyle, J. (2015). The clinical evaluation: A necessary tool for the dysphagia sleuth. *Perspectives on Swallowing and Swallowing Disorders (Dysphagia), 24*, 18–25.

Craig, A., Hancock, H., Chang, E., McCready, C., et al. (1996). A controlled clinical trial for stuttering in persons aged 9 to 14 years. *Journal of Speech and Hearing Research, 39*, 808–826.

Craig, A., & Calvert, P. (1991). Following up on treated stutterers: Studies of perception of fluency and job status. *Journal of Speech and Hearing Research, 34*, 279–284.

Craig, H. K., & Washington, J. A. (2004). Grade related changes in the production of African American English. *Journal of Speech, Language, and Hearing Research, 47*, 450–463.

Cress, C. J. (2001). Language and AAC intervention in young children: Never too early or too late to start. *American Speech-Language Hearing Association Special Interest Division 1, Language Learning and Education Newsletter, 8*(1), 3–4.

Crowe, L. K. (2003). Comparison of two reading feedback strategies in improving the oral and written language performance of children with language-learning disabilities. *American Journal of Speech-Language Pathology, 12*, 16–27.

Cruickshanks, K. J., Wiley, T. L., Tweed, T. S., Klein, B. E. K., Klein, R., Mares-Perlman, J. A., et al. (1998). Prevalence of hearing loss in older adults in Beaver Dam, Wisconsin: The epidemiology of hearing loss study. *American Journal of Epidemiology, 148*(9), 879–885.

Cummings, L. (2008). *Clinical linguistics*. Edinburgh: Edinburgh University Press.

Cunningham, A., Perry, K., Stanovich, K., & Stanovich, P. (2004). Disciplinary knowledge of K–3 teachers and their knowledge calibration in the domain of early literacy. *Annals of Dyslexia, 54*, 139–167.

Cunningham, J. W., Spadorcia, A., & Erickson, K. A. (2005). Investigating the instructional supportiveness of leveled texts. *Reading Research Quarterly, 40*(4), 410–427.

Cupples, L., & Iacono, T. (2000). Phonological awareness and oral reading skill in children with Down syndrome. *Journal of Speech, Language, and Hearing Research, 43*, 595–608.

Curenton, S. M., & Justice, L. M. (2004). African American and Caucasian preschoolers' use of decontextualized language: Literate language features in oral narratives. *Language, Speech, and Hearing Services in Schools, 35*, 240–253.

Côté, H., Payer, M., Giroux, F., & Joanette, Y. (2007). Towards a description of clinical communication impairment profiles following right-hemisphere damage. *Aphasiology, 21*, 739–749.

Dagli, M., Sati, I., Acar, A., Stone, R. E., Dursun, G., & Eryilmaz, A. (2008). Mutational falsetto: intervention outcomes in 45 patients. *The Journal of Laryngology & Otology, 122*, 277–281.

Dailey, S. (2013). Feeding and swallowing management in infants with cleft and craniofacial anomalies. *Perspectives on Speech Science and Orofacial Disorders, 23*, 62–72.

Dale, P. S., Price, T. S., Bishop, D. V. M., & Plomin, R. (2003). Outcomes of early language delay: I. Predicting persistent and transient language difficulties at 3 and 4 years. *Journal of Speech, Language, and Hearing Research, 46*, 544–560.

Dale, P. S., McMillan, A. J., Hayiou-Thomas, M. E., & Plomin, R. (2014). Illusory recovery: Are recovered children with early language delay at continuing elevated risk? *American Journal of Speech-Language Pathology, 23*, 437–447. doi:10.1044/2014_AJSLP-13-0116

Dalston, R., Warren, D., & Dalston, E. (1991). A preliminary investigation concerning the use of nasometry in identifying patients with hyponasality and/or nasal airway impairment. *Journal of Speech and Hearing Research, 34*, 11–18.

Danahauer, J., Johnson, D., Young, M., Rotan, S., Snelson, T., Stockwell, J., & McLain, M. (2012). Survey of high school students' perceptions about their iPod use, knowledge of hearing health, and need for education. *Language, Speech, and Hearing Services in Schools, 43*, 14–35.

Danahy Ebert, K., & Kohnert, K. (2011). Sustained attention in children with primary language impairment: A meta-analysis. *Journal of Speech, Language, and Hearing Research, 54*, 1372–1384.

Daniels, D., Gabel, R., & Hughes, S. (2012). Recounting the K-12 school experiences of adults who stutter: A qualitative analysis. *Journal of Fluency Disorders, 37*, 71–82.

Dark, L., & Balandin, S. (2007). Prediction and selection of vocabulary for two leisure activities. *Augmentative and Alternative Communication, 23*(4), 288–299.

Davis, S., Howell, P., & Cooke, F. (2002). Sociodynamic relationships between children who stutter and their non-stuttering classmates. *Journal of Child Psychology and Psychiatry, 43,* 939–947.

Dawson, G., Carver, L., Meltzoff, A. N., Panagiotides, H., McPartland, J., & Webb, S. J. (2002). Neural correlates of face and object recognition in young children with autism spectrum disorder, developmental delay, and typical development. *Child Development, 73,* 700–712.

Dawson, J., & Tattersall, P. (2001). *Structured Photographic Articulation Test II—Featuring Dudsberry.* DeKalb, IL: Janelle.

De Groot, B. J., Van den Bos, K. P., Van der Meulen, B. V., & Minnaert, A. E. (2015). Rapid naming and phonemic awareness in children with reading disabilities and/or specific language impairment: differentiating processes? *Journal of Speech, Language, and Hearing Research, 58,* 1538–1548. doi:10.1044/2015_JSLHR-L-14-0019

de Valenzuela, J. S., Copeland, S. R., Qi, C. H., & Park, M. (2006). Examining educational equity: Revisiting the disproportionate representation of minority students in special education. *Exceptional Children, 72,* 425–441.

Dean Qualls, C., O'Brien, R. M., Blood, G. W., & Scheffner Hammer, C. (2003). Contextual variation, familiarity, academic literacy, and rural adolescents' idiom knowledge. *Language, Speech, and Hearing Services in Schools, 34,* 69–79.

DeBonis, D., & Moncrieff, D. (2008). Auditory processing disorders: An update for speech-language pathologists. *American Journal of Speech-Language Pathology, 17,* 4–18.

DeDe, G. (2012). Effects of word frequency and modality on sentence comprehension impairments in people with aphasia. *American Journal of Speech-Language Pathology, 21,* 103–114.

DeDe, G. (2013). Reading and listening in people with aphasia: Effects of syntactic complexity. *American Journal of Speech-Language Pathology, 22,* 579–590. doi:10.1044/1058-0360(2013/12-0111)

Deem, J., & Miller, L. (2000). *Manual of voice therapy* (2nd ed.). Austin, TX: PRO-ED.

DeKosky, S. T. (2008, May 13). *Alzheimer's disease: Current and future research.* Public Policy Forum, Alzheimer's Association, Washington, DC.

Delaney, A. (2015). Special considerations for the pediatric population relating to a swallow screen versus clinical swallow or instrumental evaluation. *Perspectives on Swallowing and Swallowing Disorders (Dysphagia), 24,* 26–33.

Demmert, W.G., McCardle, P., & Leos, K. (2006). Conclusions and commentary. *Journal of American Indian Education, 45* (2), 77–88.

DePippo, K. L., Holas, M. A., & Reding, M. J. (1992). Validation of the 3-oz water swallow test for aspiration following stroke. *Archives of Neurology, 49*(12), 1259–1261.

DeRuyter, F., Fromm, D., Holland, A., & Stein, M. (2008). Aphasia resulting from left hemisphere stroke. *Treatment Efficacy Summary.* Retrieved June 28, 2009, from www.asha.org/NR/rdonlyres/4BAF3969-9ADC-4C01-B5ED-1334CC20DD3D/0/Treatment EfficacySummaries2008.pdf.

DeThorne, L. S., Petrill, S. A., Hart, S. A., Channell, R. W., Campbell, R. J., Deater-Deckard, K., Thompson, L. A., & Vandenbergh, D. J. (2008). Genetic effects on children's conversational language use. *Journal of Speech, Language, and Hearing Research, 51,* 423–435.

Deutsch, G. K., Dougherty, R. F., Bammer, R., Siok, W. T., Gabrieli, J. D., & Wandell, B. (2005). Children's reading performance is correlated with white matter structure measured by diffusion tensor imaging. *Cortex, 41,* 354–363.

Diefendorf, A. (1988). Pediatric audiology. In J. Lass, L. McReynolds, J. Northern, & D. Yoder (Eds.), *Handbook of speech language pathology and audiology* (pp. 1315–1338). Toronto: B. C. Decker.

Diehl, S. F., Ford, C., & Federico, J. (2005). The communication journey of a fully included child with an autism spectrum disorder. *Topics in Language Disorders, 25*(4), 375–387.

Dollaghan, C. A. (2004). Evidence-based practice in communication disorders: What do we know, and when do we know it? *Journal of Communication Disorders, 37,* 391–400.

Dollaghan, C. A., & Horner, E. A. (2011). Bilingual language assessment: A meta-analysis of diagnostic accuracy. *Journal of Speech, Language, and Hearing Research, 54,* 1077–1088.

Donahue, M. L., & Foster, S. K. (2004). Social cognition, conversation, and reading comprehension: How to read a comedy of manners. In C. A. Stone, E. R. Silliman, B. J. Ehren, & K. Apel (Eds.), *Handbook of language and literacy: Development and disorders* (pp. 363–379). New York: Guilford.

Dore, J., Franklin, M., Miller, R., & Ramer, A. (1976). Transitional phenomena in early language acquisition. *Journal of Child Language, 3,* 13–28.

Dorner, B. (2010). Position of the American Dietetic Association: Individualized nutrition approaches for older adults in health care communities. *Journal of American Dietary Association, 110,* 1549–1553.

Douglas, J. M. (2010). Relation of executive function to pragmatic outcome following severe traumatic brain injury. *Journal of Speech, Language, and Hearing Research, 53,* 365–382.

Downey, D., Daugherty, P., Helt, S., & Daugherty, D. (2004). Integrating AAC into the classroom. *The ASHA Leader, 9*(17), 6–7, 36.

Downey, D. M., & Snyder, L. E. (2000). College students with LLD: The phonological core as risk for failure in foreign language classes. *Topics in Language Disorder, 21*(1), 82–92.

Drager, K., Clark-Serpentine, E. A., Johnson, K. E., & Roeser, J. L. (2006). Accuracy of repetition of digitized and synthesized speech for young children in background noise. *American Journal of Speech-Language Pathology, 15*(2), 155–164.

Drager, K. D. R., Postal, V. J., Carrolus, L., Castellano, M., Gagliano, C., & Glynn, J. (2006). The effect of aided language modeling on symbol comprehension and production in 2 preschoolers with autism. *American Journal of Speech-Language Pathology, 15*, 112–125.

Drager, K. D. R., & Reichle, J. E. (2001). Effects of age and divided attention on listeners' comprehension of synthesized speech. *Augmentative and Alternative Communication, 17*, 109–119.

Duchan, J. F. (2002). What do you know about the history of speech-language pathology? And why is it important? *The ASHA Leader, 7*(23), 4–5, 29.

Duffy, J. (2005). *Motor speech disorders: Substrates, differential diagnosis, and management* (2nd ed.). St. Louis, MO: Elsevier, Mosby.

Duffy, J. (2013). *Motor speech disorders: Substrates, differential diagnosis, and management* (3rd ed.). St. Louis, MO: Elsevier, Mosby.

Eckert, M. A., Leonard, C. M., Wilke, M., Eckert, M., Richards, T., Richards, A., & Berninger, V. (2005). Anatomical signatures of dyslexia in children: Unique information from manual and voxel based morphometry brain measures. *Cortex, 41*(3), 304–315.

Easterling, C., & Robbins, E. (2008). Dementia and dysphagia. *Geriatric Nursing, 29*, 275–285.

Edmonds, L. A., & Babb, M. (2011). Effect of verb network strengthening treatment in moderate-to-severe aphasia. *American Journal of Speech-Language Pathology, 20*, 131–145.

Ehren, B. J. (2005). Looking for evidence-based practice in reading comprehension instruction. *Topics in Language Disorders, 25*, 310–321.

Ehren, B. J. (2006). Partnerships to support reading comprehension for students with language impairment. *Topics in Language Disorders, 26*, 42–54.

Ehri, L. C. (2000). Learning to read and learning to spell: Two sides of a coin. *TLD, Topics in Language Disorders, 20*(3), 19–36.

Eigsti, L., & Cicchetti, D. (2004). The impact of child maltreatment on the expressive syntax at 60 months. *Developmental Science, 7*, 88–102.

Eisenberg, S. L., McGovern Fersko, T., & Lundgren, C. (2001). The use of MLU for identifying language impairment in preschool children: A review. *American Journal of Speech-Language pathology, 10*, 323–342.

Eisenberg, S. L., Ukrainetz, T. A., Hsu, J. R., Kaderavek, J. N., Justice, L. M., & Gillam, R. B. (2008). Noun phrase elaboration in children's spoken stories. *Language, Speech, and Hearing Services in Schools, 39*, 145–157.

Ellis Weismer, S., Plante, E., Jones, M., & Tomblin, J. B. (2005): A functional magnetic resonance imaging investigation of verbal working memory in adolescents with specific language impairment. *Journal of Speech, Language, and Hearing Research, 48*, 405–425.

Ellis, L., & Beltyukova, S. (2012). Evidence-based diagnostic treatment and treatment planning for adult stuttering: A case study. *Perspectives on Fluency & Fluency Disorders, 22*, 70–87.

Englert, C. S., Raphael, T. E., Anderson, L. M., Anthony, H. M., Fear, K. L., & Gregg, S. L. (1988). A case for writing intervention: Strategies for writing informational text. *Learning Disabilities Focus, 3*(2), 98–113.

English, K. (2007). Psychosocial aspects of hearing impairment and counseling basics. In R. L. Schow & M. A. Nerbonne (Eds.), *Introduction to audiologic rehabilitation* (5th ed., pp. 245–268). Boston: Pearson.

Erickson, K. A. (2003). Reading Comprehension in AAC. *The ASHA Leader, 8*, 6–9.

Ertmer, D. J., Strong, L. M., & Sadagopan, N. (2003). Beginning to communicate after cochlear implantation: Oral language development in a young child. *Journal of Speech, Language, and Hearing Research, 46*, 328–340.

Everhart, R. (1960). Literature survey growth and developmental factors in articulation maturation. *Journal of Speech and Hearing Disorders, 25*, 59–69.

Fabiano-Smith, L., & Goldstein, B. (2010). Phonological acquisition in bilingual Spanish-English speaking children. *Journal of Speech, Language, and Hearing Research, 53*, 160–178.

Fallon, Karen A.; Light, Janice C.; Paige, Tara Kramer. American Journal of Speech-Language Pathology. Feb2001, Vol. 10 Issue 1, p81. 14p. 6 Charts., Database: Academic Search Premier

Feeney, J., & Capo, M. (2002). *Using self-advocacy videos to educate staff in TBI rehabilitation.* Paper presented at the American Speech-Language-Hearing Association national convention, Atlanta.

Feinberg, M. (1997). The effects of medications on swallowing. In B. C. Sonies (Ed.), *Dysphagia: A continuum of care.* Gaithersburg, MD: Aspen.

Feldman, H. M., Dollaghan, C. A., Campbell, T. F., Colborn, D. K., Janosky, J., Kurs-Lasky, M., Rockette, H. E., Dale, P. S., & Paradise, J. L. (2003). Parent-reported language skills in relation to otitis media during the first 3 years of life. *Journal of Speech, Language, and Hearing Research, 46*, 273–287.

Ferguson, N. F., Evans, K., & Raymer, A. M. (2012). A comparison of intention and pantomime gesture treatment for noun retrieval in people with aphasia. *American Journal of Speech-Language Pathology, 21*, 126–139.

Ferré, P., Clermont, M., Lajoie, C., Côté, H., Ferreres, A., Abusamra, V., et al. (2009). Identification of communication patterns of adults with right brain profiles. *Journal of Latin-American Neuropsychology, 1*, 32–40.

Ferré, P., Ska, B., Lajoie, C., Bleau, A., & Joanette, Y. (2011). Clinical focus on prosodic, discursive and pragmatic treatment for right hemisphere damaged adults: What's right? *Rehabilitation Research and Practice*, 1–10.

Fey, M.E., Catts, H., Proctor-Williams, K., Tomblin, B., & Zhang, X. (2004). Oral and written story composition skills of children with language impairment. *Journal of Speech, Language, and Hearing Research, 47*, 1301–1318.

Fey, M. E., Long, S. H., & Finestack, L. H. (2003). Ten principles of grammar facilitation for children with specific language impairment. *American Journal of Speech-Language Pathology, 12*, 3–15.

FHI 360 (2003). National Dissemination Center for Children with Disabilities. Accessed on March, 10, 2017 at https://www.fhi360.org/projects/national-dissemination-center-children-disabilities-nichcy.

Finestack, L. H., & Fey, M. E. (2009). Evaluation of a deductive procedure to teach grammatical inflections to children with language impairment. *American Journal of Speech-Language Pathology, 18*, 289–302.

Flax, J. F., Realpe-Bonilla, T., Hirsch, L. S., Brzustowicz, L. M., Bartlett, C. W., & Tallal, P. (2003). Specific language impairment in families: Evidence for co-occurrence with reading impairments. *Journal of Speech, Language, and Hearing Research, 46*, 530–543.

Fombonne, E. (2003). The prevalence of autism. *Journal of the American Medical Association, 289*, 87–89.

Foster, W. A., & Miller, M. (2007). Development of the literacy achievement gap: A longitudinal study of kindergarten through third grade. *Language, Speech, and Hearing Services in Schools, 38*, 173–181.

Fox, C., Boliek, C., & Ramig, L., (2006, March). The impact of intensive voice treatment (LSVT®) on speech intelligibility in children with spastic cerebral palsy. Poster presented at the Conference on Motor Speech, Austin, TX.

Fox, C., Morrison, C., Ramig, L., & Sapir, S. (2002). Current perspectives on the Lee Silverman Voice Treatment (LSVT) for individuals with idiopathic Parkinson disease. *American Journal of Speech-Language Pathology, 11*, 111–123.

Fox, C., & Boliek, C. (2012). Intensive voice treatment (LSVT LOUD) for children with spastic cerebral palsy and dysarthria. *Journal of Speech, Language, and Hearing Research, 55*, 930–945.

Fox, L. E., & Rau, M. T. (2001). Augmentative and alternative communication for adults following glossectomy and laryngectomy surgery. *Augmentative and Alternative Communication, 17*, 161–166.

Foy, J. G., & Mann, V. (2003). Home literacy environment and phonological awareness in preschool children: Differential effects for rhyme and phoneme awareness. *Applied Psycholinguistics, 24*, 59–88.

Francis, A. L., Nusbaum, H. C., & Fenn, K. (2007). Effects of training on the acoustic-phonetic representation of synthetic speech. *Journal of Speech, Language, and Hearing Research, 50*, 1445–1465.

Francis, D., Daniero, J., Hovis, K., Sathe, N., Jacobson, B., Penson, D., Feurer, I., & McPheeters, M. (2017). Voice-relate patient-reported outcome measures: A systematic review of instrument development and validation. *Journal of Speech, Language, and Hearing Research, 60*, 62–88.

Franken, M.-C., Kielstra-Van der Schalk, C. J., & Boelens, H. (2005). Experimental treatment of early stuttering: A preliminary study. Journal of Fluency Disorders, 30, 189–199.

Fridriksson, J., Moser, D., Ryalls, J., Bonilha, L., Rorden, C., & Baylis, G. (2009). Modulation of frontal lobe speech areas associated with the production and perception of speech movements. *Journal of Speech and Hearing Research, 52*, 812–819.

Fried-Oken, M., Fox, L., Rau, M. T., Tullman, J., Baker, G., Hindal, M., et al. (2006). Purposes of AAC device use for persons with ALS as reported by caregivers. *Augmentative and Alternative Communication, 22*, 209–221.

Fry, R. (2007). *The changing racial and ethnic composition of U.S. public schools*. Washington, DC: Pew Hispanic Center.

Fuchs, D., Fuchs, L. S., Thompson, A., Otaiba, S. A., Yen, L., Yang, N. J., Braun, N., & O'Connor, N. E. (2001). Is reading important in reading-readiness programs? A randomized field trial with teachers as program implementers. *Journal of Educational Psychology, 93*, 251–267.

Galaburda, A. L. (2005). Neurology of learning disabilities: What will the future bring? The answer comes from the successes of the recent past. *Journal of Learning Disabilities, 28*, 107–109.

Gallinat, E., & Spaulding, T. J. (2014). Differences in the performance of children with specific language impairment and their typically developing peers on nonverbal cognitive tests: A meta-analysis. *Journal of Speech, Language, and Hearing Research, 57*, 1363–1382. doi:10.1044/2014_JSLHR-L-12-0363

Gatlin, B., & Wanzek, J. (2015). Relations among children's use of dialect and literacy skills: A meta-analysis. *Journal of Speech, Language, and Hearing Research, 58*, 1306–1318. doi:10.1044/2015_JSLHR-L-14-0311

Gelfer, M., & Schofield, K. (2000). Comparison of acoustic and perceptual measures of voice in male-to-female transsexuals perceived as female versus those perceived as male. *Journal of Voice, 14(1)*, 22–23.

Gerber, A., & Klein, E. R. (2004). *Teacher/tutor assisted literacy learning in the primary grades, a speech-language approach to early reading: T. A. L. L. while small.* Paper presented at the annual convention of the American Speech-Language-Hearing Association, Philadelphia.

Gersten, R., & Baker, S. (2001). Teaching expressive writing to students with learning disabilities: A meta-analysis. *Elementary School Journal, 101(3)*, 251–272.

Gierut, J. A. (1998). Treatment efficacy: Functional phonological disorders in children. *Journal of Speech, Language, and Hearing Research, 41*(1), S85–S100.

Gierut, J. A. (2001). Complexity in phonological treatment: Clinical factors. *Language, Speech, and Hearing Services in Schools, 32,* 229–241.

Gierut, J. A. (2005). Phonological intervention: The how or the what? In A. Kamhi & K. Pollock (Eds.), *Phonological disorders in children: Clinical decision making in assessment and intervention* (pp. 201–210). Baltimore: Brookes.

Gierut, J. A. (2009, June 19). Phonological disorders in children. *Treatment Efficacy Summary.* Retrieved June 23, 2009, from www.asha.org/NR/rdonlyres/F251004F-005C-47D9-8A2C-B85C818F3D33/0/TESPhonologicalDisordersinChildren.pdf.

Gierut, J. A., Morrisette, M. L., Hughes, M. T., & Rowland, S. (1996). Phonological treatment efficacy and developmental norms. *Language, Speech, and Hearing Services in Schools, 27,* 215–230.

Gierut, J. (2007). Phonological complexity and language learnability. *American Journal of Speech-Language Pathology, 16,* 6–17.

Gillam, R. B., & Gorman, B. K. (2004). Language and discourse contributions to word recognition and text interpretation. In E. R. Silliman & L. C. Wilkinson (Eds.), *Language and literacy learning in schools* (pp. 63–97). New York: Guilford.

Gillon, G. T. (2000). The efficacy of phonological awareness intervention for children with spoken language impairment. *Language, Speech, and Hearing Services in Schools, 31,* 126–141.

Girolametto, L., Hoaken, L., Weitzman, E., & van Lieshout, R. (2000). Patterns of adult-child linguistic interaction in integrated day care groups. *Language, Speech, and Hearing Services in Schools, 31,* 155–168.

Girolametto, L., Weitzman, E., & Greenberg, J. (2003). Training day care staff to facilitate children's language. *American Journal of Speech-Language Pathology, 12,* 299–311.

Girolametto, L., Weitzman, E., & Greenberg, J. (2012). Facilitating emergent literacy: Efficacy of a model that partners speech-language pathologists and educators. *American Journal of Speech-Language Pathology, 21,* 47–63.

Glaspey, A., & Stoel-Gammon, C. (2007). A dynamic approach to phonological assessment. *Advances in Speech Language Pathology, 9,* 286–296.

Glattke, T. J., & Robinette, M. S. (2007). Otoacoustic emissions. In R. J. Roeser, M. Valente, & H. H. Dunn (Eds.), *Audiology: Diagnosis* (2nd ed., pp. 478–496). New York: Thieme.

Glennen, S. L., & DeCoste, C. (1997). *Handbook of augmentative communication.* San Diego, CA: Singular.

Gliklich, R., Glovsky, R., & Montgomery, W. (1999). Validation of a voice outcome survey for unilateral vocal cord paralysis. *Journal of Otolaryngology-Head and Neck Surgery, 120,* 153 – 158.

Goldman, R., & Fristoe, M. (2015). *Goldman-Fristoe test of articulation-Second edition (GFTA-2).* Circle Pines, MN: American Guidance Service.

Goldman, R., & Fristoe, M. (2015). *Goldman-Fristoe test of articulation-Third Edition (GFTA-3).* Boston: Pearson Education.

Goldstein, H., & Prelock, P. (2008). Child language disorders. *Treatment efficacy summary.* Retrieved June 28, 2009, from www.asha.org/NR/rdonlyres/4BAF3969-9ADC-4C01-B5ED-1334CC20DD3D/0/TreatmentEfficacySummaries2008.pdf.

Goldstein, B., & Iglesias, A. (2013). Language and dialectal variations. In J. Bernthal, N. Bankson, & P. Flipsen (Eds.), *Articulation and phonological disorders: Speech sound disorders in children* (7th ed., pp. 326–354). Boston: Pearson Education.

Gorham-Rowan, M., & Morris, R. (2006). Aerodynamic analysis of male-to-female transgender voice. *Journal of Voice, 20*(2), 251–262.

Gosa, M., & Dodrill, P. (2017). Pediatric dysphagia rehabilitation: Considering the evidence to support common strategies. *Perspectives of the ASHA Special Interest Groups (SIG 13), 2,* 27–35.

Gottwald, S. (2010). Stuttering prevention and early intervention: A multidimensional approach. In B. Guitar & R. J. McCauley (Eds.), *Treatment of stuttering: Established and emerging interventions* (pp. 91–117). Baltimore, MD: Lippincott Williams & Wilkins.

Granlund, M., Björck-ÄKesson, E., Wilder, J., & Ylvén, R. (2008). AAC interventions for children in a family environment: Implementing evidence in practice. *Augmentative and Alternative Communication, 24,* 207–219.

Gray, S. (2004). Word learning by preschoolers with specific language impairment: Predictors and poor learners. *Journal of Speech, Language, and Hearing Research, 47,* 1117–1132.

Greenhalgh, K. S., & Strong, C. J. (2001). Literate language features in spoken narratives of children with typical language and children with language impairments. *Language, Speech, and Hearing Services in Schools, 32,* 114–126.

Greenough, W. T. (1975). Experimental modification of the developing brain. *American Science, 63,* 37–46.

Grice, S. J., Halit, H., Farroni, T., Baron-Cohen, S., Bolton, P., & Johnson, M. H. (2005). Neural correlates of eye-gaze detection in young children with autism. *Cortex, 41,* 327–341.

Grigorenko, E. L. (2005). A conservative meta-analysis of linkage and linkage-association studies of developmental dyslexia. *Scientific Studies of Reading, 9,* 285–316.

Groher, M., & Crary, M. (2010). *Dysphagia: Clinical management in adults and children.* Maryland Heights, MO: Mosby Elsevier Inc.

Grove, N., & Dockrell, J. (2000) Multisign combinations by children with intellectual impairments: An analysis of language skills. *Journal of Speech, Language and Hearing Research, 43,* 309–323.

Grunwell, P. (1987). *Clinical phonology* (2nd ed.). London: Chapman & Hall.

Guitar, B. (2014). *Stuttering: An integrated approach to its nature and treatment* (4th ed). Baltimore, MD: Lippincott Williams & Wilkins.

Guo, L.-Y., Tomblin, J. B., & Samelson, V. (2008). Speech disruptions in the narratives of English-speaking children with specific language impairment. *Journal of Speech, Language, and Hearing Research, 51,* 722–738.

Gutierrez-Clellen, V.F., Restrepo, M.A., Bedore, L., Pena, E., & Anderson, R. (2000). Language sample analysis in Spanish-speaking children: Methodological considerations. *Language, Speech, and Hearing Services in Schools, 31,* 88–98.

Guyatt, G., & Rennie, D. (Eds.). (2002). *User's guides to the medical literature: A manual for evidence-based clinical practice.* Chicago: American Medical Association Press.

Haak, P., Lenski, M., Hidecker, M., Li, M., & Paneth, N. (2009). Cerebral palsy and aging. *Developmental Medicine & Child Neurology, 51*(Suppl. S4), 16–23.

Hadley, P. A., Simmerman, A., Long, M., & Luna, M. (2000). Facilitating language development in inner-city children: Experimental evaluation of a collaborative classroom-based intervention. *Language, Speech, and Hearing Services in Schools, 31,* 280–295.

Hall, J., McGregor, K. K., & Oleson, J. (2017). Weaknesses in lexical-semantic knowledge among college students with specific learning disabilities: Evidence from a semantic fluency task. *Journal of Speech, Language, and Hearing Research, 60,* 640–653. doi:10.1044/2016_JSLHR-L-15-0440

Hambly, C., & Riddle, L. (2002, April). *Phonological awareness training for school-age children.* Paper presented at the annual convention of the New York State Speech-Language-Hearing Association, Rochester.

Hancock, A., & Helenius, L. (2012). Adolescent male-to-female transgender voice and communication. *Journal of Communication Disorders, 45,* 313–324.

Hancock, A., & Garabedian, L. (2013). Transgender voice and communication treatment: a retrospective chart review of 25 cases. *International Journal of Communication Disorders, 48,* 54 – 65.

Hancock, A., & Garabedian, L. (2013). Transgender voice and communication treatment: A retrospective chart review of 25 cases. *International Journal of Communication Disorders, 48,* 54–65.

Hane, A. A., Feldstein, S., & Dernetz, V. H. (2003). The relation between coordinated interpersonal timing and maternal sensitivity in four-month-olds. *Journal of Psycholinguistic Research, 32,* 525–539.

Hardin-Jones, M., Chapman, K., & Scherer, N. J. (2006, June 13). Early intervention in children with cleft palate. *The ASHA Leader, 11*(8), 8–9, 32.

Hardy, E., & Robinson, N. (1999). *Swallowing disorders treatment manual* (2nd ed.). Austin (TX): PRO-ED.

Hardy, E., & Robinson, N. M. (1993). *Swallowing disorders treatment manual.* Bisbee, AZ: Imaginart.

Harlaar, N., Hayiou-Thomas, M. E., Dale, P. S., & Plomin, R. (2008). Why do preschool language abilities correlate with later reading? A twin study. *Journal of Speech, Language, and Hearing Research, 51,* 688–705.

Harris, K. R., & Graham, S. (1996). *Making the writing process work: Strategies for composition and self-regulation.* Cambridge, MA: Brookline.

Harrison, L.J., & McLeod, S. (2010). Risk and Protective Factors Associated With Speech and Language Impairment in a Nationally Representative Sample of 4- to 5-Year-Old Children. *Journal of Speech, Language, and Hearing Research, 53,* 508–529.

Hart, K. I., Fujiki, M., Brinton, B., & Hart, C. H. (2004). The relationship between social behavior and severity of language impairment. *Journal of Speech, Language, and Hearing Research, 47,* 647–662.

Hashimoto, N. (2016). The use of one or three semantic associative primes in treating anomia in aphasia. *American Journal of Speech-Language Pathology, 25,* S665–S686. doi:10.1044/2016_AJSLP-15-0085

Hayden, D., & Square, P. (1999). *Verbal motor production assessment for children.* San Antonio, TX: Psychological Corporation.

Hayiou-Thomas, M. E., Harlaar, N., Dale, S., & Plomin, R. (2010). Preschool speech, language skills, and reading at 7, 9, and 10 years: Etiology of the relationship. *Journal of Speech, Language, and Hearing Research, 53,* 311–332.

Henderson, E. H. (1990). *Teaching spelling* (2nd ed.). Boston: Houghton Mifflin.

Hewat, S., Onslow, M., Packman, A., & O'Brain, S. (2006). A phase II clinical trial of self-imposed time-out treatment for stuttering in adults and adolescents. *Disability and Rehabilitation, 28,* 33–42.

Hewlett, N. (1990). The processes of speech production and speech development. In P. Grunwell (Ed.), *Developmental speech disorders: Clinical issues and practical implications.* Edinburgh, UK: Churchill Livingstone.

Hickok G, Okada K, Barr W, Pa J, Rogalsky C, Donnelly K, et al. (2008). Bilateral capacity for speech sound processing in auditory comprehension: evidence from Wada procedures. *Brain Lang.* 107:179–184.

Hicks, C. B., Tharpe, A. M., & Ashmead, D. H. (2000). Behavioral auditory assessment of young infants: Methodologic limitations or natural lack of auditory responsiveness? *American Journal of Audiology, 9,* 124–130.

Higginbotham, D. J., Bisantz, A. M., Sunm, M., Adams, K., & Yik, F. (2009). The effect of context priming and task type on augmentative communication performance. *Augmentative and Alternative Communication, 25*(1), 19–31.

Highnam, C.L., & Bleile, K.M. (2011). Language and the cerebellum. *American Journal of Speech-Language Pathology, 20,* 337–347.

Hill, E. L. (2001). Non-specific nature of specific language impairment: A review of the literature with regard to concomitant motor impairments. *International Journal of Language & Communication Disorders, 36,* 149–171. doi:10.1080/13682820010019874

Hirano, M., Kurita, S., & Sakaguchi, S. (1989). Aging of the vibratory tissue of the human vocal folds. *Acta Otolaryngologia, 107,* 428–433.

Hixon, T., Weismer, G., & Hoit, J. (2014). *Preclinical speech science: Anatomy, physiology, acoustics, and perception* (2nd ed.). San Diego, CA: Plural.

Hixon, T., & Hoit, J. (2005). *Evaluation and management of speech breathing disorders: Principles and methods.* Tucson, AZ: Redington Brown.

Hodson, B., & Paden, E. (1991). *Targeting intelligible speech: A phonological approach to remediation* (2nd ed.). Austin, TX: PRO-ED.

Hodson, B. (2004). *Hodson assessment of phonological patterns* (3rd ed.). Austin, TX: PRO-ED.

Hodson, B. (2012). *Hodson Computerized Analysis of Phonological Patterns—4th edition (HCAPP).* Wichita, KS: PhonoComp.

Hodson, B. (2007). *Evaluation and enhancing children's phonological systems: Research and theory of practice.* Greenville, SC: Thinking Publications.

Hodson, B. (2011). Enhancing phonological patterns of young children with highly unintelligible speech. *The ASHA Leader, 16*(4), 16–19.

Hoffman, R., Norris, J., & Monjure, J. (1990). Comparison of process targeting and whole language treatment for phonologically delayed preschool children. *Language, Speech, and Hearing Services in Schools, 21,* 102–109.

Hoffman, M., Quittner, A., & Cejas, I. (2015). Comparisons of social competence in young children with and without hearing loss: A dynamic systems framework. *Journal of Deaf Studies and Deaf Education, 20*(2), 115–125.

Hogan, T., & Catts, H. W. (2004). *Phonological awareness test items: Lexical and phonological characteristics affect performance.* Paper presented at the annual convention of the American Speech-Language-Hearing Association, Philadelphia.

Hogikyan N., & Sethuraman G. (1999). Validation of an instrument to measure voice-related quality of life (V-RQOL). *Journal of Voice, 13,* 557–569.

Hoit, J., Watson, P., Hixon, K., McMahon, P., & Johnson, C. (1994). Age and velopharyngeal function during speech production. *Journal of Speech and Hearing Research, 37,* 295–302.

Hoit, J., & Weismer, G. (2018). *Foundations of speech and hearing: Anatomy and Physiology.* San Diego, CA: Plural Publishing.

Holland, A., & Fridriksson, J. (2001). Aphasia management during the early phases of recovery following stroke. *American Journal of Speech-Language Pathology, 10,* 19–28.

Homer, E., & Carbajal, P. (2015). Swallowing and feeding services in the schools: From therapy to the dinner table. *Perspectives on Swallowing and Swallowing Disorders (Dysphagia), 24,* 155–161.

Hopper, T., Bourgeois, M., Pimentel, J., Dean Qualls, C., Hickey, E., Frymark, T., & Schooling, T. (2013). An evidence-based systematic review on cognitive interventions for individuals with dementia. *American Journal of Speech-Language Pathology, 22,* 126–145.

Hopper, T. (2005, November 8). Assessment and treatment of cognitive-communication disorders in individuals with dementia. *The ASHA Leader, 10*(15), 10–11.

Hossain, S. (2012). *Cochlear implants and the Deaf culture: A transhumanist perspective.* Retrieved April 1, 2013, from http://hplusmagazine.com/2012/06/11/cochlear-implants-and-the-deaf-culture-a-transhumanist-perspective/.

Houston-Price, C., Plunkett, K., & Haris, P. (2005). Word-learning wizardry at 1;6. *Journal of Child Language, 32,* 175–189.

Howell, J., & Dean, E. (1994). *Treating phonological disorders in children: Metaphon—theory to practice* (2nd ed.). London: Whurr.

Howle, A., Baguley, I., & Brown, L. (2014). Management of dysphagia following traumatic brain injury. *Current Physical Medicine and Rehabilitation Reports, 2,* 219–230.

http://www.asha.org/NJC/AAC/;

http://www.asha.org/public/speech/disorders/AAC/)

http://www.ussaac.org/aac-devices

https://store.prentrom.com/communication-devices

https://www.ablenetinc.com/technology/speech-generating-devices

https://www.apple.com/ipad/

https://www.microsoft.com/en-us/surface

https://www.thoughtco.com/top-alternative-and-augmentative-communication-198828

https://www.tobiidynavox.com/en-us/products/devices/

Huaqing Qi, C., & Kaiser, A. P. (2004). Problem behaviors of low income children with language delays: An observation study. *Journal of Speech, Language, and Hearing Research, 47,* 595–609.

Hugdahl, K., Gundersen, H., Brekke, C., Thomsen, T., Rimol, L. M., Ersland, L., et al. (2004). fMRI brain activation in a Finnish family with specific language impairment compared with a normal control group. *Journal of Speech, Language, and Hearing Research, 47,* 162–172.

Hurst, M., & Cooper, G. (1983). Employer attitudes towards stuttering. *Journal of Fluency Disorders, 8,* 1–12.

Hustad, K., Jones, T., and Dailey, S. (2003). Implementing speech supplementation strategies: Effects on intelligibility and speech rate of individuals with chronic severe dysarthria. *Journal of Speech, Language, Hearing Research, 46,* 462–474.

Information from American Speech-Language-Hearing Association. (1994). *Functional assessment of communicative skills for adults (FACS).* Washington, DC: Author.

Ingham, R. J., Ingham, J. C., Finn, P., & Fox, P. T. (2003). Towards a functional neural systems model of developmental stuttering. *Journal of Fluency Disorders, 28,* 297–318.

Ingham, R. J., & Cordes, A. K. (1997). Self-measurement and evaluating stuttering treatment efficacy. In R. F. Curlee & G. M. Siegel (Eds.), *Nature and treatment of stuttering: New directions* (2nd ed., pp. 413–437). Boston: Allyn & Bacon.

Inglebret, E., Jones, C., & Pavel, D. M. (2008). Integrating American Indian/Alaska Native culture into shared storybook intervention. *Language, Speech, and Hearing Services in Schools,, 39,* 521–527.

Ingram, K., Bunta, F., & Ingram, D. (2004). Digital data collection and analysis: Application for clinical practice. *Language, Speech, and Hearing Services in Schools, 35,* 112–121.

Insalaco, D., Ozkurt, E., & Santiago, D. (2007). The perceptions of students in the allied health professions towards stroke rehabilitation teams and the SLP's role. *Journal of Communicatin Disorders, 40*(3), 196–214.

Inspiration Software (2017). What is visual learning and visual thinking?Accessed on October 10, 2017 at www.strokecenter.org/path/stats.htm.

Internet Stroke Center (2005). Retrieved October 22, 2012, from http://www.inspiration.com/visual-learning.

Iverach, L., & Rapee, R. (2014). Social anxiety disorder and stuttering: Current status and future directions. *Journal of Fluency Disorders, 40,* 69–82.

Jacobs, B. J., & Thompson, C. K. (2000). Cross-modality generalization effects of training noncanonical sentence comprehension and production in agrammatic aphasia. *Journal of Speech, Language, and Hearing Research, 43,* 5–20.

Jacobson, L., & Reid, R. (2007). Self-regulated strategy development for written expression: Is it effective for adolescents? *EBP Briefs, 2*(3), 1–13.

Jacobson, B., Johnson, A., Grywalski , C., Silbergleit, A., Jacobson, G., Benninger, M., & Newman, C. (1997). The Voice Handicap Index (VHI): Development and validation. *American Journal of Speech-Language Pathology, 6,* 66–70.

James, J. (1981b). Self-monitoring of stuttering: Reactivity and accuracy. *Behaviour Research and Therapy, 19,* 291–296.

Jarvis, J. (1989). Taking a Metaphon approach to phonological development: A case study. *Child Language Teaching and Therapy, 5,* 16–32.

Jerome, A. C., Fujiki, M., Brinton, B., & James, S. L. (2002). Self-esteem in children with specific language impairment. *Journal of Speech, Language, and Hearing Research, 45,* 700–714.

Johnson, C. J. (2006). Getting started in evidence-based practice for childhood speech-language disorders. *American Journal of Speech-Language Pathology, 15,* 20–35.

Johnson, C. J., Beitchman, J. H., Young, A., Escobar, M., Atkinson, L., Wilson, B., Brownlie, E. B., Douglas, L., Taback, N., Lam, I., & Wang, M. (1999). Fourteen-year follow-up of children with and without speech/language impairments: Speech/Language stability and outcomes. *Journal of Speech, Language, and Hearing Research, 42,* 744–760.

Johnson, C. J., & Yeates, E. (2006). Evidence-based vocabulary instruction for elementary students via storybook reading. *EBP Briefs, 1*(3).

Johnson, C., Danhauer, J., Ellis, B., & Jilla, A. (2016). Hearing aid benefit in patients with mild sensorineural hearing loss: A systematic review. *Journal of the American Academy of Audiology, 27*(4), 293–310.

Johnston, J. R. (2001). An alternative MLU calculation: Magnitude and variability of effects. *Journal of Speech, Language, and Hearing Research, 44,* 156–164.

Johnston, S., Reichle, J., Evans, J. (2004). Supporting augmentative and alternative communication use by beginning communicators with severe disabilities. *American Journal of Speech-Language Pathology, 13,* 20–30.

Jones, M., Onslow, M., Packman, A., O'Brian, S., Hearne, A., Williams, S., . . . Schwarz, I. (2008). Extended follow-up of a randomized controlled trial of the Lidcombe Program of early stuttering intervention. *International Journal of Language & Communication Disorders, 43,* 649–661.

Jung, T. T. K., & Hanson, J. B. (1999). Otitis media: Surgical principles based on pathogenesis. *Otolaryngologic Clinics of North America, 32,* 369–383.

Justice, L. M., Mashburn, A., Hamre, B., & Pianta, R. (2008). Quality of language and literacy instruction in preschool classrooms serving at-risk pupils. *Early Childhood Research Quarterly, 23,* 51–68.

Justice, L. M., & Ezell, H. K. (2002). Use of storybook reading to increase print awareness in at-risk children. *American Journal of Speech-Language Pathology, 11,* 17–29.

Justice, L. M., & Kaderavek, J. N. (2004). Embedded-explicit emergent literacy intervention I: Back-ground and description of approach. *Language, Speech, and Hearing Services in Schools, 35,* 201–211.

Justice, L. M., & Pence, K. (2007). Parent-implemented interactive language intervention: Can it be used effectively? *EBP Briefs, 2*(1).

Kaderavek, J. N., & Justice, L. M. (2004). Embedded-explicit emergent literacy intervention II: Goal selection and implementation in the early childhood classroom. *Language, Speech, and Hearing Services in Schools, 35,* 212–228.

Kagan, A., Black, S. E., Duchan, J. F., Simmons-Mackie, N., and Square, P. (2001). Training Volunteers as Conversation Partners Using "Supported Conversation for Adults With Aphasia" (SCA): A Controlled Trial. *Journal of Speech, Language, and Hearing Research, 44,* 624–638.

Kagohara, D. M., van der Meera, L., Ramdoss, S., O'Reilly, M. F., Lancioni, G. E., Davis, T. N., Rispolie, M., Lang, R., Marschik, P. B., Sutherland, D., Green, V. A., & Sigafoos, J. (2013). Using iPods and iPads in teaching programs for individuals with developmental disabilities: A systematic review. *Research in Developmental Disabilities, 34*(1), 147–156. doi: 10.1016/j.ridd.2012.07.027

Kahane, J., (1988). Age-related changes in the human cricoarytenoid joint. In O. Fujimura (Ed.), *Vocal physiology: Voice production, mechanisms, and functions* (pp. 145–157). New York: Raven Press.

Kamhi, A. G. (2003). The role of the SLP in improving reading fluency. *The ASHA Leader, 8*(7), 6–8.

Kamhi, A. G. (2006a). Prologue: Combining research and reason to make treatment decisions. *Language, Speech, and Hearing Services in Schools, 37,* 225–256.

Kamhi, A. G. (2006b). Treatment decisions for children with speech-sound disorders. *Language, Speech, and Hearing Services in Schools, 37,* 271–279.

Kamhi, A. G., & Catts, H. W. (2005). Language and reading: Convergences and divergences. In H. W. Catts & A. G. Kamhi (Eds.), *Language and reading disabilities* (2nd ed., pp. 1–25). Boston: Allyn & Bacon.

Kamhi, A. G., & Hinton, L. N. (2000). Explaining individual differences in spelling ability. *Topics in Language Disorders, 20*(3), 37.

Kamhi, A. (2011). What speech-language pathologists need to know about auditory processing disorder. *Language, Speech, and Hearing Services in Schools, 42,* 265–272.

Karagiannis, A., Stainback, W., & Stainback, S. (1996). Historical overview of inclusion. In S. Stainback & W. Stainback (Eds.), *Inclusion: A guide for educators.* Baltimore: Brookes.

Katz, W. F. (2003). From basic research in speech science to answers in speech-language pathology. *The ASHA Leader, 8*(1), 6–7, 20.

Kaufman, N. (1995). *Kaufman Speech Praxis Test for Children.* Detroit, MI: Wayne State University Press.

Kavrie, S., & Neils-Strunjas, J. (2002). Dysgraphia in Alzheimer's disease with mild cognitive impairment. *Journal of Medical Speech-Language Pathology, 10*(1), 73–85.

Kavé, G., & Levy, Y. (2003). Morphology in picture descriptions provided by persons with Alzheimer's disease. *Journal of Speech, Language, and Hearing Research, 46,* 341–352.

Kawashima, K., Motohashi, Y., & Fujishima, I. (2004). Prevalence of dysphagia among community-dwelling elderly individuals as estimated using a questionnaire for dysphagia screening. *Dysphagia, 19*(4), 266–271.

Kay-Raining Bird, E., Cleave, P. L., White, D., Pike, H., & Helmkay, A. (2008). Written and oral narratives of children and adolescents with Down syndrome. *Journal of speech, Language, and Hearing Research, 51,* 436–450.

Kemp, D. T. (1978). Stimulated acoustic emissions from within the human auditory system. *Journal of the Acoustical Society of American, 64,* 1386–1391.

Kemper, S., Thompson, M., & Marquis, J. (2001). Longitudinal change in language production: Effects of aging and dementia on grammatical complexity and prepositional content. *Psychology and Aging, 16,* 600–614.

Kendall, D. L., Oelke, M., Brookshire, C. E., & Nadeau, S. E. (2015). The influence of phonomotor treatment on word retrieval abilities in 26 individuals with chronic aphasia: An open trial. *Journal of Speech, Language, and Hearing Research, 58,* 798–812. doi:10.1044/2015_JSLHR-L-14-0131

Kent, R. (1981). Articulatory-acoustic perspectives on speech development. In R. Stark (Ed.), *Language behavior in infancy and childhood* (pp. 105–126). Amsterdam: Elsevier-North Holland.

Kent, R. D. (1997). *The speech sciences.* San Diego, CA: Singular.

Kent-Walsh, J,. & Mcnaughton, D. (2009). Communication partner instruction in AAC: Present practices and future directions. *Augmentative and Alternative Communication, 21*(3), 195–204. doi: 10.1080/07434610400006646

Kent-Walsh, J., Murza, K. A., Malani, M. D., & Binger, C. (2015). Effects of communication partner instruction on the communication of individuals using AAC: A meta-analysis. *Augmentative and Alternative Communication, 31*(4), 271–284. doi: 10.3109/07434618.2015.1052153

Kent, R., & Vorperian, H. (2013). Speech impairment in Down syndrome: A review. *Journal of Speech, Language, and Hearing Research, 56,* 178–210.

Kessels, R. P. C. (2003). Patients' memory for medical information. *Journal of Royal Society of Medicine, 96,* 219–222.

Ketelaars, M. P., Alphonsus Hermans, T. S., Cuperus, J., Jansonius, K., & Verhoeven, L. (2011). Semantic abilities in children with pragmatic language impairment: The case of picture naming skills. *Journal of Speech, Language, and Hearing Research, 54,* 87–98.

Keuning, K., Wieneke, G., van Wijngaarden, H., & Dejonckere, P. (2002). The correlation between nasalance and a differentiated perceptual rating of speech in Dutch patients with velopharyngeal insufficiency. *Cleft Palate-Craniofacial Journal, 39,* 277–284.

Khan, L., & Lewis, N. (2002). *Khan-Lewis Phonological Analysis—Second Edition (KLPA-2)*. Circle Pines, MN: American Guidance Service.

Khan, L., & Lewis, N. (2015). *Khan-Lewis Phonological Analysis—Third Edition (KLPA-3)*. Boston: Pearson Education.

Kirk, C., & Gillon, G. T. (2009). Integrated morphological awareness intervention as a tool for improving literacy. *Language, Speech, and Hearing Services in Schools, 40,* 341–351.

Kleim, J. A., & Jones, T. A. (2008). Principles of experience-dependent neural plasticity: Implications for rehabilitation after brain damage. *Journal of Speech, Language, and Hearing Research, 51,* S225–S239.

Klein, H. (1998, December 8). Book review of *Handbook of phonological disorders from the perspective of constraint-based nonlinear phonology* by B. Bernhardt and J. Stemberger. *ASHA Leader,* pp. 23–24.

Koppenhaver, D., & Erickson, K. (2003). Natural emergent literacy supports for preschoolers with autism and severe communication impairments. *Topics in Language Disorders, 23*(4), 283–292.

Koppenhaver, D. A. (2000). Literacy in AAC—What should be written on the envelope we push? *Augmentative and Alternative Communication, 16,* 270–279.

Koul, R., & Hester, K. (2006). Effects of repeated listening experiences on the recognition of synthetic speech by individuals with severe intellectual disabilities. *Journal of Speech, Language, and Hearing Research, 49,* 47–57.

Koul, R. K., & Corwin, M. (2010). Augmentative and alternative communication intervention for persons with chronic severe aphasia: Bringing research to practice. *EBP Briefs, 6*(2), 1–8.

Kouri, T. A., Selle, C. A., & Riley, S. A. (2006). Comparison of meaning and graphophonemic feedback strategies for guided reading instruction of children with language delays. *American Journal of Speech-Language Pathology, 15,* 236–246.

Koutsoftas, A. D., Harmon, M., & Gray, S. (2008, October 24). The effect of Tier 2 intervention for phonemic awareness in a response-to-intervention model in low-income preschool classrooms. *Language, Speech, and Hearing Services in Schools.* Retrieved June 6, 2009, from http://lshss.asha.org/cgi/rapidpdf/0161-1461_2008_07-0101v1?maxtoshow=&HITS=10&hits=10&RESULTFORMAT=&authorl=Koutsoftas&andorexactfulltext=and&searchid=1&FIRSTINDEX=0&sortspec=relevance&resourcetype.

Kristensen, H. (2000). Selective mutism and comorbidity with developmental disorder/delay, anxiety disorder, and elimination disorder. *Journal of the American Academy of Child and Adolescent Psychiatry, 39,* 249–256.

Kuehn, D., Imrey, P., Tomes, L., et al. (2002). Efficacy of continuous positive airway pressure (CPAP) treatment of hypernasality. *Cleft Palate-Craniofacial Journal, 39,* 267–276.

Kuehn, D., & Henne, L. (2003). Speech evaluation and treatment for patients with cleft palate. *American Journal of Speech-Language Pathology, 12,* 103–109.

Kuehn, D. (1991). New therapy for treating hypernasal speech using continuous positive airway pressure (CPAP) for treatment of hypernasality. *Cleft Palate-Craniofacial Journal, 39,* 267–276.

Kumin, L., Council, C., & Goodman, M. (1994). A longitudinal study of emergence of phonemes in children with Down syndrome. *Journal of Communication Disorders, 27,* 293–303.

Kumin, L. (2006). Speech intelligibility and childhood verbal apraxia in children with Down syndrome. *Down's Syndrome, Research, and Practice, 10,* 10–22.

Kummer, A., & Lee, L. (1996). Evaluation and treatment of resonance disorders. *Language, Speech, and Hearing Services in Schools, 27,* 271–281.

Kummer, A. (2011a). Perceptual assessment of resonance and velopharyngeal function. *Seminars in Speech and Language, 32,* 159–167.

Kummer, A. (2011b). Types and causes of velopharyngeal dysfunction. *Seminars in Speech and Language, 32,* 150–158.

Kummer, A. (2014). Speech and resonance disorders related to cleft palate and velopharyngeal dysfunction: A guide to evaluation and treatment. *Perspectives on School-Based Issues, 15,* 57–74.

Kummer, A. (2014). Orofacial examination. In A. Kummer (Ed.), *Cleft palate and craniofacial anomalies: The effects on speech and resonance* (3rd ed., pp. 352–386). Clifton Park, NY: Cengage Learning.

Kummer, A. W. (2014). Speech and resonance assessment. In A. Kummer (Ed.), *Cleft palate and craniofacial anomalies: The effects on speech and resonance* (3rd ed., pp. 324–351). Clifton Park, NY: Cengage Learning.

La Paro, K. M., Justice, L., Skibbe, L. E., & Pianta, R. C. (2004). Relations among maternal, child, and demographic factors and the persistence of preschool language impairment. *American Journal of Speech-Language Pathology, 13,* 291–303.

Langevin, M., Packman, A., & Onslow, M. (2009). Peer responses to stuttering in the preschool setting. *American Journal of Speech-Language Pathology, 18,* 264–276.

Langford, S., & Cooper, E. (1974). Recovery from stuttering as viewed by parents of self-diagnosed recovered stutterers. *Journal of Communication Disorders, 7,* 171–181.

Lansford, K., Borrie, S., & Bystricky L. (2016). Use of crowdsourcing to assess the ecological validity of perceptual-training paradigms in dysarthria. *American Journal of Speech-Language Pathology, 25,* 233–239.

Lanter, E., & Watson, L. R. (2008). Promoting literacy in students with ASD: The basics for the SLP. *Language, Speech, and Hearing Services in Schools, 39,* 33–43.

Lapko, L., & Bankson, N. (1975). Relationship between auditory discrimination, articulation stimulability and consistency of misarticulation. *Perceptual and Motor Skills, 40,* 171–177.

Larrivee, L., & Catts, H. (1999). Early reading achievement in children with expressive phonological disorders. *American Journal of Speech-Language Pathology, 8,* 118, 128.

Lasker, J. P., & Bedrosian, J. L. (2000). Acceptance of AAC by adults with acquired disorders. In D. Beukelman, K. Yorkston, & J. Reichle (Eds.), *Augmentative communication for adults with neurogenic and neuromuscular disabilities* (pp. 107–136). Baltimore: Brookes.

Lasker, J. P., & Bedrosian, J. L. (2001). Promoting acceptance of augmentative and alternative communication by adults with acquired communication disorders. *Augmentative and Alternative Communication, 17,* 141–153.

Lau, C. (2006). Oral feeding in the preterm infant. *Neonatal Reviews, 7,* e19–e27.

Law, J., Garrett, Z., & Nye, C. (2004). The efficacy of treatment for children with developmental speech and language delay/disorder: A meta-analysis. *Journal of Speech, Language, and Hearing Research, 47,* 924–943.

Law, J., Rush, R., Schoon, I., & Parsons, S. (2009). Modeling developmental language difficulties from school entry into adulthood: Literacy, mental health, and employment outcomes. *Journal of Speech, Language, and Hearing Research, 52,* 1401–1416.

Law, J., Boyle, J., Harris, F., Harkness, A., & Nye, C. (2000). Prevalence and natural history of primary speech and language delay: Findings from a systematic review of the literature. *International Journal of Language & Communication Disorders, 35,* 165–188. doi:10.1080/136828200247133

Lê, K., Coelho, C., Mozeiko, J., Krueger, F., & Grafman, J. (2014). Does brain volume loss predict cognitive and narrative discourse performance following traumatic brain injury? *American Journal of Speech-Language Pathology, 23,* S271–S284. doi:10.1044/2014_AJSLP-13-0095

Leder, S. (2015). Comparing simultaneous clinical swallow evaluations and fiberoptic endoscopic evaluations for swallowing: Findings and consequences. *Perspectives on Swallowing and Swallowing Disorders (Dysphagia), 24,* 12 – 17.

Lee, J., Croen, L. A., Lindan, C., Nash, K. B., Yoshida, C. K., Ferriero, D. M., et al. (2005). Predictors of outcome in perinatal arterial stroke: A population-based study. *Annals of Neurology, 58*(2), 303–308.

Lee, S. A. S., Sancibrian, S., & Ahlfinger, N. (2013). The effects of technology-assisted instruction to improve phonological awareness skills in children with reading difficulties: A systematic review. *EBP Briefs, 8*(1), 1–10.

Lehman Blake, M., Frymark, T., & Venedictov, R. (2013). An evidence-based systematic review on communication treatments for individuals with right hemisphere brain damage. *American Journal of Speech-Language Pathology, 22,* 146–160.

Lehman Blake, M., & Tompkins, C. A. (2008). Cognitive-communication disorders resulting from right hemisphere damage. *Treatment Efficacy Summary.* Retrieved June 28, 2009, from www.asha.org/NR/rdonlyres/4BAF3969-9ADC-4C01-B5ED-1334CC20DD3D/0/TreatmentEfficacySummaries2008.pdf.

Lehman Blake, M. (2006). Clinical relevance of discourse characteristics after right hemisphere brain damage. *American Journal of Speech-Language Pathology, 15,* 255–267.

Lehman Blake, M. (2007). Perspectives on treatment for communication deficits associated with right hemisphere brain damage. *American Journal of Speech-Language Pathology, 16,* 331–342.

Lehman, M. T., & Tompkins, C. (2000). Inferencing in adults with right hemisphere brain damage: An analysis of conflicting results. *Aphasiology, 14,* 485–499.

Leonard, L. B. (2011). The primacy of priming in grammatical learning and intervention: A tutorial. *Journal of Speech, Language, and Hearing Research, 54,* 608–621.

Leonard, L. B. (2014). *Children with specific language impairment* (2nd ed.). Cambridge, MA: MIT Press.

Leonard, M. A., Milich, R., & Lorch, E. P. (2011). Pragmatic language use in mediating the relation between hyperactivity and inattention and social skills problems. *Journal of Speech, Language, and Hearing Research, 54,* 567–579.

Lewis, B. A., Minnes, S., Short, E. J., Min, M. O., Wu, M., Lang, A., Weishampel, P., & Singer, L. T. (2013). Language outcomes at 12 years for children exposed prenatally to cocaine. *Journal of Speech, Language, and Hearing Research, 56,* 1662–1676. doi:10.1044/1092-4388(2013/12-0119)

Lewis, B., Freebairn, L., & Taylor, H. (2000). Follow-up of children with early expressive phonology disorders. *Journal of Learning Disabilities, 33*(5), 433–444.

Lieven, E., Behrens, H., Speares, J., & Tomasello, M. (2003). Early syntactic creativity: A usage-based approach. *Journal of Child Language, 30,* 333–370.

Light, J. (1999). Do augmentative and alternative communication interventions really make a difference?: The challenges of efficacy research. Augmentative and Alternative Communication 15 (1), 13–24.

Light, J. C., & Binger, C. (1998). *Building communicative competence with individuals who use augmentative and alternative communication.* Baltimore, Md.: P.H. Brookes.

Light, J., Drager, K. (2007). AAC technologies for young children with complex communication needs: State of the science and future research directions. *AAC: Augmentative & Alternative Communication,* Vol. 23 Issue 3, p204–216, 13p.

Light, J., & McNaughton, D. (2012). The changing face of augmentative and alternative communication: Past, present, and future challenges. *Augmentative and Alternative Communication, 28*(4), 197–204. doi: 10.3109/07434618.2012.737024.

Light, J., & McNaughton, D. (2014). Communicative competence for individuals who require augmentative and alternative communication: A new definition for a new era of communication? *Augmentative and Alternative Communication, 30*(1), 1–18. doi: 10.3109/07434618.2014.885080

Light, J.C., Roberts, B., Dimarco, R., Greiner, N. (1998). Augmentative and alternative communication to support receptive and expressive communication for people with autism. Special Issue: Autism: New Perspectives on Assessment and Intervention Journal of Communication Disorders, Vol 31(2), pp. 153–180.

Liiva, C. A., & Cleave, P. L. (2005). Roles of initiation and responsiveness in access and participation for children with specific language impairment. *Journal of Speech, Language, and Hearing Research, 48*, 868–883.

Light, J. C., Binger, C., Agate, T.L., Ramsay, K. N. (1999). Teaching partner-focused questions to individuals who use augmentative and alternative communication to enhance their communicative competence. *Journal of Speech, Language, and Hearing Research,* Vol 42(1), pp. 241–255.

Lincoln, M., & Onslow, M. (1997). Long-term outcome of early intervention for stuttering. *American Journal of Speech-Language Pathology, 6*, 51–58.

Lloyd, L. L. Fuller, D., & Arvidson, H. (1997). *Augmentative and alternative communication: A handbook of principles and practices.* Boston: Allyn & Bacon.

Lloyd, L. L., & Kangas, K. A. (1994). "Augmentative and Alternative Communication." In G. H. Shames, E. H. Wiig, & W. A. Secord (Eds.), *Human Communication Disorders* (4th ed.). Boston: Allyn & Bacon.

Logemann, J., Gensler, G., Robbins, J., Lindblad, J., et al. (2008). A randomized study of three interventions for aspiration of thin liquids in patients with dementia or Parkinson's disease. *Journal of Speech, Language, and Hearing Research, 51*, 173–183.

Logemann, J., Kahrilas, P., Kobara, M., & Vakil, N. (1989). The benefit of head rotation on pharyngeoesophageal dysphagia. *Archives of Physical Medicine Rehabilitation, 70*, 767–771.

Logemann, J. A. (1997). Structural and functional aspects of normal and disordered swallowing. In C. T. Ferrand & R. L. Bloom (Eds.), *Introduction to organic and neurogenic disorders of communication: Current scope of practice.* Boston: Allyn & Bacon.

Logemann, J. A. (1998). *Evaluation and treatment of swallowing disorders* (2nd ed.). Austin, TX: PRO-ED.

Losh, M., & Capps, L. (2003). Narrative ability in high-functioning children with autism or Asperger's syndrome. *Journal of Autism and Developmental Disorders, 33*, 239–251.

Louise-Bender, P. T., Kim, J., & Weiner, B. (2002). The shaping of individual meanings assigned to assistive technology: a review of personal factors. *Disability and Rehabilitation 24*(1-3), 5–20.

Love, R., & Webb, W. (2001). *Neurology for the speech-language pathologist* (4th ed.). Boston: Butterworth–Heinemann.

Lubinski, R., & Masters, M. G. (2001). Special populations, special settings: New and expanding frontiers. In R. Lubinski & C. Frattali (Eds.), *Professional issues in speech-language pathology and audiology* (2nd ed.). San Diego, CA: Singular.

Ludlow, C., Hoit, J., Kent, R., Ramig, L., Shrivastav, R., Strand, E., Yorkston, K., Sapienza, C. (2008). Translating principles of neural plasticity into research on speech motor control recovery and rehabilitation. *American Journal of Speech-Language Pathology, 51*, S240–S258.

Lum, J. A., Powell, M., Timms, L., & Snow, P. (2015). A meta-analysis of cross sectional studies investigating language in maltreated children. *Journal of Speech, Language, and Hearing Research, 58*, 961–976. doi:10.1044/2015_JSLHR-L-14-0056

Lund, N., & Duchan, J. (1993). *Assessing children's language in naturalistic contexts* (3rd ed.). Englewood Cliffs, NJ: Prentice Hall.

Lund, S., & Light, J. (2006). Long-term outcomes for individuals who use augmentative and alternative communication: Part I—What is a good outcome? *Augmentative and Alternative Communication, 22*, 284–299.

Lund, S., & Light, J. (2007). Long-term outcomes for individuals who use augmentative and alternative communication: Part II—What is a good outcome? *Augmentative and Alternative Communication, 23*, 1–15.

Lundgren, K., Brownell, H., Cayer-Meade, C., Milione, J., & Kearns, K. (2011). Treating metaphor interpretation deficits subsequent to right hemisphere brain damage: Preliminary results. *Aphasiology, 25*, 456–474.

Lyon, G. R., Shaywitz, S. E., & Shaywitz, B. A. (2003). Defining dyslexia, comorbidity, teachers' knowledge of language and reading: A definition of dyslexia. *Annals of Dyslexia, 53*, 1.

Maas, E., Butalla, C., & Farinella, K. (2012). Feedback frequency in treatment for childhood apraxia of speech. *American Journal of Speech-Language Pathology, 21*, 239–257.

Maas, E., Robin, D. A., Austermann Hula, S. N., Freedman, S. E., Wulf, G., & Ballard, K. J. (2008). Principles of motor learning in treatment of motor speech disorders. *American Journal of Speech-Language Pathology, 17*, 277–298.

Maas, E., & Farinella, K. (2012). Random versus blocked practice in treatment for childhood apraxia of speech.

Journal of Speech, Language, and Hearing Research, 55, 561–578.

MacArthur, C. A. (2000). New tools for writing: Assistive technology for students with writing difficulties. *Topics in Language Disorders, 20,* 85–100.

Machalicek W, Sanford A, Lang R, Rispoli M, Molfenter N, Mbeseha MK.(2010). Literacy interventions for students with physical and developmental disabilities who use aided AAC devices: a systematic review. *Journal of Developmental and Physical Disabilities; 22*(3): 219–240.

Mackie, C., & Dockrell, J. (2004). The nature of written language deficits in children with SLI. *Journal of Speech, Language, and Hearing Research, 47,* 1469–1483.

Magaziner, J., German, P., Itkin Zimmerman, S., Hebel, J. R., Burton, L., Bruber-Baldini, A. L., May, C., & Kittner, S. (2000). The prevalence of dementia in a statewide sample of new nursing home admissions aged 65 and older: Diagnosis by expert panel. *The Gerontologist, 40(6), 663–672.*

Mainela-Arnold, E., Evans, J. L., & Coady, J. A. (2008). Lexical representations in children with SLI: Evidence from a frequency-manipulated gating task. *Journal of Speech, Language, and Hearing Research, 51,* 381–393.

Mainela-Arnold, E., Evans, J. L., & Coady, J. A. (2010). Explaining lexical-semantic deficits in specific language impairment: The role of phonological similarity, phonological working memory, and lexical competition. *Journal of Speech, Language, and Hearing Research, 53,* 1742–1756.

Meinzen-Derr, J., Wiley, S., & Choo, D. (2011). Impact of early intervention on expressive and receptive language development among young children with permanent hearing loss. *American Annals of the Deaf, 155*(5), 580–591.

Mann, V., & Singson, M. (2003). Linking morphological knowledge to English decoding ability: Large effects of little suffixes. In E. Assink & D Sandra (Eds.), *Reading complex words: Cross-language studies* (pp. 1–25). Dordrecht, Netherlands: Kluwer.

Mann, W., & Lane, J. (1991). *Assistive technology for persons with disabilities: The role of occupational therapy.* Rockville, MD: American Occupational Therapy Association.

Mansson, H. (2000). Childhood stuttering: Incidence and development. *Journal of Fluency Disorders, 25,* 47–57.

Margolis, R., Killion, M., Bratt, G., & Saly, G. (2016). Validation of the Home Hearing Test. *Journal of the American Academy of Audiology, 27*(5), 416–420.

Marini, A., Boewe, A., Caltagirone, C., & Carlomagno, S. (2005). Age-related differences in the production of textual descriptions. *Journal of Psycholinguistic Research, 34,* 439–464.

Markel, N., Meisels, M., & Houck, J. (1964). Judging personality from voice quality. *Journal of Abnormal Social Psychology, 69,* 458–463.

Martin, R., & Lindamood, L. (1986). Stuttering and spontaneous recovery: Implications for the speech-language pathologist. *Language, Speech, and Hearing Services in Schools, 17,* 207–218.

Martin, R. E., Neary, M. A., & Diamant, N. E. (1997). Dysphagia following anterior cervical spine surgery. *Dysphagia, 12*(1), 2–10.

Martins, R., do Amaral, H., Tavares, E., Martins, M., Gonçalves, T., & Dias, N. (2016). Voice disorders: Etiology and diagnosis. *Journal of Voice, 16, 761.e1 – 761.e9.*

Marvin, C. A., & Wright, D. (1997). Literacy socialization in the homes of preschool children. *Language, Speech, and Hearing Services in Schools, 28,* 154–163.

Masterson, J. J., & Apel, K. (2000). Spelling assessment: Charting a path to optimal intervention. *Topics in Language Disorders, 20*(3), 50–65.

Masterson, J. J., & Bernhardt, B. (2001). *Computerized Articulation & Phonology Evaluation System (CAPES).* San Antonio, TX: Pearson.

Max, L., & Caruso, A. J. (1997). Contemporary techniques for establishing fluency in the treatment of adults who stutter. *Contemporary Issues in Communication Science and Disorders, 24,* 45–52.

McCabe, A., & Bliss, L. S. (2004–2005). Narratives from Spanish-speaking children with impaired and typical language development. *Imagination, Cognititon, and Personality, 24,* 331–346.

McCarthy, J., & Light, J. (2001). Instructional effectiveness of an integrated theatre arts program for children using augmentative and alternative communication and their nondisabled peers: Preliminary study. *Augmentative and Alternative Communication, 17,* 88–98.

McCauley, R., & Strand, E. (2008). A review of standardized tests of nonverbal oral and speech motor performance in children. *American Journal of Speech-Language Pathology, 17,* 81–91.

McCoy, K. F., Bedrosian, J. L., Hoag, L. A., & Johnson, D. E. (2007). Brevity and speed of message delivery trade-offs in augmentative and alternative communication. *Augmentative and Alternative Communication, 23,* 76–88.

McCullough, G., Pelletier, C., & Steele, C. (2003, November 4). National Dysphagia Diet: What to swallow? *The ASHA Leader.*

McDonald, E. T. (1964). *Articulation testing and treatment: A sensory-motor approach.* Pittsburgh, PA: Stanwix House.

McFadden, T. U. (1998). Sounds and stories: Teaching phonemic awareness in interactions around text. *American Journal of Speech-Language Pathology, 7*(2), 5–13.

McFarland, C., & Cacase, T. (2006). Current controversies in CAPD: From Procrustes bed to Pandora's box. In T. K. Parthasarathy (Ed.), *An introduction to auditory processing disorders in children* (pp. 247–263). Mahwah, NJ: Erlbaum.

McGinty, A., & Justice, L. M. (2009). Predictors of print knowledge in children with specific language impairment: Experiential and developmental factors. *Journal of Speech, Language, and Hearing Research, 52,* 81–97.

McGinty, A. S., & Justice, L. M. (2006). Classroom-based versus pull-out interventions: A review of the experimental evidence. *EBP Briefs, 1*(1).

McGregor, K. K. (2000). The development and enhancement of narrative skills in a preschool classroom: Toward a solution to clinician-client mismatch. *American Journal of Speech-Language Pathology, 9,* 55–71.

McGregor, K. K., Newman, R. M., Reilly, R. M., & Capone, N. C. (2002). Semantic representation and naming in children with specific language impairment. *Journal of Speech, Language, and Hearing Research, 45,* 998–1014.

McGregor, K. K., Sheng, L., & Smith, B. (2005). The precocious two-year-old: Status of the lexicon and links to the grammar. *Journal of Child Language, 32,* 563–585.

McLeod, S., & Searl, J. (2006). Adaptation to an electropalatograph palate: Acoustic, impressionistic, and perceptual data. *American Journal of Speech-Language Pathology, 15,* 192–206.

McLeod, S., & Verdon, S. (2014). A review of 30 speech assessments in 19 languages other than English. *American Journal of Speech-Language Pathology, 23,* 708–723.

McLeod, S., & Baker, E. (2017). Children's speech: An evidence-based approach to assessment and intervention. Boston: Pearson Educational.

McNaughton, D., Light, J., & Groszyk, L. (2001). "Don't give up": Employment experiences of individuals with amyotrophic lateral sclerosis who use augmentative and alternative communication. *Augmentative and Alternative Communication, 17,* 179–195.

McNeilly, L. (2005). HIV and communication. *Journal of Communication Disorders, 38,* 303–310.

Mei, C., Reilly, S., Reddihough, D., Mensah, F., & Morgan, A. (2014). Motor speech impairment, activity, and participation in children with cerebral palsy. *International Journal of Speech-Language Pathology, 16,* 427–435.

Meilijson, S. R., Kasher, A., & Elizur, A. (2004). Language performance in chronic schizophrenia: A pragmatic approach. *Journal of Speech, Language, and Hearing Research, 47,* 695–713.

Mental Health Research Association. (2007). *Childhood schizophrenia.* Retrieved July 20, 2007, from www.narsad.org/dc/childhood_disorders/schizophrenia.html.

Menzies, G., Onslow, M., Packman, A., & O'Brian, S. (2009). Cognitive behavior therapy for adults who stutter: a tutorial for speech-language pathologists. *Journal of Fluency Disorders, 34,* 187–200.

Miccio, A. W., Elbert, M., & Forrest, K. (1999). The relationship between stimulability and phonological acquisition in children with normally developing and disordered phonologies. *American Journal of Speech-Language Pathology, 8,* 347–363.

Miccio, A. W., & Ingrisano, D. (2000). The acquisition of fricatives and affricates: Evidence from a disordered phonological system. *American Journal of Speech-Language Pathology, 9,* 214–229.

Millar, D. C., Light, J. C., & Schlosser, R. W. (2006). The impact of augmentative and alternative communication intervention on the speech production of individuals with developmental disabilities: A research review. *Journal of Speech, Language, and Hearing Research, 49,* 248–264.

Millard, S., & Davis, S. (2016). The Palin parent rating scales: Parents' perspectives on childhood stuttering and its impact. *Journal of Speech, Language, and Hearing Research, 59,* 950–963.

Miller, C. A., Kail, R., Leonard, L. B., & Tomblin, J. B. (2001). Speed of processing in children with specific language impairment. *Journal of Speech, Language, and Hearing Research, 44,* 416–433.

Miller, C. A., Leonard, L. B., Kail, R. V., Zhang, X., Tomblin, J. B., & Francis, D. J. (2006). Response time in 14-year-olds with language impairment. *Journal of Speech, Language, and Hearing Research, 49,* 712–728.

Miller, C., & Madhoun, L. (2016). Feeding and swallowing issues in infants with craniofacial anomalies. *Perspectives of the ASHA Special Interest Groups (SIG 5), 1,* 13–26.

Miniutti, A. (1991). Language deficiencies in inner-city children with learning and behavioral problems. *Language, Speech, and Hearing Services in Schools, 22,* 31–38.

Mitchell, R. E., & Karchmer, M. A. (2004). Chasing the mythical ten percent: Parental hearing status of deaf and hard of hearing students in the United States. *Sign Language Studies, 4,* 138–163.

Moats, L., & Foorman, B. (2003). Measuring teachers' conversational knowledge of language and reading. *Annals of Dyslexia, 53,* 23–45.

Mok, P. L. H., Pickles, A., Durkin, K., & Conti-Ramsden, G. (2014). Longitudinal trajectories of peer relations in children with specific language impairment. *Journal of Child Psychology & Psychiatry, 55,* 516–527.

Mol, L., Krahmer, E., & van de Sandt-Koenderman, M. (2013). Gesturing by speakers with aphasia: How does it compare? *Journal of Speech, Language, and Hearing Research, 56,* 1224–1236. doi:10.1044/1092-4388(2012/11-0159)

Montgomery, J. W., & Leonard, L. B. (2006). Effects of acoustic manipulation on the real-time inflectional processing of children with specific language impairment. *Journal of Speech, Language, and Hearing Research, 49,* 1238–1256.

Montgomery, J. W. (2006). Real-time language processing in school-age children with specific language impairment. *International Journal of Language & Communication Disorders, 41,* 275–291. doi:10.1080/13682820500227987

Montgomery, J. W., & Evans, J. L. (2009). Complex sentence comprehension and working memory in children with specific language impairment. *Journal of Speech, Language, and Hearing Research, 52,* 269–288. doi:10.1044/1092-4388(2008/07-0116)

Morford, J. P., Grieve-Smith, A. B., & MacFarlane, J. (2008). Effects of language experience on the perception of American sign language. *Cognition, 109*(1), 41–53.

Morgan, P. L., Scheffner Hammer, C., Farkas, G., Hillemeier, M. M., Maczuga, S., Cook, M., & Morano, S. (2016). Who receives speech/language services by 5 years of age in the United States? *American Journal of Speech-Language Pathology, 25,* 183–199. doi:10.1044/2015_AJSLP-14-0201

Mortimer, J., & Rvachew, S. (2010). A longitudinal investigation of morpho-syntax in children with speech sounds disorders. *Journal of Communication Disorders, 43,* 61–76.

Mullins, T. (2004). Depression in older adults with hearing loss. *ASHA Leader, 21,* 12–13, 27.

Murphy, K. A., Justice, L. M., O'Connell, A. A., Pentimonti, J. M., & Kaderavek, J. N. (2016). Understanding risk for reading difficulties in children with language impairment. *Journal of Speech, Language, and Hearing Research, 59,* 1436–1447. doi:10.1044/2016_JSLHR-L-15-0110

Murphy, S. M., Faulkner, D. M., & Farley, L. R. (2014). The behaviour of young children with social communication disorders during dyadic interaction with peers. *Journal of Abnormal Child Psychology, 42*(2), 277–289.

Murray, D. S., Ruble, L. A., Willis, H., & Molloy, C. A. (2009). Parent and teacher report of social skills in children with autism spectrum disorder. *Language, Speech, and Hearing Services in Schools, 40,* 109–115.

Murray, L. L. (2012). Attention and other cognitive deficits in aphasia: presence and relation to language and communication measures. *American Journal of Speech-Language Pathology, 21,* 51–64.

Murray, E., McCabe, P., Heard, R., & Ballard, K. (2015). Differential diagnosis of children with suspected childhood apraxia of speech. *Journal of Speech, Language, and Hearing Research, 58,* 43–60.

Murray, E., McCabe, P., & Ballard, K. (2014). A systematic review of treatment outcomes for children with childhood apraxia of speech. *American Journal of Speech-Language Pathology, 17,* 1–19.

Murray, J., & Schutte, B. (2004). Cleft palate: players, pathways, and pursuits. *The Journal of Clinical Investigation, 113,* 1676–1678.

Murray, T., Carrau, R., & Chan, K. (2018). *Clinical management of swallowing disorders* (4th ed.). San Diego, CA: Plural Publishing, Inc.

Myers, P. S. (2001). Toward a definition of RHD syndrome. *Aphasiology, 15,* 913–918.

Nagaya, M., Kachi, T., Yamada, T., & Sumi, Y. (2004). Videofluorographic observations on swallowing in patients with dysphagia due to neurodegenerative diseases. *Nagoya Journal of Medical Sciences, 67,* 17–23.

Naglieri, J., & Rojahn, J. (2001). Gender differences in planning, attention, simultaneous, and successive (PASS) cognitive processes and achievement. *Journal of Educational Psychology, 93,* 430–437.

Narne, J., Prabhu, P., Chandan, H., & Deepthi, M. (2016). Gender differences in audiological findings and hearing aid benefit in 255 individuals with auditory neuropathy spectrum disorder: A retrospective study. *Journal of the American Academy of Audiology, 27*(10), 839–845.

Narayanan, U. (2012). Management of children with ambulatory cerebral palsy: An evidence-based review. *Journal of Pediatric Orthopedics, 32,* S172–S181.

Narayanan, S., & Kalappa, N. (2017) Speech, language and swallowing difficulties in a child with AIDS. *Acta Oto-Laryngologica Case Reports, 2,* 34–42.

Naremore, R. C. (2001). *Narrative frameworks and early literacy.* Seminar presented for Rochester Hearing and Speech Center and Nazareth College, Rochester, NY.

Nathan, L., Stackhouse, J., Goulandris, N., & Snowling, M. J. (2004). The development of early literacy skills among children with speech difficulties: A test of the "critical age hypothesis." *Journal of Speech, Language, and Hearing Research, 47,* 377–391.

Nation, K., Clarke, P., Marshall, C. M., & Durand, M. (2004). Hidden language impairment in children: Parellels between poor reading comprehension and Specific Language Impairment. *Journal of Speech, Language, and Hearing Research, 47,* 199–211.

Nation, K., & Norbury, C. F. (2005). Why reading comprehension fails: Insights into developmental disorders. *Topics in Language Disorders, 25*(1), 21–32.

National Center for Injury Prevention and Control. (2009). *What is traumatic brain injury?* Retrieved May 27, 2009, from www.cdc.gov/ncipc/tbi/TBI.htm.

National Dysphagia Diet Task Force. (2002). *National Dysphagia Diet: Standardization for Optimal Care.* Chicago: American Dietetic Association.

National Reading Panel. (2000). *National Reading Panel Progress Report.* Bethesda, MD: Author.

Nel, E., & Ellis, A. (2012). Swallowing abnormalities in HIV infected children: an important cause of morbidity. *BMC Pediatrics, 12,* 1–4.

Nelson Bryen, D. (2006). Job-related social networks and communication technology. *Augmentative and Alternative Communication, 22,* 1–9.

Nelson Bryen, D. (2008). Vocabulary to support socially-valued adult roles. *Augmentative and Alternative Communication, 24,* 294–301.

Nelson, N. W., & Van Meter, A. (2003, June). *Measuring written language abilities and change through the elementary years.* Poster session presented at the annual meeting of the Symposium for Research in Child Language Disorders, Madison, WI.

Nelson, N. W., & Van Meter, A. M. (2002). Assessing curriculum-based reading and writing samples. *Topics in Language Disorders, 22*(2), 35–59.

Neils-Strunjas, J., Groves-Wright, K., Mashima, P., & Harnish, S. (2006). Dysgraphia in Alzheimer's disease: A review for clinical and research purposes. *Journal of Speech, Language, and Hearing Research, 49*, 1313–1330.

New York State Department of Health. (2002). *Clinical Practice Guideline,* Publication No. 4218. Albany, NY: New York State Department of Health. Recommended by ASHA, Compendium of EBP Guidelines and Systematic Reviews. Accessed June 1, 2009, at www.asha.org/members/ebp/compendium/.

Nicolson, R., Lenane, M., Singaracharlu, S., Malaspina, D., Giedd, J. N., Hamburger, S. D., et al. (2000). Premorbid speech and language impairments in childhood-onset schizophrenia: Association with risk factors. *American Journal of Psychiatry, 157,* 794–800.

Nigam, R., Schlosser, R. W., & Lloyd, L. L. (2006). Concomitant use of the matrix strategy and the mand-model procedure in teaching graphic symbol combinations. *Augmentative and Alternative Communication, 22,* 160–177.

Nilsen, E. S., Mangal, L., & MacDonald, K. (2013) Who receives speech/language services by 5 years of age in the United States? *Journal of Speech, Language, and Hearing Research, 56,* 590–603. doi:10.1044/1092-4388(2012/12-0013)

Nippold, M., & Sun, L. (2008). Knowledge of morphologically complex words: A developmental study of older children and young adolescents. *Language, Speech, and Hearing Services in Schools, 39,* 365–373.

Nippold, M. A., Hesketh, L. J., Duthie, J. K., & Mansfield, T. C. (2005). Conversational vs. expository discourse: A study of syntactic development in children, adolescents, and adults. *Journal of Speech, Language, and Hearing Research, 48,* 1048–1064.

Nippold, M. A., Mansfield, T. C., & Billow, J. L. (2007). Peer conflict explanations in children, adolescents, and adults: Examining the development of complex syntax. *American Journal of Speech-Language Pathology, 16,* 179–186.

Nippold, M. A., Ward-Lonergan, J. M., & Fanning, J. L. (2005). Persuasive writing in children, adolescents, and adults: A study of syntactic, semantic, and pragmatic development. *Language, Speech, and Hearing Service in Schools, 36,* 125–138.

Nippold, M. A. (2014). Language intervention at the middle school: Complex talk reflects complex thought.

Language, Speech, and Hearing Services in Schools, 45, 153–156. doi:10.1044/2014_LSHSS-14-0027

Nuttall, E. V., Romero, I., & Kalesnik, J. (1992). *Assessing and Screening Preschoolers.* Boston: Allyn & Bacon.

Nye, C., Vanryckeghem, M., Schwartz, J., Herder C., Turner, H., & Howard, C. (2013). Behavioral stuttering interventions for children and adolescents: A systematic review and meta-analysis. *Journal of Speech, Language, and Hearing Research, 56,* 921–932.

O'Neal-Pirozzi, T. M. (2009). Feasibility and benefit of parent participation in a program emphasizing preschool child language development while homeless. *American Journal of Speech-Language Pathology, 12,* 229–242.

O'Neil-Pirozzi, T. M. (2003). Language functioning of residents in family homeless shelters. *American Journal of Speech-Language Pathology, 12,* 229–242.

Office of Technology Assessment. (1978). *Assessing the efficacy and safety of medical technologies.* OTA-H-75. Washington, DC: U.S. Government Printing Office.

Olazarán, J., Reisberg, B., Clare, L., Cruz, I., Peña-Casanova, J., et al. (2010). Nonpharmacological therapies in Alzheimer's disease: A systematic review of efficacy. *Dementia and Geriatric Cognitive Disorders, 30,* 161–178.

Olivier, C., Hecker, L., Klucken, J., & Westby, C. (2000). Language: The embedded curriculum in postsecondary education. *Topics in Language Disorders, 21*(1) 15–29.

Oller, J. W., Kim, K., & Choe, Y. (2001). Can instructions to nonverbal tests be given in pantomime? Additional applications of a general theory of signs. *Semiotica, 133,* 15–44.

Olson, G. (2012). Swallowing disorders vs. feeding disorders in children. Retrieved from: http://nspt4kids.com/parenting/swallowing-disorders-vs-feeding-disorders-in-children/

Olswang, L. B., Svensson, L., & Astley, S. (2010). Observation of classroom communication: Do children with Fetal Alcohol Syndrome Disorders spend their time differently than their typically developing peers? *Journal of Speech, Language, and Hearing Research, 53,* 1687–1703.

Ors, M., Ryding, E., Lindgren, M., Gustafsson, P., Blennow, G., & Rosén, I. (2005). SPECT findings in children with specific language impairment. *Cortex, 41,* 316–326.

Osser, R. W., Laubscher, E., Sorce, J., Koul, R., Flynn, S., Hotz, L., Abramson, J., Fadie, H., Shane, H. (2013). *AAC: Augmentative & Alternative Communication.* Jun 2013, Vol. 29 Issue 2, 132–145. 14p. 1 Color Photograph, 4 Charts. DOI: 10.3109/07434618.2013.784928.

Owens, R.E. (2012). *Language Development, An Introduction.* Boston: Pearson Education.

Owens, R. E. (2014). *Language disorders: A functional approach to assessment and intervention* (5th ed.). Boston: Allyn & Bacon.

Owens, R. E. (2016). *Language development, an Introduction.* Boston: Pearson Education.

Owens, R. E., & Kim, K. (2007, November). *Holistic reading and semantic investigation intervention with struggling readers.* Paper presented at the annual convention of the American Speech-Language-Hearing Association, Boston.

Özçalşkan, S., & Goldin-Meadow, S. (2010). Sex differences in language first appear in gesture. *Developmental Science, 13*(5), 752–760.

Packman, A. (2012). Therapy and therapy in stuttering: A complex relationship. *Journal of Fluency Disorders, 37,* 225–233.

Packman, A., Onslow, M., Webber, M., Harrison, E., Arnott, S., Bridgman, K., . . . Lloyd, W. (2015). *The Lidcombe Program treatment guide.* Retrieved from http://sydney.edu.au/health-sciences/asrc/docs/lp_treatment_guide_2015.pdf

Palardy, Gregory J. (2008) 'Differential school effects among low, middle, and high social class composition schools: a multiple group, multilevel latent growth curve analysis', School Effectiveness and School Improvement, 19:1, 21–49

Palasik, S., Gabel, R., Hughes, C., & Rusnak, E. (2012). Perceptions of people who stutter about occupational experiences. *Perspectives on Fluency and Fluency Disorders, 22,* 22–33.

Papaliou, C. F., & Trevarthen, C. (2006). Prelinguistic pitch patterns expressing "communication" and "apprehension". *Journal of Child Language, 33,* 163–178.

Papsin, B. K., Gysin, C., Picton, N., Nedzelski, J., & Harrison, R. V. (2000). Speech perception outcome measures in prelingually deaf children up to four years after cochlear implantation. *Annals of Otology, Rhinology & Laryngology Supplement, 185,* 38–42.

Paradis, J. (2005). Grammatical morphology in children learning English as a second language: Implications of similarities with specific language impairment. *Language, Speech, and Hearing Services in Schools, 36,* 172–187.

Paradis, J., Schneider, P., & Sorenson Duncan, T. (2013). Discriminating children with language impairment among English-language learners from diverse first-language backgrounds. *Journal of Speech, Language, and Hearing Research, 56,* 971–981. doi:10.1044/1092-4388(2012/12-0050)

Paratore, J. R. (1995). Assessing literacy: Establishing common standards in portfolio assessment. *Topics in Language Disorders, 16*(1), 67–82.

Pataraia, E., Simos, P. G., Castillo, E. M., Billingsley-Marshall, R. L., McGregor, A. L., Breier, J. I., et al. (2004). Reorganization of language-specific cortex in patients with lesions or mesial temporal epilepsy. *Neurology, 63,* 1825–1832.

Patterson, J. L. (2000). Observed and reported expressive vocabulary and word combinations in bilingual toddlers. *Journal of Speech, Language, and Hearing Research, 43,* 121–128.

Pauls, L. J., & Archibald, L. M. (2016). Executive functions in children with specific language impairment: A meta-analysis. *Journal of Speech, Language, and Hearing Research, 59,* 1074–1086. doi:10.1044/2016_JSLHR-L-15-0174

Pavelko, S. (2010). Pre-literacy interventions for preschool students. *EBP Briefs, 5*(3), 1–9.

Pavelko, S.L., & Owens, R.E. (2017). Sampling Utterances and Grammatical Analysis Revised (SUGAR): New Normative Values for Language Sample Analysis Measures. *Language, Speech, and Hearing Services in Schools, 48,* 197–215.

Peach, R. K. (2001). Further thoughts regarding management of acute aphasia following stroke. *American Journal of Speech-Language Pathology, 10,* 29–36.

Peijnenborgh, J. C., Hurks, P. M., et al. (2016). Efficacy of working memory training in children and adolescents with learning disabilities: A review study and meta-analysis. *Neuropsychological Rehabilitation, 26*(5-6), 645–672.

Pell, M. (2006). Cerebral mechanisms for understanding emotional prosody in speech. *Brain and Language, 96,* 221–234.

Pena-Brooks, A., & Hedge, M. (2007). *Assessment and treatment of articulation and phonological disorders in children* (2nd ed.). Austin, TX: PRO-ED.

Peña, E., Iglesias, A., & Lidz, C. S. (2001). Reducing test bias through dynamic assessment of children's word learning ability. *American Journal of Speech-Language Pathology, 10,* 138–154.

Peña, E. D., Gillam, R. B., Malek, M., Ruiz-Felter, R., Resendiz, M., Fiestas, C., & Sabel, T. (2006). Dynamic assessment of school-age children's narrative ability: An experimental investigation of classification accuracy. *Journal of Speech, Language, and Hearing Research, 49,* 1037–1057.

Peña, E. D., Gillam, R. B., & Bedore, L. M. (2014). Dynamic assessment of narrative ability in English accurately identifies language impairment in English language learners. *Journal of Speech, Language, and Hearing Research, 57,* 2208–2220. doi:10.1044/2014_JSLHR-L-13-0151

Pence, K. L., Justice, L. M., & Wiggins, A. K. (2008). Preschool teachers' fidelity in implementing a comprehensive language-rich curriculum. *Language, Speech, and Hearing Services in Schools, 39,* 329–341.

Perry, J., & Schenck, G. (2013). Instrumental assessment in cleft palate care. *Perspectives on Speech Science and Orofacial Disorders 23,* 49–61.

Peterson, R., Pennington, B., Shriberg, L., & Boada, R. (2009). What influences literacy outcome in children with speech sound disorder? *Journal of Speech. Language. and Hearing Research, 52,* 1175–1188.

Peterson-Falzone, S., Hardin-Jones, M., & Karnell, M. (2010). *Cleft palate speech* (4th ed.). St. Louis, MO: Mosby.

Peterson-Falzone, S. J., Trost-Cardamone, J., Karnell, M., & Hardin-Jones, M. (2006). *The clinician's guide to treating cleft palate speech*. St. Louis, MO: Mosby.

Pijnacker, J., Davids, N., van Weerdenburg, M., Verhoeven, L., Knoors, H., & van Alphen, P. (2017). Semantic processing of sentences in preschoolers with specific language impairment: Evidence from the N400 effect. *Journal of Speech, Language, and Hearing Research, 60*, 627–639. doi:10.1044/2016_JSLHR-L-15-0299

Pindzola, R. (1993). Materials for use in vocal hygiene programs for children. *Language, Speech, and Hearing Services in the Schools, 24*, 174–176.

Plante, E., Ogilvie, T., Vance, R., Aguilar, J. M., Dailey, N. S., Meyers, C., Lieser, A. M., & Burton, R. (2014). Variability in the language input to children enhances learning in a treatment context. *American Journal of Speech-Language Pathology, 23*, 530–545. doi:10.1044/2014_AJSLP-13-0038

Plexico, L. W., Manning, W. H., & DiLollo, A. (2010). Client perceptions of effective and ineffective therapeutic alliances during treatment for stuttering. *Journal of Fluency Disorders, 35*, 333–354.

Postma, A., & Kolk, H. H. J. (1993). The covert repair hypothesis: Prearticulatory repair processes in normal and stuttered disfluencies. *Journal of Speech and Hearing Research, 36*, 472–487.

Prelock, P. A. (2008). *Autism spectrum disorders. Treatment efficacy summary*. Retrieved June 28, 2009, from www.asha.org/NR/rdonlyres/4BAF3969-9ADC-4C01-B5ED-1334CC20DD3D/0/TreatmentEfficacy-Summaries2008.pdf.

Prelock, P. A., Beatson, J., Bitner, B., Broder, C., & Ducker, A. (2003). Interdisciplinary assessment of young children with autism spectrum disorder. *Language, Speech, and Hearing Services in Schools, 34*, 194–202.

Pressley, M., & Hilden, K. R. (2004). Cognitive strategies: Production deficiencies and successful strategy instruction everywhere. In D. Kuhn & R. Siegler (Eds.), *Handbook of child psychology: Vol. 2, Cognition, perception, and language* (6th edition). Hoboken, NJ: Wiley.

Pressman, H. (1992). Communication disorders and dysphagia in pediatric AIDS. *ASHA, 34*, 45–47.

Pressman, H. (2010). Dysphagia and related assessment and management in children with HIV/AIDS. In Swanepoel, D. & Louw, B. (2010). *HIV/AIDS: Related communication, hearing, and swallowing disorders*. Plural Publishing, San Diego.

Price, J. R., Roberts, J. E., Hennon, E. A., Berni, M. C., Anderson, K. L., & Sideris, J. (2008). Syntactic complexity during conversation of boys with fragile X syndrome and Down syndrome. *Journal of Speech, Language, and Hearing Research, 51*, 3–15.

Price, J. R., & Jackson, S. C. (2015). Procedures for obtaining and analyzing writing samples of school-age children and adolescents. *Language, Speech, and Hearing Services in Schools, 46*, 277–293. doi:10.1044/2015_LSHSS-14-0057

Prins, D., & Ingham, R. (2009). Evidence-based treatment and stuttering—Historical perspective. *Journal of Speech, Language, and Hearing Research, 52*, 254–263.

Prizant, B. M., Schuler, A. L., Wetherby, A. M., & Rydell, P. (1997). Enhancing language and communication: Language approaches. In D. Cohen & F. Volkmar (Eds.), *Handbook of autism and pervasive developmental disorders* (2nd ed., pp. 572–605). New York: Wiley.

Pry, R., Petersen, A., & Baghdadli, A. (2005). The relationship between expressive language level and psychological development in children with autism 5 years of age. *International Journal of Research and Practice, 9*, 179–189.

Pugh, S., & Klecan-Aker, J. S. (2004). *Effects of phonological awareness training on students with learning disabilities*. Paper presented at the annual convention of the American Speech-Language-Hearing Association, Philadelphia.

Pulvermuller, F. B., Neininger, B., Elbert, T., Mohr, B., Rockstroh, B., Koebbel, P., et al. (2001). Constraint-induced therapy of chronic aphasia after stroke. *Stroke, 32*, 1621–1626.

Punch, J., Elfenbein, J., & James, R. (2011). Targeting hearing health messages for users of personal listening devices. *American Journal of Audiology, 20*, 69–82.

Puranik, C. S., Lombardino, L. J., & Altmann, L. J. (2007). Writing through retellings: An exploratory study of language impaired and dyslexic populations. *Reading and Writing: An Interdisciplinary Journal, 20*, 251–272.

Qi, C. H., Kaiser, A. P., Milan, S. E., Yzquierdo, Z., & Hancock, T. B. (2003). The performance of low-income African American children on the Preschool Language Scale-3. *Journal of Speech, Language, and Hearing Research, 46*, 576–590.

Rackensperger, T. (2012). Family influences and academic success: The perceptions of individuals using AAC. *Augmentative and Alternative Communication, 28*(2), 106–116. doi: 10.3109/07434618.2012.677957

Rainforth, B., York, J., & MacDonald, C. (1992). *Collaborative teams for students with severe disabilities: Integrating therapy and educational services*. Baltimore: Brookes.

Raju, T., Higgins, R., Stark, A., & Leveno, K. (2006). Optimizing care and outcome for late-preterm (nearterm) infants: A summary of the workshop sponsored by the National Institute of Child Health and Human Development. *Pediatrics, 118*, 1207–1214.

Ramig, L., & Verdolini, K. (1998). Treatment efficacy: Voice disorders. *Journal of Speech-Language-Hearing Research, 41*, S101–S116.

Ramig, L. (2002). The joy of research. *The ASHA Leader, 7*(8), 6–7, 19.

Ramig, L. O., & Verdolini, K. (2009, June 19). Laryngeal-based voice disorders. *Treatment Efficacy Summary*. Retrieved June 23, 2009, from www.asha.org/NR/rdonlyres/5B211B91-9D44-42D2-82C7-55A1315D8CD6/0/TESLaryngealBasedVoiceDisorders.pdf.

Rauterkus, E. & Palmer, C. (2014). The hearing aid effect. *Journal of the American Academy of Audiology, 25*(9), 893–903.

Raymer, A. M., Beeson, P., Holland, A., Kendall, D., Mahe, L. M., Martin, N., et al. (2008). Translational research in aphasia: From neuroscience to neurorehabilitation. *Journal of Speech, Language, and Hearing Research (Neuroplasticity Supplement), 51,* S259–S275.

Redmond, S. M. (2003). Children's production of the affix -ed in past tense and past participle contexts. *Journal of Speech, Language, and Hearing Research, 46,* 1095–1109.

Redmond, S. M., & Rice, M. L. (2001). Detection of irregular verb violations by children with and without SLI. *Journal of Speech, Language, and Hearing Research, 44,* 655–669.

Rescher, B., & Rappelsberger, P. (1996). EEG changes in amplitude and coherence during a tactile task in females and males. *Journal of Psychophysiology, 10,* 161–172.

Rescorla, L. (2005). Age 13 language and reading outcomes in late talking toddlers. *Journal of Speech, Language, and Hearing Research, 48,* 459–473.

Rescorla, L. A. (2009). Age 17 language and reading outcomes in late-talking toddlers: Support for dimensional perspective on language delay. *Journal of Speech, Language, and Hearing Research, 52,* 16–30.

Rescorla, L., & Turner, H. L. (2015). Morphology and syntax in late talkers at age 5. *Journal of Speech, Language, and Hearing Research, 58,* 434–444. doi:10.1044/2015_JSLHR-L-14-0042

Reynolds, M., E., & Jefferson, L. (1999). Natural and Synthetic Speech Comprehension: Comparison of Children from Two Age Groups. *Augmentative and Alternative Communication, 15*(3), 174–182.

Rice, M. L., Cleave, P. L., & Oetting, J. B. (2000). The use of syntactic cues in lexical acquisition by children with SLI. *Journal of Speech, Language, and Hearing Research, 34,* 582–594.

Rice, M. L., Hoffman, L., & Wexler, K. (2009). Judgments of omitted BE and DO in questions as extended finiteness clinical markers of Specific Language Impairment (SLI) to 15 years: A study of growth and asymptote. *Journal of Speech, Language, and Hearing Research, 52,* 1417–1433.

Rice, M. L., Redmont, S. M., & Hoffman, L. (2006). Mean length of utterance in children with specific language impairment and in younger control children shows concurrent validity and stable and parallel growth trajectories. *Journal of Speech, Language, and Hearing Research, 49,* 793–808.

Rice, M. L., Tomblin, J. B., Hoffman, L., Richman, W. A., & Marquis, J. (2004). Grammatical tense deficits in children with SLI and nonspecific language impairment: Relationships with nonverbal IQ over time. *Journal of Speech, Language, and Hearing Research, 47,* 816–834.

Rice, M. L., & Hoffman, L. (2015). Predicting vocabulary growth in children with and without specific language impairment: A longitudinal study from 26 to 21 years of age. *Journal of Speech, Language, and Hearing Research, 58,* 345–359. doi:10.1044/2015_JSLHR-L-14-0150

Rieber, R. W., & Wollock, J. (1977). The historical roots of the theory and therapy of stuttering. *Journal of Communication Disorders, 10,* 3–24.

Riley, G. (2009). *Stuttering Severity Instrument for Children and Adults—Fourth Edition (SSI-4)*. Austin, TX: PRO-ED.

Ringo, C. C., & Dietrich, S. (1995). Neurogenic stuttering: An analysis and critique. *Journal of Medical Speech-Language Pathology, 2,* 111–122.

Rispoli, M. (2005). When children reach beyond their grasp: Why some children make pronoun case errors and others don't. *Journal of Child Language, 32,* 93–116.

Ritchie, K., & Lovenstone, S. (2002). The dementias. *The Lancet, 360,* 1759–1766.

Roark, B., Fried-Oken, M., Gibbons, C. (2015). Huffman and linear scanning methods with statistical language models. *Augmentative and Alternative Communication, 31*(1), 37–50. doi: 10.3109/07434618.2014.997890

Roberts, J. E., Long, S. H., Malkin, C., Barnes, E., Skinner, M., Hennon, E. A., et al. (2005). A comparison of phonological skills with fragile X syndrome and Down syndrome. *Journal of Speech, Language, and Hearing Research, 48,* 980–995.

Roberts, J. E., Mirrett, P., & Burchinal, M. (2001). Receptive and expressive communication development in young males with fragile X syndrome. *American Journal of Mental Retardation, 106,* 216–231.

Roberts, M. Y., & Kaiser, A. P. (2011). The effectiveness of parent-implemented language interventions: A meta-analysis. *American Journal of Speech-Language Pathology, 20,* 180–199.

Roberts, M. Y., Kaiser, A. P., Wolfe, C. E., Bryant, J. D., & Spidalieri, A. M. (2014). Effects of the teach-model-coach-review instructional approach on caregiver use of language support strategies and children's expressive language skills. *Journal of Speech, Language, and Hearing Research, 57,* 1851–1869. doi:10.1044/2014_JSLHR-L-13-0113

Robey, R. R., & Schultz, M. C. (1998). A model for conducting clinical-outcome research: An adaptation of the standard protocol for use in aphasiology. *Aphasiology, 12*(9), 787–810.

Rodermerk, K., & Galster, J. (2015). The benefits of remote microphones using four wireless protocols. *Journal of the American Academy of Audiology, 26*(8), 721–731.

Roden, D. F., Altman, K. W. (2013). Causes of dysphagia among different age groups: a systematic review of the literature. *Otolaryngologic Clinics of North America, 46*(6), 965–987. doi: 10.1016/j.otc.2013.08.008. Epub 2013 Oct 12.

Rogus-Pulia, N., & Robbins, J. (2013). Approaches to rehabilitation of dysphagia in acute poststroke patients. *Seminars in Speech and Language, 34*, 154–169.

Rommel, N., Davidson, G., Cain, T., Hebbard, G., & Omari, T. (2008). Videomanometric evaluation of pharyngooesophageal dysmotility in children with velocardiofacial syndrome. *Journal of Pediatric Gastroenterology and Nutrition, 46*, 87–91.

Romski, M. A., & Sevcik, R. A. (1996). *Breaking the speech barrier: Language development through augmented means.* Baltimore: Brookes.

Romski, M., Sevcik, R., Barton-Hulsey, A., & Whitmore, A. S. (2015). Early intervention and AAC: What a difference 30 years makes. *Augmentative and Alternative Communication, 31*(3), 181–202. doi: 10.3109/07434618.2015.1064163.

Rosenbaum, P., Paneth, N., Leviton, A., Goldstein, M., Bax, M., Damiano, D., Dan, B., Jacobson, B. (2007). A report: the definition and classification of cerebral palsy April 2006. *Developmental Medicine & Child Neurology, 49*, 8–14.

Rosenbek, J. C., Lemme, M., Ahern, M., Harris, E., & Wertz, R. (1973). A treatment for apraxia of speech in adults. *Journal of Speech and Hearing Disorders, 43*, 462–472.

Ross, K. B., & Wertz, R. T. (2003). Discriminative validity of selected measures of differentiating normal from aphasic performance. *American Journal of Speech-Language Pathology, 12*, 312–319.

Roth, F. P. (2000). Narrative writing: Development and teaching with children with writing difficulties. *Topics in Language Disorders, 20*(4), 15–28.

Roth, F. P. (2004). Word recognition assessment framework. In C. A. Stone, E. R. Silliman, B. J. Ehren, & K. Apel (Eds.), *Handbook of language and literacy: Development and disorders* (pp. 461–480). New York: Guilford.

Roth, F. P. (2011). *Treatment resource manual for speech-language pathology* (4th ed.). Clifton Park, NY: Delmar Learning.

Rowland, C., & Schweigert, P. (2000). Tangible symbols, tangible outcomes. *Augmentative and Alternative Communication, 16*, 61–78.

Roy, N., Gray, S., Simon, M., Dove, M., Dove, H., Corbin-Lewis, K., et al. (2001). An evaluation of the effects of two treatment approaches for teachers with voice disorders: A prospective randomized clinical trial. *Journal of Speech, Language, and Hearing Research, 44*, 286–296.

Roy, N. (2004). Functional voice disorders. In R. D. Kent (Ed.), *MIT encyclopedia of communication disorders* (pp. 27–30). Boston: MIT Press.

Roy, N. (2008). Assessment and treatment of musculoskeletal tension in hyperfunctional voice disorders. *International Journal of Speech-Language Pathology, 10*, 195–209.

Roy, N., Merrill, R. M., Thibeault, S., Parsa, R. A., Gray, S. D., & Smith, E. M. (2004). Prevalence of voice disorders in teachers and the general population. *Journal of Speech, Language, and Hearing Research, 47*, 281–293.

Roy, N., Merrill, R., Gray, S., & Smith, E. (2005). Voice disorders in the general population: Prevalence, risk factors, and occupational impact. *The Laryngoscope, 115*, 1988–1995.

Roy, N., Stemple, J., Merrill, R., & Thomas, L. (2007). Dysphagia in the elderly: Preliminary evidence of prevalence, risk factors, and socioemotional effects. *Annals of Otology, Rhinology, & Laryngology, 116*, 858–865.

Roy, N., Stemple, J., Merrill, R., & Thomas, L. (2007). Epidemiology of voice disorders in the elderly: Preliminary findings. *Laryngoscope, 117*, 628–633.

Rubin, K. H., Burgess, K. B., & Coplan, R. J. (2002). Social withdrawal and shyness. In P. K. Smith & C. H. Hart (Eds.), *Blackwell handbook of childhood social development* (pp. 329–352). Malden, MA: Blackwell.

Rudolph, C. D., & Link, D. T. (2002). Feeding disorders in infants and children. *Pediatric Clinics of North America, 49*(1), 97–112, vi.

Russo, M. J., Prodan, V., Meda, N. N. Carcavallo, L., Muracioli, A., Sabe, L., Bonamico, L., Allegri, R. F., & Olmos, L. (2017) High-technology augmentative communication for adults with post-stroke aphasia: a systematic review. *Expert Review of Medical Devices, 14*(5), 335–370. doi:10.1080/17434440.2017.1324291

Rvachew, S. (2006). Longitudinal predictors of implicit phonological awareness skills. *American Journal of Speech-Language Pathology, 15*, 165–176.

Rvachew, S. R., & Grawburg, M. (2006). Correlates of phonological awareness in preschoolers with speech sound disorders. *Journal of Speech, Language, and Hearing Research, 49*, 74–87.

Rvachew, S., Gaines, B. R., Cloutier, G., & Blanchet, N. (2005). Productive morphology skills of children with speech delay. *Canadian Journal of Speech-Language Pathology and Audiology, 29*, 83–89.

Ryan, B. P. (1974). *Programmed therapy for stuttering children and adults.* Springfield, IL: Charles C. Thomas.

Ryan, B. P., & Van Kirk Ryan, B. (1995). Programmed stuttering treatment for children: Comparisons of two established programs through transfer, maintenance, and follow-up. *Journal of Speech and Hearing Research, 38,* 61–75.

Saint-Exupéry, A. de (1968). *The little prince.* New York: Harcourt Brace.

Sander, E. (1972). When are speech sounds learned? *Journal of Speech and Hearing Disorders, 37,* 55–63.

Sanders, L. D., & Neville, H. J. (2000). Lexical, syntactic, and stress-pattern cues for speech segmentation. *Journal of Speech, Language, and Hearing Research, 43,* 1301–1321.

Sawyer, D. J. (2006). Dyslexia: A generation of inquiry. *Topics in Language Disorders, 26,* 95–109.

Sawyer, J., Matteson, C., Ou, H., & Nagase, T. (2017). The effects of parent-focused slow relaxed speech intervention on articulation rate, response time latency, and fluency in preschool children who stutter. *Journal of Speech, Language, and Hearing Research, 60,* 794–809.

Saxena, R., Lehmann, A., Hight, A., Darrow, K., Remenschneider, A., Kozin, E., & Lee, D. (2015). Social media utilization in the cochlear implant community. *Journal of the American Academy of Audiology, 26*(2), 197–204.

Scarpino, S., & Goldstein, B. (2012). Analysis of the speech of multilingual children with speech sound disorders. In S. McLeod & B. A. Goldstein (Eds.), *Multilingual aspects of speech sound disorders in children* (pp. 196–206). Bristol, UK: Multilingual Matters.

Scheffner Hammer, C., Morgan, P., Farkas, G., Hillemeier, M., Bitetti, D., & Maczuga, S. (2017). Late talkers: A population-based study of risk factors and school readiness consequences. *Journal of Speech, Language, and Hearing Research, 60,* 607–626. doi:10.1044/2016_JSLHR-L-15-0417

Schlosser, R. W. (2003). Outcomes measurement in AAC. In J. C. Light, D. R. Beukelman & J. Reichle (Eds.), *Communicative Competence for Individuals who use AAC: From research to effective practice* (pp. 479–508). Baltimore: Paul H. Brookes.

Schlosser, R. W., Walker, E., & Sigafoos, J. (2006). Increasing opportunities for requesting in children with developmental disabilties residing in group homes through pyramidal training. *Education and Training in Developmental Disabilties, 41*(3), 244–252.

Schlosser, R. W., & Raghavendra, P. (2004). Evidence-based practice in augmentative and alternative communication. *Augmentative and Alternative Communication, 20*(1), 1–21.

Schlosser, R. W., & Wendt, O. (2008). Effects of augmentative and alternative communication intervention on speech production in children with autism: A systematic review. *American Journal of Speech-Language Pathology, 17,* 212–230.

Schlosser, R. W., & Koul, R. K. (2015). Speech output technologies in interventions for individuals with autism spectrum disorders: A scoping review. *Augmentative and Alternative Communication, 31*(4), 285–309. doi: 10.3109/07434618.2015.1063689

Schow, R. L., & Nerbonne, M. A. (2007). *Introduction to audiologic rehabilitation.* Boston: Pearson.

Schuele, C. M. (2001). Socioeconomic influences on children's language acquisition. *Journal of Speech-Pathology and Audiology, 25*(2), 77–88.

Schuele, C. M., & Boudreau, D. (2008). Phonological awareness intervention: Beyond the basics. *Language, Speech, and Hearing Services in Schools, 39,* 3–20.

Schwartz, J. B., & Nye, C. (2006). Improving communication for children with autism: Does sign language work? *EBP Briefs, 1*(2).

Schölderle, T., Staiger, A., Lampe, R., Strecker, K., & Ziegler, W. (2016). Dysarthria in adults with cerebral palsy: Clinical presentation and impacts on communication. *Journal of Speech, Language, and Hearing Research, 59,* 216–229.

Scott, C. M. (2000). Principles and methods of spelling instruction: Applications for poor spellers. *Topics in Language Disorder, 20*(3), 66–82.

Scott, C. M., & Windsor, J. (2000). General language performance measures in spoken and written narrative and expository discourse of school-age children with language learning disabilities. *Journal of Speech, Language, and Hearing Research, 43,* 324–339.

Scott, C. M. (2014). One size does not fit all: Improving clinical practice in older children and adolescents with language and learning disorders. *Language, Speech, and Hearing Services in Schools, 45,* 145–152. doi:10.1044/2014_LSHSS-14-0014

Sebat, J., Lakshmi, B., Malhotra, D., Troge, J., Lese-Martin, C., Walsh, T., et al. (2007, April 20). Strong association of de novo copy number mutations with autism. *Science, 20,* 445–449.

Segebart DeThorne, L., Hart, S. A., Petrill, S. A., Deater-Deckard, K., Thompson, L. A., Schatschneider, C., et al. (2006). Children's history of speech-language difficulties: Genetic influences and association with reading-related measures. *Journal of Speech, Language, and Hearing Research, 49,* 1280–1293.

Segebart DeThorne, L., Petrill, S. A., Schatschneider, C., & Cutting, L. (2010). Conversational language use as a predictor of early reading development: Language history as a moderating variable. *Journal of Speech, Language, and Hearing Research, 53,* 209–223.

Sellars, C., Bowie, L., Bagg, J., et al. (2007). Risk factors for chest infection in acute stroke: A prospective cohort study. *Stroke, 38,* 2284–2291.

Sencibaugh, J. M. (2007). Meta-analysis of reading comprehension interventions for students with learning disabilities: Strategies and implications. *Reading Improvement, 44*(1), 6–22.

Serra-Prat, M., Hinojosa, G., López, D., Juan, M., Fabré, E., Voss, D. S., Calvo, M., Marta, V., Ribó, L., Palomera, E., Arreola, V., & Clavé P. (2011). Prevalence of oropharyngeal dysphagia and impaired safety and efficacy of swallow in independently living older persons. *Journal of American Geriatrics Society, 59*(1), 186–187. doi: 10.1111/j.1532-5415.2010.03227.x

Seung, H., & Chapman, R. (2000). Digit span in individuals with Down syndrome and in typically developing children: Temporal aspects. *Journal of Speech, Language, and Hearing Research, 43*, 609–620.

Shadden, B. B., & Toner, M. A. (Eds.). (1997). *Aging and communication: For clinicians by clinicians.* Austin, TX: PRO-ED.

Shaker, R., Easterling, C., Kern, M., Nitschke, T., et al. (2002). Rehabilitation of swallowing by exercise in tube-fed patients with pharyngeal dysphagia secondary to abnormal UES opening. *Gastroenterology, 122*, 1314–1321.

Shapiro, L., Hurry, J., Masterson, J., Wydell, T., & Doctor, E. (2009). Classroom implications of recent research into literacy development: From predictors to assessment. *Dyslexia, 15*, 1–2.

Shaw, G. (2012). Sign of the times: ASL comes to mobile phones. *The Hearing Journal, 65*(10), 22–26.

Sheffield, S., Jahn, K., & Gifford, R. (2015). Preserved acoustic hearing cochlear implantation improves speech perception. *Journal of the American Academy of Audiology, 26*(2), 145–154.

Shekim, L. (1990). Dementia. In L. L. LaPointe (Ed.), *Aphasia and related neurogenic language disorders* (pp. 210–220). New York: Thieme.

Sheng, L., & McGregor, K. A. (2010). Object and action naming in children with specific Language Impairment. *Journal of Speech, Language, and Hearing Research, 53*, 1704–1719.

Shipley, K., & McAfee, J. (2016). *Assessment in speech-language pathology: A resource manual* (5th ed). Boston: Cengage Learning.

Shire, S. Y., & Jones, N. (2015). Communication partners supporting children with complex communication needs: A systematic review. *Communication Disorders Quarterly, 37*(1), 3–15. doi: 10.1177/1525740114558254

Shprintzen, R. J. (1995). A new perspective on clefting. In R. J. Shprintzen & J. Bardach (Eds.), *Cleft palate speech management: A multidisciplinary approach.* St. Louis, MO: Mosby.

Shriberg, L. (1993). Four new speech and prosody-voice measures for genetics research and other studies in developmental phonological disorders. *Journal of Speech and Hearing Research, 36*, 105–140.

Shriberg, L. D., Austin, D., Lewis, B. A., McSweeney, J. L., & Wilson, D. L. (1997). The percentage of consonants correct (PCC) metric: Extensions and reliability data. *Journal of Speech, Language, and Hearing Research, 40*(4), 708–722.

Shriberg, L., Fourakis, M., Hall, S., Karlsson, H., Lohmeier, H., McSweeny, J., Potter, N., Scheer-Cohen, A., Strand, E., Tilkens, C., & Wilson, D. (2010). Extensions to the speech disorders classification system (SDCS). *Clinical Linguistics and Phonetics, 24*, 795–824.

Shriberg, L. D., & Kent, R. D. (1995). *Clinical phonetics* (2nd ed.). Boston: Allyn & Bacon.

Shriberg, L. D., & Kwiatkowski, J. (1994). Developmental phonological disorders. I: A clinical profile. *Journal of Speech and Hearing Research, 37*, 1100–1126.

Shriberg, L., Tomblin, J., & McSweeny, J. (1999). Prevalence of speech delay in 6-year old children and comorbidity with language impairment. *Journal of Speech, Language, and Hearing Research 42*, 1461–1481.

Shriberg, L., Potter, N., & Strand, E. (2011). Prevalence and phenotype of childhood apraxia of speech in youth with galactosemia. *Journal of Speech, Language, and Hearing Research, 54*, 487–519.

Shriberg, L., & Widder, C. (1990). Speech and prosody characteristics of adults with mental retardation. *Journal of Speech and Hearing Research, 33*, 627–653.

Shriberg, L., & Widder, C. (1990). Speech and prosody characteristics of adults with mental retardation. *Journal of Speech and Hearing Research, 33*, 627–653.

Shuster, L. I., & Lemieux, S. K. (2005). An fMRI investigation of covertly and overtly produced mono- and multisyllabic words. Brain and Language, *93*, 20–31.

Sigafoos, J. (2000). Creating opportunities for augmentative and alternative communication: Strategies for involving people with developmental disabilities. *Augmentative and Alternative Communication, 16*, 183–190.

Sigafoos, J., O'Reilly, M., Seely-York, S., Edrisinha, C. (2004). Teaching students with developmental disabilities to locate their AAC device. *Research in Developmental Disabilities*, Vol 25(4), pp. 371–383.

Silliman, E. R., & Wilkinson, L. C. (2004). Collaboration for language and literacy learning. In E. R. Silliman & L. C. Wilkinson (Eds.), *Language and literacy learning in schools* (pp. 3–38). New York: Guilford.

Singer, B. D., & Bashir, A. S. (2004). EmPOWER, A strategy of teaching students with language learning disabilities how to write expository text. In E. R. Silliman & L. C. Wilkinson (Eds.), *Language and literacy learning in schools* (pp. 239–272). New York: Guilford.

Singleton, N. C., & Shulman, B. B. (2014). Language development: Foundations, processes, and clinical applications (2nd ed.). Burlington, MA: Jones & Bartlett Learning.

Sitzer, D. I., Twamley, E. W., & Jeste, D. V. (2006). Cognitive training in Alzheimer's disease: A meta-analysis of the literature. *Acta Psychiatrica Scandinavica, 114*(2), 75–90.

Skarakis-Doyle, E., Dempsey, L., & Lee, C. (2008). Identifying language comprehension impairment in preschool children. *Language, Speech, and Hearing Services in Schools, 39,* 54–65.

Skebo, C. M., Lewis, B. A., Freebairn, L. A., Tag, J., Avrich Ciesla, A., & Stein, C. M. (2013). Reading skills of students with speech sound disorders at three stages of literacy development. *Language, Speech, and Hearing Services in Schools, 44,* 360–373. doi:10.1044/0161-1461(2013/12-0015)

Skibbe, L. E., Grimm, K. J., Stanton-Chapman, T. L., Justice, L. M., Pence, K. L., & Bowles, R. P. (2008). Reading trajectories of children with language difficulties from preschool through fifth grade. *Language, Speech, and Hearing Services in Schools, 39,* 475–486.

Small, J. A., & Perry, J. (2005). Do you remember? How caregivers question their spouses who have Alzheimer's disease and the impact on communication. *Journal of Speech, Language, and Hearing Research, 48*(1), 125–136.

Smit, A., Hand, B., Freilinger, J., Bernthal, J., & Bird, A. (1990). The Iowa Articulation Norms Project and its Nebraska replication. *Journal of Speech and Hearing Disorders, 55,* 779–798.

Smith, A., Sadagopan, N., Walsh, B., & Weber-Fox, C. (2010). Increasing phonological complexity reveals heightened instability in inter-articulatory coordination in adults who stutter. *Journal of Fluency Disorders, 35,* 1–18.

Smith-Myles, B., Hilgenfeld, T., Barnhill, G., Griswold, D., Hagiwara, T., & Simpson, R. (2002). Analysis of reading skills in individuals with Asperger syndrome. *Focus on Autism and Other Developmental Disabilities, 17*(1), 44–47.

Snell, M., Chen, L. Y., & Hoover, K. (2006). Teaching augmentative and alternative communication to students with severe disabilities: A review of intervention research 1997–2003. *Research and Practices for Persons with Severe Disabilities, 31,* 203–214.

Snow, C. E., Scarborough, H. S., & Burns, M. S. (1999). What speech-language pathologists need to know about early reading. *Topics in Language Disorders, 20*(1), 48–58.

Sohlberg, M. M., Ehlhardt, L., & Kennedy, M. (2005). Instructional techniques in cognitive rehabilitation: A preliminary report. *Seminars in Speech Language Pathology, 26,* 268– 279.

Soto, G., Muller, E., Hunt, P., & Goetz, L. (2001). Critical issues in the inclusion of students who use augmentative and alternative communication: An educational team perspective. *Augmentative and Alternative Communication, 17,* 62–72.

Southwood, F., & Russell, A. F. (2004). Comparison of conversation, freeplay, and story generation as methods of language elicitation. *Journal of Speech, Language, and Hearing Research, 47,* 366–376.

Spaulding, T. J, Plante, E., & Farinella, K. A. (2006). Eligibility criteria for language impairment: Is the low end of normal always appropriate? *Language, Speech, and Hearing Services in Schools, 37,* 61–72.

Spaulding, T. J., Plante, E., & Vance, R. (2008). Sustained selective attention skills of preschool children with specific language impairment: Evidence for separate attentional capacities. *Journal of Speech, Language, and Hearing Research, 51,* 16–34. doi:10.1044/1092-4388(2008/002)

Spencer, E., Schuele, C. N., Guillot, K., & Lee, M. (2008). Phonological awareness skill of speech-language pathologists and other educators. *Language, Speech, and Hearing Services in Schools, 39,* 512–520.

Stadskleiv, K. (2017). Experiences from a support group for families of preschool children in the expressive AAC user group. *Augmentative and Alternative Communication, 33*(1), 3–13. doi:10.1080/07434618.2016.1276960

Starkweather, W. (1987). *Fluency and stuttering.* Englewood Cliffs, NJ: Prentice Hall.

Starkweather, W. (1997). Therapy for younger children. In R. F. Curlee & G. M. Siegel (Eds.), *Nature and treatment of stuttering: New directions* (2nd ed., pp. 143–166). Boston: Allyn & Bacon.

Starmer, H. (2017). Swallowing exercises in head and neck cancer. *Perspectives of the ASHA Special Interest Groups (SIG 13), 2,* 21–26.

Starmer, H., Gourin, C., Lua, L., & Burkhead, L. (2011). Pretreatment swallowing assessment in head and neck cancer patients. *Laryngoscope, 121,* 1208–1211.

Stemple, J. (2007). *Principles of physiologic voice therapy.* Short Course. Tempe, AZ: Arizona State University.

Stemple, J., Roy, N., & Klaben, B. (2014). *Clinical Voice Pathology: Theory and Management* (5th ed). San Diego, CA: Plural Publishing, Inc.

Stillman, R., & Battle, C. (1984). Developing prelanguage communication in the severely handicapped: An interpretation of the Van Dijk method. *Seminars in Speech-Language Pathology, 5,* 159–170.

Stoicheff, M. (1981). Speaking fundamental frequency characteristics of nonsmoking female adults. *Journal of Speech and Hearing Research, 24,* 437–441.

Story, B. (2002). An overview of the physiology, physics, and modeling of the sound source for vowels. *Acoustical Science and Technology, 23,* 195–206.

Strand, E., Stoeckel, R., & Baas, B. (2006). Treatment of severe childhood apraxia of severe childhood apraxia of speech: A treatment efficacy study. *Journal of Medical Speech Pathology, 14,* 297–307.

Strand, E., & Skinder, A. (1999). Treatment of developmental apraxia of speech: Integral stimulation methods. In A. Caruso & E. Strand (Eds.), *Clinical management of motor speech disorders in children* (pp. 109–148). New York: Thieme.

Strand, E. A., & McCauley, R. (1997, November). *Differential diagnosis of phonological impairment and developmental apraxia of speech*. Paper presented at the American Speech-Language-Hearing Association annual convention, Boston.

Strand, E. (2010). *An overview of dynamic temporal and tactile cueing for childhood apraxia of speech and other motor speech disorders* [video]. (Available from Childhood Apraxia of Speech Association of North America, 416 Lincoln Avenue 2nd Fl., Pittsburgh, PA 15209).

Strange, W., & Broen, P. (1980). Perception and production of approximant consonants by 3-year-olds: A first study. In G. Yeni-Komshian, J. Kavanaugh, & C. A. Ferguson (Eds.), *Child phonology: Vol. 2. Perception*. New York: Academic Press.

Streb, J., Hemighausen, E., & Rösler, F. (2004). Different anaphoric expressions are investigated by event-related brain potentials. *Journal of Psycholinguistic Research, 33*, 175–201.

Striano, T., Rochat, P., & Legerstee, M. (2003). The role of modeling and request type on symbolic comprehension of objects and gestures in young children. *Journal of Child Language, 30*, 27–45.

Suggate, S. P. (2014) A meta-analysis of the long-term effects of phonemic awareness, phonics, fluency, and reading comprehension interventions. *Journal of Learning Disabilities*.

Suiter, D., & Leder, S. (2008). Clinical utility of the 3-ounce water swallow test. *Dysphagia, 23*, 244–250.

Sullivan, P. (2008). Gastrointestinal disorders in children with neurodevelopmental disabilities. *Developmental Disabilities Research Reviews, 14*, 128–136.

Sura, L., Madhavan, A., Carnaby, G., & Crary, M. (2012). Dysphagia in the elderly: management and nutritional considerations. *Clinical Interventions in Aging, 7*, 287–298.

Suttrup, I., & Warnecke, T. (2016). Dysphagia in Parkinson's disease. *Dysphagia, 31*, 24–32.

Swanson, H. L., & Beebe-Frankenberger, M. (2004). The relationship between working memory and mathematical problem solving in children at risk and not at risk for math disabilities. *Journal of Educational Psychology, 96*, 471–491.

Sweetow, R., & Sabes, J. (2006). The need for and development of an adaptive Listening and Communication Enhancement (LACE) program. *Journal of the American Academy of Audiology, 17*(8), 538–558.

Szacka, K., Potulska-Chromik, A., Fronczewska-Wieniawska, K., Spychała, A., Kròlicki, L., & Kuźma-Kozakiewicz, M. (2016). Scintigraphic evaluation of mild to moderate dysphagia in motor neuron disease. *Clinical Nuclear Medicine, 41*, e175–e180.

Tager-Flusberg, H., Paul, R., & Lord, C. E. (2005). Language and communication in autism. In F. Volkmar, R. Paul, A. Klin & D. J. Cohen (Eds.), *Handbook of autism and pervasive developmental disorder: Vol. 1* (3rd ed., pp. 335–364). New York: Wiley.

Tattersall, P., & Dawson, J., (2016). *Structured Photographic Articulation Test III—Featuring Dudsberry (SPAT- D 3)*. DeKalb, IL: Janelle Publications, Inc.

Tattershall, S. (2004). *SLPs contributing to and learning within the writing process*. Paper presented at the annual convention of the American Speech-Language-Hearing Association, Philadelphia.

Templeton, S. (2003). The spelling/meaning connection. *Voices from the Middle, 10*(3), 56–57.

Templeton, S. (2004). Instructional approaches to spelling: The window on students' word knowledge in reading and writing. In E. R. Silliman & L. C. Wilkinson (Eds.), *Language and literacy learning in schools* (pp. 273–291). New York: Guilford.

Terre, R, & Mearin, F. (2007). Prospective evaluation of oro-pharyngeal dysphagia after severe traumatic brain injury. *Brain Injury, 21*(13–14), 1411–1417.

Terry NP. Examining relationships among dialect variation and emergent literacy skills. Communication Disorders Quarterly. 2010 doi: 10.1177/1525740110368846.

Terry, N. P. (2012). Examining relationships among dialect variation and emergent literacy skills. *Communication Disorders Quarterly. 33*(2), 67–77.

Thal, D., Jackson-Maldonado, D., & Acosta, D. (2000). Validity of a parent-report measure of vocabulary and grammar for Spanish-speaking toddlers. *Journal of Speech, Language, and Hearing Research, 43*, 1087–1100.

The International Classification of Functioning. (ICF; http://www.who.int/classifications/icf/en/)

Therrien, M. C., Light, J., & Pope, L. (2016). Systematic review of the effects of interventions to promote peer interactions for children who use aided AAC. *Augmentative and Alternative Communication, 32*(2), 81–93. doi:10.3109/07434618.2016.1146331

Thibeault, S., Merrill, R., Roy, N., Gray, S., & Smith, E. (2004). Occupational risk factors associated with voice disorders among teachers. *Annals of Epidemiology, 14*, 786–792.

Thiemann, K. S., & Goldstein, H. (2004). Effects of peer training and written text cueing on social communication of school-age children with pervasive developmental disorder. *Journal of Speech, Language, and Hearing Research, 47*, 126–144.

Thiemann-Bourque, K., Brady, N., McGuff, S., Stump, K., & Naylor, A. (2016). Picture Exchange Communication System and pals: A peer-mediated augmentative and alternative communication intervention for minimally verbal preschoolers with autism. *Journal of Speech, Language, and Hearing Research, 59*, 1133–1145. doi:10.1044/2016_JSLHR-L-15-0313

Thistle, J. J., & Wilkinson, K. (2009). The effects of color cues on typically developing preschoolers' speed of locating a target line drawing: Implications for augmentative and alternative communication display design. *American Journal of Speech-Language Pathology, 18*(3), 231–240.

Thistle, J., Wilkinson, K. (2017) Effects of background color and symbol arrangement cues on construction of multi-symbol messages by young children without disabilities: implications for aided AAC design. AAC: Augmentative & Alternative Communication, Sep2017, Vol. 33 Issue 3, p160–169.

Thomas, L. (1979). *The medusa and the snail: More notes of a biology watcher.* New York: Viking.

Thomas, L., & Stemple, J. (2007). Voice therapy: Does science support the art? *Communicative Disorders Review, 1,* 49–77.

Thomason, K. M., Gorman, B. K., & Summers, C. (2007). English literacy development for English Language Learners: Does Spanish instruction promote or hinder? *EBP Briefs, 2*(2), 1–15.

Thompson, C. K. (2004). Neuroimaging: Applications for studying aphasia. In L. L. LaPointe (Ed.), *Aphasia and related disorders* (pp. 19–38). New York: Thieme.

Thompson, C. K., Shapiro, L. P., Kiran, S., & Sobecks, J. (2003). The role of syntactic complexity in treatment of sentence deficits in agrammatic aphasia: The Complexity Account of Treatment Efficacy (CATE). *Journal of Speech, Language, and Hearing Research, 46,* 591–607.

Thordardottir, E. T., & Ellis Weismer, S. (2002). Verb argument structure weakness in specific language impairment in relation to age and utterance length. *Clinical Linguistics & Phonetics, 16,* 233–250. doi:10.1080/02699200110116462

Thunstam, L. (2004). *Social networks and communication for children with deafness and additional impairments.* Unpublished master's thesis, Mälardalens University, Sweden.

Tierney, L. M., Jr., McPhee, S. J., & Papadakis, M. A. (2000). *Current medical diagnosis and treatment* (39th ed.). New York: Lange Medical Books/ McGraw-Hill.

Timler, G. R., Vogler-Elias, D., & McGill, K. F. (2007). Strategies for promoting generalization of social communication skills in preschoolers and school-aged children. *Topics in Language Disorders, 27,* 167–181.

Titze, I. R. (1994). *Principles of voice production.* Englewood Cliffs, NJ: Prentice Hall.

Titze, I., Lemke, J., & Montequin, D. (1997). Populations in the U.S. workforce who rely on voice as a primary tool of trade: A preliminary report. *Journal of Voice, 11,* 254–259.

Tjaden, K., and Liss, J. (1995). The influence of familiarity on judgments of treated speech. *American Journal of Speech-Language Pathology, 4,* 38–39.

Tomblin, J. B., Zhang, X., Buckwalter, P., & O'Brien, M. (2003). The stability of primary language disorder: Four years after kindergarten diagnosis. *Journal of Speech, Language, and Hearing Research, 46,* 1283–1296.

Tomes, L. A., Kuehn, D. P., & Peterson-Falzone, S. J. (1997). Behavioral treatment of velopharyngeal impairment. In K. R. Bzoch (Ed.), *Communicative disorders related to cleft lip and palate* (4th ed.; pp. 529–562). Austin, TX: PRO-ED.

Tompkins, C., Blake, M. T., Wambaugh, J., & Meigh, K. (2011). A novel, implicit treatment for language comprehension processes in right hemisphere brain damage: Phase I data. *Aphasiology, 25,* 789–799.

Tompkins, C., Fassbinder, W., Blake, M., Baumgaertner, A., & Jayaram, N. (2004). Inference generation during text comprehension by adults with right hemisphere brain damage: Activation failure vs. multiple activation? *Journal of Speech, Language, and Hearing Research, 47,* 1380–1395.

Tompkins, C., Klepousniotou, E., & Scott, G. (2013). Treatment of right hemisphere disorders. In I. Papathanasiou, P. Coppens, & C. Potagas (Eds.), *Aphasia and related neurogenic communication disorders* (pp. 345–364). Sudbury, MA: Jones and Bartlett.

Tompkins, C., Scharp, V., Meigh, K., & Fassbinder, W. (2008). Coarse coding and discourse comprehension in adults with right hemisphere brain damage. *Aphasiology, 22,* 204–223.

Tompkins, C., Lehman-Blake, M., Baumgaertner, A., & Fassbinder, W. (2001). Mechanisms of discourse comprehension impairment after right hemisphere brain damage: Suppression in inferential ambiguity resolution. *Journal of Speech, Language, and Hearing Research, 44,* 400–415.

Tompkins, C. A., Baumgaertner, A., Lehman, M. T., & Fassbinder, W. (2000). Mechanisms of discourse comprehension impairment after right hemisphere brain damage: Suppression of lexical ambiguity resolution. *Journal of Speech, Language, and Hearing Research, 43,* 62–78.

Torgesen, J. K. (2000). Individual difference in response to early interventions in reading: The lingering problem of treatment resisters. *Learning Disabilities Research and Practice, 15,* 55–64.

Torgesen, J. K. (2005). Recent discoveries from research on remedial interventions for children with dyslexia. In M. Snowling & C. Hulme (Eds.), *The science of reading: A handbook* (pp. 521–537). Oxford, UK: Blackwell.

Towey, M., Whitcomb, J., & Bray, C. (2004). *Print-sound-story-talk, a successful early reading first program.* Paper presented at the annual convention of the American Speech-Language-Hearing Association, Philadelphia.

Trapl, M., Enderle, P., Nowotny, M., Teuschl, Y., Matz, K., Dachenhausen, A., & Brainin, M. (2007). Dysphagia bedside screening for acute-stroke patients: the Gugging Swallowing Screen. *Stroke, 38,* 2948–2952.

Treffert, D. A. (2009). *Hyperlexia: Reading precociousness or savant skill?* Wisconsin Medical Society. Retrieved June 6, 2009, from www.wisconsinmedicalsociety .org/savant_syndrome/savant_articles/hyperlexia.

Troche, M., & Mishra, A. (2017). Swallowing exercises in patients with neurodegenerative disease: What is the current evidence? *Perspectives of the ASHA Special Interest Groups (SIG 13), 2,* 13–20.

Truong, K., & Cunningham, L. (2011, July/August). Is a temporary threshold shift harmless? *Audiology Today.*

Tsao, F., Liu, H., & Kuhl, P. K. (2004). Speech perception in infancy predicts language development in the second year of life: A longitudinal study. *Child Development, 75,* 1067–1084.

Tye-Murray, N. (2009). *Foundations of aural rehabilitation: Children, adults, and their family members* (3rd ed.). Clifton Park, NY: Delmar Cengage Learning.

U.S. Census Bureau. (2013). *Language Use in the United States.* Washington, DC: U.S. Government.

U.S. Department of Health and Human Services. (2007). *Child maltreatment, 2007.* Retrieved June 12, 2007, from www.acf.hhs.gov/programs/cb/pubs/cm07/summary.htm.

Ukrainetz, T. A., Harpell, S., Walsh, C., & Coyle, C. (2000). A preliminary investigation of dynamic assessment with Native American kindergarteners. *Language, Speech, and Hearing Services in Schools, 31,* 142–154.

Valian, V., & Aubry, S. (2005). When opportunity knocks twice: two-year-olds' repetition of sentence subjects. *Journal of Child Language, 32,* 617–641.

Valian, V., & Casey, L. (2003). Young children's acquisition of wh- questions: The role of structured input. *Journal of Child Language, 30,* 117–143.

Van Borsel, J., De Cuypere, G., Rubens, R., & Destaerke, B. (2000). Voice problems in female-to-male transsexuals. *International Journal of Language and Communication Disorders, 35,* 427–442.

Van den Berg, J. (1958). Myoelastic-aerodynamic theory of voice production. *Journal of Speech and Hearing Research, 1,* 227–244.

Van der Merwe, A. (2004). The voice use reduction program. *American Journal of Speech-Language Pathology, 13,* 208–218.

Van Kleeck, A., Vander Woude, J., & Hammett, L. (2006). Fostering literal and inferential language skills in Head Start preschoolers with language impairment using scripted book-sharing discussions. *American Journal of Speech-Language Pathology, 15,* 85–95.

Van Kleeck, A., & Schuele, C. M. (2010). Historical perspectives on literacy in early childhood. *American Journal of Speech-Language Pathology, 19,* 341–355.

Van Lancker Sidtis, D., Choi, J., Alken, A., & Sidtis, J. J. (2015). Formulaic language in Parkinson's disease and Alzheimer's disease: Complementary effects of subcortical and cortical dysfunction. *Journal of Speech, Language, and Hearing Research, 58,* 1493–1507. doi:10.1044/2015_JSLHR-L-14-0341

Van Meter, A. M., Nelson, N. W., & Ansell, P. (2004). *Developing spelling and vocabulary skills in curriculum writing activities.* Paper presented at the annual convention of the American Speech-Language-Hearing Association, Philadelphia.

Van Riper, C., & Emerick, L. (1984). *Speech correction: An introduction to speech pathology and audiology* (7th ed.). Englewood Cliffs, NJ: Prentice Hall.

Van Riper, C. (1982). *The nature of stuttering.* Englewood Cliffs, NJ: Prentice Hall.

Van Riper, C. (1992). *The nature of stuttering* (2nd ed.). Prospect Heights, IL: Waveland Press.

Van Stan, J., Roy, N., Awan, S., Stemple, J., & Hillman, R. (2015). A taxonomy of voice therapy. *American Journal of Speech-Language Pathology, 24,* 101–125.

Vanderheiden, G., & Yoder, D. E. (1986). *Overview.* Rockville, MD: American Speech-Language-Hearing Association.

Vanryckeghem, M., Brutten, G., & Hernandez, L. (2005). A comparative investigation of the speech-associated attitude of preschool and kindergarten children who do and do not stutter. *Journal of Fluency Disorders, 30,* 307–318.

Vanryckeghem, M., & Brutten, G. (2006). *KiddyCAT Communication Attitude Test for Preschool and Kindergarten Children Who Stutter.* San Diego, CA: Plural Publishing, Inc.

Vaughn, S., & Klingner, J. (2004). Teaching reading comprehension to students with learning disabilities. In C. A. Stone, E. R. Silliman, B. J. Ehren, & K. Apel (Eds.), *Handbook of language and literacy: Development and disorders* (pp. 541–555). New York: Guilford.

Venkatagiri, H. S. (1999). Efficient Keyboard Layouts for Sequential Access in Augmentative and Alternative Communication. *Augmentative and Alternative Communication, 15*(2).

Verdolini, K. (1998). *Resonant voice therapy.* Iowa City, IA: The National Center for Voice and Speech.

Verdolini, K., Rosen, C., & Branski, R. (2006). *Classification manual for voice disorders-I.* Mahwah, NJ: Lawrence Erlbaum Associates.

Victorino, K. R., & Schwartz, R. G. (2015). Control of auditory attention in children with specific language impairment. *Journal of Speech, Language, and Hearing Research, 58,* 1245–1257. doi:10.1044/2015_JSLHR-L-14-0181

Vogel, I., Verschuure, H., Van der Ploeg, C., Brug, J., & Raat, H.(2010). Estimating adolescent risk for hearing loss based on data from a large school-based survey. *American Journal of Public Health, 100*(6), 1095–1100.

Vugs, B., Hendriks, M., Cuperus, J., & Verhoeven, L. (2014). Working memory performance and executive function behaviors in young children with SLI. *Research in Developmental Disabilities, 35,* 62–74. doi:10.1016/j.ridd.2013.10.022

Wahlberg, T., & Magliano, J. P. (2004). The ability of high-functioning individuals with autism to comprehend written discourse. *Discourse Processes,* *38*(1), 119–144.

Waite, M. C., Theodoros, D. G., Russell, T. G., & Cahill, L. M. (2010). Internet-based telehealth assessment of language using the CELF-4. *Language, Speech, and Hearing Services in Schools, 41,* 445–458.

Waltzman, S. B., & Roland, J. T. (2005). Cochlear implantation in children younger than 12 months. *Pediatrics, 116,* e487–e493.

Wambaugh, J., & Bain, B. (2002). Make research methods an integral part of your clinical practice. *The ASHA Leader, 7*(21), 1, 10–13.

Wambaugh, J. et al. (2013). Advances in the treatment of acquired apraxia of speech. *Perspectives on Neurophysiology and Neurogenic Speech and Language Disorders, 23,* 112–119.

Wang, P., & Spillane, A. (2009). Evidence-based social skills interventions for children with autism: A meta-analysis. *Education and Training in Developmental Disabilities, 44*(3), 318–342.

Weismer, S. E., Tomblin, J. B., Zhang, X., Buckwalter, P., Gaura Chynoweth, J., & Jones, M. (2000). Nonword repetition performance in school-age children with and without language impairment. *Journal of Speech, Language, and Hearing Research, 43,* 865–878.

Wendt, O., & Miller, B. (2013). Systematic review documents emerging empirical support for certain applications of iPods® and iPads® in intervention programs for individuals with developmental disabilities, but these are not a "one-size-fits-all" solution. *Evidence-Based Communication Assessment & Intervention, 7*(3), 91–96. doi: 10.1080/17489539.2014.884986

Westby, C. E. (2004). A language perspective on executive functioning, metacognition, and self-regulation in reading. In C. A. Stone, E. R. Silliman, B. J. Ehren, & K. Apel (Eds.), *Handbook of language and literacy: Development and disorders* (pp. 398–427). New York: Guilford.

Westby, C. E. (2005). Assessing and remediating text comprehension problems. In H. W. Catts & A. G. Kamhi (Eds.), *Language and reading disabilities* (2nd ed., pp. 157–232). Boston: Allyn & Bacon.

Wheeler-Hegland, K., Frymark, T., Schooling, T., McCabe, D., Ashford, J., Mullen, R., Smith Hammond, C., Musson, N. (2009). Evidence-based systematic review: Oropharyngeal dysphagia behavioral treatments. Part V—Applications for clinicians and researchers. *Journal of Rehabilitation & Development, 46,* 215–222.

Whitehurst, G. J., & Lonigan, C. J. (2001). Emergent readers: Development from prereaders to readers. In S. B. Neuman & D. K. Dickinson (Eds.), *Handbook of early literacy research* (pp. 11–29). New York: Guilford.

Whitmire, K. A. (2000). Adolescence as a developmental phase: A tutorial. *Topics in Language Disorders, 20*(2), 1–14.

Wiig, E. H., Zureich, P. Z., & Chan, H. H. (2000). A clinical rationale for assessing rapid automatized naming with language disorders. *Journal of Learning Disabilities, 33,* 359–374.

Wilcox, K., & Morris, S. (1999). *Children's speech intelligibility measure.* San Antonio, TX: Psychological Corporation.

Wilder, J., & Granlund, M. (2006). Presymbolic children in Sweden: Interaction, family accommodation and social networks. In *Proceedings from the 12th ISAAC Research Conference, Düsseldorf, August.*

Wilkinson, K., Carlin, M., & Thistle, J. (2008). The role of color cues in facilitating accurate and rapid location of aided symbols by children with and without Down syndrome. *American Journal of Speech-Language Pathology, 17,* 179–193.

Williams-Sanchez, V., McArdle, R., Wilson, R., Kidd, G., Wilson, C., & Bourne, A. (2014). Validation of a screening tests of auditory function using the telephone. *Journal of the American Academy of Audiology, 25*(10), 937–951.

Williams, A. (2000). Multiple oppositions: Theoretical foundations for an alternative contrastive intervention approach. *American Journal of Speech-Language Pathology, 9,* 282–288.

Williams, A. (2000a). Multiple oppositions: Case studies of variables in phonological intervention. *American Journal of Speech-Language Pathology, 9,* 282–288.

Windsor, J., Scott, C. M., & Street, C. K. (2000). Verb and noun morphology in the spoken and written language of children with language learning disabilities. *Journal of Speech, Language, and Hearing Research, 43,* 1322–1336.

Wise, R. J. S., Scott, S. K., Blank, S. C., Mummery, C. J., Murphy, K., & Warburton, E. A. (2001). Separate neural subsystems within "Wernicke's area". Brain, *124,* 83–95.

Wisenburn, B., & Mahoney, K. (2009). A meta-analysis of word-finding treatments for aphasia. *Aphasiology, 23*(11), 1338–1352.

Wolf, M., & Katzir-Cohen, T. (2001). Reading fluency and its intervention. *Scientific Studies in Reading, 5,* 211–239.

Wolfe, J., Morais, M., & Schaefer, E. (2015). Improving hearing performance for cochlear implant recipients with use of a digital, wireless, remote-microphone, audio-streaming accessory. *Journal of the American Academy of Audiology, 26*(6), 532–539.

Woll, B., & Morgan, G. (2012). Language impairments in the development of sign: Do they reside in a specific modality or are they modality-independent deficits? *Bilingualism: Language and Cognition, 15*(1), 75–87.

Wolter, J. A., Wood, A., & D'zatko, K. W. (2009). The influence of morphological awareness on the literacy development of first-grade children. *Language, Speech, and Hearing Services in Schools, 40,* 286–298.

Wolter, J. A., & Pike, K. (2015). Dynamic assessment of morphological awareness and third-grade literacy success. *Language, Speech, and Hearing Services in Schools, 46*, 112–126. doi:10.1044/2015_LSHSS_14_0037

Won, J., & Rubinstein, J. (2012). CI performance in prelingually deaf children and postlingually deaf adults. *The Hearing Journal, 65*(9), 32–34.

Wong, B. Y. (2000). Writing strategies instruction for expository essays for adolescents with and without learning disabilities. *Topics in Language Disorders, 20*(4), 244.

Wong, B. Y., Butler, D. L., Ficzere, S. A., & Kuperis, S. (1996). Teaching low achievers and students with learning disabilities to plan, write, and revise opinion essays. *Journal of Learning Disabilities, 29*(2), 197–212.

Woods, E. K. (1995). The influence of posture and positioning on oral motor development and dysphagia. In S. R. Rosenthal, J. J. Sheppard, & M. Lotze (Eds.), *Dysphagia and the child with developmental disabilities: Medical, clinical, and family interventions*. San Diego, CA: Singular.

Woods, J. J., & Wetherby, A. M. (2003). Early identification of and intervention for infants and toddlers who are at risk for autism spectrum disorder. *Language, Speech, and Hearing Services in Schools, 34*, 180–193.

World Health Organization. (2001). *The world health report 2001—Mental illness: New understanding, new hope*. Geneva: Author. from www.whoint/whr/en/.

World Health Organization. (2016). Preterm birth. Retrieved May 13, 2017, from http://www.who.int/mediacentre/factsheets/fs363/en/

World Health Organization. (WHO; http://www.who.int/mediacentre/factsheets/fs300/en/)

Wright, C. A., Kaiser, A. P., Reikowsky, D. I., & Roberts, M. Y. (2013). Effects of a naturalistic sign intervention on expressive language of toddlers with Down syndrome. *Journal of Speech, Language, and Hearing Research, 56*, 994–1008. doi:10.1044/1092-4388(2012/12-0060)

Xue, S. A., & Hao, G. J. (2003). Changes in the human vocal tract due to aging and the acoustic correlates of speech production: A pilot study. *Journal of Speech, Language, and Hearing Research, 46*, 689–701.

Yairi, E., Ambrose, N., & Nierman, B. (1993). The early months of stuttering: A developmental study. *Journal of Speech and Hearing Research, 36*, 521–528.

Yairi, E., Watkins, R., Ambrose, N., et al. (2001). What is stuttering? [Letter to the editor]. *Journal of Speech, Language, and Hearing Research, 44*, 585–592.

Yairi, E., & Ambrose, N. (1992a). A longitudinal study of children: A preliminary report. *Journal of Speech and Hearing Research, 35*, 755–760.

Yairi, E., & Ambrose, N. (1992b). Onset of stuttering in preschool children: Selected factors. *Journal of Speech and Hearing Research, 35*, 782–788.

Yairi, E., & Ambrose, N. (2004). Stuttering: Recent developments and future directions. *The ASHA Leader, 18*, 4–5, 14–15.

Yairi, E. (1981). Disfluencies of normally speaking 2-year-old children. *Journal of Speech Language, and Hearing Research, 24*, 301–307.

Yairi, E. (1982). Longitudinal studies of disfluencies in 2-year-old children. *Journal of Speech and Hearing Research, 25*, 402–404.

Yairi, E. (1983). The onset of stuttering in 2- and 3-year-old children: A preliminary report. *Journal of Speech and Hearing Disorders, 48*, 171–177.

Yairi, E. (2004). The formative years of stuttering: A changing portrait. *Contemporary Issues in Communication Science and Disorders, 31*, 92–104.

Yairi, E., Ambrose, N., & Cox, N. (1996). Genetics of stuttering: A critical review. *Journal of Speech and Hearing Research, 39*, 771–784.

Yairi, E., & Ambrose, N. (1999). Early childhood stuttering I: Persistency and recovery rates. *Journal of Speech, Language, and Hearing Research, 42*(5), 1097–1112.

Yairi, E., & Ambrose, N. (2013). Epidemiology of stuttering: 21st century advances. *Journal of Fluency Disorders, 38*(2), 66–87.

Yang, H. & Gray, S. (2017). Executive function in preschoolers with primary language impairment. *Journal of Speech, Language, and Hearing Research, 60*, 379–392. doi:10.1044/2016_JSLHR-L-15-0267

Yaruss, J. S. (1997). Clinical measurement of stuttering behaviors. *Contemporary Issues in Communication Science and Disorders, 24*, 33–44.

Yaruss, J. S., & Pelczarski, K. M. (2007). Evidence-based practice for school-age stuttering: Balancing existing research with clinical practice. *EBP Briefs, 2*(4), 1–8.

Yaruss, J., Lee, J., Kikani, K., Leslie, P., Herring, C., Ramachandar, S., Tichenor, S., Quesal, R., & McNeil, M. (2017). Update on didactic and clinical education in fluency disorders: 2013–2014. *American Journal of Speech-Language Pathology, 26*, 124–137.

Yaruss, S., Coleman, C., & Quesal, R. (2012). Stuttering in school-age children: A comprehensive approach to treatment. *Language, Speech, and Hearing Services in Schools, 43*, 536–548.

Yavas, M., & Goldstein, B. (1998). Phonological assessment and treatment of bilingual speakers. *American Journal of Speech-Language Pathology, 7*(2), 49–60.

Yavas, M. (1998). *Phonology: Development and disorders*. San Diego, CA: Singular.

Ylvisaker, M., & DeBonis, D. (2000). Executive function impairment in adolescence: TBI and ADHD. *Topics in Language Disorders, 20*(2), 29–57.

Ylvisaker, M., & Feeney, T. J. (1998). *Collaborative brain injury intervention: positive everyday routines*. San Diego, CA: Singular.

Yoder, P. J., Molfese, D., & Gardner, E. (2011). Initial mean length of utterance predicts the relative efficacy of two grammatical treatments in preschoolers with specific language impairment. *Journal of speech, Language, and Hearing Research, 54*, 1170–1181.

Yont, K. M., Hewitt, L. E., & Miccio, A. W. (2000). A coding system for describing conversational breakdowns in preschool children. *American Journal of Speech Language Pathology, 9,* 300–309.

Yorkston, K., Beukelman, D., Strand, E., & Hakel, M. (2010). *Management of motor speech disorders in children and adults* (3rd ed.). Austin, TX: PRO-ED.

Yorkston, K. M., Smith, E., & Beukelman, D. R. (1990). Extended communication samples of augmentative communicators: I. A comparison of individualized versus standard single-word vocabularies. *Journal of Speech and Hearing Disorders, 55,* 217–224.

Yorkston, K., Miller, R., & Strand, E. (2004). *Management of Speech and Swallowing in Degenerative Diseases* (2nd ed.). Austin, TX: PRO-ED.

Yorkston, K., & Beukelman, D. (2013). Evidence supporting dysarthria intervention: An update of systematic reviews. *Perspectives on Neurophysiology and Neurogenic Speech and Language Disorders, 23,* 105–111.

Yoshinaga-Itano, C., Sedley, A. L., Coulter, D. K., & Mehl, A. L. (1998). Language of early and later identified children with hearing loss. *Pediatrics, 102,* 1161–1171.

Zajac, D. (1997). Velopharyngeal function in young and older adult speakers: Evidence from aerodynamic studies. *Journal of the Acoustical Society of America, 102,* 1846–1852.

Zebrowski, P., & Wolf, A. (2011). Working with teenagers who stutter: Simple suggestions for a complex challenge. *Perspectives on Fluency and Fluency Disorders, 21,* 37–42.

Zemlin, W. R. (1998). *Speech and hearing sciences: Anatomy and physiology* (4th ed.). Boston: Allyn & Bacon.

Zhao X., Leotta, A., Kustanovich, V., Lajonchere, C., Geschwind, D. H., Law, K., et al. (2007, July 31). A unified genetic theory for sporadic and inherited autism. *Proceedings of the National Academy of Science, 31,* 12831–12836.

Zumach, A., Gerrits, E., Chenault, M., & Antenuis, L. (2010). Long-term effects of early-life otitis media on language development. *Journal of Speech, Language, and Hearing Research, 53,* 1, 34–43.

SUBJECT INDEX